PLAYING THE MARKET CAN BE RISKY BUSINESS— BUT *SHOPPING* THE MARKET DOESN'T HAVE TO BE!

Take the uncertainty out of choosing the best buys available with *THE SUPERMARKET NUTRITION COUNTER*. If you're among the 60 percent of American shoppers who rely on the new nutrition labels to make your food shopping choices, you may not be getting all the facts you need to ensure that your family eats balanced meals and healthful snacks. In this all-new, revised second edition, nutrition experts and best-selling authors Annette B. Natow and Jo-Ann Heslin provide more than 18,000 entries in more than 350 food categories, making this essential guide more comprehensive than ever before. Also included are food storage tips, shopping strategies for navigating the typical supermarket, the top three reasons why a consumer selects a food, how men and women differ in shopping the aisles, and other information to help you get more for your money every time you shop.

ANNETTE B. NATOW, Ph.D., R.D., and JO-ANN HESLIN, M.A., R.D., are the authors of twenty-one books on nutrition. Both are former faculty members of Adelphi University and the State University of New York, Downstate Medical Center. They are editors of the *Journal of Nutrition for the Elderly*, serve as editorial board members for the *Environmental Nutrition Newsletter*, and are frequent contributors to magazines and journals.

THE

SUPERMARKET NUTRITION COUNTER

SECOND EDITION
Fully Revised and Updated

Annette B. Natow, Ph.D., R.D.
and Jo-Ann Heslin, M.A., R.D.

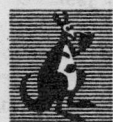

POCKET BOOKS
New York   London   Toronto   Sydney   Tokyo   Singapore

An *Original* Publication of POCKET BOOKS

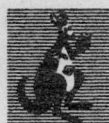

POCKET BOOKS, a division of Simon & Schuster Inc.
1230 Avenue of the Americas, New York, NY 10020

ISBN 0-671-89473-0

First Pocket Books printing April 1997

10 9 8 7 6 5 4 3 2 1

POCKET and colophon are registered trademarks of Simon & Schuster Inc.

Cover design by Tom McKeveny

Printed in the U.S.A.

To our families who support us through every project: Harry, Allen, Irene, Sarah, Meryl, Laura, Marty, George, Emily, Steven, Joe, Kristen and Karen

ACKNOWLEDGMENTS

———◇———

Without the tireless cooperation of Steven and Stephen, *The Supermarket Counter* would never have been completed. Our thanks to the National Live Stock and Meat Board and the Food Marketing Institute for providing research material and resources. A special thanks to our editor, Peter Wolverton, and our agent, Nancy Trichter.

"We are all inclined to think the foods which we like are good for us, and appearance and flavor attract or repel very quickly; but as far as real nourishment goes, these things are second hand and the [shopper] must be able to discriminate between real nutritive value and other factors, in order to spend . . . money to the best advantage."

Mary Swartz Rose, Ph.D.
Feeding the Family
The Macmillan Company, 1919

CONTENTS

———◇———

CONTENTS

SOURCES OF DATA

———◇———

Values in this counter have been obtained from the Composition of Foods, United States Department of Agriculture, Agricultural Handbooks: No. 8-1, Dairy and Egg Products; No. 8-2, Spices and Herbs; No. 8-3, Baby Foods; No. 8-4, Fats and Oils; No. 8-5, Poultry Products; No. 8-6, Soups, Sauces and Gravies; No. 8-7, Sausages and Luncheon Meats; No. 8-8, Breakfast Cereals; No. 8-9, Fruit and Fruit Juices; No. 8-10, Pork Products; No. 8-11, Vegetables and Vegetable Products; No. 8-12, Nut and Seed Products; No. 8-13, Beef Products; No. 8-14, Beverages; No. 8-15, Finfish and Shellfish Products; No. 8-16, Legumes and Legume Products; No. 8-17, Lamb, Veal and Game Products; No. 8-18, Baked Products; No. 8-19, Snacks and Sweets; No. 8-20, Cereal Grains and Pasta; No. 8-21, Fast Foods; Supplements 1989, 1990, 1991, 1992.

"Nutritive Value of Foods." United States Department of Agriculture, Home and Garden Bulletin No. 72.

J. Davies and J. Dickerson, *Nutrient Content of Food Portions*. Cambridge, UK: The Royal Society of Chemistry, 1991.

G. A. Leveille, M. E. Zabik, K. J. Morgan, *Nutrients in Foods*. Cambridge, MA: The Nutrition Guild, 1983.

A. Moller, E. Saxholt, B.E. Mikkelsen. *Food Composition Tables: Amino Acids, Carbohydrates and Fatty Acids in Danish Foods,* 1991.

Souci, Fachmann, and Kraut, *Food Composition and Nutrition Tables*. Stuttgart: Wissenschaftliche Verlagsgesellschaft MbH, 1989.

Information from food labels, manufacturers and processors. The values are based on research conducted through 1996. Manufacturers' ingredients are subject to change, so current values may vary from those listed in the book.

INTRODUCTION

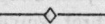

It's hard to believe but the average supermarket carries 30,000 separate items and over half of these are foods. No wonder grocery shopping takes so long. And when you try to compare the nutrients in different products to ensure the healthiest menu, it takes even longer. Recent surveys show that over 60% of Americans are concerned about the nutritional value in the foods they buy. You want to make good choices, but you may not have enough time to spend comparing the labels of five or more pasta sauces, rice mixes or frozen dinners. That's where *The Supermarket Nutrition Counter* lends a hand. Now you have a chance to compare these products before you get near the supermarket.

The Supermarket Nutrition Counter will show you how to navigate the supermarket to find the best choices in each section as you push your cart up and down the aisles. You'll also learn how to interpret the nutrition facts on labels, use cents-off coupons, make use of storage tips to preserve the nutrients in the foods you buy and even how to stock your kitchen so there will always be a quick something to eat.

Fast fact
Nearly 20% of the new products introduced in supermarkets are low-fat, low-cholesterol items.

Fast fact
In the United States, there are 131,000 grocery stores with over $401 billion in sales.

TRAVELING THROUGH THE SUPERMARKET

The first step to efficient, healthy shopping is getting to know the layout of the supermarket where you shop. Grocery stores tend to be organized in similar layouts, and there are a few tricks to getting the most out of your shopping time. Wheel your cart around the outside aisles first. You'll be passing the fresh dairy products, fruits, vegetables, breads and meat, fish and poultry. These foods are the ones that are emphasized in the Food Guide Pyramid. Load your basket with these.

Navigating the Supermarket Aisles

Supermarkets are set up to encourage shoppers to buy more. For instance, milk, which is usually bought on every shopping trip, is placed in the rear of the store to encourage spontaneous shopping on the way to the dairy case. Marketers know we expect to find sale items at the end of the aisle. Placing not-on-sale items here or at the checkout counter results in increased sales. Salad dressings placed near the lettuce in the produce section are more likely to be bought than others shelved separately, as are items placed at eye level on store shelves. Studies show that placing a product at eye level can increase sales by 50%. Being aware of these practices can start you on the road to savvy shopping.

Fast fact ───────────────────────────────

A supermarket shopping cart travels 30,000 miles in its lifetime and on an average shopping trip carries 20 items.

FOOD GUIDE PYRAMID
A Guide to Daily Food Choices

The Pyramid is an outline of what to eat each day. It's not a rigid prescription, but a general guide that lets you choose a healthful diet that's right for you. The Pyramid calls for eating a variety of foods to get the nutrients you need and at the same time the right amount of calories to maintain a healthy weight.

Fats & Sweets
USE SPARINGLY

Milk, Yogurt, & Cheese Group
2-3 SERVINGS

Meat, Poultry, Fish, Dry Beans, Eggs, & Nuts Group
2-3 SERVINGS

Vegetable Group
3-5 SERVINGS

Fruit Group
2-4 SERVINGS

Bread, Cereal, Rice, & Pasta Group
6-11 SERVINGS

The Food Guide Pyramid emphasizes foods from the five food groups shown in the three lower sections of the Pyramid.

Each of these food groups provides some, but not all, of the nutrients you need. Foods in one group can't replace those in another. No one food group is more important than another; for good health, you need them all.

Source: U.S. DEPARTMENT OF AGRICULTURE and the U.S. DEPARTMENT OF HEALTH AND HUMAN SERVICES.

Provided by: the Education Department of the NATIONAL LIVE STOCK AND MEAT BOARD.

Fast fact _____

According to a Food Marketing Institute survey, taste, convenience and nutrition are the basic selling points for new food products. 20,076 new food products were introduced in 1994. Most of these, over 90%, were variations of existing products, such as new flavors, and less than 10% were truly new items. The failure rate among new products runs between 80% and 94%.

Shopping Strategies

Shop with a list whenever you can. Surveys show that 55% of shoppers make a list before going to the supermarket. They tend to buy twice as many items as are on their list, but the list reminds them of needed items and helps to direct purchases.

Larger sizes are usually, but not always, a better value. A half gallon of milk costs less than two quart containers, but it's a bargain only if you'll use it up before it spoils.

Prices on store brands may be as much as 50% less than the least expensive brand-name competitor but usually result in savings of 10 to 25%. Check this out by comparing the unit cost (price per ounce or per pound) of the store brand and your favorite. Also check out the quality of store brands. You may find them improved over the last time you used them.

Watch out for sale items, especially in the case of produce. You may not be able to use them up before they spoil. Other sale items with freshness dates may be near the end of their shelf life.

Get familiar with the layout of the store you shop in most often. Grocery shoppers spend an average of $1.33 for every minute they remain in the store. Up to a point, the more time spent looking for an item, the more they will buy.

It pays to stoop down to lower shelves when grocery shopping. The high-profit items are at eye level, and you'll find the lower markup products down below.

Cents-off coupons can save you money if they don't encourage you to buy items you wouldn't ordinarily use. Manufacturers offer cents-off coupons to promote use of their products. If you use them when the supermarket doubles the value or when an item is on sale, you can save even more. You will be seeing more and more of point-of-purchase coupons. Look for them in shelf dispensers or at the checkout counter.

Remember that you pay for convenience. Unsliced Italian bread costs less than one that is sliced and has a garlic-flavored spread. You may be willing to pay for preparation time saved, but on the other hand, you may prefer to slice and flavor the bread yourself and save money.

Convenience foods like canned vegetables, frozen juice concentrates and packaged mixes for muffins and cakes **can be real time-savers** and save you from having to keep on hand supplies of ingredients you rarely use.

Fast fact _____

The greatest number of coupons distributed are for cereals and breakfast foods. Grocery shoppers saved $4.2 billion in 1994 by redeeming coupons. Even though only a small percentage of coupons are redeemed, a recent study showed that merely seeing a coupon in a newspaper insert can boost sales. Cents-off coupons you get as inserts in newspapers have a redemption rate of 2 to 3%. Those distributed in shelf dispensers have redemption rates of 17%.

Fast fact _____

Canned chicken noodle soup is the No. 1 selling food item in supermarkets. Three hundred and fifty million cans are purchased each year.

Men and Women in the Supermarket

Although male shoppers in the supermarket are still in the minority, their numbers are increasing. A 1993 report by *Progressive Grocer* magazine found 19% of the men surveyed said they were the primary grocery shopper compared with 14% in 1988. Other studies report that as many as one-third of the weekend shoppers are men.

Men and women tend to buy different items. Men, especially younger ones, buy beer, cupcakes, ice cream and hot dogs. Women buy more cottage cheese, refrigerated yogurt and salad dressing. Single male shoppers and men who head families grocery shop more times a week than women. They also tend to shop at the last minute and when they are hungry so that they are more susceptible to impulse buying. And men are less likely to use cents-off coupons—50% of men compared to 67% of women.

FOOD LABELING

In May 1994, the current food labeling law took effect but Americans have always been label conscious. According to a 1994 survey done by the Calorie Control Council, 62% of adults said they always try to check nutrition labels of foods to determine the fat content. Almost as many check for calorie content. In the 1996 Trends: Consumer Attitudes and the Supermarket survey conducted by the Food Marketing Institute, more than half of all supermarket shoppers said they always read the nutrition label when they buy a food for the first time. Almost half of these shoppers found the wording and format of the nutrition facts panel very useful.

The expanded nutrition label called Nutrition Facts is found on almost all packaged foods. The labels are designed to show how

Food Label at a Glance

Serving sizes are now more consistent across product lines, are stated in both household and metric measures, and reflect the amounts people actually eat.

The list of nutrients covers those most important to the health of today's consumers, most of whom need to worry about getting too much of certain nutrients (fat, for example), rather than too few vitamins or minerals, as in the past.

The label of larger packages may now tell the number of calories per gram of fat, carbohydrate, and protein.

Nutrition Facts

Serving Size 1 cup (228g)
Servings Per Container 2

Amount Per Serving

Calories 260   Calories from Fat 120

	% Daily Value*
Total Fat 13g	**20%**
Saturated Fat 5g	**25%**
Cholesterol 30mg	**10%**
Sodium 660mg	**28%**
Total Carbohydrate 31g	**10%**
Dietary Fiber 0g	**0%**
Sugars 5g	
Protein 5g	

Vitamin A 4%	•	Vitamin C 2%
Calcium 15%	•	Iron 4%

* Percent Daily Values are based on a 2,000 calorie diet. Your daily values may be higher or lower depending on your calorie needs:

	Calories:	2,000	2,500
Total Fat	Less than	65g	80g
Sat Fat	Less than	20g	25g
Cholesterol	Less than	300mg	300mg
Sodium	Less than	2,400mg	2,400mg
Total Carbohydrate		300g	375g
Dietary Fiber		25g	30g

Calories per gram:
Fat 9 • Carbohydrate 4 • Protein 4

New title signals that the label contains the newly required information.

Calories from fat are now shown on the label to help consumers meet dietary guidelines that recommend people get no more than 30 percent of the calories in their overall diet from fat.

% Daily Value shows how a food fits into the overall daily diet.

Daily Values are also something new. Some are maximums, as with fat (65 grams or less); others are minimums, as with carbohydrate (300 grams or more). The daily values for a 2,000- and 2,500-calorie diet must be listed on the label of larger packages.

This label is only a sample. Exact specifications are in the final rules.
Source: Food and Drug Administration, 1994

a food fits into the daily diet. They also make it easier to compare one food with another. The amount of calories in a serving (serving size closely reflects the amounts people actually eat) and the calories from fat are given in numbers. Total fat, cholesterol, sodium, total carbohydrate and dietary fiber are given both as numbers and as percentages of Daily Value (DV).

Daily values are the label reference numbers. These numbers are set by the government and are based on current nutrition recommendations. The percent daily values are based on a 2,000-calorie diet; values can also be given for an optional 2,500-calorie diet. Although these calorie levels cover the average intakes of most people, they do not cover everybody. The nutrients listed on the label are the ones that are important for good health; too much of some and too little of others may lead to increased risk for certain diseases. It really isn't necessary to worry about nutrition values for each food you eat or even each meal you eat. What you should aim for is those foods that give you more carbohydrate, vitamins and minerals and less sodium, fat, saturated fat and cholesterol most of the time.

The Daily Values for total fat, saturated fat, cholesterol and sodium set upper limits on the amount to eat each day to stay healthy. Other Daily Values help you identify the best levels to aim for each day. This applies to total carbohydrate, fiber, vitamins and minerals.

Loopholes in the Labels

Although the labels can help guide consumers in making better food choices, they are not perfect. So many issues were involved in formulating labels that accurately represent the nutritional value of different foods that even with the concerted effort of experts there remain some gray areas.

Because of an exemption, 2% milk may continue to call itself "low fat" even though it doesn't meet the new Food and Drug

Administration (FDA) definition that limits this designation to 3 grams of fat in a serving. A glass of 2% milk may contain up to 5 grams of fat.

Trans-fatty acids are formed when liquid oils are hardened (hydrogenated) to form solid shortenings. These trans-fatty acids are found in margarine, chips, crackers, cookies and other processed foods made from hardened fat. Trans fats are included in the "total fat" category on nutrition labels. Under the labeling law, the manufacturer must list the amount of total fat, saturated fat and cholesterol in a food but not the amount of trans fat. Recent research suggests that trans fat could be responsible for 30,000 deaths from heart disease each year in the United States because it raises blood cholesterol the same way saturated fats do. Some experts, however, believe that more studies are needed to clarify the dangers of trans-fatty acids.

Fruits and vegetables and fresh meats and poultry are not required to have individual nutrition labels. However, the meat industry is participating in a voluntary program in which supermarkets will display posters showing nutrition information on the most popular cuts.

Rules about the use of the word *healthy* on food labels went into effect in 1996. To be labeled as *healthy*, foods will have to contain low levels of fat and saturated fat, limited amounts of sodium and cholesterol and at least some amount of a beneficial nutrient, like vitamin C.

Businesses that produce 600,000 or fewer units of food a year are exempt from nutrition labeling rules. These are generally local businesses like a cider mill or small regional bakery. That number will drop to 100,000 units in a few years.

Foods in small packages like Life Savers and snack-size candies don't need nutrition labels but must list a telephone number or address where consumers can get the required information. Also exempt are food products like coffee, tea, some spices and flavorings that contain no significant amounts of any nutrient. Ready-to-eat foods from the deli or bakery prepared on site and take-out foods also do not need labeling.

What the Label Claims Really Mean

The FDA required labels mean you'll no longer have to guess what it means when you see a nutrition claim like low sodium or fat free on a package. These claims can only be used when the food meets strict government definitions.

LABEL LANGUAGE

Label Claim	Definition*
Calorie Free	Less than 5 calories
Low Calorie	40 calories or less
Light or Lite	50% or less fat content than previous standard for the product; fat content must be reduced by 50% or more
Light in Sodium	50% less sodium than previous standard for the product
Less Sodium or Reduced in Sodium	25% less sodium than previous standard for the product
Fat Free	Less than ½ gram fat
Low Fat	3 grams or less fat (except milk can contain 5 grams)
Reduced Fat	25% less fat than previous standard for the product
Cholesterol Free	Less than 2 milligrams cholesterol and 2 grams or less saturated fat
Low Cholesterol	20 milligrams or less cholesterol and 2 grams or less saturated fat

Label Claim	Definition*
Sodium Free and Salt Free	Less than 5 milligrams sodium
Very Low Sodium	35 milligrams or less sodium
Low Sodium	140 milligrams or less sodium
High Fiber	5 grams or more fiber
Excellent or High source of a nutrient	Must supply at least 20% of the Daily Value of the nutrient
Good source of a nutrient	Must supply between 10 and 19% of the Daily Value of the nutrient
Lean meat, poultry, seafood, packaged meals	Less than 10 grams of fat, 4 grams of saturated fat, 95 milligrams of cholesterol
Extra Lean meat, poultry seafood, packaged meals	Less than 5 grams of fat, 2 grams of saturated fat and 95 milligrams of cholesterol

*Per Reference Amount (standard serving size). Some claims have higher nutrient levels for main dish products and meal products such as frozen entrees and dinners.

Health Claims

In the past you may have seen health claims on labels suggesting that a product could help prevent a specific disease. Today health claims on food labels are regulated. A food must meet certain nutrient levels to make a health claim and only seven types of health claims are allowed when research supports a link between the nutrient and the disease.

HEALTH CLAIMS ALLOWED ON LABELS

Calcium and osteoporosis (adult bone loss)
Sodium and high blood pressure (hypertension)
Dietary fat and cancer
Dietary saturated fat and cholesterol and risk of coronary heart disease
Fruits and vegetables and cancer

Fiber-containing grain products, fruits and vegetables and cancer

Fruits, vegetables and grain products that contain fiber and risk of coronary heart disease

A label may not make a health claim for a specific nutrient in a food if the food also contains other nutrients that would lessen the health benefits. So that while a container of skim milk can make a health claim for its calcium content, a container of whole milk cannot, because even though it contains calcium, it also has a lot of fat, which increases the risk for other diseases. Foods that have more than 13 grams of fat, 4 grams of saturated fat, 60 milligrams of cholesterol or 480 milligrams of sodium per serving and have a nutrient claim for a different nutrient must carry the following statement: "See [appropriate panel] for information about [nutrient requiring disclosure] and other nutrients." Because of the complex rules governing putting health claims on labels, experts believe they will not be widely used.

Summing Up: Although the new food labels may not be perfect, they are beneficial because so many foods will now be required to display them and serving sizes are now standardized to make comparisons easier. Rather than trying to interpret every fact, concentrate on what is important. The values for carbohydrate, fiber, vitamins A and C, calcium and iron should be high, while the values for total fat, saturated fat, cholesterol and sodium should be low.

Fast fact _____

The American Dietetic Association's National Center for Nutrition and Dietetics has a consumer hot line for food-labeling information and materials. Call (800) 366-1655.

SUPERMARKET SECTIONS

The Bread Box

The experts urge us to eat whole grains. They have all the vitamins, minerals and fiber originally found in grain. Many of these important nutrients are lost when the grains are refined. Some nutrients, vitamins B_1 (thiamin), B_2 (riboflavin), niacin and the mineral iron, are added to refined grains, which are then called "enriched." Refined, enriched wheat is the kind usually used to make white bread.

What Kinds of Bread Do We Use?

A recent study shows that half of U. S. households use white bread. This is down from three-fourths just ten years ago. Americans have expanded their tastes in bread:

49.2% use white bread
43.8% use whole wheat
16.4% use 100% whole grain
16.4% use French/Italian
12.2% use low-calorie/light
11.9% use rye/pumpernickle
10.6% use raisin
10.5% use sourdough
9.3% use fiber/high fiber
8.7% use oat/oat bran

Tortillas, not bagels, are the most-eaten ethnic bread. It is estimated that Americans eat 50 billion tortillas a year!

You can't always tell by color whether or not bread is made with whole grains. Some wheat breads look toasty brown, but the color is not from whole wheat flour. Caramel (browned sugar), molasses or raisin juice can add rich brown color. The ingredient list on the label will tell you which grains are in the bread. The one listed first is the major grain in the bread, cereal or cracker.

Bread labeled 100% whole wheat contains only whole wheat flour. But even when a bread is not 100% whole wheat, it can still be nutritious. Wheat germ, cracked wheat, oatmeal, sprouted wheat, bran breads and enriched breads are also good sources of nutrients. You may enjoy the flavor of pumpernickel and rye breads, which are mixtures of white flour and smaller amounts of whole grains.

Cereals

Cereals can be hot, cooked in a pan or in the microwave, or cold, ready to eat. They're rich in nutrients, fill you up and are usually low in fat too. If your favorites have a lot of sugar added (you can tell when you see sugar listed as one of the first ingredients), mix it with cereal that contains less sugar.

Note: Some cereals that contain fruit or fruit juice and have more than 4 grams (1 teaspoon) of sugar in a serving may still be good choices. They may look like they're high in sugar, but the sugars in the dried fruit or juice are counted in on the label with the added sugar.

Crackers

The cracker shelf is one of the largest and most varied shelves in the supermarket. For a healthy snack, try some of the new reduced-fat and fat-free varieties like cracked pepper, flavorful without fat. Rice cakes (spicy Mexican style is great), bagel chips, bread sticks, saltines and soda crackers are usually good low-fat choices, but don't forget old-fashioned graham crackers for a sweet treat.

Other Grains

There are many types of delicious grains. Besides regular white enriched rice, you'll find long grain, short grain, wild rice (not really rice at all), barley, buckwheat (kasha), bulgur, cracked wheat, millet, cornmeal, and quinoa to name some of the most usual grains available. All can be cooked in an hour or less. If you start soaking them early in the day, you can often cut the cooking time. Package labels give cooking directions.

Summing Up: The Food Guide Pyramid (p. xvii), the U.S. Department of Agriculture and U.S. Department of Health and Human Services' guide for choosing a good diet, recommends eating six to eleven servings from the bread and cereal group each day. A serving is one slice of bread; four crackers; 1 ounce of ready-to-eat cereal; or ½ cup of hot cereal, pasta, rice, bulgur or other grains. Studies show that only 5% of Americans eat the minimum six grain servings recommended.

Fast fact

The average American ate 19 pounds of pasta in 1991, up 48% from 1989. It is estimated that consumption will reach 30 pounds per person by the year 2000.

The Dairy Case

Choose lowfat or skim milk. Sales of skim milk have tripled in the last ten years. It has all the vitamins and minerals you get in whole milk minus the fat. Whole milk is best for children under two or three. The same holds true for yogurt with low-fat or fat-free versions best for everyday use. Even though yogurt is still more popular in Europe, it's estimated that four out of ten of us eat it regularly.

Milk is 93% water, so it is easy for bacteria, yeasts and molds to grow in it. That's why milk should be kept cold at all times. Keep the milk container or bottle in the refrigerator. Ultrapasteurized milk is treated at an ultrahigh temperature to kill off the bacteria that cause spoilage, and therefore it lasts longer. Shelf-stable milk is now available so that you can always have a supply of milk on hand.

Also in the dairy case is a large selection of reduced-fat cheeses. Try them to see which ones you like best as an alternative to regular cheese, which is high in fat and should be used in smaller amounts.

Pick Up Some Culture

Bacterial cultures are what causes milk to ferment and make yogurt yogurt. Research suggests that yogurt containing live bacteria has health benefits. These bacteria seem to boost the immune system, helping to prevent colon cancer. Yogurt has also been shown to help prevent diarrhea and canker sores. The types with active cultures are well tolerated by some people who cannot handle the sugar in milk (lactose) and is therefore a good source of calcium. Some yogurt makers pasteurize yogurt after the bacteria is added, killing the cultures and eliminating any possible health benefits.

If you want live cultures, look for a label that states "active yogurt cultures," "live yogurt cultures" or "cultured after pasteurization."

Summing Up: The Food Guide Pyramid recommends two or three servings from the milk, yogurt and cheese group. Teens, young adults and women who are pregnant or breastfeeding need three servings. The average American has only one serving a day. A serving is 1 cup of milk, buttermilk or yogurt; 1½ cups ice milk, 1½ ounces hard cheese or 2 ounces processed cheese. It takes 2 cups of cottage cheese to equal the calcium in 1 cup of milk, so it's not the best milk replacement.

Fruits and Vegetables

Even though fresh fruits and vegetables account for only about 10% of grocery sales, surveys show that customers often decide where to shop based on the quality of the produce section. Fruits and vegetables are no longer seasonal. You can now buy almost all kinds year round. At any one time your supermarket may stock apples from New Zealand, grapes from Chile, melons from Israel and mangoes from Peru.

But remember, buying fruits and vegetables in season means lower prices and better quality. Medium-sized fruits are a better buy than larger sizes, and you pay a premium price for jumbo because they are scarce.

Prepared produce like precut melons, prewashed salad ingredients, or celery and carrot sticks cost much more. A pound of whole carrots may cost as little as 35 cents, the price of precut carrot sticks climbs to almost $2.00 a pound, but the time saved may be well worth the cost.

Note: The Nutrition Facts Panel on dried fruit may lead you to believe that prunes, for example, contain a lot of added sugar. In fact, there is no added sugar. The 11 grams of sugar (almost 3 teaspoons) in six prunes is all natural sugar. The nutrition label does not distinguish between added sugar and natural sugar. Read the ingredient listing to see if there is any sugar added. When no sugar is listed, all the sugar is natural to the food.

Fruit and vegetable juices are good sources of vitamins and minerals, but they do not contain all the fiber from the original fruit. They are available as frozen concentrates, ready to use from the dairy case, and in shelf-stable containers (box drinks). Don't confuse pure juice with juice drinks. They are not the same. Pure juice contains 100% fruit juice, while juice drinks can contain as little as 10 to 30% real juice. In addition, these drinks contain water and added sugar.

The federal labeling law requires that the percentage of actual fruit juice or vegetable juice in a drink, punch, ade or cocktail be shown on the label. You will find it on the side nutrition panel of juice packages. Because it is not on the front and it may be in small print, you might have to look carefully to find it, but don't let that stop you. Higher percentages of fruit and vegetable juices mean a healthier beverage, richer in vitamins and minerals with less water and usually less sweeteners. Many juice drinks cost the same or even more than pure (100%) juice even though sugar and water cost less.

Note: Some 100% juice drinks contain a large percentage of apple or grape juice in addition to more exotic juices, like guava or papaya, that lend their names to the beverage.

Summing Up: The Food Guide Pyramid recommends five or more servings of fruit and vegetables a day. Some surveys show that many Americans may not eat even one. It is much easier to meet this guideline if you stock up on ready-to-use fruits and vegetables when you shop.

A serving of fruit is one-half grapefruit; one medium apple, banana or orange; one peach; one pear; two plums; twelve cherries; two raw figs; ½ cup cooked or canned fruit; ½ cup berries, pineapple or melon chunks; ¼ cup dried fruit or ¾ cup of fruit juice.

A serving of vegetables is one small potato, ½ cup of cooked vegetables, one small ear of corn, one cup raw, leafy vegetables or ¾ cup of vegetable juice.

Fast fact
Potatoes that are sprouting can still be used as long as the potatoes are firm. Simply break off the sprouts and peel before cooking.

Does Sex Really Count?

You may have heard the claim that some eggplants are female and others male. This is determined by the shape of the scarlike depression at the blossom end of the vegetable, opposite the stem end. If the scar is round, the eggplant is male, if it's elongated, the eggplant is female. Don't bother examining your eggplant because experts say gender has no effect on the quality of the vegetable.

Variety in the Salad Bowl

Supermarkets now stock a variety of salad greens, in salad bars, prewashed in bags or as heads of lettuce. Iceberg lettuce has always been popular because of its crispness, but if you want greener, leafier or tastier choices that are more nutrient-rich, try arugula, Belgian endive, butterhead, radicchio, romaine, chicory, escarole, spinach or watercress.

Arugula—Slender green leaves with a peppery flavor; younger, smaller leaves are milder.

Belgian endive—Bullet-shaped heads are yellow colored, so it really is not a green; it is crisp, mildly sharp and flavorful.

Butterhead—Includes Boston and Bibb, has soft buttery texture with a mild, sweet flavor.

Radicchio—Colorful red leaves that look like little red cabbages; not as crisp as endive, which it stars with in tricolored salads.

Chicory—Also called curly endive, its thin, curly leaves are fairly bitter; can be used raw or cooked.

Escarole—Leaves are wider and flatter than chicory; slightly bitter but the inner leaves tend to be milder; popular in soups; can be used raw.

Romaine—Very nutritious green often used in Caesar salads.

Watercress—Small, dark green leaves with a sharp, peppery flavor; used in salads and sandwiches and as a garnish.

Meat Case (and Beans Too)

The meat group in the Food Guide Pyramid includes meat, poultry, fish, dry beans, eggs and nuts. Protein is found in all the foods in this group along with iron and other minerals and vitamins. Animal protein foods also supply vitamin B_{12}, while beans are a good source of fiber.

Chickens Up

Americans almost doubled their annual intake of chicken between 1975 and 1992. We eat about 48 pounds of chicken a year. It is estimated that this will increase to 94 pounds per person by the year 2005.

In 1994, according to the Department of Agriculture, Americans ate per person:

  63.7 pounds of beef
  49.5 pounds of pork
  48.2 pounds of chicken
  14.9 pounds of fish and shellfish
  14.3 pounds of turkey
   0.9 pound of lamb
   0.8 pound of veal

Poultry is often thought of as low in fat, but some, like duck and goose, are high in fat and should be eaten only once in a while. Although chicken is low in fat, the skin is loaded with it. Research shows that cooking chicken with the skin on keeps the meat moist without adding fat, but always remove the skin before you eat it.

Choosing Lower-Fat Protein Foods

High-fat option	Low-fat option
Porterhouse steak	Flank steak
Rib roast	Eye round
Regular hamburger	Ground meat, 10% or less fat
Spareribs	Center cut pork loin
Frozen breaded fish	Frozen plain fish
Sardines packed in oil	Sardines in mustard sauce
Tuna packed in oil	Tuna packed in water
Refried beans	Plain beans with salsa
Bluefish, mackerel	Scrod, halibut, tuna
Fried chicken	Baked chicken

Note: You can find reduced-fat versions of bologna, salami, hot dogs and bacon, but the original varieties are high in fat and salt. Both types, regular and reduced fat, usually contain nitrites that combine with substances found naturally in some foods and in the stomach to form carcinogens (cancer causing) called *nitrosamines.* Use these kinds of processed meats once in a while. Nuts and seeds, other members of the meat group, are good sources of protein, but they are high in fat. Eat small amounts of these.

Four ounces of lean, boneless meat, fish or poultry will give 3 ounces cooked, about the size of a deck of cards. That's plenty, even though it's less than what you usually get in a restaurant.

The mandatory nutrition labeling requirements established by the labeling act do not apply to fresh meat, including ground beef, poultry and seafood. The meat industry is participating in the voluntary nutrition labeling program in which brochures and

posters in supermarkets will offer consumers the same information for fresh meat that is required on packaged foods. In this
supplementary material, nutrition information (Nutri-Facts) will
be available for forty-five commonly consumed meat and poultry
cuts and twenty seafood items.

There is a proposal to allow percentages of lean and fat in
ground beef to be listed on the package label, provided that nutrition information is available at the point of sale (Nutri-Facts).
Nutrition information for three blends of ground beef, ranging
from 10% to 27% fat, will be included in the charts. They will be
noted as percentage lean and percentage fat, so that the ground
meat with 10% fat will be labeled as 90% lean, 10% fat. In a
survey, four out of ten shoppers chose labels with full descrip-
tions such as ground beef 70% lean/30% fat.

Summing Up: The Food Guide Pyramid recommends two or
three servings from the meat, poultry, fish, dry beans, eggs and
nuts group. The average American eats more than two servings
from the meat group a day. A serving is equal to 3 ounces of
cooked, lean meat, fish or poultry. One-half cup cooked beans
or lentils, 2 ounces of tofu, 2 tablespoons of peanut butter, ⅓
cup nuts or one egg can fill in for 1 ounce of meat.

Fast fact
Ham, unlike beef, does not have a lot of marbling. So once
the visible fat is trimmed away, you've gotten rid of most
of it.

Fast fact
The average American ate 14.9 pounds of seafood in 1994.
Tuna remained the favorite. The other top nine in order of
consumption were shrimp, Alaska pollack (surimi),
salmon, cod, catfish, clams, flatfish, crabs and scallops.

Why Not Try Tofu?

Ounce for ounce, tofu has just as much protein as meat, and is cholesterol free and very low in saturated fat. Because tofu is made from soybeans, it has all the health giving properties of soy—cholesterol lowering and cancer preventing—that scientists are beginning to learn about.

Tofu can be found in most supermarkets and green grocers. It is versatile, picking up the flavors of foods it's cooked with. Soft tofu, called *silken* on the package, can be mashed and used as a substitute for cottage cheese, or it can be blended until creamy in a food processor or blender and then substituted for sour cream or mayonnaise in dips. Firm tofu can be sliced and marinated in soy sauce, garlic, sesame oil and ginger (try 2 tablespoons of salt-reduced soy sauce, 1 teaspoon of sesame oil, 1 clove of minced garlic and a sprinkle of ginger) and then stir-fried or, even tastier, broiled for a flavorful meat substitute.

Snacks

Many snacks fall into the fats, oils and sweets food group. This group makes up the tip, the smallest part of the Food Guide Pyramid. Instead of a recommended number of servings, the advice given is to use these foods sparingly. Most of us enjoy high-sugar, high-fat snacks like soda, chips, cookies, cake, ice cream and candy. Considered fun foods, they are often used as a treat or reward, as a cure for boredom, as well as a quick way to satisfy hunger. Americans are such eager snackers that over 300 new snack items are introduced every year!

Eating these foods is not the issue; the amount you eat is. Have a snack-size candy bar, not a regular size. Try an ice cream bar or small cup instead of a soup bowl full of ice cream, an individual bag of chips rather than the giant economy size, a cupcake instead of a large slice of cake.

Chips and pretzels are popular snack foods. In 1994, Americans ate, on the average, 22 pounds of salty snacks like potato chips, popcorn, pretzels and tortilla chips. Pretzels usually are lower in fat than regular chips and are also available lightly salted or unsalted. Americans prefer chips, eating three times as many potato chips and twice as many tortilla chips as pretzels.

Choose cookies that snap instead of bend or fruit bars for low-fat choices, air-popped popcorn or pretzels rather than chips. Lower-fat and no-fat versions of your favorite chips are becoming available; look for them.

Americans love candy. We each eat an average of 23.9 pounds a year! That's 34% more than in 1983. Try some licorice, jelly beans, candy corn or marshmallows. These are all sweet, low-fat treats. Hard candies and lollipops provide long-lasting, low-fat, sweet snacking.

Ice cream should be a sometimes food. Although it does contain some calcium, it also has lots of fat, saturated fat and cholesterol. Look for lower-fat or fat-free varieties. Or look for lower-fat frozen desserts like ice milk or frozen yogurt. But don't think of ice milk or frozen yogurt as equivalent to milk or regular yogurt. Most frozen flavors are higher in sugar and fat and lower in calcium. Sorbet and ices are refreshing alternatives, but don't count on them for calcium.

Pastries like pies, Danish pastries, croissants and donuts can be very high in fat. They're all once-in-a-while snacks. Even muffins, often thought of as a healthy substitute for pastries, can be high in fat. Look for muffins that are labeled low fat or have a bagel with jelly instead.

Americans drink a lot of soda, $47.3 billion worth a year. This is almost three times the amount spent on milk. One ounce of soda contains about 1 teaspoon of sugar, so the usual 12 ounces contains 12 teaspoons. Colas, the most popular soda, and some fruit-flavored soda often contain caffeine too. Instead of soda, try plain sparkling water (mixed half and half with fruit juice), mineral water or iced tea for a change.

Fast fact _____

Each package of Mars M&M's contains exactly the same percentage of each color: 30% brown, 20% yellow, 20% red, 10% orange, 10% green, 10% blue. In 1995, in response to consumer input, tan M&M's were replaced by blue.

Fast fact _____

A national poll conducted by an ice cream company found that 88% of Americans reached for ice cream during times of stress. Chocolate was the favorite of those age 24 to 54 and butter pecan and other nut flavors were preferred by those over 55. Three-fourths of those polled chose ice cream—vanilla for men, chocolate for women—after an amorous interlude.

Fast fact _____

Bird's Eye frozen vegetables got their start back in 1929 when the old Postum Company, now Kraft, acquired quick-freezing machinery from a former fur trader, Clarence Birdseye.

Fast fact _____

Frozen dinners have come a long way since they were introduced as TV dinners in 1954. In fact, the name TV dinner is no longer used on the package, and the packaging now is microwaveable instead of the original sectioned aluminum tray.

Deep Freeze

Frozen fruits and vegetables are a quick and convenient way to add vitamins and minerals to meals. Most of the time, stay away from those that are sauced, buttered and sugared. You can add your own flavorings and toppings, as little or as much as you like, suiting your taste and saving money at the same time. Frozen potatoes are popular. Here's where label reading is important because many are high in fat and should be reserved for occasional use.

Instead of complete dinners, use frozen entrees—pasta dishes, pizza, tacos, chicken or fish, pancakes or waffles—convenience foods you can use as the base for a quick meal. Simply add a salad or fresh fruit, some bread and a beverage.

SO THAT THERE'S ALWAYS SOMETHING TO EAT

Sometimes you just may be too tired to eat out or even take in or order in. Even though there are no leftovers from yesterday, you can easily put together a quick, satisfying meal when you keep your refrigerator and cabinets stocked with foods we used to call staples.

Use the following list for a start, adding your own special favorites. You'll never have to complain again about there being nothing to eat.

Freezer

Bread: sliced loaf, tortillas or pita
  Made in minutes: bagel pizza, salad pita, grilled cheese
Vegetables: green peas, mixed vegetables, corn
  Made in minutes: peas and pasta
Fruit: strawberries, raspberries
  Made in minutes: fruit cup, topping for angel food cake

Frozen juice and juice drinks
Frozen lowfat yogurt
Meat and poultry: hamburger or turkey patties, chicken pieces, boneless chicken breast
  Made in minutes: creamed chicken (use canned cream soup)

Fast fact

In a study of daily activities of over 10,000 people, cooking ranked seventh among the sixteen common activities. It was outranked only by love-making, socializing, talking, eating, engaging in sports and shopping.

Refrigerator

Cheese: your favorite hard cheese, grated cheese
Eggs
Butter or other spread
Vegetables, onions, carrots

Cupboard

Canned tomatoes: crushed, stewed, sauce
Pasta, rice
Canned beans: chickpeas, black beans, blackeye peas, baked beans
Oil: olive and another vegetable like corn or canola
Vinegar: try flavored*
Catsup
Soy sauce
Salsa*
Anchovy or sun-dried tomato paste*
Bread crumbs

*A small amount of these add a punch of flavor.

Dried fruit: raisins, prunes, apricots
Nuts: walnuts or your favorites
Shelf-stable or evaporated milk
Dried mushrooms*
Spices: cinnamon, ginger, oregano, paprika, curry powder, dried
  garlic, seasoned pepper
Bouillon cubes
Canned soup: chicken broth, cream soup*
Cereal: Oatmeal and ready-to-eat
Jam or jelly
Sugar
Popcorn, unpopped
Tea
Coffee

Fast fact _____

You love garlic, know that its good for you, but hate the
thought of garlic breath? Try chewing on fresh parsley,
roasted coffee beans, fresh mint or cardamom or caraway
seeds.

_____

Fast fact _____

For a healthful meal, fill three-quarters of your plate with
vegetables, beans, lentils, bread, pasta, rice, grains and
fruits, and the other quarter fill with lean meat, fish, poultry or protein alternatives, like nuts, eggs or tofu.

_____

HANDLING FOOD SAFELY

To keep food at its best in flavor and nutrition and avoid food
poisoning, it must be handled and stored carefully. When you're
loading your cart in the supermarket, it's a good idea to pick up
cold and frozen foods last. Cold food should feel cold, and frozen

food should be solid. Pack them together in one double bag so they have less chance to thaw out on the way home. And get them home fast. Canned foods should be free of dents, rust, cracks and bulges, which can indicate food spoilage. Look for the use-by date on packaged foods, and don't buy any that you can't use by this time.

Be sure the temperatures of your refrigerator and freezer are kept cold enough. Refrigerators should be at 40°F, as cold as possible without freezing milk or vegetables. The freezer should be at 0°F, keeping the contents frozen hard. Unpack and refrigerate or freeze as soon as you get home. If you can't use meat, poultry or fish within two days, freeze immediately.

Fast fact

Forget the myth that dishes prepared with mayonnaise are more likely to spoil in the heat. Foods with mayonnaise are actually safer because of its high acid level.

There is a time limit for storage of all foods. Even canned foods that look like they last forever are best when used within one year. Rotate canned and frozen foods so that the older ones are used up first. You may have noticed that more packaged foods now show a date on their label. Sometimes only a date appears, as on milk and juice containers; other times the statement "best when purchased by [date]" or "sell by [date]" is on condiments, salad dressings and bakery goods. "Use by" is on box drinks, jelly and cereals. Some products have expiration dates, which indicate the end of their shelf life. Depending on the product, there is a reasonable time to use it after the sell date before it stales or spoils. Of course, the way the food has been handled before it is sold in the store will affect the length of time it remains usable. It's always best to buy food in a store that has a rapid turnover of products.

A good food rule is, "When in doubt, throw it out." When you see mold on cottage cheese or other soft cheeses, sour cream, yogurt, bread, cake and other baked goods, grains, cooked dried beans or peas or corn on the cob, toss them. Small, moldy spots can be cut away from hard cheese, firm fruits and vegetables like carrots, peppers and cabbage. When you cut the mold away, cut at least one inch around and below the spot. Store the food in a clean container and use it as soon as you can. You can also scoop out tiny spots of mold from jellies. Be careful to scoop out a larger amount around the mold. Pure maple syrup that has become moldy can simply be boiled and used.

The high temperatures of cooking will kill most of the bacteria that cause food-borne illness. Ground meat must be cooked thoroughly until it is gray, not pink, in the middle, particularly if children, elderly persons or people with compromised immune systems will be eating the meat. Several deaths of children have been reported recently that were due to eating undercooked, ground meat from cattle carrying a deadly strain of E. coli bacteria. Thorough cooking of the ground meat will kill the bacteria.

Once cooked, keep the food hot (above 140°F) until it is served. Don't keep cooked foods at room temperature for longer than two hours. Don't cool warm leftovers on the kitchen counter before refrigerating. Thaw perishable foods in the refrigerator or microwave, not at room temperature.

Fast fact _____
The Food Marketing Institute reports that only 3% of Americans pay attention to product expiration dates when shopping at the grocery store.

Fast fact _____
Hot seafood cocktail sauce was found to disinfect the raw oysters it was served on. Horseradish and lemon juice also killed off some bacteria but were not as effective as Tabasco and other hot sauces.

SAFE TIME LIMITS FOR REFRIGERATOR OR FREEZER STORAGE

Food	Cabinet	Refrigerator	Freezer
Berries		1–2 days	
Brownie and Cake mixes	9 months		
Chicken, fresh		1–2 days	9 months
Canned foods	12 months		
Dried peas and beans	12 months		
Egg substitutes, opened		3 days	Don't freeze
Eggs		3 weeks	Don't freeze
Fish (cod, sole)		1–2 days	6 months
Fish (salmon)		1–2 days	2–3 months
Flour	6–8 months		
Frozen dinners			3–4 months
Ground meat		1–2 days	3–4 months
Half & half		10 days	
Ham slices		3–4 days	1–2 months
Herbs, dried	6 months		
Hot dogs, luncheon meat, unopened		1 week	1–2 months
Jellies			
Unopened	12 months		
Opened		3 months	
Mayonnaise			
Unopened	2–3 months		
Opened		2 months	
Meat leftovers		3–4 days	
Milk		5 days	
Pasta	2 years		
Popcorn kernels	2 years		

(continued)

Food	Cabinet	Refrigerator	Freezer
Potatoes	2–3 months		
Rice, white	2 years		
Salad dressing			
Unopened	10–12 months		
Opened		3 months	
Salad oil, opened	1–3 months		
Sauce and gravy mix	6–12 months		
Shrimp			
Fresh		1 day	
Frozen			12 months
Soups and stews		3–4 days	2–3 months
Spices (basil, cinnamon, thyme, chili powder, parsley flakes, paprika, etc.)	1 year		
Steaks, chops		3–5 days	6–9 months
Sugar			
White	2 years		
Brown	4 months		
Syrup	12 months		
Tea bags	18 months		

Fast fact

Although hot dogs are processed meat, they should not be eaten uncooked. A study found that 20% of major brand hot dogs contained bacteria that could lead to serious illness in children, pregnant women, the elderly and people with weak immune systems. Cooking the hot dogs until they are steaming hot throughout will kill the bacteria.

Food Poisoning

Every year more than 7 million Americans have food poisoning. Symptoms include nausea, vomiting, diarrhea, fever and cramps. They can begin anywhere from 30 minutes to as long as 2 weeks after the bad food was eaten, but most times symptoms occur within 4 to 48 hours. Sometimes symptoms are very severe. If the person is very young, pregnant or already ill, call a doctor or go to an emergency room right away.

Safe Handling Instructions for Fresh Meat and Poultry

The U.S. Department of Agriculture requires fresh meat and poultry to be labeled with safe handling instructions. The safe handling instruction label was developed to help consumers prevent food-borne illness at home. It covers four safety guidelines: safety, cross-contamination, cooking and handling leftovers.

Safe Handling Instructions

This product was prepared from inspected and passed meat and/or poultry. Some food products may contain bacteria that could cause illness if the product is mishandled or cooked improperly. For your protection, follow these safe handling instructions.

 Keep refrigerated or frozen.
Thaw in refrigerator or microwave.

 Keep raw meat and poultry separate from other foods. Wash working surfaces (including cutting boards), utensils, and hands after touching raw meat or poultry.

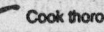 Cook thoroughly.

 Keep hot foods hot. Refrigerate leftovers immediately or discard.

USING YOUR SUPERMARKET
NUTRITION COUNTER

Shoppers average just over two trips a week to the supermarket. It doesn't matter if you shop at Safeway, Kroger, A&P, Publix, Associated, Winn-Dixie, Grand Union or Balducci's in New York, this book lists the calories, fat, cholesterol, sodium and fiber of most of the 16,000 foods you'll find there. For the first time, information about these nutrient values is at your fingertips. Now you will find it easy to follow a healthy diet. Before *The Supermarket Nutrition Counter,* it was impossible to compare so many foods at one time. For example, when you want to select bread, look up the bread category on page 49. You will find over 250 different breads listed so you can see which one is the best source of carbohydrate and fiber.

The Supermarket Nutrition Counter lists the calories, fat, carbohydrate, sodium and fiber values. These are key nutrients for good health. Fat and sodium should be limited, whereas carbohydrate and fiber should be increased. The 1990 Food Labeling Act has established guidelines for nutrient intakes. It recommends that a diet of 2,000 calories a day should include at least 300 grams of carbohydrate and 25 grams of dietary fiber and less than 65 grams of total fat and 2,400 milligrams of sodium.

In *The Supermarket Nutrition Counter,* foods are listed alphabetically. For each group, you will find brand-name foods listed first in alphabetical order followed by an alphabetical listing of unbranded (generic) foods. The unbranded listing will help to determine nutrition values for foods when you do not find your favorite brand listed. They also help you to evaluate unbranded and store brands. Large categories are divided into subcategories such as canned, fresh, frozen, and ready-to-use to make it easier to find what you are looking for. Many categories have take-out and home recipe subcategories. Look there for foods you buy at the supermarket that have been prepared there and so do not need to be nutrition labeled. One out of eight shoppers (12%) buys take-out foods. *The Supermarket Nutrition Counter* has over 400 take-out items for you to choose from to make it easier for you to evaluate these foods.

Most foods are listed alphabetically. But in some cases, foods are grouped by category. For example, pasta dinners, like spaghetti and meatballs, lasagne and manicotti, are all found under the category PASTA DISHES. Other group categories include

Fast fact ——————————————————————————
Although Orville Redenbacher and Sara Lee are real people, as was the late Duncan Hines, there is no Betty Crocker, Mrs. Paul or Chef Boyardee.
————————————————————————————————

DEFINITIONS

as prep (as prepared): refers to food that has been prepared according to package directions

home recipe: describes homemade dishes; those included can be used as a guide to the nutrient values of similar products you may prepare or take-out food you buy ready-to-eat

lean and fat: describes meat with some fat on its edges that is not cut away before cooking or poultry prepared with skin and fat as purchased

lean only: lean portion, trimmed of all visible fat

shelf stable: refers to prepared products found on the supermarket shelf that are ready to be heated or eaten and do not require refrigeration

takeout: describes prepared dishes that you purchase ready-to-eat; those included serve as a guide to the nutrient and calorie values of similar products you may purchase

trace (tr): value used when a food contains less than one calorie, less than one gram (g) of fat, carbohydrate or fiber or less than one milligram (mg) of sodium

ABBREVIATIONS

—◇—

avg	=	average
diam	=	diameter
frzn	=	frozen
g	=	gram
lb	=	pound
lg	=	large
med	=	medium
mg	=	milligram
oz	=	ounce
pkg	=	package
prep	=	prepared
pt	=	pint
qt	=	quart
reg	=	regular
serv	=	serving
sm	=	small
sq	=	square
tbsp	=	tablespoon
tr	=	trace
tsp	=	teaspoon
w/	=	with
w/o	=	without
in	=	inch
<	=	less than

EQUIVALENT MEASURES

——◇——

1 tablespoon	=	3 teaspoons
4 tablespoons	=	¼ cup
8 tablespoons	=	½ cup
12 tablespoons	=	¾ cup
16 tablespoons	=	1 cup
1000 milligrams	=	1 gram
28 grams	=	1 ounce

Liquid Measurements

2 tablespoons	=	1 ounce
¼ cup	=	2 ounces
½ cup	=	4 ounces
¾ cup	=	6 ounces
1 cup	=	8 ounces
2 cups	=	1 pint
4 cups	=	1 quart

Dry Measurements

4 ounces	=	¼ pound
8 ounces	=	½ pound
12 ounces	=	¾ pound
16 ounces	=	1 pound

NOTES

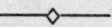

Discrepancies in figures are due to rounding, product reformulation and reevaluation. The labeling law allows rounding of values. Most of the data are analysis data obtained directly from manufacturers, not from labels. In some cases, our values may not be exactly the same as label information because they have not been rounded.

All total fat, carbohydrate (CARB.) and fiber* (FIB.) values are given in grams (g).

All sodium (SOD.) values are given in milligrams (mg).

A dash (—) indicates data not available.

---

*All fiber values are dietary fiber. Except for sweets, foods that are high in carbohydrate (pasta, bread, cereals, fruit, and vegetables) also provide dietary fiber. Animal products—eggs, milk, cheese, meat, fish, poultry—are not sources of fiber. The fiber values indicated for these foods come from added ingredients.

FOOD	PORTION	CAL.	FAT	SOD.	CARB.	FIB.
ABALONE						
fresh fried	3 oz	161	6	502	9	—
raw	3 oz	89	1	255	5	—
ACEROLA						
acerola	1	2	tr	0	tr	—
ACEROLA JUICE						
juice	1 cup	51	1	7	12	—
ADZUKI BEANS						
CANNED						
Eden						
Organic	½ cup (4.1 oz)	100	0	10	18	5
sweetened	1 cup	702	tr	646	163	—
DRIED						
cooked	1 cup	294	tr	18	57	—
READY-TO-USE						
yokan sliced	3¼ in slices	112	tr	36	26	—
AKEE						
fresh	3½ oz	223	20	—	5	—
ALE						
(*see* BEER AND ALE, AND MALT)						
ALFALFA						
sprouts	1 tbsp	1	tr	0	tr	—
sprouts	1 cup	40	tr	2	1	—
ALLIGATOR						
tail cooked	3½ oz	143	3	—	1	—
ALLSPICE						
ground	1 tsp	5	tr	1	1	—
ALMONDS						
Beer Nuts						
Almonds	1 pkg (1 oz)	180	14	51	7	—
Dole						
Blanched Slivered	1 oz	170	14	4	5	—
Blanched Whole	1 oz	170	14	4	5	—
Chopped Natural	1 oz	170	14	4	5	—
Sliced Natural	1 oz	170	14	4	5	—
Whole Natural	1 oz	170	14	4	5	—
Erewhon						
Almond Butter	1 tbsp (16 g)	90	8	18	2	—

FOOD	PORTION	CAL.	FAT	SOD.	CARB.	FIB.
Hain						
Almond Butter Natural Raw	2 tbsp	190	18	120	3	—
Almond Butter Toasted	2 tbsp	220	19	210	3	—
Lance						
Smoked	1 pkg (0.7 oz)	120	11	130	3	—
Nutella						
Spread	1 tbsp (0.5 oz)	85	5	5	9	—
Planters						
Almonds	1 oz	170	15	0	5	3
Gold Measure Slivered	1 pkg (2 oz)	340	31	0	11	4
Honey Roasted	1 oz	160	14	190	7	2
almond butter honey & cinnamon	1 tbsp	96	8	2	4	—
almond butter w/ salt	1 tbsp	101	9	75	3	—
almond butter w/o salt	1 tbsp	101	10	2	3	—
almond meal	1 oz	116	5	2	8	—
almond paste	1 oz	127	8	3	12	—
dried blanched	1 oz	166	15	3	5	—
dried unblanched	1 oz	167	15	3	6	—
dry roasted unblanched	1 oz	167	15	3	7	—
dry roasted unblanched salted	1 oz	167	15	260	7	—
oil roasted blanched	1 oz	174	16	3	5	3
oil roasted blanched salted	1 oz	174	16	3	5	—
oil roasted unblanched	1 oz	176	16	3	5	—
toasted unblanched	1 oz	167	14	3	7	3

AMARANTH

(*see also* CEREAL, COOKIES)

FOOD	PORTION	CAL.	FAT	SOD.	CARB.	FIB.
Arrowhead						
Seeds	¼ cup (1.6 oz)	170	2	0	29	3
Health Valley						
Amaranth Cereal With Bananas	½ cup (1 oz)	110	2	5	20	4
Amaranth Crunch With Raisins	¼ cup (1 oz)	110	3	10	20	3
Amaranth Flakes 100% Organic	½ cup (1 oz)	90	tr	5	21	3
Fast Menu Amaranth With Garden Vegetables	7½ oz	140	3	140	16	8
cooked	½ cup	59	tr	14	3	—
uncooked	½ cup	366	6	21	65	—

FOOD	PORTION	CAL.	FAT	SOD.	CARB.	FIB.
ANASAZI BEANS						
DRIED						
Arrowhead	¼ cup (1.5 oz)	150	1	0	27	9
Bean Cuisine	½ cup	115	1	5	—	5
ANCHOVY						
CANNED						
in oil	5	42	2	734	0	—
in oil	1 can (1.6 oz)	95	4	1651	0	—
FRESH						
fillets	3 (0.4 oz)	21	1	—	tr	—
raw	3 oz	62	4	88	0	—
ANGLERFISH						
raw	3½ oz	72	1	109	0	—
ANISE						
seed	1 tsp	7	tr	tr	1	—
ANTELOPE						
roasted	3 oz	127	2	46	0	—
APPLE						
CANNED						
Luck's						
Fried Apples	8 oz	190	0	—	—	—
White House						
Escalloped Apples	4 oz	120	0	10	28	1
Sliced	4 oz	55	0	10	15	1
Spiced Apple Rings	1 ring	25	0	0	6	tr
sliced sweetened	1 cup	136	1	7	34	—
DRIED						
Del Monte						
Sliced	⅓ cup (1.4 oz)	80	0	310	23	5
Mariani						
Apples	¼ cup	150	0	—	—	—
Sonoma						
Pieces	10-12 pieces (1.4 oz)	110	0	0	29	4
cooked w/ sugar	½ cup	116	tr	27	29	—
cooked w/o sugar	½ cup	172	tr	26	20	—
rings	10	155	tr	56	42	—
FRESH						
Dole	1	80	1	0	18	5
apple	1	81	tr	1	21	3
w/o skin sliced	1 cup	62	tr	0	16	2

FOOD	PORTION	CAL.	FAT	SOD.	CARB.	FIB.
w/o skin sliced & cooked	1 cup	91	tr	1	23	—
w/o skin sliced & microwaved	1 cup	96	tr	1	25	—
FROZEN						
Mrs. Paul's						
Apple Fritters	2	270	9	500	35	—
Stouffer's						
Escalloped	1 cup (6 oz)	180	3	70	37	3
sliced w/o sugar	½ cup	41	tr	3	11	—

APPLE JUICE

FOOD	PORTION	CAL.	FAT	SOD.	CARB.	FIB.
After The Fall						
Organic	1 bottle (10 oz)	110	0	25	28	—
Vermont Apple	1 bottle (10 oz)	110	0	24	27	—
Vermont Apple	1 bottle (8 oz)	90	0	20	22	—
Vermont Harvest Moon Sparkling Apple Cider	8 fl oz	110	0	5	27	—
Apple & Eve						
Cider	6 fl oz	80	0	0	16	—
Juice	6 fl oz	80	0	0	16	—
Nothin' But Juice	6 fl oz	78	0	0	18	—
Bruce						
Lite	½ cup	88	0	25	20	—
Hi-C						
Jammin' Apple	8 fl oz	130	0	30	31	—
Hood						
Select Cider	1 cup (8 oz)	120	0	2	30	—
Minute Maid						
Box	8.45 fl oz	120	0	30	29	—
Juices To Go	1 bottle (10 fl oz)	110	0	30	28	—
Juices To Go	1 bottle (11.5 fl oz)	140	0	35	35	—
Juices To Go	1 can (16 fl oz)	160	0	40	40	—
Naturals	8 fl oz	110	0	30	28	—
Mott's						
From Concentrate as prep	8 fl oz	120	0	20	29	—
Fruit Basket Cocktail as prep	8 fl oz	120	0	5	29	—
Natural	8 fl oz	120	0	20	29	0
Ocean Spray						
Juice	8 fl oz	110	0	35	28	0
Odwalla						
Live Apple	8 fl oz	140	0	25	34	0
Red Cheek						
From Concentrate	8 fl oz	120	0	20	29	0

FOOD	PORTION	CAL.	FAT	SOD.	CARB.	FIB.
Red Cheek (CONT.)						
Natural	8 fl oz	120	0	20	29	0
S&W						
100% Unsweetened	6 oz	85	0	5	20	—
Seneca						
Clarified frzn, as prep	8 fl oz	120	0	24	30	0
Granny Smith frzn as prep	8 fl oz	120	0	24	30	0
Natural frzn as prep	8 fl oz	120	0	24	30	0
Sippin' Pak						
100% Pure	8.45 fl oz	110	0	25	28	—
Sipps						
Juice	8.45 oz	130	0	—	—	—
Snapple						
Apple Crisp	10 fl oz	140	0	30	36	—
Tree Of Life						
East Coast Apple	8 fl oz	120	0	25	30	—
Tree Top						
Cider	6 oz	90	0	10	22	—
Cider frzn as prep	6 oz	90	0	10	22	—
Frzn as prep	6 oz	90	0	10	22	—
Juice	6 oz	90	0	10	22	—
Sparkling Juice	6 oz	90	0	—	22	—
Unfiltered	6 oz	90	0	10	22	—
Unfiltered frzn as prep	6 oz	90	0	10	22	—
w/ Vitamin C	6 oz	90	0	10	22	—
Tropicana						
Season's Best	1 container (10 fl oz)	140	0	15	35	—
Season's Best	1 bottle (7 fl oz)	100	0	10	24	—
Season's Best	8 fl oz	110	0	10	28	—
Season's Best	1 bottle (10 fl oz)	140	0	15	35	—
Season's Best	1 container (6 fl oz)	80	0	5	21	—
Season's Best	1 container (8 fl oz)	110	0	10	28	—
Season's Best	1 can (11.5 fl oz)	160	0	25	40	—
Veryfine						
100%	8 oz	107	0	<10	27	—
White House						
Juice	6 oz	90	0	0	22	0
frzn as prep	1 cup	111	tr	17	28	—
frzn not prep	6 oz	349	1	54	87	—
juice	1 cup	116	tr	7	29	tr
APPLESAUCE						
Eden	½ cup (4.3 oz)	50	0	15	15	2

FOOD	PORTION	CAL.	FAT	SOD.	CARB.	FIB.
Mott's						
Chunky	5 oz	110	0	0	26	2
Cinnamon	5 oz	120	0	0	29	1
Fruit Snacks Apple Spice	4 oz	70	0	0	18	1
Fruit Snacks Cinnamon	4 oz	90	0	0	23	1
Fruit Snacks Strawberry	4 oz	80	0	5	19	1
Fruit Snacks Sweetened	4 oz	90	0	0	22	1
Sweetened	5 oz	110	0	0	28	1
S&W						
Diet	½ cup	55	0	10	14	—
Gravenstein Sweetened	½ cup	90	0	10	24	—
Gravenstein Unsweetened	½ cup	55	0	5	14	—
Sweetened	½ cup	55	0	10	14	—
Unsweetened	½ cup	25	2	5	2	—
Seneca						
Cinnamon	½ cup	100	0	0	24	3
Golden Delicious	½ cup	100	0	0	24	3
McIntosh	½ cup	100	0	0	24	3
Natural	½ cup	60	0	0	15	3
Regular	½ cup	100	0	0	24	3
Tree Top						
Cinnamon	½ cup	80	0	0	21	—
Natural	½ cup	60	0	0	15	—
Original	½ cup	80	0	0	21	—
White House						
Chunky	4 oz	80	0	5	22	1
Cinnamon	4 oz	100	0	5	25	1
Natural Packed w/ Apple Juice	4 oz	60	0	5	14	1
Regular	4 oz	80	0	5	22	1
Unsweetened	4 oz	50	0	0	12	2
sweetened	½ cup	97	tr	4	25	2
unsweetened	½ cup	53	tr	2	14	2

APRICOT JUICE

FOOD	PORTION	CAL.	FAT	SOD.	CARB.	FIB.
Del Monte						
Nectar	8 fl oz	140	0	15	35	1
Kern's						
Nectar	6 fl oz	110	0	0	27	—
Libby						
Nectar	1 can (11.5 fl oz)	220	0	10	52	—
S&W						
Nectar	6 oz	35	0	20	12	—
nectar	1 cup	141	tr	9	36	2

FOOD	PORTION	CAL.	FAT	SOD.	CARB.	FIB.
APRICOTS						
CANNED						
Del Monte						
Halves Unpeeled In Heavy Syrup	½ cup (4.5 oz)	100	0	10	26	1
Halves Unpeeled Lite	½ cup (4.3 oz)	60	0	10	16	1
Libby						
Halves Unpeeled Lite	½ cup (4.4 oz)	60	0	10	13	1
S&W						
Halves Diet	½ cup	35	0	5	9	—
Halves Unpeeled In Heavy Syrup	½ cup	110	0	15	28	—
Halves Unsweetened	½ cup	35	0	5	9	—
Whole Peeled Diet	½ cup	28	0	5	7	—
Whole Peeled In Heavy Syrup	½ cup	100	0	15	26	—
halves heavy syrup pack w/ skin	1 cup (9.1 oz)	214	tr	10	55	—
halves water pack w/ skin	1 cup (8.5 oz)	65	tr	7	16	—
halves water pack w/o skin	1 cup (8 oz)	51	tr	25	12	—
heavy syrup w/ skin	3 halves	70	tr	3	18	—
juice pack w/ skin	3 halves	40	tr	3	10	—
light syrup w/ skin	3 halves	54	tr	3	14	—
puree from heavy syrup pack w/ skin	¾ cup (9.1 oz)	214	tr	10	55	—
puree from light pack w/ skin	¾ cup (8.9 oz)	160	tr	10	42	—
puree from water pack w/ skin	¾ cup (8.5 oz)	65	tr	7	16	—
puree juice pack w/ skin	1 cup (8.7 oz)	119	tr	9	31	—
water pack w/ skin	3 halves	22	tr	2	5	—
water pack w/o skin	4 halves	20	tr	10	5	—
DRIED						
Sonoma						
10 pieces (1.4 oz)		120	0	0	31	1
Del Monte						
Sun Dried	⅓ cup (1.4 oz)	80	0	5	25	6
Mariani						
Whole	¼ cup	140	0	—	—	—
halves	10	83	tr	3	22	3
halves cooked w/o sugar	½ cup	106	tr	4	27	—
FRESH						
apricots	3	51	tr	1	12	—
FROZEN						
sweetened	½ cup	119	tr	5	30	—

FOOD	PORTION	CAL.	FAT	SOD.	CARB.	FIB.
ARROWHEAD						
fresh boiled	1 med (⅓ oz)	9	tr	2	2	—
ARROWROOT						
flour	1 cup	457	tr	2	113	4
ARTICHOKE						
CANNED						
S&W						
Hearts Marinated	½ cup	225	26	15	6	—
FRESH						
Dole	1 lg	23	tr	65	5	3
boiled	1 med (4 oz)	60	tr	114	13	—
hearts cooked	½ cup	42	tr	80	9	—
sunchoke raw sliced	½ cup	57	tr	—	13	—
FROZEN						
Birds Eye						
Hearts Deluxe	½ cup	30	0	40	7	3
cooked	1 pkg (9 oz)	108	1	127	22	—
ARUGULA						
raw	½ cup	2	tr	3	tr	—
ASPARAGUS						
CANNED						
Del Monte						
Salad Tips Tender Green	½ cup (4.4 oz)	20	0	420	3	1
Spears Cut Tender Green	½ cup (4.4 oz)	20	0	420	3	1
Spears Extra Long Tender Green	½ cup (4.4 oz)	20	0	420	3	1
Spears Tender Green	½ cup (4.4 oz)	20	0	420	3	1
Tips Tender Green	½ cup (4.4 oz)	20	0	420	3	1
Owatonna						
Spears Cut	½ cup	20	0			
S&W						
Points Water Pack	½ cup	17	0	10	3	—
Spears Colossal Fancy	½ cup	20	0	320	4	—
Spears Fancy	½ cup	18	0	320	3	—
Seneca						
Asparagus	½ cup	20	0	264	3	2
spears	½ cup	24	1	—	3	—
FRESH						
Dole	5 spears	18	0	0	2	2
cooked	4 spears	14	tr	7	3	—
cooked	½ cup	22	tr	10	4	—
raw	½ cup	16	tr	2	3	—
raw	4 spears	14	tr	1	3	—

FOOD	PORTION	CAL.	FAT	SOD.	CARB.	FIB.
FROZEN						
Big Valley	5-6 spears (3 oz)	20	0	0	3	1
Birds Eye						
Cut	½ cup	23	0	5	4	—
Spears	½ cup	25	0	0	4	—
Green Giant						
Harvest Fresh Cuts	½ cup	25	0	60	4	2
cooked	4 spears	17	tr	2	3	—
cooked	1 pkg (10 oz)	82	1	12	14	—

AVOCADO
FRESH

FOOD	PORTION	CAL.	FAT	SOD.	CARB.	FIB.
California Avocado	½	153	14	—	—	—
California Avocado mashed	1 cup	407	36	—	—	—
avocado	1	324	31	21	15	—
puree	1 cup	370	35	24	17	—

BABY FOOD
Nutritional guidelines for infants are different from those recommended for older children and adults. Check with a pediatrician for advice on feeding children under the age of 2.

BAKED SELECTIONS
Gerber

FOOD	PORTION	CAL.	FAT	SOD.	CARB.	FIB.
Chunky Animal Cookies	2 (0.5 oz)	60	2	—	10	—
Chunky Biter Biscuits	1 (0.4 oz)	50	1	—	9	—
Chunky Zwieback Toast	2 (0.5 oz)	70	2	—	10	—
Graduates Animal Crackers Cinnamon	2 (0.2 oz)	30	1	—	5	—
Graduates Arrowroot Cookies	2 (0.4 oz)	50	2	—	8	—
Graduates Pretzels	2 (0.4 oz)	45	0	—	10	—

CEREAL
Beech-Nut

FOOD	PORTION	CAL.	FAT	SOD.	CARB.	FIB.
Stage 1 Barley	½ oz	60	0	10	12	1
Stage 1 Oatmeal	½ oz	60	2	15	11	1
Stage 1 Oatmeal & Apples	1 jar (4 oz)	70	0	0	16	1
Stage 1 Rice	½ oz	60	0	0	13	0
Stage 2 Mixed	½ oz	50	1	10	12	tr
Stage 2 Mixed & Apples	1 jar (4 oz)	70	0	0	16	1
Stage 2 Oatmeal & Chiquita Bananas	½ oz	60	1	0	12	1
Stage 2 Rice & Apples	1 jar (4 oz)	70	0	0	16	1
Stage 2 Rice & Chiquita Bananas	½ oz	60	0	0	13	0

FOOD	PORTION	CAL.	FAT	SOD.	CARB.	FIB.
Beech-Nut (CONT.)						
Stage 2 Rice & Golden Delicious Apples	½ oz	60	0	0	14	0
Earth's Best						
Brown Rice	5 tbsp (0.5 oz)	60	0	0	12	—
Mixed Grain	5 tbsp (0.5 oz)	60	0	0	11	—
Peach Oatmeal Banana	1 jar (4.5 fl oz)	60	0	10	12	—
Prunes & Oatmeal	1 jar (4.5 fl oz)	100	0	20	24	—
Gerber						
1st Foods Barley	4 tbsp (0.5 oz)	60	1	—	11	—
1st Foods Oatmeal	4 tbsp (0.5 oz)	50	1	—	9	—
1st Foods Rice	4 tbsp (0.5 oz)	60	1	—	11	—
2nd Foods High Protein	4 tbsp (0.5 oz)	50	1	—	6	—
2nd Foods Mixed	4 tbsp (0.5 oz)	60	1	—	11	—
2nd Foods Mixed With Applesauce & Bananas	1 jar (4 oz)	90	1	—	20	—
2nd Foods Mixed With Banana	4 tbsp (0.5 oz)	60	1	—	11	—
2nd Foods Oatmeal With Applesauce & Bananas	1 jar (4 oz)	90	1	—	20	—
2nd Foods Oatmeal With Bananas	4 tbsp (0.5 oz)	60	1	—	10	—
2nd Foods Rice With Applesauce & Bananas	1 jar (4 oz)	90	0	—	21	—
2nd Foods Rice With Bananas	4 tbsp (0.5 oz)	60	1	—	11	—
3rd Foods Mixed With Applesauce & Bananas	1 jar (6 oz)	140	1	—	31	—
3rd Foods Oatmeal With Applesauce & Bananas	1 jar (6 oz)	140	1	—	28	—
3rd Foods Rice With Mixed Fruit	1 jar (6 oz)	130	0	—	31	—
Tropical Foods Corn Cereal	4 tbsp (0.5 oz)	60	1	—	12	—
Tropical Foods Rice With Mango	4 tbsp (0.5 oz)	50	0	—	12	—
Health Valley						
Brown Rice 100% Organic	1 tbsp (0.5 oz)	60	1	5	10	1

FOOD	PORTION	CAL.	FAT	SOD.	CARB.	FIB.
Health Valley (CONT.)						
Sprouted Baby Cereal 100% Organic	1 tbsp (0.5 oz)	60	1	5	10	—
DESSERT						
Beech-Nut						
Stage 2 Apple & Strawberry Dessert	1 jar (4 oz)	100	0	0	23	1
Stage 2 Apple Peach & Strawberry Dessert	1 jar (4 oz)	100	0	0	22	1
Stage 2 Apple Yogurt Dessert	1 jar (4 oz)	100	1	25	22	0
Stage 2 Banana Pineapple Dessert	1 jar (4 oz)	100	0	15	23	0
Stage 2 Banana Pudding (Spanish Label)	1 jar (4 oz)	110	0	0	26	0
Stage 2 Banana Yogurt Dessert	1 jar (4 oz)	120	2	25	24	0
Stage 2 Cottage Cheese With Pears Dessert	1 jar (4 oz)	120	1	15	24	1
Stage 2 Dutch Apple Dessert	1 jar (4 oz)	100	0	10	22	0
Stage 2 Flan De Vanilla	1 jar (4 oz)	120	3	60	23	0
Stage 2 Flan De Banana	1 jar (4 oz)	110	0	0	26	0
Stage 2 Fruit Dessert	1 jar (4 oz)	80	0	0	19	1
Stage 2 Frutas Islenas Dessert	1 jar (4 oz)	100	0	10	23	0
Stage 2 Guava Tropical Fruit Dessert	1 jar (4 oz)	90	0	10	22	2
Stage 2 Mango Tropical Fruit Dessert	1 jar (4 oz)	110	0	10	26	1
Stage 2 Mixed Fruit Yogurt Dessert	1 jar (4 oz)	100	0	15	21	1
Stage 2 Papaya Tropical Fruit Dessert	1 jar (4 oz)	100	0	10	22	0
Stage 2 Vanilla Custard Pudding	1 jar (4 oz)	120	3	60	23	0
Stage 3 Cottage Cheese With Pears	1 jar (6 oz)	180	2	20	37	1
Stage 3 Fruit Dessert	1 jar (6 oz)	120	0	0	28	2
Stage 3 Mixed Fruit Yogurt Dessert	1 jar (6 oz)	170	0	30	39	1
Stage 3 Vanilla Custard Pudding	1 jar (6 oz)	190	6	85	32	0

FOOD	PORTION	CAL.	FAT	SOD.	CARB.	FIB.
Gerber						
2nd Foods Banana Apple Dessert	1 jar (4 oz)	80	0	—	19	—
2nd Foods Banana Yogurt Dessert	1 jar (4 oz)	90	0	—	21	—
2nd Foods Cherry Vanilla Pudding	1 jar (4 oz)	80	0	—	19	—
2nd Foods Dutch Apple	1 jar (4 oz)	100	2	—	20	—
2nd Foods Fruit Dessert	1 jar (4 oz)	100	0	—	23	—
2nd Foods Hawaiian Delight	1 jar (4 oz)	90	0	—	22	—
2nd Foods Mixed Fruit Yogurt Dessert	1 jar (4 oz)	90	0	—	21	—
2nd Foods Peach Cobbler	1 jar (4 oz)	90	0	—	21	—
2nd Foods Peach Yogurt Dessert	1 jar (4 oz)	90	0	—	21	—
2nd Foods Vanilla Custard Pudding	1 jar (4 oz)	100	1	—	21	—
3rd Foods Dutch Apple	1 jar (6 oz)	130	2	—	29	—
3rd Foods Fruit Dessert	1 jar (6 oz)	120	0	—	30	—
3rd Foods Hawaiian Delight	1 jar (6 oz)	150	0	—	35	—
3rd Foods Peach Cobbler	1 jar (6 oz)	130	0	—	31	—
3rd Foods Vanilla Custard Pudding	1 jar (6 oz)	150	2	—	31	—
Tropical Foods Banana Vanilla Dessert	1 jar (4 oz)	100	1	—	21	—
Tropical Foods Guava With Tapioca	1 jar (4 oz)	80	0	—	21	—
Tropical Foods Mango Banana Passion Fruit	1 jar (4 oz)	80	0	—	20	—
Tropical Foods Mango With Tapioca	1 jar (4 oz)	80	0	—	21	—
Tropical Foods Papaya Pineapple Dessert	1 jar (4 oz)	90	0	—	22	—
Tropical Foods Papaya With Tapioca	1 jar (4 oz)	70	0	—	17	—
Tropical Foods Peaches Mango	1 jar (4 oz)	80	0	—	19	—
Tropical Foods Pineapple Banana Dessert	1 jar (4 oz)	90	0	—	22	—

FOOD	PORTION	CAL.	FAT	SOD.	CARB.	FIB.
Gerber (CONT.)						
Tropical Foods Tropical Fruits Medley	1 jar (4 oz)	70	0	—	18	—
DINNER						
Beech-Nut						
Stage 2 Beef & Egg Noodle	1 jar (4 oz)	100	6	50	8	2
Stage 2 Beef Supreme	1 jar (4 oz)	130	9	45	8	1
Stage 2 Chicken & Rice	1 jar (4 oz)	80	3	70	9	1
Stage 2 Chicken Noodle	1 jar (4 oz)	70	4	45	7	2
Stage 2 Chicken Soup	1 jar (4 oz)	90	4	50	8	1
Stage 2 Turkey Supreme	1 jar (4 oz)	90	4	45	9	1
Stage 2 Vegetable Beef	1 jar (4 oz)	80	4	45	8	1
Stage 2 Vegetable Chicken	1 jar (4 oz)	80	4	40	8	1
Stage 2 Vegetable Ham	1 jar (4 oz)	80	3	30	9	1
Stage 2 Vegetable Lamb	1 jar (4 oz)	80	3	55	9	1
Stage 2 Vegetables Turkey Rice	1 jar (4 oz)	70	3	50	8	1
Stage 3 Beef & Egg Noodle	1 jar (6 oz)	130	6	50	13	2
Stage 3 Chicken Noodle	1 jar (6 oz)	110	4	55	14	1
Stage 3 Macaroni & Beef	1 jar (6 oz)	130	6	60	14	2
Stage 3 Spaghetti & Beef	1 jar (6 oz)	130	6	70	16	1
Stage 3 Turkey Rice	1 jar (6 oz)	100	3	60	13	2
Stage 3 Vegetable Beef	1 jar (6 oz)	130	6	60	14	2
Stage 3 Vegetable Chicken	1 jar (6 oz)	110	4	55	14	1
Table Time Chicken & Stars	1 bowl (6 oz)	150	6	170	17	1
Table Time Macaroni & Cheese	1 bowl (6 oz)	200	12	320	21	0
Table Time Seashells In Tomato Sauce	1 bowl (6 oz)	150	4	170	25	1
Table Time Spaghetti Rings In Meat Sauce	1 bowl (6 oz)	160	6	180	20	0
Table Time Turkey Stew With Rice	1 bowl (6 oz)	150	4	200	14	1
Table Time Vegetable Stew With Beef	1 bowl (6 oz)	110	3	170	16	1
Earth's Best						
Corn Rice & Cheese Dinner	1 jar (4.5 fl oz)	120	5	45	13	—
Macaroni & Cheese	1 jar (4.5 oz)	100	4	10	12	—

FOOD	PORTION	CAL.	FAT	SOD.	CARB.	FIB.
Earth's Best (CONT.)						
Pasta Dinner	1 jar (4.5 fl oz)	90	3	20	13	—
Potato & Green Bean Dinner	1 jar (4.5 fl oz)	100	3	25	13	—
Rice & Lentil Dinner	1 jar (4.5 fl oz)	80	2	25	13	—
Summer Vegetable Dinner	1 jar (4.5 oz)	90	3	15	12	—
Gerber						
2nd Foods Apples & Chicken	1 jar (4 oz)	70	2	—	12	—
2nd Foods Apples & Ham	1 jar (4 oz)	70	1	—	14	—
2nd Foods Apples & Turkey	1 jar (4 oz)	80	2	—	13	—
2nd Foods Beef Egg Noodle	1 jar (4 oz)	80	3	—	10	—
2nd Foods Broccoli & Chicken	1 jar (4 oz)	50	2	—	4	—
2nd Foods Carrots & Beef	1 jar (4 oz)	70	3	—	7	—
2nd Foods Chicken Noodle	1 jar (4 oz)	70	2	—	11	—
2nd Foods Green Beans & Turkey	1 jar (4 oz)	70	2	—	9	—
2nd Foods Macaroni Cheese	1 jar (4 oz)	80	2	—	10	—
2nd Foods Macaroni Tomato Beef	1 jar (4 oz)	70	2	—	11	—
2nd Foods Turkey Rice	1 jar (4 oz)	70	3	—	9	—
2nd Foods Vegetable Bacon	1 jar (4 oz)	90	5	—	10	—
2nd Foods Vegetable Beef	1 jar (4 oz)	70	3	—	10	—
2nd Foods Vegetable Chicken	1 jar (4 oz)	70	2	—	11	—
2nd Foods Vegetable Ham	1 jar (4 oz)	70	3	—	10	—
2nd Foods Vegetable Turkey	1 jar (4 oz)	60	2	—	9	—
3rd Foods Beef Egg Noodle	1 jar (6 oz)	110	4	—	15	—
3rd Foods Chicken Noodle	1 jar (6 oz)	100	3	—	15	—
3rd Foods Macaroni Tomato Beef	1 jar (6 oz)	110	2	—	19	—

FOOD	PORTION	CAL.	FAT	SOD.	CARB.	FIB.
Gerber (cont.)						
3rd Foods Spaghetti Tomato Sauce Beef	1 jar (6 oz)	120	3	—	19	—
3rd Foods Turkey Rice	1 jar (6 oz)	100	3	—	14	—
3rd Foods Vegetable Bacon	1 jar (6 oz)	130	6	—	17	—
3rd Foods Vegetable Beef	1 jar (6 oz)	120	4	—	16	—
3rd Foods Vegetable Chicken	1 jar (6 oz)	100	3	—	15	—
3rd Foods Vegetable Ham	1 jar (6 oz)	110	4	—	16	—
3rd Foods Vegetable Turkey	1 jar (6 oz)	100	3	—	15	—
Chunky Homestyle Noodles & Beef	1 jar (6 oz)	150	6	—	18	—
Chunky Macaroni Alphabets With Beef & Sauce	1 jar (6.3 oz)	140	4	—	20	—
Chunky Noodles & Chicken With Carrots & Peas	1 jar (6 oz)	110	3	—	16	—
Chunky Rice With Beef & Tomato Sauce	1 jar (6.3 oz)	140	4	—	21	—
Chunky Saucy Rice With Chicken	1 jar (6 oz)	120	3	—	19	—
Chunky Spaghetti Tomato Sauce Beef	1 jar (6.3 oz)	150	4	—	22	—
Chunky Vegetables & Beef	1 jar (6.3 oz)	130	5	—	16	—
Chunky Vegetables & Chicken	1 jar (6.3 oz)	140	5	—	17	—
Chunky Vegetables & Ham	1 jar (6.3 oz)	130	5	—	16	—
Chunky Vegetables & Turkey	1 jar (6.3 oz)	110	3	—	15	—
Graduates Chicken Stew With Noodles	1 bowl (6 oz)	120	4	—	15	—
Graduates Macaroni & Beef in Sauce	1 bowl (6 oz)	150	4	—	20	—
Graduates Spaghetti With Mini Meatballs & Sauce	1 bowl (6 oz)	160	5	—	21	—
Graduates Tomato Sauce With Beef Ravioli	1 bowl (6 oz)	170	4	—	28	—

FOOD	PORTION	CAL.	FAT	SOD.	CARB.	FIB.
Gerber (CONT.)						
Graduates Tomato Sauce With Cheese Ravioli	1 bowl (6 oz)	170	4	—	28	—
Graduates Turkey Stew With Rice	1 bowl (6 oz)	100	2	—	13	—
Graduates Vegetable Stew With Beef	1 bowl (6 oz)	130	3	—	15	—
Tropical Foods Beans & Rice	1 jar (4 oz)	60	2	—	9	—
Tropical Foods Chicken & Rice	1 jar (4 oz)	60	2	—	8	—
FRUIT						
Beech-Nut						
Stage 1 Applesauce Golden Delicious	1 jar (4 oz)	70	0	0	15	1
Stage 1 Applesauce Golden Delicious	1 jar (2.5 oz)	50	0	0	12	1
Stage 1 Bananas Chiquita	1 jar (2.5 oz)	70	0	0	16	1
Stage 1 Bananas Chiquita	1 jar (4 oz)	110	0	0	24	1
Stage 1 Chiquita Bananas With Pears & Apples	1 jar (4 oz)	90	0	0	21	1
Stage 1 Peaches Yellow Cling	1 jar (2.5 oz)	45	0	0	11	2
Stage 1 Peaches Yellow Cling	1 jar (4 oz)	70	0	0	14	3
Stage 1 Pears Bartlett	1 jar (4 oz)	70	0	0	18	3
Stage 1 Pears Bartlett	1 jar (2.5 oz)	50	0	0	12	2
Stage 2 Apples & Apricots	1 jar (4 oz)	70	0	0	17	1
Stage 2 Apples & Bananas	1 jar (4 oz)	60	0	0	14	1
Stage 2 Apples & Blueberries	1 jar (4 oz)	70	0	0	17	1
Stage 2 Apples & Cherries	1 jar (4 oz)	80	0	0	18	1
Stage 2 Apples & Pears	1 jar (4 oz)	80	0	0	19	1
Stage 2 Apples Pears & Bananas	1 jar (4 oz)	90	0	0	20	1
Stage 2 Apricots With Pears & Apples	1 jar (4 oz)	90	0	0	20	2
Stage 2 Bartlett Pears & Pineapple	1 jar (4 oz)	70	0	0	17	3

FOOD	PORTION	CAL.	FAT	SOD.	CARB.	FIB.
Beech-Nut (CONT.)						
Stage 2 Peaches & Bananas	1 jar (4 oz)	70	0	0	15	3
Stage 2 Plums With Apples & Rice	1 jar (4 oz)	90	0	10	18	1
Stage 2 Prunes With Pears	1 jar (4 oz)	110	0	10	24	3
Stage 3 Apples & Bananas	1 jar (6 oz)	90	0	0	21	1
Stage 3 Apples & Cherries	1 jar (6 oz)	110	0	0	26	1
Stage 3 Applesauce	1 jar (6 oz)	100	0	0	23	2
Stage 3 Apricots With Pears & Apples	1 jar (6 oz)	130	0	0	32	—
Stage 3 Bananas Chiquita	1 jar (6 oz)	160	0	0	33	3
Stage 3 Peaches	1 jar (6 oz)	100	0	0	21	4
Stage 3 Pears Bartlett	1 jar (6 oz)	110	0	0	27	5
Earth's Best						
Apples	1 jar (4.5 oz)	70	0	10	17	—
Apples & Apricots	1 jar (4.5 fl oz)	70	0	5	17	—
Apples & Blueberries	1 jar (4.5 fl oz)	70	0	10	17	—
Apples & Plums	1 jar (4.5 fl oz)	70	0	10	17	—
Bananas	1 jar (4.5 oz)	90	0	0	20	—
Pears	1 jar (4.5 fl oz)	60	0	10	14	—
Plums Bananas & Rice	1 jar (4.5 fl oz)	90	1	10	19	—
Gerber						
1st Foods Applesauce	1 jar (2.5 oz)	25	0	—	9	—
1st Foods Bananas	1 jar (2.5 oz)	70	0	—	17	—
1st Foods Peaches	1 jar (2.5 oz)	30	0	—	7	—
1st Foods Pears	1 jar (2.5 oz)	40	0	—	10	—
1st Foods Prunes	1 jar (2.5 oz)	70	0	—	17	—
2nd Foods Apple Blueberry	1 jar (4 oz)	50	0	—	13	—
2nd Foods Applesauce	1 jar (4 oz)	60	0	—	14	—
2nd Foods Applesauce Apricot	1 jar (4 oz)	60	0	—	14	—
2nd Foods Apricots With Tapioca	1 jar (4 oz)	80	0	—	19	—
2nd Foods Banana With Pineapple & Tapioca	1 jar (4 oz)	60	0	—	14	—
2nd Foods Banana With Tapioca	1 jar (4 oz)	90	0	—	21	—
2nd Foods Peaches	1 jar (4 oz)	70	0	—	17	—

FOOD	PORTION	CAL.	FAT	SOD.	CARB.	FIB.
Gerber (CONT.)						
2nd Foods Pear Pineapple	1 jar (4 oz)	60	0	—	15	—
2nd Foods Pears	1 jar (4 oz)	60	0	—	15	—
2nd Foods Plums With Tapioca	1 jar (4 oz)	80	0	—	20	—
2nd Foods Prunes With Tapioca	1 jar (4 oz)	90	0	—	21	—
JUICE						
Beech-Nut						
Stage 1 Apple	4 fl oz	60	0	10	15	0
Stage 1 Pear	4 fl oz	60	0	0	15	0
Stage 1 White Grape	4 fl oz	100	0	10	23	0
Stage 2 Apple Banana	4 fl oz	70	0	0	16	0
Stage 2 Apple Cherry	4 fl oz	70	0	10	17	0
Stage 2 Apple Cranberry	4 fl oz	60	0	10	15	0
Stage 2 Apple Grape	4 fl oz	70	0	15	18	0
Stage 2 Juice Plus Grape	4 fl oz	100	0	10	23	0
Stage 2 Mango Nectar (Spanish Label)	4 fl oz	80	0	0	18	0
Stage 2 Mixed Fruit	4 fl oz	70	0	10	15	0
Stage 2 Papaya Nectar (Spanish Label)	4 fl oz	80	0	10	20	0
Stage 2 Tropical Blend	4 fl oz	90	0	5	15	0
Stage 2 Tropical Blend Nectar (Spanish Label)	4 fl oz	90	0	5	19	0
Stage 3 Orange	4 fl oz	60	0	0	15	0
Earth's Best						
Apple	1 bottle (4.2 fl oz)	60	0	20	14	—
Apple Banana	1 bottle (4.2 fl oz)	60	0	20	14	—
Apple Grape	1 bottle (4.2 fl oz)	60	0	15	14	—
Apples & Bananas	1 jar (4.5 fl oz)	80	0	20	18	—
Pear	1 bottle (4.2 fl oz)	60	0	0	15	—
Gerber						
1st Foods Apple	4 fl oz	60	0	—	14	—
1st Foods Pear	4 fl oz	60	0	—	14	—
1st Foods Red Grape	4 fl oz	80	0	—	20	—
1st Foods White Grape	4 fl oz	80	0	—	19	—
2nd Foods Apple Banana	4 fl oz	60	0	—	15	—
2nd Foods Apple Cherry	4 fl oz	60	0	—	14	—
2nd Foods Apple Grape	4 fl oz	60	0	—	15	—
2nd Foods Apple Peach	4 fl oz	60	0	—	14	—
2nd Foods Apple Plum	4 fl oz	60	0	—	15	—

FOOD	PORTION	CAL.	FAT	SOD.	CARB.	FIB.
Gerber (CONT.)						
2nd Foods Apple Prune	4 fl oz	60	0	—	16	—
2nd Foods Apple With Yogurt	4 fl oz	100	2	—	18	—
2nd Foods Banana With Yogurt	4 fl oz	110	2	—	21	—
2nd Foods Mixed Fruit	4 fl oz	60	0	—	14	—
2nd Foods Mixed Fruit With Yogurt	4 fl oz	100	2	—	18	—
2nd Foods Orange	4 fl oz	60	0	—	13	—
2nd Foods Pear Peach With Yogurt	4 fl oz	90	1	—	18	—
3rd Foods Apple Carrot	4 fl oz	50	0	—	12	—
3rd Foods Apple Sweet Potato	4 fl oz	60	0	—	14	—
3rd Foods Orange Carrot	4 fl oz	50	0	—	12	—
3rd Foods Pineapple Carrot	4 fl oz	60	0	—	13	—
Graduates Apple	4 fl oz	80	0	—	21	—
Graduates Apple Banana	4 fl oz	90	0	—	23	—
Graduates Apple Cherry	4 fl oz	80	0	—	21	—
Graduates Apple Grape	4 fl oz	90	0	—	22	—
Tropical Foods Guava With Mixed Fruit	4 fl oz	70	0	—	18	—
Tropical Foods Mango With Mixed Fruit	4 fl oz	70	0	—	18	—
Tropical Foods Papaya With Mixed Fruit	4 fl oz	70	0	—	18	—
MEAT						
Beech-Nut						
Stage 1 Beef & Broth	1 jar (2.5 oz)	90	6	40	0	0
Stage 1 Chicken & Broth	1 jar (2.5 oz)	70	3	55	0	0
Stage 1 Lamb & Broth	1 jar (2.5 oz)	60	3	50	0	0
Stage 1 Turkey & Broth	1 jar (2.5 oz)	90	6	40	0	0
Stage 1 Veal & Broth	1 jar (2.5 oz)	60	2	50	0	0
Gerber						
2nd Foods Beef	1 jar (2.5 oz)	80	4	—	0	—
2nd Foods Chicken	1 jar (2.5 oz)	90	6	—	0	—
2nd Foods Egg Yolks	1 jar (2.5 oz)	130	11	—	1	—
2nd Foods Ham	1 jar (2.5 oz)	90	6	—	0	—
2nd Foods Lamb	1 jar (2.5 oz)	80	4	—	0	—
2nd Foods Turkey	1 jar (2.5 oz)	80	5	—	0	—
2nd Foods Veal	1 jar (2.5 oz)	70	4	—	0	—
3rd Foods Beef	1 jar (2.5 oz)	80	4	—	0	—

FOOD	PORTION	CAL.	FAT	SOD.	CARB.	FIB.
Gerber (cont.)						
3rd Foods Chicken	1 jar (2.5 oz)	90	6	—	0	—
3rd Foods Ham	1 jar (2.5 oz)	90	6	—	0	—
3rd Foods Turkey	1 jar (2.5 oz)	90	5	—	0	—
3rd Foods Veal	1 jar (2.5 oz)	80	4	—	0	—
Graduates Chicken Sticks	1 jar (2.5 oz)	110	7	—	2	—
Graduates Meat Sticks	1 jar (2.5 oz)	110	7	—	2	—
Graduates Turkey Sticks	1 jar (2.5 oz)	120	8	—	2	—
VEGETABLE						
Beech-Nut						
Stage 1 Butternut Squash	1 jar (2.5 oz)	30	0	10	7	2
Stage 1 Butternut Squash	1 jar (4 oz)	50	0	10	11	3
Stage 1 Carrots Tender Sweet	1 jar (2.5 oz)	30	0	80	7	2
Stage 1 Green Beans (Spanish Label)	1 jar (2.5 oz)	20	0	0	4	2
Stage 1 Green Beans Tender Young	1 jar (4 oz)	35	0	0	6	3
Stage 1 Peas Tender Sweet	1 jar (4 oz)	60	0	0	11	5
Stage 1 Peas Tender Sweet	1 jar (2.5 oz)	40	0	0	7	3
Stage 1 Sweet Potatoes Tender Golden	1 jar (4 oz)	80	0	10	17	0
Stage 1 Sweet Potatoes Tender Golden	1 jar (2.5 oz)	50	0	10	10	0
Stage 2 Carrots & Peas	1 jar (4 oz)	50	0	25	10	3
Stage 2 Creamed Corn	1 jar (4 oz)	90	0	20	18	2
Stage 2 Garden Vegetables	1 jar (4 oz)	50	0	10	9	3
Stage 2 Mixed Vegetables	1 jar (4 oz)	45	0	10	9	3
Stage 3 Carrots	1 jar (6 oz)	70	0	240	15	5
Stage 3 Green Beans	1 jar (6 oz)	50	0	0	10	4
Stage 3 Sweet Potatoes	1 jar (6 oz)	110	0	15	25	1
Earth's Best						
Carrots	1 jar (4.5 fl oz)	40	0	70	8	—
Carrots & Parsnips	1 jar (4.5 fl oz)	60	0	30	14	—
Corn & Butternut Squash	1 jar (4.5 fl oz)	90	2	0	15	—

FOOD	PORTION	CAL.	FAT	SOD.	CARB.	FIB.
Earth's Best (CONT.)						
Garden Vegetables	1 jar (4.5 fl oz)	70	0	15	15	—
Green Beans & Rice	1 jar (4.5 fl oz)	40	1	15	6	—
Peas & Brown Rice	1 jar (4.5 fl oz)	80	0	10	16	—
Spinach & Potatoes	1 jar (4.5 fl oz)	60	2	25	8	—
Sweet Potatoes	1 jar (4.5 fl oz)	60	1	15	12	—
Winter Squash	1 jar (4.5 fl oz)	50	0	10	12	—
Gerber						
1st Foods Carrots	1 jar (2.5 oz)	25	0	—	5	—
1st Foods Green Beans	1 jar (2.5 oz)	25	0	—	5	—
1st Foods Peas	1 jar (2.5 oz)	30	0	—	6	—
1st Foods Squash	1 jar (2.5 oz)	25	0	—	5	—
1st Foods Sweet Potatoes	1 jar (2.5 oz)	45	0	—	10	—
2nd Foods Beets	1 jar (4 oz)	45	0	—	10	—
2nd Foods Carrots	1 jar (4 oz)	30	0	—	7	—
2nd Foods Creamed Corn	1 jar (4 oz)	80	1	—	15	—
2nd Foods Creamed Spinach	1 jar (4 oz)	50	1	—	8	—
2nd Foods Garden Vegetables	1 jar (4 oz)	45	1	—	7	—
2nd Foods Green Beans	1 jar (4 oz)	35	0	—	7	—
2nd Foods Mixed Vegetables	1 jar (4 oz)	50	1	—	9	—
2nd Foods Peas	1 jar (4 oz)	60	1	—	9	—
2nd Foods Squash	1 jar (4 oz)	35	0	—	8	—
2nd Foods Sweet Potatoes	1 jar (4 oz)	70	0	—	16	—
3rd Foods Broccoli Carrots Cheese	1 jar (6 oz)	80	2	—	12	—
3rd Foods Carrots	1 jar (6 oz)	50	0	—	11	—
3rd Foods Creamed Green Beans	1 jar (6 oz)	80	1	—	16	—
3rd Foods Mixed Vegetables	1 jar (6 oz)	70	0	—	15	—
3rd Foods Peas	1 jar (6 oz)	80	1	—	14	—
3rd Foods Squash	1 jar (6 oz)	60	1	—	12	—
3rd Foods Sweet Potatoes	1 jar (6 oz)	100	0	—	24	—
Graduates Carrots	1 jar (4.5 oz)	30	0	—	6	—
Graduates Green Beans	1 jar (4.5 oz)	30	0	—	6	—
Graduates Peas	1 jar (4.5 oz)	60	0	—	11	—

FOOD	PORTION	CAL.	FAT	SOD.	CARB.	FIB.
Gerber (CONT.)						
Graduates Potatoes	1 jar (4.5 oz)	50	0	—	11	—

BACON
(*see also* BACON SUBSTITUTES)

FOOD	PORTION	CAL.	FAT	SOD.	CARB.	FIB.
Armour						
Lower Salt cooked	1 strip	38	3	—	—	—
Star cooked	1 strip	38	3	185	—	—
Black Label						
Center Cut cooked	3 slices (0.5 oz)	70	6	240	0	0
Cooked	2 slices (0.5 oz)	80	7	330	0	0
Low Salt cooked	2 slices (0.5 oz)	80	7	210	0	0
Hormel						
Bacon Bits	1 tbsp (7 g)	30	2	250	0	0
Bacon Pieces	1 tbsp (7 g)	25	2	170	0	0
Microwave cooked	2 slices (0.5 oz)	70	5	230	0	0
Jones						
Sliced	1 slice	130	13	150	tr	—
Nathan's						
Beef cooked	3 slices	100	7	310	tr	—
Old Smokehouse						
Cooked	2 slices (0.5 oz)	80	7	280	0	0
Oscar Mayer						
Bacon Bits	1 tbsp (7 g)	25	2	220	0	0
Center Cut cooked	3 slices (0.5 oz)	70	6	320	tr	0
Cooked	2 slices (0.4 oz)	60	5	290	0	0
Lower Sodium cooked	2 slices (0.5 oz)	60	5	180	0	0
Thick Cut cooked	1 slice (0.4 oz)	50	4	250	0	0
Range Brand						
Cooked	2 slices (0.7 oz)	100	9	460	0	0
Red Label						
Cooked	2 slices (0.5 oz)	80	7	330	0	0
Shannon						
Irish	1 oz	70	5	—	0	—
breakfast strips cooked	3 strips (34 g)	156	12	—	—	—
breakfast strips beef cooked	3 strips (34 g)	153	12	766	tr	—
cooked	3 strips	109	9	303	tr	—
gammon lean & fat grilled	4.2 oz	274	15	—	0	0
grilled	2 slices (1.7 oz)	86	4	719	1	—

BACON SUBSTITUTES

FOOD	PORTION	CAL.	FAT	SOD.	CARB.	FIB.
Bac-Os						
	2 tsp (5 g)	25	1	90	2	—
Harvest Direct						
Bacon Bits	3.5 oz	320	15	2000	24	17

FOOD	PORTION	CAL.	FAT	SOD.	CARB.	FIB.
Lightlife						
Fakin' Bacon	3 strips (2 oz)	79	3	233	6	—
Louis Rich						
Turkey Bacon	1 slice (0.5 oz)	30	3	190	0	0
McCormick						
Bac'n Pieces	2 tsp	20	tr	140	1	—
Morningstar Farms						
Breakfast Strips	3 (25 g)	80	6	350	4	—
Worthington						
Stripples	4 strips (33 g)	120	9	460	6	—
bacon substitute	1 strip	25	2	117	1	—

BAGEL
(*see also* CRACKER)

FRESH

Alvarado St. Bakery

FOOD	PORTION	CAL.	FAT	SOD.	CARB.	FIB.
Sprouted Wheat	1 (3.3 oz)	260	1	400	54	2
Sprouted Wheat Cinnamon/Raisin	1 (3.3 oz)	280	1	270	59	3
Sprouted Wheat Onion/ Poppyseed	1 (3.3 oz)	320	2	410	66	2
Sprouted Wheat Sesame	1 (3.3 oz)	320	4	410	64	2
cinnamon raisin	1 (3½ in)	194	1	229	39	—
cinnamon raisin toasted	1 (3½ in)	194	1	229	39	—
egg	1 (3½ in)	197	2	359	38	—
egg toasted	1 (3½ in)	197	2	358	38	—
oat bran	1 (3½ in)	181	1	360	38	—
oat bran toasted	1 (3½ in)	181	1	360	38	—
onion	1 (3½ in)	195	1	379	38	2
plain	1 (3½ in)	195	1	379	38	2
plain toasted	1 (3½ in)	195	1	379	38	2
poppy seed	1 (3½ in)	195	1	379	38	2

FROZEN

Great Starts

FOOD	PORTION	CAL.	FAT	SOD.	CARB.	FIB.
Ham & Cheese On A Bagel	3 oz	240	8	600	28	—
Lender's						
Cinnamon'N Raisin	1 (2.5 oz)	200	1	310	40	1
Egg	1 (2 oz)	150	1	360	29	—
Onion	1 (2 oz)	160	1	290	31	1
Plain	1 (2 oz)	150	1	320	30	—
Sara Lee						
Cinnamon Raisin	1 (3 oz)	240	2	280	48	—
Cinnamon Raisin	1 (2.5 oz)	200	2	230	39	—

FOOD	PORTION	CAL.	FAT	SOD.	CARB.	FIB.
Sara Lee (CONT.)						
Egg	1 (2.5 oz)	200	2	360	38	—
Egg	1 (3 oz)	250	2	450	48	—
Oat Bran	1 (2.5 oz)	180	1	360	38	—
Oat Bran	1 (3 oz)	220	1	450	47	—
Onion	1 (3 oz)	230	1	560	45	—
Onion	1 (2.5 oz)	190	1	450	37	—
Plain	1 (3 oz)	230	1	580	46	—
Plain	1 (2.5 oz)	190	1	460	38	—
Poppy Seed	1 (3 oz)	230	1	560	46	—
Poppy Seed	1 (2.5 oz)	190	1	450	37	—
Sesame Seed	1 (3 oz)	240	2	550	46	—
Sesame Seed	1 (2.5 oz)	190	1	440	37	—
Tree Of Life						
Onion	1 (3 oz)	210	0	115	44	0
Plain	1 (3 oz)	210	0	115	44	0
Poppy	1 (3 oz)	210	0	115	44	0
Raisin	1 (3 oz)	210	0	115	45	tr
Sesame	1 (3 oz)	210	0	115	44	0
Weight Watchers						
Bagel Sandwich Ham And Cheese	1 (3 oz)	210	6	469	28	—

BAKING POWDER

FOOD	PORTION	CAL.	FAT	SOD.	CARB.	FIB.
Calumet	1 tsp	3	tr	—	—	—
Clabber Girl	1 tsp	0	0	435	1	—
Davis	1 tsp	6	0	450	2	—
Watkins	¼ tsp (1 g)	0	0	150	0	0
baking powder	1 tsp	2	0	488	1	—
low sodium	1 tsp	5	0	4	2	—

BAKING SODA

FOOD	PORTION	CAL.	FAT	SOD.	CARB.	FIB.
Arm & Hammer	1 tsp	0	0	1368	0	—
baking soda	1 tsp	0	0	1259	0	—

BALSAM PEAR

FOOD	PORTION	CAL.	FAT	SOD.	CARB.	FIB.
leafy tips cooked	½ cup	10	tr	4	2	—
leafy tips raw	½ cup	7	tr	3	1	—
pods cooked	½ cup	12	tr	4	3	—

BAMBOO SHOOTS

FOOD	PORTION	CAL.	FAT	SOD.	CARB.	FIB.
CANNED						
Empress						
Sliced	2 oz	14	0	10	3	—
Ka-Me						
Sliced	½ cup (4.5 oz)	15	0	10	3	1
sliced	1 cup	25	1	9	4	—

FOOD	PORTION	CAL.	FAT	SOD.	CARB.	FIB.
FRESH						
cooked	½ cup	15	tr	5	2	—
raw	½ cup	21	tr	3	1	—
BANANA						
banana chips	1 oz	147	10	2	17	2
DRIED						
powder	1 tbsp	21	tr	0	5	—
FRESH						
Chiquita						
Fresh	1 (3½ oz)	110	0	—	—	—
Dole						
banana	1	120	1	0	28	3
banana	1	105	tr	1	27	2
mashed	1 cup	207	1	2	53	4
BANANA JUICE						
Libby						
Nectar	1 can (11.5 fl oz)	190	0	35	47	—
BARBECUE SAUCE						
(*see also* SAUCE)						
Bull's Eye						
Original	2 tbsp	50	0	—	—	—
Hain						
Honey	1 tbsp	14	1	120	1	—
Healthy Choice						
Hickory	2 tbsp (1.1 oz)	25	0	230	6	0
Hot & Spicy	2 tbsp (1.1 oz)	25	0	230	6	0
Original	2 tbsp (1.1 oz)	25	0	230	6	0
Heinz						
Select	1 oz	40	0	275	9	—
Select Hickory	1 oz	35	0	260	8	—
Thick & Rich Cajun Style	1 oz	35	0	360	8	—
Thick & Rich Chunky	1 oz	30	0	380	6	—
Thick & Rich Hawaiian Style	1 oz	40	0	210	10	—
Thick & Rich Hickory Smoke	1 oz	35	0	380	8	—
Thick & Rich Mesquite Smoke	1 oz	30	0	380	7	—
Thick & Rich Mushroom	1 oz	30	0	460	6	—
Thick & Rich Old Fashioned	1 oz	35	0	350	8	—
Thick & Rich Onion	1 oz	30	0	420	7	—
Thick & Rich Original	1 oz	35	0	390	8	—

FOOD	PORTION	CAL.	FAT	SOD.	CARB.	FIB.
Heinz (CONT.)						
Thick & Rich Texas Hot	1 oz	30	0	390	7	—
House Of Tsang						
Hong Kong	1 tbsp (0.6 oz)	10	0	150	2	0
Hunt's						
Country Style	1 tbsp	20	tr	140	5	tr
Homestyle	1 tbsp	20	tr	170	6	tr
Honey Mustard	1 tbsp (1.2 oz)	50	0	450	11	<1
Kansas City Style	1 tbsp	20	tr	85	5	tr
New Orleans Style	1 tbsp	20	tr	150	5	tr
Original	2 tbsp (1.2 oz)	40	0	410	9	1
Southern Style	1 tbsp	20	tr	170	5	tr
Texas Style	1 tbsp	25	tr	150	6	tr
Western Style	1 tbsp	20	tr	170	5	tr
Kraft						
Char-Grill	2 tbsp (1.2 oz)	60	1	440	12	0
Extra Rich Original	2 tbsp (1.2 oz)	50	0	360	12	0
Garlic	2 tbsp (1.2 oz)	40	0	420	9	0
Hickory Smoke	2 tbsp (1.2 oz)	40	0	440	10	0
Hickory Smoke Onion Bits	2 tbsp (1.2 oz)	50	0	340	11	tr
Honey	2 tbsp (1.2 oz)	50	0	320	13	0
Hot	2 tbsp (1.2 oz)	40	0	540	9	0
Hot Hickory Smoke	2 tbsp (1.2 oz)	40	0	360	9	0
Italian Seasonings	2 tbsp (1.2 oz)	45	1	280	10	0
Kansas City Style	2 tbsp (1.2 oz)	45	0	280	11	tr
Mesquite Smoke	2 tbsp (1.2 oz)	40	0	410	9	0
Onion Bits	2 tbsp (1.2 oz)	50	0	340	11	0
Original	2 tbsp (1.2 oz)	40	0	460	10	0
Teriyaki	2 tbsp (1.2 oz)	60	1	430	12	0
Thick'N Spicy Hickory Smoke	2 tbsp (1.2 oz)	50	0	440	12	0
Thick'N Spicy Honey	2 tbsp (1.2 oz)	60	0	350	13	0
Thick'N Spicy Kansas City Style	2 tbsp (1.2 oz)	60	0	228	13	tr
Thick'N Spicy Mesquite Smoke	2 tbsp (1.2 oz)	50	0	440	12	0
Thick'N Spicy Original	2 tbsp (1.2 oz)	50	0	440	12	0
Lawry's						
Dijon Honey	¼ cup	203	1	1768	27	tr
Maull's						
Beer Non-Alcholic	3.5 oz	128	2	—	—	—
Regular	3.5 oz	123	2	—	—	—
Smoky	3.5 oz	124	tr	—	—	—

FOOD	PORTION	CAL.	FAT	SOD.	CARB.	FIB.
Maull's (CONT.)						
Sweet-N-Mild	3.5 oz	167	2	—	—	—
Sweet-N-Smoky	3.5 oz	160	tr	—	—	—
With Onion Bits	3.5 oz	126	2	—	—	—
Red Wing						
"K" Sauce	2 tbsp (1.2 oz)	45	0	410	9	0
Watkins						
Bold	2 tsp (0.4 oz)	25	0	290	5	0
Honey	2 tsp (0.4 oz)	25	0	290	6	0
Mesquite	2 tsp (0.4 oz)	25	0	300	5	0
Original	2 tsp (0.4 oz)	25	0	300	5	0
Smokehouse	2 tsp (0.4 oz)	25	0	300	5	0
barbecue	1 cup	188	5	2038	32	—
BARLEY						
Arrowhead	¼ cup (1.7 oz)	170	1	0	37	6
Hulless	¼ cup (1.6 oz)	140	1	0	35	6
Quaker						
Medium Pearled	¼ cup	172	1	0	36	5
Quick Pearled	¼ cup	172	1	0	36	5
Scotch						
Medium Pearled	¼ cup	172	1	0	36	5
Quick Pearled	¼ cup	172	1	0	36	5
pearled cooked	½ cup	97	tr	2	30	—
pearled uncooked	½ cup	352	1	9	78	16
BASIL						
Watkins						
Liquid Spice	1 tbsp (0.5 oz)	120	14	0	0	0
fresh chopped	2 tbsp	1	tr	0	tr	—
ground	1 tsp	4	tr	tr	1	—
leaves fresh	5	1	tr	0	tr	—
BASS						
freshwater raw	3 oz	97	3	59	0	—
sea cooked	3 oz	105	2	74	0	—
sea raw	3 oz	82	2	58	0	—
striped baked	3 oz	105	3	75	0	—
BAY LEAF						
Watkins						
¼ tsp (0.5 g)		0	0	0	0	0
crumbled	1 tsp	2	tr	tr	tr	—
BEAN SPROUTS						
(*see also* INDIVIDUAL BEAN NAMES)						
CANNED						
La Choy	⅔ cup	8	tr	20	1	tr

FOOD	PORTION	CAL.	FAT	SOD.	CARB.	FIB.

BEANS
(see also INDIVIDUAL NAMES)

CANNED

Allen

Baked	½ cup (4.5 oz)	150	1	350	29	8

B&M

Barbeque Baked Beans	8 oz	260	6	1000	48	11
Honey Baked	8 oz	240	2	940	50	11
Hot N Spicy Baked	8 oz	240	3	990	50	12
Maple Baked	8 oz	240	2	890	52	11
Tomato Baked Beans	8 oz	230	3	1010	48	—
Vegetarian Baked	8 oz	230	3	370	50	—

Brick Oven

Baked Beans	½ cup	160	2	560	28	—

Brown Beauty

Mexican Beans With Jalapeno	½ cup (4.5 oz)	120	1	370	21	7

Bush's

Baked	½ cup (4.6 oz)	150	1	550	29	7
Baked With Onions	½ cup (4.6 oz)	150	2	500	26	6
Homestyle Baked	½ cup (4.6 oz)	160	2	480	28	8
Vegetarian	½ cup (4.6 oz)	140	1	550	24	6

Campbell

Barbecue Beans	½ can (7⅞ oz)	210	4	900	43	—
Home Style Beans	½ can (8 oz)	220	4	820	48	—
Hot Chili Beans	½ can (7¾ oz)	180	4	870	38	—
Old Fashioned Beans In Molasses & Brown Sugar Sauce	½ can (8 oz)	230	3	730	49	—
Pork & Beans In Tomato Sauce	½ can (8 oz)	200	3	770	43	—
Vegetarian	½ can (7¾ oz)	170	1	780	40	—

Casa Fiesta

Refried	3.5 oz	110	2	299	17	—

Chi-Chi's

Ranchero Beans	½ cup (4.3 oz)	100	1	540	18	1
Refried	½ cup (4.2 oz)	130	6	570	16	4

Crest Top

Pork And Beans	½ cup (4.5 oz)	130	1	330	21	6

Friends

Maple Baked	8 oz	240	2	890	52	11

Gebhardt

Chili	4 oz	115	1	580	21	5

FOOD	PORTION	CAL.	FAT	SOD.	CARB.	FIB.
Gebhardt (CONT.)						
Refried	4 oz	100	2	490	20	7
Refried Jalapeno	4 oz	115	2	270	19	7
Green Giant						
Pork And Beans In Tomato Sauce	½ cup	90	1	420	21	6
Three Bean Salad	½ cup	70	tr	470	18	3
Hanover						
Four Bean Salad	½ cup	80	0	—	—	—
Health Valley						
Boston Baked	7½ oz	190	tr	300	41	5
Boston Baked No Salt Added	7.5 oz	190	tr	20	41	5
Fast Menu Honey Baked Organic Beans With Tofu Weiner	7½ oz	150	4	140	15	16
Vegetarian With Miso	7½ oz	180	1	60	38	5
Hormel						
Beans & Wieners	1 can (7.5 oz)	290	13	1270	32	6
Hunt's						
Big John's Beans 'n Fixin's	4 oz	170	6	490	26	6
Pork And Beans	4 oz	135	1	430	26	8
Kid's Kitchen						
Beans & Weiners	1 cup (7.5 oz)	310	13	760	37	8
Little Pancho						
Refried & Green Chili	½ cup	80	0	330	15	—
Luck's						
Cut Green & Shelled Beans Seasoned w/ Pork	7.25 oz	200	6	—	—	—
Mixed Beans Seasoned w/ Pork	7.25 oz	200	5	—	—	—
McIlhenny						
Spicy	1 oz	7	tr	19	1	1
Old El Paso						
Mexe-Beans	½ cup	163	1	627	31	13
Refried	4 oz	80	2	430	15	5
Refried Fat Free	½ cup	90	0	360	17	—
Refried Vegetarian	4 oz	70	1	590	15	5
Refried With Cheese	¼ cup	130	3	470	17	5
Refried With Green Chilies	¼ cup	49	tr	252	8	3
Refried With Sausages	¼ cup	180	8	300	8	—

FOOD	PORTION	CAL.	FAT	SOD.	CARB.	FIB.
Rosarita						
Refried	4 oz	100	2	480	18	6
Refried Spicy	4 oz	100	2	500	19	6
Refried Vegetarian	4 oz	100	2	480	18	6
Refried With Bacon	4 oz	110	2	560	20	6
Refried With Green Chilies	4 oz	90	2	460	18	6
Refried With Nacho Cheese	4 oz	110	2	490	20	6
Refried With Onions	4 oz	110	2	490	21	6
S&W						
Barbecue Beans Texas Style	½ cup	135	1	550	24	—
Maple Sugar Beans	½ cup	150	1	586	28	—
Mixed Bean Salad Marinated	½ cup	90	1	730	17	—
Pork 'N Beans	½ cup	130	2	135	22	—
Smokey Ranch	½ cup	130	2	569	20	—
Trappey						
Mexi-Beans With Jalapeno	½ cup (4.5 oz)	130	2	460	22	8
Pork And Beans	½ cup (4.5 oz)	110	1	710	21	7
Pork And Beans With Jalapeno	½ cup (4.5 oz)	130	2	610	24	6
Van Camp's						
Baked Beans Fat Free	½ cup (4.6 oz)	130	0	430	28	5
Baked Beans Premium	½ cup (4.6 oz)	140	1	520	29	5
Beanee Weenee	1 cup (9 oz)	320	14	1240	35	8
Beanee Weenee Baked Flavor	1 cup (9 oz)	410	14	1210	58	10
Beanee Weenee Barbeque	1 cup (9 oz)	340	14	1150	43	8
Brown Sugar Beans	½ cup (4.6 oz)	170	3	410	31	6
Mexican Style Chili Beans	½ cup (4.6 oz)	110	2	430	21	8
Pork And Beans	½ cup (4.6 oz)	110	2	490	24	6
Vegetarian In Tomato Sauce	½ cup (4.6 oz)	110	1	400	23	5
Wagon Master						
Pork And Beans	½ cup (4.5 oz)	110	1	710	21	7
baked beans plain	½ cup	118	1	504	26	10
baked beans vegetarian	½ cup	118	1	504	26	10
baked beans w/ beef	½ cup	161	5	632	22	—
baked beans w/ franks	½ cup	182	8	551	20	9

FOOD	PORTION	CAL.	FAT	SOD.	CARB.	FIB.
baked beans w/ pork	½ cup	133	2	522	25	7
baked beans w/ pork & sweet sauce	½ cup	140	2	423	26	7
baked beans w/ pork & tomato sauce	½ cup	123	1	554	24	7
refried beans	½ cup	134	1	534	23	—
FROZEN						
Hanover						
Romano Bean Medley	½ cup	25	0	—	—	—
MIX						
Bean Cuisine						
Florentine Beans With Bow Ties	½ cup	199	7	450	27	—
Pasta & Beans Country French With Gemelli	½ cup	214	8	369	27	—
TAKE-OUT						
baked beans	½ cup	190	6	532	27	—
barbecue beans	3.5 oz	120	tr	460	26	—
four bean salad	3.5 oz	100	tr	280	20	—
refried beans	½ cup	43	2	104	5	—
three bean salad	¾ cup	230	11	500	31	1

BEAR

simmered	3 oz	220	11	—	0	—

BEAVER

roasted	3 oz	140	6	50	0	—
simmered	3 oz	141	5	39	0	—

BEECHNUTS

dried	1 oz	164	14	—	10	—

BEEF

(*see also* BEEF DISHES, VEAL)
(Beef is graded according to its marbling, the little flecks of fat in the muscle. Beef graded "Prime" has the highest percentage of fat, followed by "Choice" with less fat and "Select" with the least fat.)

CANNED
Armour

Chopped Beef	2 oz	170	15	810	2	—
Corned Beef	2 oz	120	7	490	1	—
Potted Meat	¼ cup (2.2 oz)	90	6	600	0	—
Potted Meat	1 can (3 oz)	120	8	820	0	—
Roast Beef In Gravy	½ cup (4.6 oz)	150	4	640	3	—
Tripe	3 oz	90	2	100	0	—

FOOD	PORTION	CAL.	FAT	SOD.	CARB.	FIB.
Hormel						
Corned Beef	2 oz	120	7	490	0	0
Potted Meat	4 tbsp (2 oz)	60	7	580	1	0
Roast Beef With Gravy	2 oz	60	2	280	1	0
Treet						
50% Less Fat	2 oz	120	8	750	4	—
Underwood						
Roast Beef	2.08 oz	140	11	360	tr	—
Roast Beef Mesquite Smoked	2.08 oz	126	11	300	tr	—
Roast Beef Light	2.08 oz	90	6	210	2	—
corned beef	1 oz	71	4	—	—	—
corned beef	3 oz	85	5	—	0	—
DRIED						
Hormel						
Pillow Pack	10 slices (1 oz)	45	1	810	1	0
Sliced	10 slices (1 oz)	50	2	1240	1	0
FRESH						

(Note that the values for cooked beef may differ slightly from values for raw beef. When meat is cooked some moisture and fat is lost, changing the nutrition value slightly. As a rule of thumb it can be assumed that a 4 oz raw portion will equal a 3 oz cooked portion of meat.)

FOOD	PORTION	CAL.	FAT	SOD.	CARB.	FIB.
Dakota Lean						
Chuck Roast raw	3 oz	80	2	—	1	—
Eye Round raw	3 oz	80	2	—	0	—
Flank Steak raw	3 oz	80	1	—	1	—
Ground raw	3 oz	88	2	—	0	—
Outside Round raw	3 oz	80	1	—	0	—
Ribeye raw	3 oz	90	2	—	1	—
Sirloin Tip raw	3 oz	90	3	—	1	—
Strip Loin raw	3 oz	90	2	—	1	—
Tenderloin raw	3 oz	70	1	—	1	—
Top Round raw	3 oz	80	1	—	1	—
Double J						
Filet	3.5 oz	130	4	54	—	—
NY Strip	3.5 oz	133	4	57	—	—
Rib Eye	3.5 oz	134	5	55	—	—
Top Butt	3.5 oz	136	5	55	—	—
Healthy Choice						
Ground Extra Lean	4 oz	130	4	230	2	0
Laura's Lean						
Eye Of Round	4 oz	150	5	85	0	—
Flank Steak	4 oz	160	7	75	0	—

FOOD	PORTION	CAL.	FAT	SOD.	CARB.	FIB.
Laura's Lean (CONT.)						
Ground	4 oz	180	10	75	0	—
Ground Round	4 oz	160	7	75	0	—
Ribeye Steak	4 oz	150	5	60	0	—
Sirloin Tip Round	4 oz	140	5	65	0	—
Sirloin Top Butt	4 oz	140	5	90	0	—
Strip Steak	4 oz	150	5	85	0	—
Tenderloins	4 oz	150	6	75	0	—
Top Round	4 oz	140	4	80	0	—
bottom round lean & fat trim 0 in Choice braised	3 oz	193	26	43	0	—
bottom round lean & fat trim 0 in Choice roasted	3 oz	172	8	56	0	—
bottom round lean & fat trim 0 in Select braised	3 oz	171	6	43	0	—
bottom round lean & fat trim 0 in Select roasted	3 oz	150	24	56	0	—
bottom round lean & fat trim 1/4 in Choice braised	3 oz	241	15	42	0	—
bottom round lean & fat trim 1/4 in Choice roasted	3 oz	221	14	53	0	—
bottom round lean & fat trim 1/4 in Select braised	3 oz	220	13	42	0	—
bottom round lean & fat trim 1/4 in Select roasted	3 oz	199	11	54	0	—
brisket flat half lean & fat trim 0 in braised	3 oz	183	8	53	0	—
brisket flat half lean & fat trim 1/4 in braised	3 oz	309	24	48	0	—
brisket point half lean & fat trim 0 in braised	3 oz	304	24	57	0	—
brisket point half lean & fat trim 1/4 in braised	3 oz	343	29	55	0	—
brisket whole lean & fat trim 0 in braised	3 oz	247	17	55	0	—
brisket whole lean & fat trim 1/4 in braised	3 oz	327	27	52	0	—
chuck arm pot roast lean & fat trim 0 in braised	3 oz	238	14	53	0	—
chuck arm pot roast lean & fat trim 1/4 in braised	3 oz	282	20	51	0	—
chuck blade roast lean & fat trim 0 in braised	3 oz	284	21	56	0	—
chuck blade roast lean & fat trim 1/4 in braised	3 oz	293	22	55	0	—

FOOD	PORTION	CAL.	FAT	SOD.	CARB.	FIB.
corned beef brisket cooked	3 oz	213	16	964	tr	—
eye of round lean & fat trim 0 in Choice roasted	3 oz	153	5	53	0	—
eye of round lean & fat trim 0 in Select roasted	3 oz	137	4	53	0	—
eye of round lean & fat trim ¼ in Choice roasted	3 oz	205	12	50	0	—
eye of round lean & fat trim ¼ in Select roasted	3 oz	184	10	51	0	—
flank lean & fat trim 0 in braised	3 oz	224	14	60	0	—
flank lean & fat trim 0 in broiled	3 oz	192	11	69	0	—
ground extra lean broiled medium	3 oz	217	14	59	0	—
ground extra lean broiled well done	3 oz	225	14	70	0	—
ground extra lean fried medium	3 oz	216	14	59	0	—
ground extra lean fried well done	3 oz	224	14	69	0	—
ground extra lean raw	4 oz	265	19	75	0	—
ground lean broiled medium	3 oz	231	16	65	0	—
ground lean broiled well done	3 oz	238	15	76	0	—
ground regular broiled medium	3 oz	246	18	70	0	—
ground regular broiled well done	3 oz	248	17	79	0	—
ground low-fat w/ carrageenan raw	4 oz	160	7	70	tr	—
porterhouse steak lean & fat trim ¼ in Choice broiled	3 oz	260	19	52	0	—
porterhouse steak lean only trim ¼ in Prime broiled	3 oz	185	9	56	0	—
rib eye small end lean & fat trim 0 in Choice broiled	3 oz	261	19	54	0	—
rib large end lean & fat trim 0 in roasted	3 oz	300	24	55	0	—
rib large end lean & fat trim ¼ in broiled	3 oz	295	24	54	0	—
rib large end lean & fat trim ¼ in roasted	3 oz	310	25	54	0	—

FOOD	PORTION	CAL.	FAT	SOD.	CARB.	FIB.
rib small end lean & fat trim 0 in broiled	3 oz	252	18	54	0	—
rib small end lean & fat trim ¼ in broiled	3 oz	285	22	53	0	—
rib small end lean & fat trim ¼ in roasted	3 oz	295	24	53	0	—
rib whole lean & fat trim ¼ in Choice broiled	3 oz	306	25	53	0	—
rib whole lean & fat trim ¼ in Choice roasted	3 oz	320	27	53	0	—
rib whole lean & fat trim ¼ in Prime roasted	3 oz	348	30	54	0	—
rib whole lean & fat trim ¼ in Select broiled	3 oz	274	21	54	0	—
rib whole lean & fat trim ¼ in Select roasted	3 oz	286	23	54	0	—
shank crosscut lean & fat trim ¼ in Choice simmered	3 oz	224	12	52	0	—
short loin top loin lean & fat trim 0 in Choice broiled	1 steak (5.4 oz)	353	19	104	0	—
short loin top loin lean & fat trim 0 in Choice broiled	3 oz	193	10	57	0	—
short loin top loin lean & fat trim 0 in Select broiled	1 steak (5.4 oz)	309	14	104	0	—
short loin top loin lean & fat trim ¼ in Choice braised	3 oz	253	18	54	0	—
short loin top loin lean & fat trim ¼ in Choice broiled	1 steak (6.3 oz)	536	38	114	0	—
short loin top loin lean & fat trim ¼ in Prime broiled	1 steak (6.3 oz)	582	43	114	0	—
short loin top loin lean & fat trim ¼ in Select broiled	1 steak (6.3 oz)	473	31	114	0	—
short loin top loin lean only trim 0 in Choice broiled	1 steak (5.2 oz)	311	14	101	0	—
short loin top loin lean only trim ¼ in Choice broiled	1 steak (5.2 oz)	314	15	100	0	—

FOOD	PORTION	CAL.	FAT	SOD.	CARB.	FIB.
short ribs lean & fat Choice braised	3 oz	400	36	43	0	—
t-bone steak lean & fat trim ¼ in Choice broiled	3 oz	253	18	52	0	—
t-bone steak lean only trim ¼ in Choice broiled	3 oz	182	9	56	0	—
tenderloin lean & fat trim 0 in Select broiled	3 oz	194	11	52	0	—
tenderloin lean & fat trim ¼ in Choice broiled	3 oz	259	19	50	0	—
tenderloin lean & fat trim ¼ in Choice roasted	3 oz	288	22	55	0	—
tenderloin lean & fat trim ¼ in Choice broiled	3 oz	208	12	52	0	—
tenderloin lean & fat trim ¼ in Prime broiled	3 oz	270	20	50	0	—
tenderloin lean & fat trim ¼ in Select roasted	3 oz	275	21	48	0	—
tenderloin lean only trim 0 in Select broiled	3 oz	170	7	54	0	—
tenderloin lean only trim ¼ in Choice broiled	3 oz	188	10	54	0	—
tenderloin lean only trim ¼ in Select broiled	3 oz	169	7	54	0	—
tip round lean & fat trim 0 in Choice roasted	3 oz	170	8	54	0	—
tip round lean & fat trim 0 in Select roasted	3 oz	158	6	55	0	—
tip round lean & fat trim ¼ in Choice roasted	3 oz	210	13	53	0	—
tip round lean & fat trim ¼ in Prime roasted	3 oz	233	15	53	0	—
tip round lean & fat trim ¼ in Select roasted	3 oz	191	10	53	0	—
top round lean & fat trim 0 in Choice braised	3 oz	184	6	38	0	—
top round lean & fat trim 0 in Select braised	3 oz	170	5	38	0	—
top round lean & fat trim ¼ in Choice braised	3 oz	221	11	38	0	—
top round lean & fat trim ¼ in Choice broiled	3 oz	190	9	51	0	—
top round lean & fat trim ¼ in Choice fried	3 oz	235	13	58	0	—

FOOD	PORTION	CAL.	FAT	SOD.	CARB.	FIB.
top round lean & fat trim ¼ in Prime broiled	3 oz	195	9	51	0	—
top round lean & fat trim ¼ in Select braised	3 oz	175	7	51	0	—
top round lean & fat trim ¼ in Select braised	3 oz	199	8	38	0	—
top sirloin lean & fat trim 0 in Choice broiled	3 oz	194	10	55	0	—
top sirloin lean & fat trim 0 in Select broiled	3 oz	166	6	55	0	—
top sirloin lean & fat trim ¼ in Choice broiled	3 oz	228	14	53	0	—
top sirloin lean & fat trim ¼ in Choice fried	3 oz	277	19	59	0	—
top sirloin lean & fat trim ¼ in Select broiled	3 oz	208	12	54	0	—
tripe raw	4 oz	111	4	52	0	—
FROZEN						
patties broiled medium	3 oz	240	17	66	0	—
READY-TO-USE						
Healthy Choice						
Deli-Thin Roast Beef	6 slices (2 oz)	60	2	520	1	0
Fresh-Trak Roast Beef	1 slice (1 oz)	30	1	260	0	0
Oscar Mayer						
Deli-Thin Roast Beef	4 slices (1.8 oz)	60	2	530	1	0
Weight Watchers						
Deli Thin Oven Roasted Cured	5 slices (⅓ oz)	10	tr	85	tr	—
TAKE-OUT						
roast beef medium	2 oz	70	2	210	0	—
roast beef rare	2 oz	70	2	210	0	—

BEEF DISHES
CANNED
Armour

FOOD	PORTION	CAL.	FAT	SOD.	CARB.	FIB.
Corned Beef Hash	1 cup (8.3 oz)	440	30	840	23	—
Roast Beef Hash	1 cup (8.4 oz)	400	25	1460	23	—
Stew	1 cup (8.6 oz)	220	12	1250	21	—
Dinty Moore						
American Classics Beef Stew	1 bowl (10 oz)	260	13	1160	21	3
American Classics Meatloaf With Mashed Potatoes	1 bowl (10 oz)	300	13	1060	27	3

FOOD	PORTION	CAL.	FAT	SOD.	CARB.	FIB.
Dinty Moore (CONT.)						
American Classics Roast Beef With Mashed Potatoes	1 bowl (10 oz)	240	5	860	25	2
American Classics Salisbury Steak	1 bowl (10 oz)	310	14	1090	22	3
Beef Stew	1 can (7.5 oz)	190	10	870	15	2
Beef Stew	1 cup (8.3 oz)	230	14	950	16	2
Meatball Stew	1 cup (8.4 oz)	260	16	1110	16	3
Microwave Cup Beef Stew	1 cup (7.5 oz)	190	10	870	15	2
Microwave Cup Corned Beef Hash	1 cup (7.5 oz)	350	22	850	19	2
Microwave Cup Hearty Burger Stew	1 cup (7.5 oz)	240	13	930	19	3
Microwave Cup Meatball Stew	1 cup (7.5 oz)	240	15	990	14	2
Sliced Potatoes & Beef	1 can (7.5 oz)	230	9	1050	28	4
Hormel						
Beef Goulash	1 can (7.5 oz)	230	11	1040	19	3
Corned Beef Hash	1 cup (8.3 oz)	390	24	930	22	2
Roast Beef Hash	1 cup (8.3 oz)	390	24	790	22	2
Manwich						
Mexican as prep	1 sandwich	310	13	690	30	2
Sloppy Joe as prep	1 sandwich	310	13	620	31	1
Mary Kitchen						
Corned Beef Hash	1 can (7.5 oz)	350	22	850	19	2
Roast Beef Hash	1 can (7.5 oz)	348	21	707	21	2
Micro Cup Meals						
Beef Stew	1 cup (7.5 oz)	180	9	880	15	2
Wolf Brand						
Beef Stew	1 cup	179	8	1043	18	—
corned beef hash	3 oz	155	10	—	9	—
FROZEN						
Chefwich						
Beef w/ Barbecue Sauce	1	340	10	—	—	—
Hot Pocket						
Stuffed Sandwich Barbecue	1 (4.5 oz)	340	12	850	45	1
Stuffed Sandwich Beef & Cheddar	1 (4.5 oz)	360	18	830	36	tr
Stuffed Sandwich Beef Fajita	1 (4.5 oz)	360	17	780	39	5

FOOD	PORTION	CAL.	FAT	SOD.	CARB.	FIB.
Lean Pockets						
Stuffed Sandwich Beef & Broccoli	1 (4.5 oz)	250	7	710	37	7
Luigino's						
Creamed Sauce Shaved Cured Beef With Croutons	1 pkg (8 oz)	360	20	810	29	3
Egg Noodles Rich Gravy Swedish Meatballs	1 cup (7.5 oz)	280	12	690	30	3
Egg Noodles Rich Gravy Swedish Meatballs	1 pkg (9 oz)	340	15	820	36	3
Ovenstuffs						
Beef/Cheddar Deli Melt	1 (4.75 oz)	390	22	820	28	—
Tyson						
Microwave BBQ Sandwich	1 sandwich	200	3	600	29	—
MIX						
Casbah						
Gyro as prep	1 patty (2 oz)	145	5	456	12	tr
Hamburger Helper						
Beef Noodle as prep	1 cup	330	15	920	29	—
Beef Romanoff as prep	1 cup	350	16	1070	31	—
Beef Taco as prep	1 cup	330	14	970	33	—
Cheddar 'n Bacon as prep	1 cup	380	19	970	30	—
Cheeseburger Macaroni as prep	1 cup	370	19	1030	28	—
Cheesy Italian as prep	1 cup	370	18	1040	29	—
Chili Macaroni as prep	1 cup	330	14	960	32	—
Hamburger Hash as prep	1 cup	320	15	1020	27	—
Hamburger Stew as prep	1 cup	300	14	1010	26	—
Lasagne as prep	1 cup	340	14	910	33	—
Meat Loaf as prep	5 oz	360	22	710	14	—
Nacho Cheese as prep	1 cup	360	15	1050	35	—
Pizza Dish as prep	1 cup	360	14	1010	27	—
Pizzabake as prep	⅙ pkg (4.5 oz)	320	14	840	29	—
Potatoes Au Gratin as prep	1 cup	350	18	900	27	—
Potatoes Stroganoff as prep	1 cup	330	16	990	26	—
Rice Oriental as prep	1 cup	340	14	1120	38	—
Sloppy Joe Bake as prep	5 oz	340	15	1100	33	—
Spaghetti as prep	1 cup	340	14	1100	32	—
Stroganoff as prep	1 cup	390	20	870	30	—

FOOD	PORTION	CAL.	FAT	SOD.	CARB.	FIB.
Hamburger Helper (CONT.)						
Tacobake as prep	⅙ pkg (5.75 oz)	320	15	940	31	—
Zesty Italian as prep	1 cup	340	13	980	35	—
Lipton						
Microeasy Hearty Beef Stew	¼ pkg	71	1	729	14	—
Microeasy Homestyle Meatloaf	¼ pkg	87	2	630	15	—
Manwich						
Seasoning Mix as prep	1 sandwich	320	13	590	31	2
SHELF-STABLE						
Lunch Bucket						
Beef Stew	1 pkg (7.5 oz)	180	11	870	13	—
TAKE-OUT						
bubble & squeak	5 oz	186	13	—	16	3
cornish pasty	1 (8 oz)	847	52	—	79	3
irish stew	1 cup (7 oz)	280	16	—	10	—
kebab indian	1 (5.4 oz)	553	40	—	2	—
kheena	6.7 oz	781	71	—	1	tr
koftas	5	280	22	—	3	tr
roast beef sandwich plain	1	346	14	792	33	—
roast beef sandwich w/ cheese	1	402	18	1634	27	—
roast beef submarine sandwich w/ tomato lettuce & mayonnaise	1	411	13	845	44	—
samosa	2 (4 oz)	652	62	—	20	2
shepherds pie	6 oz	196	10	—	15	1
steak & kidney pie w/ top crust	1 slice (5 oz)	400	26	—	23	1
steak sandwich w/ tomato lettuce salt & mayonnaise	1	459	14	798	52	—
stew	6 oz	208	13	—	6	1
stew w/ vegetables	1 cup	220	11	292	15	—
stroganoff	¾ cup	260	19	503	43	—
swiss steak	4.6 oz	214	9	139	10	2
toad in the hole	1 (4.7 oz)	383	29	—	23	1

BEEFALO

FOOD	PORTION	CAL.	FAT	SOD.	CARB.	FIB.
roasted	3 oz	160	5	70	0	—

BEER AND ALE

FOOD	PORTION	CAL.	FAT	SOD.	CARB.	FIB.
Coors	12 oz	132	0	10	30	—
Coors Extra Gold	12 oz	147	0	10	32	—

FOOD	PORTION	CAL.	FAT	SOD.	CARB.	FIB.
Hamm's	12 oz	137	0	—	12	—
Killian's	12 oz	212	0	10	29	—
Old Milwaukee	12 oz	145	0	25	13	—
Olympia	12 oz	143	0	—	12	—
Pabst	12 oz	143	0	—	12	—
Schaefer	12 oz	138	0	23	13	—
Schlitz	12 oz	145	0	23	13	—
Signature	12 oz	150	0	21	13	—
Stroh	12 oz	142	0	23	13	—
Winterfest	12 oz	167	0	11	38	—
LIGHT						
Amstel	12 oz	95	0			
Anheuser Busch						
Natural	12 oz	110	0	—		
Bud	12 oz	108	0	—	—	
Coors	12 oz	101	0	10	13	—
Michelob	12 oz	134	0	—	—	
Miller	12 oz	96	0			
Molson	12 oz	109	0	—		
Old Milwaukee	12 oz	122	0	18	9	—
Piels	12 oz	136	0	—		
Schaefer	12 oz	111	0	16	8	—
Schlitz	12 oz	99	0	9	3	—
Schmidts	12 oz	96	0	—	—	
Stroh	12 oz	115	0	11	7	—
ale brown	10 oz	77	0	—	8	0
ale pale	10 oz	88	0	—	12	0
beer light	12 oz can	100	0	10	5	—
beer regular	12 oz can	146	0	19	13	—
lager	10 oz	80	0	—	4	0
pilsner lager beer	7 fl oz	85	tr	4	13	—
stout	10 oz	102	0	—	6	0
NONALCOHOLIC						
Hamm's	12 oz	55	0	—	12	—
Kingsbury	12 fl oz	60	0	—	—	
Pabst	12 oz	55	0	—	12	—
Spirit	12 oz	80	0	—	16	—
Guiness						
Kaliber	12 oz	43	0	—	—	
alcohol free beer	7 fl oz	50	tr	3	11	—
BEET JUICE						
juice	3½ oz	36	0	200	8	—

FOOD	PORTION	CAL.	FAT	SOD.	CARB.	FIB.

BEETS
CANNED
Del Monte

FOOD	PORTION	CAL.	FAT	SOD.	CARB.	FIB.
Pickled Crinkle Style Sliced	½ cup (4.5 oz)	80	0	380	19	2
Sliced	½ cup (4.3 oz)	35	0	290	8	2
Whole	½ cup (4.3 oz)	35	0	290	8	2
Whole Tiny	½ cup (4.3 oz)	35	0	290	8	2

S&W

FOOD	PORTION	CAL.	FAT	SOD.	CARB.	FIB.
Diced Tender	½ cup	40	0	270	9	—
Julienne French Style	½ cup	40	0	270	9	—
Pickled Whole Extra Small	½ cup	70	0	215	16	—
Pickled w/ Red Wine Vinegar Sliced	½ cup	70	0	215	16	—
Sliced Small Premium	½ cup	40	0	270	9	—
Sliced Water Pack	½ cup	35	0	40	9	—
Whole Small	½ cup	40	0	270	9	—

Seneca

FOOD	PORTION	CAL.	FAT	SOD.	CARB.	FIB.
Cut	½ cup	35	0	264	9	2
Diced	½ cup	35	0	264	9	2
Harvard	½ cup	90	0	144	21	1
Pickled	2 tbsp	20	0	48	6	0
Pickled With Onions	2 tbsp	20	0	48	6	0
Sliced	½ cup	35	0	264	9	2
Whole	½ cup	35	0	264	9	2
harvard	½ cup	89	tr	199	22	—
pickled	½ cup	75	tr	301	19	—
sliced	½ cup	27	tr	—	6	—

FRESH

FOOD	PORTION	CAL.	FAT	SOD.	CARB.	FIB.
greens cooked	½ cup	20	tr	173	4	—
greens raw	½ cup	4	tr	38	1	—
greens raw chopped	½ cup	4	tr	38	1	—
raw sliced	½ cup (2.4 oz)	29	tr	53	7	—
sliced cooked	½ cup (3 oz)	38	tr	65	9	—
whole cooked	2 (3.5 oz)	44	tr	77	10	—
whole raw	2 (5.7 oz)	70	tr	126	16	—

BEVERAGES

(see BEER AND ALE, CHAMPAGNE, COFFEE, DRINK MIXERS, FRUIT DRINKS, MALT, MINERAL WATER/BOTTLED WATER, LIQUOR/LIQUEUR, SODA, TEA/ HERBAL TEA, WINE, WINE COOLER)

BISCUIT
FROZEN
Great Starts

FOOD	PORTION	CAL.	FAT	SOD.	CARB.	FIB.
Egg Canadian Bacon & Cheese	5.2 oz	420	22	1845	37	—

FOOD	PORTION	CAL.	FAT	SOD.	CARB.	FIB.
Great Starts (CONT.)						
Sausage	4.7 oz	410	22	1180	36	—
Jimmy Dean						
Chicken Twin	2 (3.2 oz)	280	13	870	32	2
Sausage Twin	2 (3.4 oz)	330	21	900	25	2
Steak Twin	2 (3.2 oz)	270	13	660	26	2
Rudy's Farm						
Ham Twin	2 (3 oz)	160	3	790	23	1
Sausage & Cheese Twin	2 (3 oz)	290	18	570	22	1
Sausage Twin	2 (2.7 oz)	296	18	580	22	1
Weight Watchers						
Sausage Biscuit	3 oz	220	11	560	19	—
HOME RECIPE						
buttermilk	1 (2 oz)	212	10	348	27	—
oatcakes	2 (4 oz)	115	5	—	16	1
plain	1 (2 oz)	212	10	348	27	—
MIX						
Bisquick	½ cup (2 oz)	240	8	700	37	—
Reduced Fat	½ cup (2 oz)	210	4	660	39	—
Health Valley						
Buttermilk Biscuit Mix not prep	1 oz	100	1	170	20	3
Jiffy						
As prep	1	150	7	384	30	2
Biscuit	¼ cup (1.1 oz)	130	5	320	22	1
Buttermilk as prep	1	170	4	380	29	tr
buttermilk	1 (2 oz)	191	7	544	28	1
plain	1 (2 oz)	191	7	544	28	1
READY-TO-EAT						
Arnold						
Old Fashioned	1	60	3	100	8	—
REFRIGERATED						
1869 Brand						
Baking Powder	1	100	5	310	12	—
Buttermilk	1	100	5	310	12	—
Butter Tastin'	1	100	5	300	12	—
Ballard						
Ovenready	1	50	1	180	10	—
Ovenready Buttermilk	1	50	1	180	10	—
Big Country						
Southern Style	1	100	4	320	14	—
Hungry Jack						
Butter Tastin' Flaky	1	90	4	280	11	—
Buttermilk Flaky	1	90	4	300	12	—
Buttermilk Fluffy	1	90	4	280	12	—

FOOD	PORTION	CAL.	FAT	SOD.	CARB.	FIB.
Hungry Jack (CONT.)						
Extra Rich Buttermilk	1	50	1	180	9	—
Flaky	1	80	4	300	12	—
Honey Tastin' Flaky	1	90	4	290	13	—
Pillsbury						
Big Country Butter Tastin'	1	100	4	320	14	—
Big Country Buttermilk	1	100	4	320	14	—
Butter	1	50	1	180	10	—
Buttermilk	1	50	1	180	10	—
Country	1	50	1	180	10	—
Deluxe Heat N' Eat Buttermilk	2	170	5	530	27	—
Good'N Buttery Fluffy	1	90	5	270	11	—
Hearty Grains Multi-Grain	1	80	2	230	15	—
Hearty Grains Oatmeal Raisin	1	90	2	210	16	—
Heat N' Eat Big Premium	2	280	15	610	32	—
Tender Layer Buttermilk	1	50	1	170	9	—
Roman Meal						
Honey Nut Oat Bran	1 (1.5 oz)	131	5	278	21	1
buttermilk	1 (1 oz)	98	4	341	14	—
plain	1 (1 oz)	98	4	341	14	tr
TAKE-OUT						
buttermilk	1	127	6	368	17	—
plain	1 (35 g)	276	34	584	13	—
w/ egg	1	315	20	655	24	—
w/ egg & bacon	1	457	31	999	29	—
w/ egg & sausage	1	582	39	1142	41	—
w/ egg & steak	1	474	28	888	37	—
w/ egg cheese & bacon	1	477	31	1261	33	—
w/ ham	1	387	18	1433	44	—
w/ sausage	1	485	32	1071	40	—
w/ steak	1	456	26	795	44	—

BISON

FOOD	PORTION	CAL.	FAT	SOD.	CARB.	FIB.
roasted	3 oz	122	2	48	0	—

BLACK BEANS
CANNED

FOOD	PORTION	CAL.	FAT	SOD.	CARB.	FIB.
Allen						
Seasoned	½ cup (4.5 oz)	120	2	410	20	7
Eden						
Organic	½ cup (4.3 oz)	100	0	15	17	6

FOOD	PORTION	CAL.	FAT	SOD.	CARB.	FIB.
Health Valley						
Fast Menu Organic Black Beans With Tofu Weiners	7½ oz	150	1	170	20	15
Fast Menu Western Black Beans With Garden Vegetable	7½ oz	160	5	250	14	14
Trappey						
Seasoned	½ cup (4.5 oz)	120	2	410	20	7
DRIED						
cooked	1 cup	227	1	1	41	—
MIX						
Bean Cuisine						
Black Turtle	½ cup	115	1	5	—	5
Pasta & Beans Black Beans With Fusilli	½ cup	174	4	453	27	—
Mahatma						
Black Beans & Rice	1 cup	200	2	850	39	6

BLACKBERRIES
CANNED

FOOD	PORTION	CAL.	FAT	SOD.	CARB.	FIB.
Allen-Wolco	½ cup (5.3 oz)	60	1	20	13	9
in heavy syrup	½ cup	118	tr	3	30	—
FRESH						
blackberries	½ cup	37	tr	0	9	3
FROZEN						
Big Valley	⅔ cup (4.9 oz)	70	0	0	15	4
unsweetened	1 cup	97	1	2	24	—

BLACKEYE PEAS
CANNED

FOOD	PORTION	CAL.	FAT	SOD.	CARB.	FIB.
Allen	½ cup (4.5 oz)	110	1	340	18	4
Allen						
Fresh Shell	½ cup (4.4 oz)	120	1	350	21	6
With Bacon	½ cup (4.5 oz)	105	2	390	20	5
With Snaps	½ cup (4.4 oz)	120	1	420	20	5
Dorman						
Fresh Shell	½ cup (4.4 oz)	120	1	350	21	6
East Texas Fair						
Fresh Shell	½ cup (4.4 oz)	120	1	350	21	6
With Snaps	½ cup (4.4 oz)	120	1	420	20	5
Homefolks						
Fresh Shell	½ cup (4.4 oz)	120	1	350	21	6
With Jalapeno	½ cup (4.4 oz)	120	1	580	20	5
With Snaps	½ cup (4.4 oz)	120	1	420	20	5

FOOD	PORTION	CAL.	FAT	SOD.	CARB.	FIB.
Luck's						
Seasoned w/ Pork	7.25 oz	200	6	—	—	—
Sunshine						
With Bacon	½ cup (4.5 oz)	105	2	390	20	5
Trappey						
With Bacon	½ cup (4.5 oz)	120	2	350	19	5
With Bacon & Jalapeno	½ cup (4.4 oz)	110	2	470	19	5
w/pork	½ cup	199	4	840	40	—
DRIED						
cooked	1 cup	198	1	6	36	16
FROZEN						
Fresh Like	3.5 oz	138	1	6	24	1

BLINTZE

FOOD	PORTION	CAL.	FAT	SOD.	CARB.	FIB.
Empire						
Apple	2 (4.4 oz)	220	6	260	36	5
Blueberry	2 (4.4 oz)	190	4	260	36	2
Cheese	2 (4.4 oz)	200	6	310	29	3
Cherry	2 (4.4 oz)	200	4	280	38	3
Potato	2 (4.4 oz)	190	6	530	32	3
Golden						
Apple Raisin	1 (2.25 oz)	80	2	145	16	—
Blueberry	1 (2.25 oz)	90	1	150	18	—
Cheese	1 (2.25 oz)	80	2	135	13	—
Cherry	1 (2.25 oz)	95	1	145	18	—
Potato	1 (2.25 oz)	90	4	170	15	—
TAKE-OUT						
cheese	2	186	6	268	18	tr

BLUEBERRIES

FOOD	PORTION	CAL.	FAT	SOD.	CARB.	FIB.
CANNED						
S&W						
In Heavy Syrup	½ cup	111	0	—	30	—
in heavy syrup	1 cup	225	1	9	56	—
DRIED						
Sonoma	¼ cup (1.3 oz)	140	0	0	33	5
FRESH						
blueberries	1 cup	82	1	9	20	—
FROZEN						
Big Valley	¾ cup (4.9 oz)	70	0	0	12	4
unsweetened	1 cup	78	1	1	19	—

BLUEBERRY JUICE

FOOD	PORTION	CAL.	FAT	SOD.	CARB.	FIB.
After The Fall						
Maine Coast	1 cup (8 oz)	90	0	20	25	0

FOOD	PORTION	CAL.	FAT	SOD.	CARB.	FIB.
BLUEFIN						
fillet baked	4.1 oz	186	6	90	0	—
BLUEFISH						
fresh baked	3 oz	135	5	65	0	—
BOAR						
wild roasted	3 oz	136	4	—	0	—
BOK CHOY						
Dole						
Shredded	½ cup	5	tr	23	1	—
BORAGE						
fresh chopped cooked	3½ oz	25	1	88	4	—
raw chopped	½ cup	9	tr	35	1	—
BOYSENBERRIES						
in heavy syrup	1 cup	226	tr	9	57	—
unsweetened frzn	1 cup	66	tr	2	16	—
BOYSENBERRY JUICE						
Smucker's						
Juice	8 oz	120	0	10	30	—
Juice Sparkler	10 oz	130	tr	5	31	—
BRAINS						
Armour						
Pork Brains In Milk Gravy	⅔ cup (5.5 oz)	150	5	550	10	—
beef pan-fried	3 oz	167	13	134	0	—
beef simmered	3 oz	136	11	102	0	—
lamb braised	3 oz	124	9	114	0	—
lamb fried	3 oz	232	19	133	0	—
pork braised	3 oz	117	8	77	0	—
veal braised	3 oz	115	8	133	0	—
veal fried	3 oz	181	14	150	0	—
BRAN						
Arrowhead						
Oat Bran	⅓ cup (1.4 oz)	150	3	0	23	7
Wheat Bran	¼ cup (0.6 oz)	30	1	0	7	6
Good Shepherd						
Wheat Bran	1 oz	80	1	5	18	3
H-O						
Super Bran	⅓ cup	110	2	0	18	3
Health Valley						
Fast Menu Oat Bran Pilaf With Garden Vegetables	7½ oz	210	7	330	30	15

FOOD	PORTION	CAL.	FAT	SOD.	CARB.	FIB.
Hodgson Mill						
Oat	¼ cup (1.3 oz)	120	3	3	23	6
Wheat	¼ cup (0.5 oz)	30	1	0	10	7
Kretschmer						
Toasted Wheat	⅓ cup	57	2	2	15	3
Mother's						
Oat	½ cup	150	3	0	24	6
Quaker						
Oat	½ cup	150	3	0	24	6
Unprocessed	2 tbsp	8	tr	0	4	3
Roman Meal						
Oat	1 oz	94	3	3	13	5
Stone-Buhr						
Oat	⅓ cup (1 oz)	90	2	0	20	4
corn	⅓ cup	56	tr	2	21	21
oat cooked	½ cup	44	tr	1	13	—
oat dry	½ cup	116	3	1	31	7
rice dry	⅓ cup	88	6	1	14	6
wheat dry	½ cup	65	1	1	19	13

BRAZIL NUTS

FOOD	PORTION	CAL.	FAT	SOD.	CARB.	FIB.
dried unblanched	1 oz	186	19	0	4	—

BREAD

(*see also* BAGEL, BISCUIT, BREADSTICK, CROISSANT, ENGLISH MUFFIN, MUFFIN, ROLL, SCONE)

FOOD	PORTION	CAL.	FAT	SOD.	CARB.	FIB.
CANNED						
B&M						
Brown Bread	½ in slice (1.6 oz)	92	0	345	21	4
Brown Bread Raisins	½ in slice (1.6 oz)	94	0	320	22	4
Friends						
Brown Bread	1 slice (1.6 oz)	92	0	345	21	2
Brown Bread w/ Raisin	1 slice (1.6 oz)	94	0	320	22	2
S&W						
Brown Bread New England Recipe	2 slices	76	0	172	17	—
boston brown	1 slice (1.6 oz)	88	1	284	20	2
FROZEN						
Kineret						
Challah	⅛ loaf (2 oz)	150	4	220	25	1
HOME RECIPE						
banana	1 slice (2 oz)	195	6	181	33	—
cornbread as prep w/ 2% milk	1 piece (2.3 oz)	173	5	428	28	—
cornbread as prep w/ whole milk	1 piece (2.3 oz)	176	5	428	28	—

FOOD	PORTION	CAL.	FAT	SOD.	CARB.	FIB.
datenut	½ in slice	92	3	63	15	—
irish soda bread	1 slice (2 oz)	174	3	239	34	—
pita whole wheat	1 (6 in diam)	247	1	—	—	—
pumpkin	1 slice (1 oz)	94	4	89	15	—
white as prep w/ nonfat dry milk	1 slice	78	1	95	15	—
white as prep w/ 2% milk	1 slice	81	2	104	14	—
white as prep w/ whole milk	1 slice	82	2	104	14	—
whole wheat	1 slice	79	2	98	15	—
MIX						
Aunt Jemima						
Corn Bread Easy Mix	⅓ cup (1.3 oz)	150	4	450	26	1
Ballard						
Corn Bread	⅛ bread	140	3	570	25	—
Dromedary						
Corn Bread	1 piece (2 in x 2 in)	130	3	480	20	—
Natural Ovens						
Cracked Wheat	2 slices (2.4 oz)	140	1	140	38	4
English Muffin Bread	2 slices (2.4 oz)	140	1	140	35	2
Executive Fitness Sunny Millet	2 slices (2.6 oz)	160	2	70	37	4
Garden Bread	1 oz	50	1	100	14	1
Glorious Cinnamon & Raisin Fat Free	2 slices (2.1 oz)	110	1	140	30	3
Honey 'N Flax	2 slices (2.5 oz)	140	1	140	30	4
Hunger Filler Bread	2 slices (2.1 oz)	110	2	140	28	5
Light Wheat	2 slices (2.2 oz)	84	1	140	30	5
Nutty Natural Wheat Bread	2 slices (2.5 oz)	140	2	140	32	6
Seven Grain Herb	2 slices (2.5 oz)	140	1	140	30	4
Soft Hearth Whole Wheat	2 slices (2 oz)	100	2	140	30	4
Soft Sandwich Very Low Fat	2 slices (2.3 oz)	110	1	140	26	2
Stay Slim	2 slices (2 oz)	100	2	140	20	4
Zia Foods						
Cornbread Blue Cornmeal	1 piece (1.2 oz)	110	6	—	—	—
cornbread	1 piece (2 oz)	189	6	467	29	1
READY-TO-EAT						
Alvarado St. Bakery						
Barley	1 slice (1.2 oz)	70	1	140	15	2
California Style	1 slice (1.2 oz)	60	1	150	10	2

FOOD	PORTION	CAL.	FAT	SOD.	CARB.	FIB.
Alvarado St. Bakery (CONT.)						
French	1 slice (1.2 oz)	80	1	125	15	2
Multi-Grain	1 slice (1.2 oz)	60	1	160	11	2
Multi-Grain No-Salt	1 slice (1.2 oz)	60	1	0	11	2
Oat Berry	1 slice (1.2 oz)	70	1	150	13	2
Raisin	1 slice (1.1 oz)	80	1	105	15	2
Rye Seed	1 slice (1.2 oz)	60	1	150	11	2
Sourdough	1 slice (1.2 oz)	80	1	125	15	2
Wheat	1 slice (1.3 oz)	90	1	170	18	3
America's Own						
Wheat Cottage	1 slice	70	1	—	—	—
White Cottage	1 slice	70	1	—	—	—
Arnold						
12 Grain Natural	1 slice (0.8 oz)	60	0	100	10	1
Augusto Pan De Aqua	1 oz	80	1	150	14	1
Bran'nola Country Oat	1 slice (1.3 oz)	90	3	130	16	3
Bran'nola Dark Wheat	1 slice (1.3 oz)	90	3	150	15	3
Bran'nola Hearty Wheat	1 slice (1.3 oz)	100	3	160	15	3
Bran'nola Nutty Grains	1 slice (1.3 oz)	90	2	120	14	3
Bran'nola Original	1 slice (1.3 oz)	90	2	150	16	3
Cinnamon Chip	1 slice	80	2	90	13	tr
Cinnamon Raisin	1 slice (0.9 oz)	70	1	85	13	1
Country Bran Bakery Light	1 slice (0.8 oz)	40	tr	80	7	3
Cranberry	1 slice (0.9 oz)	70	1	80	14	1
French Stick Francisco	1 slice (1 oz)	70	2	110	12	—
French Stick Savoni	1 oz	80	tr	—	15	1
French Twin Loaves Francisco	2 slices (2 oz)	150	2	280	27	—
Italian Bakery Light	1 slice (0.7 oz)	40	tr	90	7	2
Italian Francisco	1 slice (1 oz)	70	1	110	12	—
Italian Stick Francisco	1 oz	90	1	110	17	—
Oatmeal Bakery	1 slice	60	1	95	12	2
Oatmeal Bakery Light	1 slice	40	tr	100	8	2
Oatmeal Raisin	1 slice (0.9 oz)	60	tr	90	12	2
Pita Wheat	½ pocket (1 oz)	71	0	—	16	—
Pita White	½ pocket (0.5 oz)	71	0	—	16	—
Pumpernickel	1 slice (1.1 oz)	70	1	200	15	1
Rye Bakery Soft Light	1 slice (1.1 oz)	40	tr	90	7	2
Rye Bakery Soft Seeded	1 slice (1.1 oz)	70	1	170	14	1
Rye Bakery Soft Unseeded	1 slice (1.1 oz)	70	1	170	14	1
Rye Dill	1 slice (1.1 oz)	60	1	140	10	1
Rye Real Jewish Dijon	1 slice	70	tr	210	15	1

FOOD	PORTION	CAL.	FAT	SOD.	CARB.	FIB.
Arnold (cont.)						
Rye Real Jewish Melba Thin	1 slice (0.7 oz)	40	tr	95	9	1
Rye Real Jewish Unseeded	1 slice	80	tr	180	16	1
Rye Real Jewish With Caraway	1 slice	80	tr	180	16	1
Rye Real Jewish Without Seeds	1 slice (1.1 oz)	70	tr	150	15	1
Sourdough Francisco	1 slice	90	1	250	19	1
Wheat Berry Honey	1 slice (1.1 oz)	80	2	140	13	2
Wheat Brick Oven	1 slice (0.8 oz)	60	2	100	9	2
Wheat Golden Light	1 slice (0.8 oz)	40	tr	90	7	2
Wheat Natural	1 slice (1.3 oz)	80	1	180	15	2
White Brick Oven	1 slice (0.8 oz)	60	1	130	11	1
White Country	1 slice (1.3 oz)	100	2	200	18	1
White Extra Fiber Brick Oven	1 slice (0.9 oz)	50	tr	90	10	2
White Light Brick Oven	1 slice (0.8 oz)	40	tr	95	10	2
White Premium Light	1 slice	40	tr	90	7	2
White Thin Sliced Brick Oven	1 slice	40	tr	75	7	tr
Whole Wheat 100% Light Brick Oven	1 slice (0.8 oz)	40	tr	85	6	3
Whole Wheat 100% Stoneground	1 slice (0.8 oz)	50	1	100	8	2
August Bros.						
Pumpernickel	1 slice (24 oz loaf)	90	1	220	18	1
Pumpernickel	1 slice	80	1	210	14	1
Rye N' Pump	1 slice	90	1	220	18	1
Rye Onion	1 slice	80	1	210	14	1
Rye Thin Unseeded	1 slice	40	—	110	8	1
Rye With Seeds	1 slice (1 lb loaf)	80	1	210	14	1
Rye With Seeds	1 slice (24 oz loaf)	90	1	210	18	1
Rye Without Seeds	1 slice (24 oz loaf)	90	—	220	18	1
Rye Without Seeds	1 slice	80	1	210	14	1
Beefsteak						
Pumpernickel	1 slice (1 oz)	70	1	180	13	1
Rye Hearty	1 slice (1 oz)	70	1	170	13	1
Rye Light	2 slices (1.6 oz)	70	1	250	17	5
Rye Mild	2 slices (1.4 oz)	90	1	240	18	2
Rye Soft	1 slice (1 oz)	70	1	180	13	1
Wheat Hearty	1 slice (1 oz)	70	1	160	13	1
Wheat Soft	1 slice (1 oz)	70	1	150	13	tr

FOOD	PORTION	CAL.	FAT	SOD.	CARB.	FIB.
Beefsteak (CONT.)						
White Robust	1 slice (1 oz)	70	1	140	13	tr
Bread Du Jour						
Austrian Wheat	3 in slice (1 oz)	130	2	280	26	2
French	3 in slice (1 oz)	130	1	300	26	1
Brownberry						
Bran'nola Country Oat	1 slice	90	2	166	18	3
Bran'nola Hearty Wheat	1 slice	88	2	197	17	3
Bran'nola Nutty Grains	1 slice	85	2	144	17	3
Bran'nola Original	1 slice	85	1	137	18	3
Health Nut	1 slice	71	3	158	12	3
Oatmeal Natural	1 slice	63	1	144	13	1
Oatmeal Soft	1 slice	48	1	82	10	2
Raisin Bran	1 slice	61	1	108	12	2
Raisin Cinnamon	1 slice	66	1	107	12	1
Raisin Walnut	1 slice	68	3	96	11	2
Wheat Apple Honey	1 slice	69	2	148	11	2
Wheat Soft	1 slice	74	2	127	12	1
Cedar's						
Mountain Bread Six Grain	1 piece (2.4 oz)	200	4	380	35	4
Damascus Bakeries						
Mountain Shepard Lahvash	⅓ loaf (2 oz)	135	0	90	28	2
Dicarlo's						
Focaccia	⅛ bread (2 oz)	130	2	260	25	1
French Parisian	2 slices (1 oz)	70	1	150	14	tr
Freihofer's						
Country Potato	1 slice (1.3 oz)	100	1	200	19	1
Country White	1 slice (1.3 oz)	100	1	220	19	tr
Wheat	1½ slices	70	1	—	—	2
White Light	2 slices (1.6 oz)	80	1	210	18	4
Whole Wheat 100%	1 slice (1.3 oz)	90	2	160	16	2
Home Pride						
Hearty Buttermilk & Biscuit White	1 slice (1.3 oz)	100	2	280	18	tr
Hearty Deli Rye	1 slice (2 oz)	140	2	350	26	3
Hearty Golden Honey Wheat	1 slice (1.3 oz)	90	2	210	18	2
Hearty Honey Oats & Cracked Wheat	1 slice (1.4 oz)	100	2	210	19	2
Hearty Seven Grain Multi Grain	1 slice (1.3 oz)	100	2	200	17	2
Honey Wheat	1 slice (1 oz)	70	1	150	13	1

FOOD	PORTION	CAL.	FAT	SOD.	CARB.	FIB.
Home Pride (CONT.)						
Seven Grain	1 slice (0.9 oz)	60	1	130	12	1
Wheat	1 slice (0.9 oz)	70	1	140	13	1
Wheat Light	3 slices (2.1 oz)	110	2	300	25	6
White	1 slice (0.9 oz)	70	1	160	13	0
White Grain	1 slice (1 oz)	60	1	140	13	2
White Light	3 slices (0.9 oz)	110	2	320	25	6
Whole Wheat Hearty 100% Stoneground	1 slice (1.4 oz)	90	2	250	18	3
Malsovit						
Raisin	1 slice	77	1	146	12	3
Matthew's						
9 Grain & Nut	1 slice	80	3	100	9	2
Cinnamon	1 slice	70	1	100	13	2
Golden	1 slice	70	1	125	14	1
Oat Bran	1 slice	65	0	110	12	2
Pita Whole Wheat	1	210	2	390	45	7
Sodium Free	1 slice	70	1	<5	12	2
Whole Wheat	1 slice	70	1	130	12	2
Mediterranean Magic						
Focaccia	⅕ loaf (1.8 oz)	140	2	550	27	tr
Monks' Bread						
Hi-Fibre	1 slice	50	1	110	13	—
Raisin	1 slice	70	2	85	10	—
Sunflower & Bran	1 slice	70	1	80	12	2
White	1 slice	60	1	95	10	—
Whole Wheat 100% Stoneground	1 slice	70	1	110	13	—
Parisian						
French Stick Extra Sour	2 oz	150	1	311	27	—
French Stick Sweet	2 oz	154	2	331	27	—
Pepperidge Farm						
7 Grain Hearty Slice	2 slices	180	2	340	36	2
Cinnamon	1 slice	90	3	110	15	2
Cracked Wheat	1 slice	70	1	140	13	1
Crunchy Oat	2 slices (1½ lb loaf)	190	4	290	34	3
Date Walnut	1 slice	90	3	110	14	2
French Fully Baked	2 oz	150	2	320	28	1
French Twin	1 oz	80	1	160	15	0
Honey Bran	1 slice	90	1	160	18	1
Italian Brown & Serve	1 oz	80	1	150	14	0
Italian Sliced	1 slice	70	1	125	12	—
Oatmeal	1 slice	70	1	160	12	1
Oatmeal	1 slice (1½ lb loaf)	90	1	200	17	1

FOOD	PORTION	CAL.	FAT	SOD.	CARB.	FIB.
Pepperidge Farm (CONT.)						
Oatmeal Light	1 slice	45	0	95	9	1
Oatmeal Very Thin Sliced	1 slice	40	1	80	8	—
Pumpernickel Family	1 slice	80	1	230	15	2
Pumpernickel Party	4 slices	60	1	160	12	1
Raisin With Cinnamon	1 slice	90	2	100	16	1
Rye Dijon	1 slice	50	1	180	9	1
Rye Dijon Thick Sliced	1 slice	70	1	260	15	2
Rye Family	1 slice (32 g)	80	1	220	16	2
Rye Party	4 slices	60	1	250	12	1
Rye Seedless Family	1 slice	80	1	210	16	2
Rye Soft	1 slice	70	1	120	12	—
Sesame Wheat	2 slices	190	3	340	36	3
Sprouted Wheat	1 slice	70	2	100	11	2
Vienna Light	1 slice	45	0	100	10	1
Vienna Thick Sliced	1 slice	70	1	125	13	0
Wheat	1 slice (1½ lb loaf)	90	2	190	18	2
Wheat Family	1 slice	70	1	130	13	2
Wheat Light	1 slice	45	0	90	9	1
Wheat Very Thin Sliced	1 slice	35	0	75	7	0
White Country	2 slices	190	2	340	38	2
White Large Family Thin Slice	1 slice	70	1	150	13	0
White Sandwich	2 slices	130	2	260	24	0
White Thin Slice	1 slice	80	2	130	14	0
White Toasting	1 slice	90	1	200	17	1
White Very Thin Sliced	1 slice	40	0	80	8	0
Whole Wheat Thin Slice	1 slice	60	1	110	12	2
Roman Meal						
Brown & Serve Mini Loaf	½ loaf (2 oz)	136	2	275	24	1
Cracked Wheat	1 slice (1.4 oz)	92	2	129	15	2
Hearty Wheat Light	1 slice (0.8 oz)	42	tr	102	7	2
Honey Nut Oat Bran	1 slice (1 oz)	72	2	129	11	1
Honey Oat Bran	1 slice (1 oz)	70	1	132	12	1
Oat	1 slice (1 oz)	69	1	100	12	1
Oat Bran	1 slice (1 oz)	68	1	136	12	1
Oat Bran Light	1 slice (0.8 oz)	42	tr	100	7	2
Round Top	1 slice (1 oz)	67	1	142	12	1
Sandwich	1 slice (0.8 oz)	55	1	115	10	1
Seven Grain	1 slice (1 oz)	67	1	142	12	1
Seven Grain Light	1 slice (0.8 oz)	42	1	101	7	3
Sourdough Light	1 slice (0.8 oz)	41	tr	115	7	3
Sourdough Whole Grain Light	1 slice (0.8 oz)	40	tr	104	7	3

FOOD	PORTION	CAL.	FAT	SOD.	CARB.	FIB.
Roman Meal (CONT.)						
Sun Grain	1 slice (1 oz)	70	2	135	11	1
Twelve Grain	1 slice (1 oz)	70	2	140	11	1
Twelve Grain Light	1 slice (0.8 oz)	42	tr	104	7	3
Wheat Light	1 slice (0.8 oz)	41	tr	102	7	3
Wheatberry Honey	1 slice (1 oz)	67	1	139	12	1
Wheatberry Light	1 slice (0.8 oz)	42	tr	102	7	2
White Light	1 slice (0.8 oz)	41	tr	105	7	3
Whole Grain 100%	1 slice (1.4 oz)	91	1	198	16	2
Whole Grain Sourdough	1 slice (1 oz)	66	1	141	12	1
Whole Wheat 100%	1 slice (1 oz)	64	1	141	11	2
Whole Wheat 100% Light	1 slice (0.8 oz)	42	tr	102	7	2
Sahara						
Pita Oat Bran	½ pocket (1 oz)	66	tr	163	14	2
Pita White	½ pocket	78	1	147	16	—
Stroehmann						
White Whole Special Recipe	1 slice	70	1	160	13	—
White Whole Special Recipe Kids	1 slice	60	tr	150	12	—
Sunmaid						
Raisin	1 slice	70	tr	85	13	1
Tree Of Life						
100% Spelt	1 slice (1.8 oz)	130	3	290	22	3
Millet	1 slice (1.8 oz)	130	2	240	25	2
Rye Sour Dough	1 slice (1.8 oz)	110	0	30	24	5
Sprouted Seven Grain	1 slice (1.8 oz)	110	2	140	20	2
Weight Watchers						
Italian	1 slice (0.8 oz)	38	tr	99	7	2
Multi-Grain	1 slice (0.8 oz)	41	1	98	7	2
Oat	1 slice (0.8 oz)	42	1	102	7	2
Raisin	1 slice (0.9 oz)	55	tr	95	11	1
Rye	1 slice (0.8 oz)	38	tr	100	7	2
Wheat	1 slice (0.8 oz)	40	tr	99	7	2
White	1 slice (0.8 oz)	40	tr	96	7	2
Wonder						
Calcium Enriched	1 slice (1 oz)	70	1	150	12	tr
Cinnamon Raisin	1 slice (1 oz)	70	1	100	14	tr
Cracked Wheat	1 slice (1 oz)	70	1	150	14	1
French	1 slice (1 oz)	80	2	160	15	tr
French Light	2 slices (1.6 oz)	80	1	210	18	5
Granola	1 slice (1.5 oz)	100	2	210	19	2
Honey Bran Light	2 slices (1.6 oz)	80	1	190	18	6

FOOD	PORTION	CAL.	FAT	SOD.	CARB.	FIB.
Wonder (CONT.)						
Italian	1 slice (1.1 oz)	80	1	190	15	tr
Italian Family	1 slice (1 oz)	70	1	170	13	tr
Italian Light	2 slices (1.6 oz)	80	1	230	18	5
Kid	1 slice (0.9 oz)	70	1	150	13	tr
Light Calcium Enriched	2 slices (1.6 oz)	80	1	240	18	5
Nine Grain Light	2 slices (1.6 oz)	80	1	230	18	6
Oatmeal Light	2 slices (1.6 oz)	90	0	230	19	4
Rye	1 slice (1 oz)	70	1	170	13	1
Rye Light	2 slices (1.6 oz)	70	1	220	17	5
Sourdough	1 slice (1.2 oz)	90	2	180	17	tr
Sourdough Light	2 slices (1.6 oz)	80	1	250	18	5
Texas Toast	1 slice (1.4 oz)	100	1	220	19	1
Vienna	1 slice (1 oz)	70	1	170	13	tr
Wheat Calcium Light	2 slices (1.6 oz)	80	1	240	18	6
Wheat Family	1 slice (0.9 oz)	70	1	150	13	tr
Wheat Golden Country Style	2 slices (1.4 oz)	100	2	220	19	1
Wheat Light	2 slices (1.6 oz)	80	1	230	18	6
White	1 slice (0.9 oz)	70	1	150	13	tr
White Calcium	2 slices (1.6 oz)	100	1	240	20	1
White Calcium Light	2 slices (1.6 oz)	80	1	260	18	5
White Light	2 slices (1.6 oz)	80	1	230	18	5
White With Buttermilk	1 slice (1 oz)	80	1	180	14	tr
Whole Wheat 100%	1 slice (1 oz)	70	1	180	12	2
Whole Wheat 100% Soft	2 slices (1.6 oz)	110	2	240	21	1
Whole Wheat 100% Stoneground	1 slice (1.2 oz)	80	2	190	14	2
cracked wheat	1 slice	65	1	135	12	1
egg	1 slice (1.4 oz)	115	2	197	19	—
french	1 loaf (1 lb)	1270	18	2633	230	—
french	1 slice (1 oz)	78	1	172	15	1
gluten	1 slice	47	tr	104	8	—
italian	1 loaf (1 lb)	1255	4	2656	256	—
italian	1 slice (1 oz)	81	1	175	15	1
navajo fry	1 (5 in diam)	296	9	625	48	—
navajo fry	1 (10.5 in diam)	527	15	1112	85	—
oat bran	1 slice	71	1	122	12	1
oat bran reduced calorie	1 slice	46	1	81	10	—
oatmeal	1 slice	73	1	162	13	1
oatmeal reduced calorie	1 slice	48	1	89	10	—
pita	1 reg (2 oz)	165	1	322	33	1
pita	1 sm (1 oz)	78	tr	152	16	1
pita whole wheat	1 reg (2 oz)	170	2	340	35	5

FOOD	PORTION	CAL.	FAT	SOD.	CARB.	FIB.
pita whole wheat	1 sm (1 oz)	76	1	151	16	2
protein	1 slice	47	tr	104	8	—
pumpernickel	1 slice	80	1	215	15	2
raisin	1 slice	71	1	101	14	—
rice bran	1 slice	66	1	119	12	—
rye	1 slice	83	1	211	16	2
rye reduced calorie	1 slice	47	1	93	9	—
seven grain	1 slice	65	1	127	12	2
sourdough	1 slice (1 oz)	78	1	172	15	1
vienna	1 slice (1 oz)	78	1	172	15	1
wheat reduced calorie	1 slice	46	1	117	10	3
wheat berry	1 slice	65	1	132	12	1
wheat bran	1 slice	89	1	175	17	3
wheat germ	1 slice	74	1	157	14	—
white	1 slice	67	1	135	12	1
white reduced calorie	1 slice	48	1	104	10	2
white toasted	1 slice	67	1	136	13	—
white cubed	1 cup	80	1	154	15	—
whole wheat	1 slice	70	1	149	13	2
REFRIGERATED						
Pillsbury						
Crusty French Loaf	1 in slice	60	tr	120	11	—
Hearty Grains Country Oatmeal Twists	1	80	2	120	15	—
Hearty Grains Cracked Wheat Twists	1	80	2	120	14	—
Pipin'Hot Wheat Loaf	1 in slice	70	2	170	12	—
Pipin'Hot White Loaf	1 in slice	70	2	170	12	—
Roman Meal						
Loaf	1 slice (1 oz)	85	3	199	13	1
Stefano's						
Stuffed Bread Broccoli & Cheese	½ bread (6 oz)	450	17	830	54	7
TAKE-OUT						
chapatis as prep w/ fat	1 (2½ oz)	230	9	—	34	5
chapatis as prep w/o fat	1 (2½ oz)	141	1	—	31	5
cornbread	2 in x 2 in (1.4 oz)	107	2	276	18	—
cornstick	1 (1.3 oz)	101	4	195	13	tr
focaccia onion	1 piece (4.6 oz)	282	10	536	43	2
focaccia rosemary	1 piece (3.5 oz)	251	7	535	40	2
focaccia tomato olive	1 piece (4.7 oz)	270	8	683	42	2
naan	1 (6 oz)	571	21	—	85	4
papadums fried	2 (1.5 oz)	81	4	—	9	2
paratha	1 (4.4 oz)	403	18	—	54	5

FOOD	PORTION	CAL.	FAT	SOD.	CARB.	FIB.
BREAD COATING						
Don's Chuck Wagon						
All Purpose Mix	¼ cup (1 oz)	100	0	580	20	1
Fish & Chips Mix	¼ cup (1 oz)	100	0	740	21	1
Fish Mix	¼ cup (1 oz)	95	0	940	21	1
Frying Mix Chicken	¼ cup (1 oz)	95	0	850	21	1
Frying Mix Seafood Seasoned	¼ cup (1 oz)	95	1	990	21	1
Mushroom Mix	¼ cup (1 oz)	95	0	990	21	1
Onion Ring Mix	¼ cup (1 oz)	100	0	690	21	1
Golden Dipt						
Breading Frying Mix	1 oz	90	0	630	20	—
Chicken Frying Mix	1 oz	90	0	1430	20	—
Onion Ring Mix	1 oz	100	0	570	22	—
Ka-Me						
Tempura Batter Mix	1 oz	100	0	5	22	0
Little Crow						
Fryin' Magic	0.5 oz	43	tr	542	8	—
Mrs. Dash						
Crispy Coating	0.5 oz	63	1	3	10	—
Oven Fry						
Homestyle Flour Recipe For Chicken	¼ pkg	85	2	971	15	—
Shake 'N Bake						
Extra Crispy Oven Fry For Pork	¼ pkg (1 oz)	120	3	688	21	—
Italian Herb Recipe	¼ pkg (½ oz)	77	1	618	14	—
Original Barbecue For Chicken	¼ pkg (½ oz)	93	2	841	18	—
Original Barbecue For Pork	¼ pkg (½ oz)	38	1	351	7	—
Original Country Mild	¼ pkg (½ oz)	76	4	501	10	—
Original For Chicken	¼ pkg (½ oz)	75	2	451	14	—
Original For Fish	¼ pkg (½ oz)	73	1	406	14	—
Original For Pork	¼ pkg (½ oz)	41	1	301	8	—
BREAD MACHINE MIX						
Dromedary						
Country White	½ in slice (2 oz)	140	1	230	28	1
Italian Herb	½ in slice (1.8 oz)	140	3	250	25	1
Stoneground Wheat	½ in slice (1.8 oz)	140	2	200	26	2
Pillsbury						
Cracked Wheat	1/12 pkg (1.3 oz)	130	2	260	25	2
Sassafras						
Apricot Oatmeal	1 slice (1.4 oz)	140	1	190	29	2

FOOD	PORTION	CAL.	FAT	SOD.	CARB.	FIB.
Wanda's						
Dried Tomato Cheddar	¼ cup mix per serv (1.2 oz)	140	0	230	22	3
European White	¼ cup mix per serv (1.2 oz)	130	0	115	26	1
Oatmeal	¼ cup mix per serv (1.2 oz)	120	0	350	24	1
Oatmeal Cinnamon	¼ cup mix per serv (1.2 oz)	120	0	280	19	1
Old World Rye	¼ cup mix per serv (1.9 oz)	90	0	300	27	3
Onion	¼ cup mix per serv (1.2 oz)	120	0	270	25	1
Orange Cinnamon	¼ cup mix per serv (1.3 oz)	130	0	90	28	1
Oregano Garlic	¼ cup mix per serv (1.2 oz)	130	1	270	25	2
Rosemary Basil	¼ cup mix per serv (1.2 oz)	130	0	250	26	1
Rye	¼ cup mix per serv (1.2 oz)	120	0	270	25	1
Rye Caraway	¼ cup mix per serv (1.2 oz)	120	0	270	25	1
Sourdough	¼ cup mix per serv (1.2 oz)	120	0	160	25	1
Sunflower Sesame Poppyseed	¼ cup mix per serv (1.2 oz)	120	0	310	25	2
Ten Grain	¼ cup mix per serv (1.4 oz)	140	0	160	27	3
Wheat	¼ cup mix per serv (1.2 oz)	130	0	270	26	2
White	¼ cup mix per serv (1.2 oz)	130	0	250	26	1
Whole Wheat	¼ cup mix per serv (1.3 oz)	130	0	330	26	4

BREADCRUMBS
4C

FOOD	PORTION	CAL.	FAT	SOD.	CARB.	FIB.
Salt Free	1 tbsp (0.5 oz)	50	1	0	10	—
Seasoned	1 tbsp (0.5 oz)	50	1	270	10	—
Toasted	1 tbsp (0.5 oz)	50	1	110	10	—
Toasted Salt Free	1 tbsp (0.5 oz)	50	1	0	10	—
Arnold						
Italian	½ oz	50	tr	200	8	tr

FOOD	PORTION	CAL.	FAT	SOD.	CARB.	FIB.
Arnold (CONT.)						
Plain	½ oz	50	tr	80	8	tr
Contadina						
Plain	⅓ cup	100	2	700	19	1
Devonsheer						
Italian Style	1 oz	104	1	408	20	1
Plain	1 oz	108	1	272	21	1
Friday's						
Seasoned	1 oz	56	tr	—	—	—
Jaclyn's						
Organic Whole Wheat Plain	½ oz	28	1	5	13	—
Organic Whole Wheat Italian Style	½ oz	28	1	5	13	—
Progresso						
Italian Style	2 tbsp	60	tr	240	11	—
Plain	2 tbsp	60	tr	110	11	—
dry	1 cup	426	6	930	78	5
dry seasonsed	1 cup (4 oz)	441	3	3180	85	5
fresh	⅔ cup	76	1	153	14	1

BREADFRUIT

breadfruit	3.5 oz	109	tr	—	—	—
fresh	¼ small	99	tr	2	26	—
seeds cooked	1 oz	48	1	—	9	—
seeds raw	1 oz	54	2	—	8	—
seeds roasted	1 oz	59	tr	—	11	—

BREADNUTTREE SEEDS

dried	1 oz	104	tr	—	23	—

BREADSTICKS

Angonoa						
Cheese	5 (1 oz)	120	3	270	20	1
Cheese Mini	16 (1 oz)	120	3	120	20	1
Garlic	6 (1 oz)	120	2	390	21	1
Italian Style Plain	5 (1 oz)	120	3	280	20	1
Low Sodium With Sesame Seed	6 (1 oz)	130	4	65	19	2
Onion	6 (1 oz)	120	2	200	21	2
Pizza Mini	26 (1 oz)	120	2	180	21	1
Sesame Mini	16 (1 oz)	130	4	220	19	2
Sesame Royale	6 (1 oz)	130	4	210	18	2
Whole Wheat Mini	14 (1 oz)	130	4	220	19	3
Bread Du Jour						
Italian	1 (1.9 oz)	130	2	280	25	1

FOOD	PORTION	CAL.	FAT	SOD.	CARB.	FIB.
Bread Du Jour (CONT.)						
Sourdough	1 (1.9 oz)	130	1	280	25	1
J.J. Cassone						
Garlic	1 (1.6 oz)	150	3	—	26	2
Keebler						
Garlic	2	30	tr	20	6	—
Onion	2	30	tr	25	6	—
Plain	2	30	tr	30	6	—
Sesame	2	30	1	30	5	—
Lance						
Cheese	2	20	0	40	4	—
Garlic	2	30	0	40	5	—
Plain	2	30	0	50	5	—
Sesame	2	30	0	50	4	—
Pillsbury						
Soft Bread Sticks	1	100	2	230	17	—
Roman Meal						
Brown & Serve Soft	1 (2.7 oz)	181	3	275	32	3
Refrigerated	1 (1.4 oz)	117	4	274	18	1
Stella D'Oro						
Deli Garlic Fat Free	5	60	0	120	12	—
Deli Original Fat Free	5	60	0	130	12	—
Garlic	1	35	1	55	6	—
Grissini Garlic Fat Free	3	60	0	120	12	—
Grissini Original Fat Free	3	60	0	130	12	—
Onion	1	40	1	38	6	—
Regular	1	40	1	40	7	—
Regular Sodium Free	2	80	2	0	14	—
Sesame Low Fat	2	70	1	90	14	—
Sesame Sodium Free	1	50	3	0	7	—
Traditional Garlic Fat Free	2	70	0	150	15	—
Traditional Original Fat Free	2	70	0	150	15	—
Wheat	1	40	1	20	6	—
onion poppyseed home recipe	1	64	1	69	11	—
plain	1 sm	25	1	66	4	—
plain	1	41	1	66	7	—

BREAKFAST BAR

(*see also* BREAKFAST DRINKS, NUTRITIONAL SUPPLEMENTS)

FOOD	PORTION	CAL.	FAT	SOD.	CARB.	FIB.
Carnation						
Chewy Chocolate Chip	1 (1.26 oz)	150	6	80	22	tr

FOOD	PORTION	CAL.	FAT	SOD.	CARB.	FIB.
Carnation (CONT.)						
Chewy Peanut Butter Chocolate Chip	1 (1.26 oz)	140	5	90	21	tr
Glenny's						
Sunrise Bee Pollen	1 (1.5 oz)	190	8	—	22	—
Sunrise Ginseng	1 (1.5 oz)	160	7	—	24	—
Sunrise Spirulina	1 (1.5 oz)	140	5	—	21	—
Nutri-Grain						
Apple Cinnamon	1 (1.3 oz)	140	3	60	27	1
Blueberry	1 (1.3 oz)	140	3	60	27	1
Raspberry	1 (1.3 oz)	140	3	60	27	1
Strawberry	1 (1.3 oz)	140	3	60	27	1

BREAKFAST DRINKS

(*see also* BREAKFAST BAR, NUTRITIONAL SUPPLEMENTS)

FOOD	PORTION	CAL.	FAT	SOD.	CARB.	FIB.
Carnation						
Instant Breakfast Cafe Mocha	1 pkg + skim milk (9 fl oz)	220	1	216	39	1
Instant Breakfast Cafe Mocha	1 pkg	130	1	100	28	1
Instant Breakfast Cafe Mocha	1 can (10 fl oz)	220	3	210	35	0
Instant Breakfast Classic Chocolate Malt	1 pkg	130	2	130	26	1
Instant Breakfast Classic Chocolate Malt	1 pkg + skim milk (9 fl oz)	220	1	240	39	1
Instant Breakfast Creamy Milk Chocolate	8 fl oz	220	3	220	36	1
Instant Breakfast Creamy Milk Chocolate	1 can (10 fl oz)	220	3	230	37	1
Instant Breakfast Creamy Milk Chocolate	1 pkg + skim milk (9 fl oz)	220	1	240	39	1
Instant Breakfast Creamy Milk Chocolate	1 pkg	130	1	100	28	1
Instant Breakfast French Vanilla	1 pkg + skim milk (9 fl oz)	220	1	240	39	0
Instant Breakfast French Vanilla	1 pkg	130	0	110	27	0
Instant Breakfast No Sugar Added Classic Chocolate	1 pkg + skim milk (9 fl oz)	160	2	240	24	1

FOOD	PORTION	CAL.	FAT	SOD.	CARB.	FIB.
Carnation (CONT.)						
Instant Breakfast No Sugar Added Classic Chocolate	1 pkg	70	2	120	11	1
Instant Breakfast No Sugar Added Creamy Milk Chocolate	1 pkg + skim milk (9 fl oz)	160	1	216	24	1
Instant Breakfast No Sugar Added Creamy Milk Chocolate	1 pkg	70	1	90	12	1
Instant Breakfast No Sugar Added French Vanilla	1 pkg + skim milk (9 fl oz)	150	1	216	24	0
Instant Breakfast No Sugar Added French Vanilla	1 pkg	70	0	90	12	0
Instant Breakfast No Sugar Added Strawberry Creme	1 pkg + skim milk (9 fl oz)	150	1	216	24	0
Instant Breakfast No Sugar Added Strawberry Creme	1 pkg	70	0	90	12	0
Instant Breakfast Strawberry Creme	1 pkg + skim milk (9 fl oz)	220	1	288	39	0
Instant Breakfast Strawberry Creme	1 pkg	130	0	160	28	0
Pillsbury						
Instant Breakfast Chocolate Malt as prep w/ whole milk	1 serving	290	9	310	38	—
Instant Breakfast Chocolate as prep w/ whole milk	1 serving	290	9	310	38	—
Instant Breakfast Strawberry as prep w/ whole milk	1 serving	290	9	300	39	—
Instant Breakfast Vanilla as prep w/ whole milk	1 serving	300	9	330	41	—
orange drink powder	3 rounded tsp	93	0	4	24	—
orange drink powder as prep w/water	6 oz	86	0	9	22	—

BROAD BEANS

canned	1 cup	183	1	1161	32	—

FOOD	PORTION	CAL.	FAT	SOD.	CARB.	FIB.
dried cooked	1 cup	186	1	8	33	—
fresh cooked	3½ oz	56	tr	41	10	—

BROCCOLI

FRESH

Dole						
1 med spear	40	1	75	4	5
chopped cooked	½ cup	22	tr	20	4	2
raw chopped	½ cup	12	tr	12	2	1
FROZEN						
Big Valley						
Chopped	¾ cup (3 oz)	25	0	20	4	2
Cuts	¾ cup (3 oz)	25	0	20	4	2
Birds Eye						
Baby Spears Deluxe	⅔ cup	30	0	15	5	3
Chopped	⅔ cup	25	0	15	5	3
Farm Fresh Spears	¾ cup	30	0	25	7	2
Florets Deluxe	½ cup	25	0	20	5	3
Polybag Cuts	½ cup	25	0	25	4	3
Polybag Deluxe Florets	⅔ cup	25	0	15	4	3
Spears	⅔ cup	25	0	20	5	3
With Cheese Sauce	½ pkg	110	5	520	9	1
Fresh Like						
Spear	3.5 oz	26	tr	32	5	1
Green Giant						
Cut	½ cup	16	0	95	3	2
Cuts	½ cup	12	0	15	3	2
Harvest Fresh Spears	½ cup	20	0	115	4	2
In Butter Sauce	½ cup	40	2	350	6	—
In Cheese Sauce	½ cup	60	2	530	9	2
Mini Spears Select	4–5 spears	18	0	25	5	3
One Serve Cuts In Butter Sauce	1 pkg	45	2	10	7	3
One Serve Cuts In Cheese Sauce	1 pkg	70	3	660	11	3
Valley Combinations Broccoli Fanfare	½ cup	80	2	340	14	—
Hanover						
Cut	½ cup	25	0	—	—	—
Florets	½ cup	30	0	—	—	—
Pepperidge Farm						
Broccoli With Cheese In Pastry	1	230	16	380	18	—
chopped cooked	½ cup	25	tr	22	5	—
spears cooked	10 oz pkg	69	tr	60	13	4
spears cooked	½ cup	25	tr	22	5	3

FOOD	PORTION	CAL.	FAT	SOD.	CARB.	FIB.

BROWNIE
FROZEN
Pepperidge Farm

FOOD	PORTION	CAL.	FAT	SOD.	CARB.	FIB.
Monterey Hot Fudge Chocolate Chunk Brownie	1	480	26	200	56	—
Newport Hot Fudge Brownie	1	400	20	160	50	—
Weight Watchers						
Brownie Ala Mode	1	180	4	150	35	—
Chocolate Brownie	1 (1.25 oz)	100	3	150	16	—
Mint Frosted	1 (1.23 oz)	100	5	130	18	—
HOME RECIPE						
plain	1 (0.8 oz)	112	7	82	12	1
w/nuts	1 (0.8 oz)	95	6	51	11	—
MIX						
Betty Crocker						
Brownie With Hot Fudge MicroRave Single	1	350	12	260	55	—
Frosted MicroRave	1	180	7	120	21	—
Fudge Family Size	1	150	5	100	22	—
Fudge Light	1	100	1	90	21	—
Fudge MicroRave	1	150	6	110	22	—
Fudge Regular Size	1	150	6	105	23	—
Supreme Caramel	1	120	4	115	21	—
Supreme Frosted	1	160	6	120	26	—
Supreme German Chocolate	1	160	7	110	24	—
Supreme Original	1	140	6	80	21	—
Supreme Party	1	160	6	110	26	—
Supreme Walnut	1	140	7	80	18	—
Walnut MicroRave	1	160	7	95	21	—
Estee						
Lite	2	100	4	0	23	1
Jiffy						
Fudge as prep	1	160	4	150	28	tr
Pillsbury						
Deluxe Family-Size Fudge Brownie	2 in sq	150	7	95	20	—
Deluxe Fudge Brownie	2 in sq	150	6	100	21	—
Deluxe Fudge Brownie With Walnuts	2 in sq	150	8	90	19	—
Fudge Microwave	1	190	9	105	25	—

FOOD	PORTION	CAL.	FAT	SOD.	CARB.	FIB.
Pillsbury (CONT.)						
The Ultimate Carmel Fudge Chunk Brownie	2 in sq	170	7	105	25	—
The Ultimate Chunky Triple Fudge Brownie	2 in sq	170	7	105	25	—
The Ultimate Double Fudge Brownie	2 in sq	160	6	105	24	—
The Ultimate Rockey Road Fudge Brownie	2 in sq	170	8	95	24	—
plain	1 (1.2 oz)	139	7	83	20	1
plain low calorie	1 (0.8 oz)	84	2	21	16	1
READY-TO-EAT						
Lance	1 pkg (78 g)	320	12	210	52	—
Frito Lay						
Fudge Nut	3 oz	360	14	225	56	—
Greenfield						
Brownie HomeStyle	1 (1.4 oz)	120	0	65	29	1
Hostess						
Brownie Bites	5 (2 oz)	260	14	125	32	2
Brownie Bites Walnut	5 (2 oz)	270	15	140	31	2
Little Debbie						
Fudge	1 pkg (2.5 oz)	310	15	190	44	1
Fudge	1 pkg (2.1 oz)	270	13	170	39	1
Fudge	1 pkg (3.6 oz)	450	21	280	65	2
Fudge	1 pkg (2.9 oz)	360	17	230	52	1
Pepperidge Farm						
Charlotte Fudgey Brownie	1	220	11	105	28	2
Tahoe Milk Chocolate Pecan	1	210	10	100	30	1
Westport Fudgey Brownies w/ Walnuts	1	220	11	105	28	2
Tastykake						
Brownie	1 (85 g)	340	14	220	53	5
plain	1 lg (2 oz)	227	9	175	36	1
plain	1 sm (1 oz)	115	5	88	18	1
w/ nuts	1 (1 oz)	100	4	59	16	—
w/o nuts	1 (2 oz)	243	10	153	39	—

BRUSSELS SPROUTS

FRESH

Dole	½ cup	19	tr	11	4	2
cooked	1 sprout	8	tr	4	2	—
cooked	½ cup	30	tr	17	7	3

FOOD	PORTION	CAL.	FAT	SOD.	CARB.	FIB.
raw	½ cup	19	tr	11	4	—
raw	1 sprout	8	tr	5	2	1
FROZEN						
Big Valley						
Whole	5-8 pieces (3 oz)	35	0	9	6	1
Birds Eye						
Brussels Sprouts	½ cup	35	0	15	7	3
Green Giant						
In Butter Sauce	½ cup	40	1	280	8	—
Hanover						
Brussels Sprouts	½ cup	40	0	—	—	—
cooked	½ cup	33	tr	18	6	—

BUCKWHEAT
Wolff's

FOOD	PORTION	CAL.	FAT	SOD.	CARB.	FIB.
Brown Groats Roasted	1 cup (8 oz)	900	4	—	188	—
Flour	1 cup (8 oz)	860	5	—	170	—
Kasha Coarse cooked	¼ cup (1.6 oz)	170	2	10	35	2
Kasha Fine cooked	¼ cup (1.6 oz)	170	2	10	35	2
Kasha Medium cooked	¼ cup (1.6 oz)	170	2	10	35	2
Kasha Whole cooked	¼ cup (1.6 oz)	170	2	10	35	2
White Grits	1 cup (8 oz)	840	3	—	173	—
flour whole groat	1 cup	402	4	—	85	—
groats roasted cooked	½ cup	91	tr	4	20	—
groats roasted uncooked	½ cup	283	2	9	61	—

BUFFALO

FOOD	PORTION	CAL.	FAT	SOD.	CARB.	FIB.
water roasted	3 oz	111	2	48	0	—

BULGUR

FOOD	PORTION	CAL.	FAT	SOD.	CARB.	FIB.
Good Shepherd	¼ cup (43 g)	150	1	0	33	1
Hodgson Mill	¼ cup (1.4 oz)	120	1	0	24	1
cooked	½ cup	76	tr	5	17	—
uncooked	½ cup	239	tr	12	53	—

BURBOT (FISH)

FOOD	PORTION	CAL.	FAT	SOD.	CARB.	FIB.
fresh baked	3 oz	98	1	106	0	—

BURDOCK ROOT

FOOD	PORTION	CAL.	FAT	SOD.	CARB.	FIB.
cooked	1 cup	110	tr	5	26	—
raw	1 cup	85	tr	6	20	—

BUTTER
(*see also* BUTTER BLENDS, BUTTER SUBSTITUTES, MARGARINE)
STICK

FOOD	PORTION	CAL.	FAT	SOD.	CARB.	FIB.
Cabot	1 tsp	35	4	41	0	—
Unsalted	1 tsp	35	4	0	0	—

FOOD	PORTION	CAL.	FAT	SOD.	CARB.	FIB.
Crystal						
Salted	1 tbsp (0.5 oz)	102	11	89	tr	0
Unsalted	1 tbsp (0.5 oz)	102	11	1	tr	0
Land O'Lakes						
Butter	1 tbsp (0.5 oz)	100	11	85	0	—
Light	1 tbsp	50	6	70	0	—
Light Unsalted	1 tbsp	50	6	5	0	—
Unsalted	1 tbsp (0.5 oz)	100	11	0	0	—
butter	1 pat	36	4	41	tr	—
butter	1 stick (4 oz)	813	92	937	tr	—
clarified butter	3½ oz	876	99	—	0	—
TUB						
Land O'Lakes						
Unsalted	1 tbsp	60	7	0	0	—
Whipped	1 tbsp (0.3 oz)	70	7	55	0	—
whipped	4 oz	542	61	625	tr	—
whipped	1 pat	27	3	31	tr	—

BUTTER BEANS

CANNED

Allen						
Baby	½ cup (4.5 oz)	120	1	460	22	6
Large	½ cup (4.5 oz)	120	1	290	20	7
Hanover						
Butter Beans	½ cup	80	0	—	—	—
In Sauce	½ cup	100	0	—	—	—
Luck's						
Speckled Seasoned w/ Pork	7.5 oz	230	8	—	—	—
S&W						
Tender Cooked	½ cup	100	0	440	19	—
Trappey						
Baby White With Bacon	½ cup (4.5 oz)	130	2	350	21	6
Large White With Bacon	½ cup (4.5 oz)	110	1	300	21	6

BUTTER BLENDS

(*see also* BUTTER, BUTTER SUBSTITUTES, MARGARINE)

STICK

Blue Bonnet						
Better Blend	1 tbsp	90	11	95	0	—
Better Blend Unsalted	1 tbsp	90	11	0	0	—
Country Morning						
Blend	1 tbsp	100	11	90	0	—
Blend Light	1 tbsp (0.5 oz)	50	6	110	0	—
Blend Unsalted	1 tbsp	100	11	0	0	—
butter blend	1 stick	811	91	1013	1	—

FOOD	PORTION	CAL.	FAT	SOD.	CARB.	FIB.
TUB						
Blue Bonnet						
Better Blend	1 tbsp	90	11	95	0	—
Country Morning						
Blend Light	1 tbsp (0.5 oz)	50	6	90	0	—
Blend Tub	1 tbsp	100	11	80	0	—
Downey's						
Cinnamon Honey-Butter	1 tbsp	52	1	5	—	—
Original Honey-Butter	1 tbsp	52	1	5	—	—
Le Slim Cow						
Tub	1 tbsp	40	4	15	—	—
Touch of Butter	1 tbsp (0.5 oz)	60	7	110	0	0

BUTTER SUBSTITUTES

(*see also* BUTTER BLENDS, MARGARINE)

FOOD	PORTION	CAL.	FAT	SOD.	CARB.	FIB.
Butter Buds						
Mix	1 tsp (2 g)	5	0	75	2	—
Sprinkles	1 tsp (2 g)	5	0	120	2	—
Molly McButter						
w/ Bacon	½ tsp (1 g)	4	tr	62	1	—
w/ Cheese	½ tsp (0.9 g)	4	tr	55	tr	—
w/ Sour Cream	½ tsp (1.1 g)	4	tr	69	1	—
Watkins						
Butter Sprinkles	1 tsp (2 g)	5	0	170	1	0
Imitation Butter Flavored Mist	1 tbsp (0.5 oz)	120	14	0	0	0

BUTTERBUR

FOOD	PORTION	CAL.	FAT	SOD.	CARB.	FIB.
canned fuki chopped	1 cup	3	tr	5	tr	—
fresh fuki raw	1 cup	13	tr	7	3	—

BUTTERFISH

FOOD	PORTION	CAL.	FAT	SOD.	CARB.	FIB.
baked	3 oz	159	9	97	0	—
fillet baked	1 oz	47	3	29	0	—

BUTTERNUTS

FOOD	PORTION	CAL.	FAT	SOD.	CARB.	FIB.
dried	1 oz	174	16	0	3	—

BUTTERSCOTCH

(*see also* CANDY)

FOOD	PORTION	CAL.	FAT	SOD.	CARB.	FIB.
Nestle						
Morsels Butterscotch	1 tbsp	80	4	15	10	—

CABBAGE

FRESH

FOOD	PORTION	CAL.	FAT	SOD.	CARB.	FIB.
Dole						
	1/12 med head	18	0	30	3	2
Napa shredded	½ cup	6	tr	3	1	tr

FOOD	PORTION	CAL.	FAT	SOD.	CARB.	FIB.
Fresh Express						
Cole Slaw	1½ cups (3 oz)	25	0	25	6	2
chinese pak-choi raw shredded	½ cup	5	tr	23	1	—
chinese pak-choi shredded cooked	½ cup	10	tr	29	2	—
chinese pe-tsai raw shredded	1 cup	12	tr	7	2	—
chinese pe-tsai shredded cooked	1 cup	16	tr	11	3	—
danish raw	1 head (2 lbs)	228	2	164	49	18
danish raw shredded	½ cup (1.2 oz)	9	tr	6	2	tr
danish shredded cooked	½ cup (2.6 oz)	17	tr	6	3	1
green raw	1 head (2 lbs)	228	2	164	49	18
green raw shredded	½ cup (1.2 oz)	9	tr	6	2	tr
green shredded cooked	½ cup (2.6 oz)	17	tr	6	3	1
red raw shredded	½ cup	10	tr	4	2	1
red shredded cooked	½ cup	16	tr	6	3	—
savoy raw shredded	½ cup	10	tr	10	2	—
savoy shredded cooked	½ cup	18	tr	17	4	—
HOME RECIPE						
coleslaw w/ dressing	¾ cup	147	11	267	13	—
TAKE-OUT						
coleslaw w/ dressing	½ cup	42	2	14	7	—
stuffed cabbage	1 (6 oz)	373	22	1007	18	—
sweet & sour red cabbage	4 oz	61	3	—	8	3
vinegar & oil coleslaw	3.5 oz	150	9	480	16	—

CAKE

(see also BROWNIE, COOKIE, DANISH PASTRY, DOUGHNUT, PIE)

FROSTING/ICING

Betty Crocker						
Butter Pecan Ready-to-Spread	1/12 tub	170	7	50	26	—
Cherry Ready-to-Spread	1/12 tub	160	6	50	27	—
Chocolate Chip Ready-to-Spread	1/12 tub	170	7	30	27	—
Chocolate Fudge as prep	1/12 mix	180	6	70	30	—
Chocolate Light Ready-to-Spread	1/12 tub	130	2	60	28	—
Chocolate Ready-to-Spread	1/12 tub	160	7	60	24	—
Chocolate With Candy Coated Chocolate Chips Ready-to-Spread	1/12 tub	160	7	60	24	—

FOOD	PORTION	CAL.	FAT	SOD.	CARB.	FIB.
Betty Crocker (CONT.)						
Chocolate With Dinosaurs Ready-to-Spread	1/12 tub	160	7	60	24	—
Chocolate With Turbo Racers Ready-to-Spread	1/12 tub	160	7	60	24	—
Coconut Pecan as prep	1/12 mix	180	8	50	19	—
Coconut Pecan Ready-to-Spread	1/12 tub	160	9	80	20	—
Cream Cheese Ready-to-Spread	1/12 tub	170	7	70	26	—
Creamy Milk Chocolate as prep	1/12 mix	170	5	40	29	—
Creamy Vanilla as prep	1/12 mix	170	5	50	32	—
Dark Dutch Fudge Ready-to-Spread	1/12 tub	160	7	70	22	—
Lemon Ready-to-Spread	1/12 tub	170	6	70	28	—
Milk Chocolate Light Ready-to-Spread	1/12 tub	140	2	50	29	—
Milk Chocolate Ready-to-Spread	1/12 tub	160	6	55	25	—
Rainbow Chip Ready-to-Spread	1/12 tub	170	7	30	27	—
Sour Cream Chocolate Ready-to-Spread	1/12 tub	160	7	100	23	—
Sour Cream White Ready-to-Spread	1/12 tub	160	6	50	27	—
Vanilla Light Ready-to-Spread	1/12 tub	140	2	30	30	—
Vanilla Ready-to-Spread	1/12 tub	160	6	30	27	—
Vanilla With Teddy Bears Ready-to-Spread	1/12 tub	160	6	25	27	—
White Fluffy as prep	1/12 mix	70	0	40	16	—
Duncan Hines						
Chocolate Creamy Homestyle	1 oz	130	5	95	20	2
Milk Chocolate Creamy Homestyle	1 oz	130	5	95	20	1
Vanilla Creamy Homestyle	1 oz	140	5	60	22	1
Estee						
Lite Frosting as prep	3 tbsp (0.7 oz)	100	3	0	20	0

FOOD	PORTION	CAL.	FAT	SOD.	CARB.	FIB.
Jiffy						
Fudge	¼ cup (1.2 oz)	150	4	150	28	tr
White	¼ cup (1.2 oz)	150	5	150	27	0
Pillsbury						
Cake & Cookie Decorator Chocolate	1 tbsp	60	2	0	11	—
Cake & Cookie Decorator all colors except chocolate	1 tbsp	70	2	0	12	—
Chocolate Fudge	for ⅛ cake	110	5	65	17	—
Coconut Almond Frosting Mix	for 1/12 cake	160	10	85	16	—
Coconut Pecan Frosting Mix	for 1/12 cake	150	7	105	20	—
Fluffy White Frosting Mix	for 1/12 cake	60	0	65	15	—
Frost It Hot Chocolate	for ⅛ cake	50	0	50	12	—
Frost It Hot Fluffy White	for ⅛ cake	50	0	50	12	—
Frosting Supreme Caramel Pecan	for 1/12 cake	160	8	70	21	—
Frosting Supreme Chocolate Chip	for 1/12 cake	150	5	70	27	—
Frosting Supreme Chocolate Fudge	for 1/12 cake	150	6	80	24	—
Frosting Supreme Chocolate Mint	for 1/12 cake	150	7	80	24	—
Frosting Supreme Coconut Almond	for 1/12 cake	150	9	60	17	—
Frosting Supreme Coconut Pecan	for 1/12 cake	160	10	60	17	—
Frosting Supreme Cream Cheese	for 1/12 cake	160	6	115	26	—
Frosting Supreme Double Dutch	for 1/12 cake	140	6	45	22	—
Frosting Supreme Lemon	for 1/12 cake	160	6	80	26	—
Frosting Supreme Milk Chocolate	for 1/12 cake	150	6	60	23	—
Frosting Supreme Mocha	for 1/12 cake	150	6	60	24	—
Frosting Supreme Sour Cream Vanilla	for 1/12 cake	160	6	80	27	—
Frosting Supreme Strawberry	for 1/12 cake	160	6	75	26	—
Frosting Supreme Vanilla	for 1/12 cake	160	6	75	26	—

FOOD	PORTION	CAL.	FAT	SOD.	CARB.	FIB.
Pillsbury (CONT.)						
Funfetti Chocolate Fudge	½₁₂ can	140	6	80	22	—
Funfetti Vanilla Pink	½₁₂ can	150	6	70	24	—
Funfetti Vanilla White	½₁₂ can	150	6	70	24	—
Vanilla	for ⅛ cake	120	5	60	19	—
chocolate as prep w/ butter	½₁₂ box (1.5 oz)	161	6	63	30	—
chocolate as prep w/ butter	1 box (13.7 oz)	1908	65	754	357	—
chocolate as prep w/ butter home recipe	½₁₂ recipe (1.8 oz)	200	6	95	39	—
chocolate as prep w/ butter home recipe	1 recipe (21.1 oz)	2409	69	1144	467	—
chocolate as prep w/ margarine	½₁₂ box (1.5 oz)	161	6	69	30	—
chocolate as prep w/ margarine	1 box (13.7 oz)	1909	65	819	357	—
chocolate as prep w/ margarine home recipe	½₁₂ recipe (1.8 oz)	200	6	103	39	—
chocolate as prep w/ margarine home recipe	1 recipe (21.1 oz)	2411	69	1235	468	—
chocolate ready-to-use	1 pkg (16 oz)	1834	81	845	292	—
chocolate ready-to-use	½₁₂ pkg (1.3 oz)	151	7	70	24	—
coconut ready-to-use	1 pkg (16 oz)	1903	111	899	244	—
coconut ready-to-use	½₁₂ pkg (1.3 oz)	157	9	74	20	—
cream cheese ready-to-use	½₁₂ pkg (1.3 oz)	157	7	90	25	—
cream cheese ready-to-use	1 pkg (16 oz)	1906	80	1094	308	—
glaze home recipe	1 recipe (11.5 oz)	1173	26	307	240	—
glaze home recipe	½₁₂ recipe (1 oz)	97	2	25	20	—
seven minute home recipe	½₁₂ recipe (1.1 oz)	102	0	55	26	—
seven minute home recipe	1 recipe (13.6 oz)	1231	0	859	312	—
sour cream ready-to-use	½₁₂ pkg (1.3 oz)	157	7	78	26	—
sour cream ready-to-use	1 pkg (16 oz)	1904	80	943	312	—
vanilla as prep w/ butter	½₁₂ pkg (1.5 oz)	182	7	90	30	—
vanilla as prep w/ butter	1 pkg (14.5 oz)	2188	86	1082	366	—
vanilla as prep w/ butter home recipe	1 recipe (20.1 oz)	1972	24	366	448	—
vanilla as prep w/ butter home recipe	½₁₂ recipe (1.7 oz)	165	2	31	38	—
vanilla as prep w/ margarine	½₁₂ pkg (1.5 oz)	182	7	96	30	—
vanilla as prep w/ margarine	1 pkg (14.5 oz)	2190	86	1149	366	—
vanilla as prep w/ margarine home recipe	1 recipe (20.1 oz)	2326	62	1175	454	—

FOOD	PORTION	CAL.	FAT	SOD.	CARB.	FIB.
vanilla as prep w/ margarine home recipe	1/12 recipe (1.7 oz)	195	5	98	38	—
vanilla ready-to-use	1/12 pkg (1.3 oz)	159	6	34	26	—
vanilla ready-to-use	1 pkg (16 oz)	1936	78	418	321	—
white as prep w/ water	1 pkg (11.1 oz)	770	0	490	197	—
white as prep w/ water	1/12 pkg (0.9 oz)	64	0	40	16	—
FROZEN						
Pepperidge Farm						
Amhurst Apple Crumb Coffee Cake	1	220	11	150	30	—
Apple 'N Spice Bake Dessert Lights	1 piece (4¼ oz)	170	2	105	37	—
Apple Turnover	1	300	17	210	34	—
Berkshire Apple Crisp	1	250	8	130	43	1
Blueberry Turnovers	1	310	19	230	32	—
Boston Cream Supreme	1 piece (2⅞ oz)	290	14	190	39	—
Butter Pound	1 slice (1 oz)	130	7	150	16	—
Carrot Classic	1 cake	260	16	280	32	—
Carrot w/ Cream Cheese Icing	1 slice (1½ oz)	150	9	160	19	—
Charleston Peach Melba Shortcake	1	220	5	170	41	—
Cherries Supreme Dessert Lights	1 piece (3¼ oz)	170	11	35	38	—
Cherry Turnover	1	310	19	280	32	—
Chocolate Supreme	1 piece (2⅞ oz)	300	16	140	37	—
Chocolate Fudge Large Layer	1 slice (1⅝ oz)	180	10	140	23	—
Chocolate Fudge Strip Large Layer	1 piece (1⅝ oz)	170	9	140	20	—
Chocolate Mousse Cake Dessert Lights	1 piece (2½ oz)	190	9	260	25	—
Cholesterol Free Pound	1 slice (1 oz)	110	6	85	13	—
Coconut Classic	1 cake	230	11	160	31	—
Coconut Large Layer	1 slice (1⅝ oz)	180	8	120	24	—
Devil's Food Large Layer	1 slice (1⅝ oz)	180	9	135	24	—
Double Chocolate Classic	1 cake	250	13	180	31	—
Fruit Squares Apple	1	220	12	170	27	—
Fruit Squares Cherry	1	230	12	180	28	—
Fudge Golden Classic	1 cake	260	14	160	34	—
German Chocolate Classic	1 cake	250	13	230	29	—

FOOD	PORTION	CAL.	FAT	SOD.	CARB.	FIB.
Pepperidge Farm (CONT.)						
German Chocolate Large Layer	1 slice (1⅝ oz)	180	10	170	22	—
Golden Large Layer	1 slice (1⅝ oz)	180	9	110	24	—
Lemon Cake Supreme Dessert Lights	1 piece (2¾ oz)	170	5	100	26	—
Lemon Coconut Classic Cake	3 oz	280	13	—	—	—
Lemon Coconut Supreme	1 piece (3 oz)	280	13	220	38	—
Lemon Cream Supreme	1 piece (1⅝ oz)	170	9	120	21	—
Manhattan Strawberry Cheesecake	1	300	9	250	49	—
Peach Melba Supreme	1 (3⅛ oz)	270	7	135	50	—
Peach Parfait Dessert Lights	1 piece (4¼ oz)	150	5	70	24	—
Peach Turnover	1	310	18	260	34	—
Pineapple Cream Supreme	1 piece (2 oz)	190	7	130	28	—
Raspberry Turnovers	1	310	17	260	36	—
Raspberry Vanilla Swirl Dessert Lights	1 piece (3¼ oz)	160	5	140	25	—
Strawberry Shortcake Dessert Lights	1 piece (3 oz)	170	5	50	30	1
Strawberry Cream Supreme	1 piece (2 oz)	190	7	120	30	—
Strawberry Strip Large Layer	1 piece (1½ oz)	160	8	120	21	—
Vanilla Fudge Swirl Classic	1 cake	250	11	160	33	—
Vanilla Large Layer	1 slice (1⅝ oz)	190	8	120	25	—
Pet-Ritz						
Cobbler Apple	⅙ cake (4.33 oz)	290	9	—	50	—
Cobbler Blackberry	⅙ cake (4.33 oz)	250	10	—	39	—
Cobbler Blueberry	⅙ cake (4.33 oz)	270	12	—	50	—
Cobbler Cherry	⅙ cake (4.33 oz)	280	10	—	46	—
Cobbler Peach	⅙ cake (4.33 oz)	260	10	—	46	—
Cobbler Strawberry	⅙ cake (4.33 oz)	290	9	—	50	—
Sara Lee						
Apple Crisp Light	1 (3 oz)	150	2	130	31	—
Banana Single Layer Iced	1 slice (1.7 oz)	170	6	160	28	—
Black Forest Light	1 slice (3.6 oz)	170	5	85	34	—
Black Forest Two Layer	1 slice (2.5 oz)	190	8	100	28	—

FOOD	PORTION	CAL.	FAT	SOD.	CARB.	FIB.
Sara Lee (CONT.)						
Carrot Light	1 slice (2.5 oz)	170	4	75	30	—
Carrot Single Layer Iced	1 slice (2.4 oz)	250	13	240	30	—
Cheesecake Original Strawberry	1 slice (3.2 oz)	222	8	171	34	—
Cheesecake Original Cherry	1 slice (3.2 oz)	243	8	164	35	—
Cheesecake Original Plain	1 slice (2.8 oz)	230	11	153	27	—
Chocolate Free & Light	1 slice (1.7 oz)	110	0	140	26	—
Coffee Cake All Butter Butter Streusel	1 slice (1.4 oz)	160	7	160	20	—
Coffee Cake All Butter Cheese	1 slice (2 oz)	210	11	220	25	—
Coffee Cake All Butter Pecan	1 slice (1.4 oz)	160	8	180	19	—
Double Chocolate Light	1 (2.5 oz)	150	5	65	23	—
Double Chocolate Three Layer	1 slice (2.2 oz)	220	11	130	26	—
French Cheese	1 slice (2.9 oz)	250	16	120	23	—
French Cheesecake Light	1 (3.2 oz)	150	4	90	24	—
Lemon Cream Light	1 (3.2 oz)	180	6	60	29	—
Pound All Butter Family Size	1 slice (1 oz)	130	7	85	14	—
Pound All Butter Original	1 slice (1 oz)	130	7	85	14	—
Pound Free & Light	1 slice (1 oz)	70	0	105	17	—
Strawberry French Cheesecake Light	1 (3.5 oz)	150	2	65	29	—
Strawberry Shortcake Two Layer	1 slice (2.5 oz)	190	8	90	26	—
Strawberry Yogurt Dessert Free & Light	1 slice (2.2 oz)	120	1	90	26	—
Weight Watchers						
Apple Crisp	1 (3.5 oz)	190	5	190	40	—
Brownie Cheesecake	1 (3.5 oz)	200	5	260	34	—
Cheese Sweet Roll	1 (2.25 oz)	180	4	—	32	—
Cherries And Cream Cake	1 (3 oz)	150	2	200	30	—
Chocolate	1 (2.5 oz)	180	5	250	31	—
Chocolate Eclair	1 (2.1 oz)	120	4	110	19	—
Coffee Cake With Cinnamon Streusel	1 (2.25 oz)	160	4	—	27	—
Double Fudge	1 piece (2.75 oz)	190	4	150	34	—
Strawberry Cheesecake	1 piece (3.9 oz)	180	4	210	28	—

FOOD	PORTION	CAL.	FAT	SOD.	CARB.	FIB.
boston cream pie	⅙ cake (3.2 oz)	232	8	132	40	1
eclair w/ chocolate icing & custard filling	1	205	10	—	—	—
HOME RECIPE						
angelfood	1/12 cake (1.9 oz)	142	tr	96	32	1
apple crisp	1 recipe 6 serv (29.6 oz)	1377	31	1537	273	—
apple crisp	½ cup (5 oz)	230	5	257	46	—
boston cream pie	⅙ cake (3.3 oz)	293	12	309	43	1
carrot w/ cream cheese icing	1/12 cake (3.9 oz)	484	29	273	52	—
carrot w/ cream cheese icing	1 cake 10 in diam	6175	328	4470	775	—
cheesecake	1/12 cake (4.5 oz)	456	9	362	32	—
cheesecake w/ cherry topping	1/12 cake (5 oz)	359	23	254	33	—
chocolate cupcake creme filled w/ frosting	1 (1.8 oz)	188	7	213	30	—
chocolate w/o frosting	1/12 cake (3.3 oz)	340	14	299	51	—
chocolate w/o frosting	2 layers (39.9 oz)	4067	172	3581	608	—
coffeecake creme-filled chocolate frosting	⅙ cake (3.2 oz)	298	10	290	49	2
coffeecake crumb topped cinnamon	1/12 cake (2.1 oz)	240	12	233	30	2
cream puff shell	1 (2.3 oz)	239	17	368	15	—
cream puff w/ custard filling	1 (4.6 oz)	336	20	444	30	—
eclair	1 (3 oz)	262	16	337	24	—
fruitcake	1/36 cake (2.9 oz)	302	10	121	54	3
fruitcake dark	1 cake 7½ in x 2¼ in	5185	228	2123	738	—
gingerbread	1/9 cake (2.6 oz)	264	12	242	36	2
pineapple upside down	1/9 cake (4 oz)	367	14	367	58	—
pound	1 loaf 8½ in x 3½ in	1935	94	1645	265	—
pound cake	1 slice (1 oz)	120	5	96	15	—
sheet cake w/ white frosting	1 cake 9 in sq	4020	129	2488	694	—
sheet cake w/ white frosting	1/9 cake	445	14	275	77	—
sheet cake w/o frosting	1 cake 9 in sq	2830	108	2331	434	—
sheet cake w/o frosting	1/9 cake	315	12	258	48	—
shortcake	1 (2.3 oz)	225	9	329	32	—
sponge	1/12 cake (2.2 oz)	140	2	107	27	—
white w/ coconut frosting	1/12 cake (3.9 oz)	399	12	318	71	—

FOOD	PORTION	CAL.	FAT	SOD.	CARB.	FIB.
white w/o frosting	1/12 cake (2.6 oz)	264	9	242	42	—
yellow w/o frosting	2 layers (28.7 oz)	2947	119	2803	433	—
yellow w/o frosting	1/12 cake (2.4 oz)	245	10	233	36	—
MIX						
Aunt Jemima						
Coffee Cake Easy Mix	1/3 cup (1.4 oz)	170	5	240	30	1
Betty Crocker						
Angel Food Confetti	1/12 cake	150	0	300	34	—
Angel Food Lemon Custard	1/12 cake	150	0	300	34	—
Angel Food Traditional	1/12 cake	130	0	170	30	—
Angel Food White	1/12 cake	150	0	300	34	—
Apple Streusel MicroRave	1/6 cake	240	11	190	33	—
Apple Streusel MicroRave No Cholesterol Recipe	1/6 cake	210	8	200	33	—
Butter Chocolate	1/12 cake	280	14	400	35	—
Butter Pecan No Cholesterol Recipe	1/12 cake	220	7	320	35	—
Butter Pecan SuperMoist	1/12 cake	250	11	320	35	—
Butter Yellow	1/12 cake	260	11	340	37	—
Carrot	1/12 cake	250	10	300	36	—
Carrot No Cholesterol Recipe	1/12 cake	210	6	300	36	—
Cherry Chip	1/12 cake	190	3	270	37	—
Chocolate Chocolate Chip	1/12 cake	260	12	400	34	—
Chocolate Chip	1/12 cake	290	15	300	35	—
Chocolate Chip No Cholesterol Recipe	1/12 cake	220	8	300	35	—
Chocolate Fudge	1/12 cake	260	12	450	35	—
Chocolate Pudding Classic Dessert	1/6 cake	230	5	250	44	—
Cinnamon Pecan Streusel Microwave	1/6 cake	280	12	220	40	—
Cinnamon Pecan Streusel Microwave No Cholesterol	1/6 cake	230	7	220	40	—
Devil's Food	1/12 cake	260	12	430	35	—
Devil's Food Chocolate Frosting MicroRave	1/6 cake	310	17	250	37	—
Devil's Food No Cholesterol Recipe	1/12 cake	220	7	430	35	—

FOOD	PORTION	CAL.	FAT	SOD.	CARB.	FIB.
Betty Crocker (CONT.)						
Devil's Food SuperMoist Light	1/12 cake	200	4	340	36	—
Devil's Food SuperMoist Light No Cholesterol Recipe	1/12 cake	180	3	370	36	—
Devil's Food With Chocolate Frosting MicroRave Single	1	440	18	480	64	—
German Chocolate	1/12 cake	260	12	420	35	—
German Chocolate Chocolate Frosting MicroRave	1/6 cake	320	18	250	37	—
German Chocolate No Cholesterol Recipe	1/12 cake	220	8	420	35	—
Gingerbread Classic Dessert	1/9 cake	220	7	330	35	—
Gingerbread Classic Dessert No Cholesterol Recipe	1/9 cake	210	6	330	35	—
Golden Pound Classic Dessert	1/12 cake	200	9	170	28	—
Golden Vanilla	1/12 cake	280	14	270	36	—
Golden Vanilla No Cholesterol Recipe	1/12 cake	220	7	270	36	—
Golden Vanilla Rainbow Chip Frosting MicroRave	1/6 cake	320	18	230	40	—
Lemon	1/12 cake	260	11	280	37	—
Lemon Chiffon Classic Dessert	1/12 cake	200	5	200	36	—
Lemon No Cholesterol Recipe	1/12 cake	220	7	280	37	—
Lemon Pudding Classic Dessert	1/6 cake	230	5	270	45	—
Marble	1/12 cake	260	11	290	36	—
Marble No Cholesterol Recipe	1/12 cake	220	7	290	36	—
Milk Chocolate	1/12 cake	260	12	340	34	—
Milk Chocolate No Cholesterol Recipe	1/12 cake	210	7	340	34	—
Pineapple Upsidedown Classic Dessert	1/9 cake	250	10	210	39	—
Rainbow Chip	1/12 cake	250	11	320	35	—

FOOD	PORTION	CAL.	FAT	SOD.	CARB.	FIB.
Betty Crocker (CONT.)						
Sour Cream Chocolate	1/12 cake	260	12	430	35	—
Sour Cream Chocolate No Cholesterol Recipe	1/12 cake	220	8	430	35	—
Sour Cream White	1/12 cake	180	3	290	36	—
Spice	1/12 cake	260	11	320	36	—
Spice No Cholesterol Recipe	1/12 cake	220	7	320	36	—
White	1/12 cake	240	9	270	36	—
White No Cholesterol Recipe	1/12 cake	220	7	270	36	—
White SuperMoist Light	1/12 cake	180	3	330	37	—
Yellow	1/12 cake	260	11	300	36	—
Yellow Chocolate Frosting MicroRave	1/6 cake	300	17	220	36	—
Yellow No Cholesterol Recipe	1/12 cake	220	7	300	36	—
Yellow SuperMoist Light	1/12 cake	200	4	310	37	—
Yellow SuperMoist Light No Cholesterol Recipe	1/12 cake	190	3	330	37	—
Yellow With Chocolate Frosting MicroRave Single	1	440	19	500	64	—
Bisquick						
Reduced Fat	1/2 cup (2 oz)	210	4	660	39	—
Dromedary						
Carrot	1/12 cake	232	15	292	23	—
Cobbler Apple Crumb	1/6 cake	237	6	490	41	—
Cobbler Cherry Crumb	1/6 cake	231	6	160	42	—
Date Nut	1/12 cake	183	8	248	26	—
Date Nut Roll	1/2 in slice	80	2	160	13	—
Gingerbread	1 piece (2 in x 2 in)	100	2	190	19	—
Pound	1/2 in slice	150	6	160	21	—
Duncan Hines						
Angel Food	1/12 pkg (1.3 oz)	140	0	115	30	1
Cupcake Yellow With Chocolate Frosting	1	180	0	140	29	—
Devil's Food Moist Deluxe	1/12 cake (1.5 oz)	290	15	390	34	1
French Vanilla Moist Deluxe	1/12 cake (1.5 oz)	250	11	270	36	0
Fudge Marble Moist Deluxe	1/12 cake (1.5 oz)	250	11	270	36	0
Lemon Supreme Moist Deluxe	1/12 cake (1.5 oz)	250	11	270	36	0

FOOD	PORTION	CAL.	FAT	SOD.	CARB.	FIB.
Duncan Hines (CONT.)						
Yellow Moist Deluxe	1/12 cake (1.5 oz)	250	11	270	36	—
Estee						
Lite White as prep	1/8 cake (1.7 oz)	200	4	170	38	tr
Lite Chocolate	1/8 cake (1.7 oz)	190	4	264	36	1
Lite Pound as prep	1/8 cake (1.7 oz)	200	4	170	38	tr
Hain						
Whole Wheat Baking Mix	1½ oz	150	1	680	30	5
Jell-O						
Cheesecake	1/8 cake	277	13	349	36	—
Cheesecake New York Style	1/8 cake	283	12	421	38	—
Jiffy						
Devil's Food as prep	1/5 cake	220	6	528	40	1
Golden Yellow as prep	1/5 cake	220	5	340	41	1
White as prep	1/5 cake	210	5	320	41	tr
Pillsbury						
Apple Cinnamon Coffee Cake	1/8 cake	240	7	150	40	—
Banana Quick Bread	1/12 loaf	170	6	200	27	—
Blueberry Nut Quick Bread	1/12 loaf	150	4	150	26	—
Butter Recipe	1/12 cake	260	12	370	34	—
Cherry Nut Quick Bread	1/12 loaf	180	5	150	29	—
Chocolate Chip	1/12 cake	270	14	290	33	—
Chocolate Microwave	1/8 cake	210	12	260	23	—
Chocolate With Chocolate Frosting	1/8 cake	300	17	310	35	—
Chocolate With Vanilla Frosting	1/8 cake	300	17	300	36	—
Cranberry Quick Bread	1/12 loaf	160	4	200	30	—
Date Quick Bread	1/12 loaf	160	2	150	32	—
Devil's Food	1/12 cake	270	14	370	32	—
Double Chocolate Supreme Microwave	1/8 cake	330	19	340	39	—
Double Lemon Supreme Microwave	1/8 cake	300	15	210	40	—
Fudge Marble	1/12 cake	270	12	300	36	—
German Chocolate	1/12 cake	250	11	—	—	—
Gingerbread	3 in sq	190	4	310	36	—
Lemon	1/12 cake	250	11	290	34	—
Lemon Microwave	1/8 cake	220	13	180	23	—
Lemon With Lemon Frosting	1/8 cake	300	17	220	37	—

FOOD	PORTION	CAL.	FAT	SOD.	CARB.	FIB.
Pillsbury (CONT.)						
Nut Quick Bread	1/12 loaf	170	6	190	28	—
Strawberry	1/12 cake	260	11	300	37	—
Streusel Swirl Cinnamon	1/16 cake	260	11	200	38	—
Streusel Swirl Cinnamon Microwave	1/8 cake	240	11	180	33	—
Streusel Swirl Lemon	1/16 cake	270	11	340	39	—
Tunnel of Fudge Bundt	1/16 cake	270	12	—	—	—
Tunnel of Fudge Bundt Microwave	1/8 cake	290	17	320	36	—
White	1/12 cake	240	10	290	35	—
Yellow	1/12 cake	260	12	300	36	—
Yellow Microwave	1/8 cake	220	13	170	23	—
Yellow With Chocolate Frosting	1/8 cake	300	17	220	36	—
Royal						
Cheese Cake Lite No-Bake	1/8 pie	130	3	230	22	—
Cheese Cake Real No-Bake	1/8 pie	160	3	250	29	—
Wanda's						
Double Chocolate	1/4 cup mix per serv (1.4 oz)	170	2	460	35	2
angelfood	1/12 cake (1.8 oz)	129	tr	255	29	1
angelfood	10 in cake (20.9 oz)	1535	2	3036	350	9
carrot w/o frosting	1/12 cake (2.5 oz)	239	11	249	33	—
carrot w/o frosting	2 layers (29.6 oz)	2886	133	3001	395	—
cheesecake no-bake	1/8 cake (3.5 oz)	271	13	377	35	2
chocolate pudding type w/o frosting	1/12 cake (2.7 oz)	270	14	402	34	—
chocolate pudding type w/o frosting	2 layers (32.4 oz)	3234	172	4815	409	—
chocolate w/o frosting	1/12 cake (2.3 oz)	198	8	370	32	—
chocolate w/o frosting	2 layers (26.8 oz)	2393	92	4464	384	—
chocolate w/o frosting low sodium	1/10 cake (1.3 oz)	116	3	130	23	—
coffeecake crumb topped cinnamon	1/8 cake (2 oz)	178	5	236	30	2
devil's food w/ chocolate frosting	1 cake 9 in diam	3755	136	2900	645	—
devil's food w/ chocolate frosting	1/16 cake	235	8	181	40	—
devil's food w/o frosting	1/12 cake (2.3 oz)	198	8	370	32	—
fudge w/o frosting	1/12 cake (2.3 oz)	198	8	370	32	—

FOOD	PORTION	CAL.	FAT	SOD.	CARB.	FIB.
german chocolate pudding type w/ coconut nut frosting	1/12 cake (3.9 oz)	404	21	369	55	—
gingerbread	1 cake 8 in sq	1575	39	1733	291	—
gingerbread	1/9 cake (2.4 oz)	207	7	307	34	2
lemon w/o frosting no sugar low sodium	1/10 cake (1.3 oz)	118	3	83	23	—
marble pudding type w/o frosting	2 layers (30.6 oz)	3021	148	2884	412	—
marble pudding type w/o frosting	1/12 cake (2.6 oz)	253	12	242	35	—
white pudding type w/o frosting	1/12 cake (2.4 oz)	244	10	305	36	—
white pudding type w/o frosting	2 layers (29 oz)	2915	123	3654	427	—
white w/o frosting	2 layer cake (26 oz)	2265	57	3593	410	—
white w/o frosting	1/12 cake (2.2 oz)	190	5	301	34	—
white w/o frosting no sugar low sodium	1/10 cake (1.3 oz)	118	3	83	23	—
yellow pudding-type w/o frosting	2 layers (31 oz)	3084	139	3800	421	—
yellow pudding-type w/o frosting	1/12 cake (2.6 oz)	257	12	317	35	—
yellow w/ chocolate frosting	1/16 cake	235	8	157	40	—
yellow w/ chocolate frosting	1 cake 9 in diam	3895	175	3080	620	—
yellow w/o frosting	2 layers (26.5 oz)	2415	71	3580	411	—
yellow w/o frosting	1/12 cake (2.2 oz)	202	6	299	34	—
READY-TO-EAT						
Baker Maid						
Creole Royal Pineapple Apricot	3 slices (5 oz)	270	3	230	61	4
Creole Royal Pineapple Apricot	1 slice (1.7 oz)	90	1	75	20	1
Dutch Mill						
Dessert Shells Chocolate Covered	1 (0.5 oz)	80	5	—	8	0
Entenmann's						
Apple Puffs	1 (3 oz)	280	13	320	39	—
Apple Strudel Old Fashioned	1 serving (1.5 oz)	120	5	110	17	—
Cheese Topped Buns	1 (2.3 oz)	240	12	240	29	—
Cinnamon Buns	1 (2.1 oz)	230	10	200	31	—

FOOD	PORTION	CAL.	FAT	SOD.	CARB.	FIB.
Entenmann's (CONT.)						
Cinnamon Filbert Ring	1 serving (1.5 oz)	190	12	160	19	—
Coffee Cake Cheese	1 serving (1.6 oz)	150	7	140	20	—
Coffee Cake Cheese Filled Crumb	1 serving (1.4 oz)	130	6	140	18	—
Coffee Cake Crumb	1 serving (1.3 oz)	160	7	160	21	—
Danish Ring	1 serving (1.5 oz)	180	10	160	18	—
Danish Ring Pecan	1 serving (1.5 oz)	190	12	130	19	—
Danish Ring Walnut	1 serving (1.5 oz)	190	12	130	19	—
Danish Twist Lemon	1 serving (1.2 oz)	140	7	140	17	—
Danish Twist Raspberry	1 serving (1.2 oz)	140	7	120	18	—
Devil's Food Cake Fudge Iced	1 serving (1.2 oz)	130	5	120	19	—
French Crumb Cake All Butter	1 serving (1.6 oz)	180	8	220	26	—
Louisiana Crunch Cake	1 serving (1.7 oz)	180	8	180	27	—
Pound Loaf All Butter	1 serving (1 oz)	110	5	150	15	—
Pound Loaf Sour Cream	1 serving (1 oz)	120	7	90	14	—
Thick Fudge Golden Cake	1 serving (1.2 oz)	130	6	120	20	—
Freihofer's						
Angel Food	⅕ cake (2 oz)	150	0	410	35	0
Cinnamon Swirl Buns	1 (2.8 oz)	290	9	250	47	1
Coffee Cake Cinnamon Pecan	⅛ cake (2 oz)	220	9	160	33	1
Crumb	⅛ cake (2 oz)	240	11	260	33	1
Homestyle Golden Loaf	⅛ cake (1.8 oz)	200	9	190	28	0
Pound	⅕ cake (2.8 oz)	330	17	330	41	0
Hostess						
Angel Food Ring	⅙ cake (1.6 oz)	150	3	220	29	0
Fruit Cake Holiday	⅙ cake (5.3 oz)	490	14	410	93	3
Pound Cake	⅕ cake (3.2 oz)	350	16	360	48	1
Perugina						
Pannettone Au Beurre	⅙ cake (2.9 oz)	310	12	140	47	2
Sinbad						
Baklava	1 piece (2 oz)	337	20	153	44	2
Thomas'						
Date Nut Loaf	1 oz	90	2	170	18	1
angelfood	1⁄12 cake (1 oz)	73	tr	212	16	1
angelfood	1 cake (11.9 oz)	876	3	2548	197	5
bakewell tart	1 slice (3 oz)	410	27	—	39	2
battenburg cake	1 slice (2 oz)	204	10	—	28	1
cheesecake	1 cake 9 in diam	3350	213	2464	317	—
cheesecake	⅙ cake (2.8 oz)	256	18	165	20	2

FOOD	PORTION	CAL.	FAT	SOD.	CARB.	FIB.
cherry fudge w/ chocolate frosting	1/8 cake (2.5 oz)	187	9	160	27	—
chocolate w/ chocolate frosting	1/8 cake (2.2 oz)	235	11	213	35	2
coffeecake cheese	1/6 cake (2.7 oz)	258	12	257	38	1
coffeecake crumb topped cheese	1/6 cake (2.7 oz)	258	12	257	38	1
coffeecake crumb topped cinnamon	1/9 cake (2.2 oz)	263	15	221	29	2
coffeecake fruit	1/8 cake (1.8 oz)	156	5	192	26	—
crumpets toasted	2 (4 oz)	119	1	—	26	2
eccles cake	1 slice (2 oz)	285	16	—	36	1
eclair	1 (1.4 oz)	149	10	—	15	tr
fruitcake	1 piece (1.5 oz)	139	4	116	27	—
madeira cake	1 slice (1 oz)	98	4	—	15	1
panettone dal forno	1/9 cake (1.9 oz)	212	8	120	31	0
pound	1/10 cake (1 oz)	117	6	119	15	—
pound	1 cake (8½ x 3½ x 3 in)	1935	94	1857	257	—
pound	1 slice (1 oz)	110	12	108	15	—
pound fat free	1 oz	80	tr	96	17	—
pound fat free	1 cake (12 oz)	961	4	1158	208	—
sour cream pound	1/10 cake (1 oz)	117	5	120	16	tr
sponge	1/12 cake (1.3 oz)	110	1	93	23	—
strudel apple	1 piece (2½ oz)	195	8	191	29	2
tiramisu	1 cake (4.4 lbs)	5732	421	1107	439	3
tiramisu	1 piece (5.1 oz)	409	30	79	31	tr
treacle tart	1 slice (2.5 oz)	258	10	—	42	1
vanilla slice	1 slice (2½ oz)	248	13	—	30	1
white w/ white frosting	1 cake 9 in diam	4170	148	2827	670	—
white w/ white frosting	1/16 cake	260	9	176	42	—
yellow w/ chocolate frosting	1/8 cake (2.2 oz)	242	11	216	36	1
yellow w/ chocolate frosting	1 cake 9 diam	3895	175	3080	620	—
yellow w/ vanilla frosting	1/8 cake (2.2 oz)	239	9	220	38	—
REFRIGERATED						
Baby Watson						
Cheesecake	1 slice (3.8 oz)	390	30	330	23	2
Cheesecake Light	1/16 cake (3.9 oz)	280	16	270	24	3
Pillsbury						
Apple Turnovers	1	170	8	330	23	—
Cherry Turnovers	1	170	8	320	23	—
Coffee Cake Cinnamon Swirl	1/8 of cake	180	9	170	22	—

FOOD	PORTION	CAL.	FAT	SOD.	CARB.	FIB.
Pillsbury (CONT.)						
Coffee Cake Pecan Struesel	⅛ of cake	180	9	170	21	—
Pastry Pockets	1	240	13	520	25	—
SNACK						
Drake's						
Coffee Cake	1 (1.1 oz)	140	6	90	18	—
Coffee Cake Chocolate Crumb	1 (2.5 oz)	245	9	206	38	—
Coffee Cake Cinnamon Crumb	½₂ cake (1.3 oz)	150	6	110	22	—
Coffee Cake Small	1 (2 oz)	220	9	160	33	—
Devil Dog	1 (1.5 oz)	160	6	135	24	—
Funny Bones	1 (1.25 oz)	150	8	110	18	—
Light & Fruity Apple	1 (1.2 oz)	90	1	110	20	—
Light & Fruity Blueberry	1 (1.2 oz)	90	1	95	20	—
Light & Fruity Cinnamon Raisin	1 (1.2 oz)	90	1	105	19	—
Pound Cake	1	110	5	70	16	—
Ring Ding	1 (1.5 oz)	180	10	115	23	—
Ring Ding Mint	1 (1.5 oz)	190	11	115	22	—
Sunny Doodle	1 (1 oz)	100	3	100	16	—
Yankee Doodle	1 (1 oz)	100	4	110	16	—
Yodel's	1 (1 oz)	150	9	65	16	—
Greenfield						
Blondie Apple Spice	1 (1.4 oz)	120	0	65	28	0
Blondie Chocolate Chip	1 (1.4 oz)	120	0	65	29	0
Hostess						
Apple Twist	1 (2.5 oz)	220	4	270	42	tr
Baseball Yellow Cakes	1 (1.6 oz)	160	3	160	32	0
Choco-Diles	1 (1.8 oz)	210	10	160	31	1
Choco Licious	1 (1.5 oz)	170	6	190	28	1
Cinnaminis Original	5 (2.4 oz)	300	17	230	37	2
Cinnamon Roll	1 (2.3 oz)	220	6	260	39	1
Crumb Cake	1 (1.9 oz)	210	8	135	33	1
Crumb Cake Light	1 (1.8 oz)	150	1	190	35	tr
Cup Cakes Chocolate	1 (1.6 oz)	170	5	160	28	tr
Cup Cakes Chocolate Light	1 (1.4 oz)	120	2	170	26	tr
Cup Cakes Orange	1 (1.5 oz)	160	5	160	28	0
Dessert Cups	1 (1 oz)	90	2	170	18	0
Ding Dongs	1 (1.3 oz)	160	9	110	21	tr
Fruit Loaf	1 (3.8 oz)	350	10	290	67	2
Ho Ho's	1 (1 oz)	130	6	75	17	tr

FOOD	PORTION	CAL.	FAT	SOD.	CARB.	FIB.
Hostess (CONT.)						
Holiday Cakes	1 (1.6 oz)	160	3	160	32	0
Honey Bun Glazed	1 (2.7 oz)	320	19	90	35	2
Honey Bun Iced	1 (3.4 oz)	390	20	220	49	2
Hopper Cakes	1 (1.6 oz)	160	3	160	32	0
Lil Angels	1 (1 oz)	90	2	130	17	0
Pecan Spinners	1 (1 oz)	110	5	65	15	tr
Sno Balls	1 (1.6 oz)	160	5	180	29	1
Suzy Q's	1 (2 oz)	220	9	270	35	2
Suzy Q's Banana	1 (2 oz)	220	10	280	32	tr
Swirls Caramel Pecan	1 (2 oz)	140	15	55	25	1
Tiger Tails	1 (1.5 oz)	160	6	150	26	tr
Twinkies	1 (1.4 oz)	140	4	180	25	0
Twinkies Banana	2 (2.7 oz)	300	13	370	42	tr
Twinkies Devil Food	2 (2.7 oz)	300	12	360	47	2
Twinkies Lights	1 (1.4 oz)	120	2	200	24	0
Twinkies Strawberry Fruit 'n Creme	1 (1.6 oz)	150	3	200	30	tr
Kellogg's						
Pop-Tarts Apple Cinnamon	1 (1.8 oz)	210	5	170	38	1
Pop-Tarts Blueberry	1 (1.8 oz)	210	7	210	36	1
Pop-Tarts Brown Sugar Cinnamon	1 (1.8 oz)	220	9	210	32	1
Pop-Tarts Cherry	1 (1.8 oz)	200	5	220	37	1
Pop-Tarts Chocolate Graham	1 (1.8 oz)	210	6	220	36	1
Pop-Tarts Frosted Blueberry	1 (1.8 oz)	200	5	210	37	1
Pop-Tarts Frosted Brown Sugar Cinnamon	1 (1.8 oz)	210	7	180	34	1
Pop-Tarts Frosted Cherry	1 (1.8 oz)	200	5	220	37	1
Pop-Tarts Frosted Chocolate Fudge	1 (1.8 oz)	200	5	220	37	1
Pop-Tarts Frosted Chocolate Vanilla Creme	1 (1.8 oz)	200	5	230	37	1
Pop-Tarts Frosted Grape	1 (1.8 oz)	200	5	200	38	1
Pop-Tarts Frosted Raspberry	1 (1.8 oz)	210	6	210	37	1
Pop-Tarts Frosted S'mores	1 (1.8 oz)	200	5	200	37	1
Pop-Tarts Frosted Strawberry	1 (1.8 oz)	200	5	170	38	1

FOOD	PORTION	CAL.	FAT	SOD.	CARB.	FIB.
Kellogg's (CONT.)						
Pop-Tarts Minis Frosted Chocolate	1 pkg (1.5 oz)	170	4	200	30	1
Pop-Tarts Minis Frosted Grape	1 pkg (1.5 oz)	170	4	180	32	0
Pop-Tarts Minis Frosted Strawberry	1 pkg (1.5 oz)	170	4	180	32	0
Pop-Tarts Strawberry	1 (1.8 oz)	200	5	180	37	1
Rice Krispies Treats	1 (0.8 oz)	90	2	75	18	0
Lance						
Apple Oatmeal	1 pkg (51 g)	200	9	210	35	—
Dunking Sticks	1 (39 g)	190	10	130	22	—
Fig Cake	1 pkg (60 g)	210	3	90	43	—
Honey Buns	1 (85 g)	330	14	210	48	—
Oatmeal Cake	1 (57 g)	240	11	250	35	—
Pecan Twirls	1 pkg (57 g)	220	8	190	34	—
Raisin Cake	1 (57 g)	230	10	200	35	—
Little Debbie						
Apple Delights	1 pkg (1.2 oz)	140	5	115	24	1
Apple-Roos	1 pkg (1.5 oz)	150	3	80	32	1
Banana Nut Muffin Loaves	1 pkg (1.9 oz)	210	9	210	30	1
Banana Twins	1 pkg (2.2 oz)	250	10	180	40	0
Be My Valentine	1 pkg (2.2 oz)	280	14	150	39	1
Cherry Cordials	1 pkg (1.3 oz)	160	8	100	23	1
Choco-Cakes	1 pkg (2.1 oz)	250	13	170	35	1
Choco-Cakes	1 pkg (2.2 oz)	240	12	180	35	1
Choc-o-Jel	1 pkg (1.2 oz)	150	7	95	21	1
Chocolate	1 pkg (3 oz)	360	17	220	52	1
Chocolate Chip	1 pkg (2.4 oz)	290	15	190	42	1
Chocolate Twins	1 pkg (2.4 oz)	240	9	280	42	1
Christmas Tree Cakes	1 pkg (1.5 oz)	190	9	90	27	0
Coconut	1 pkg (2.4 oz)	300	14	200	42	0
Coconut	1 pkg (2.1 oz)	270	13	180	38	1
Coconut Rounds	1 pkg (1.2 oz)	140	7	85	22	1
Coffee Cake Apple	1 pkg (1.9 oz)	220	7	190	36	1
Coffee Cake Apple Streusel	1 pkg (2 oz)	220	7	200	37	1
Devil Cremes	1 pkg (3.2 oz)	380	17	310	57	1
Devil Cremes	1 pkg (1.6 oz)	190	8	160	28	0
Devil Squares	1 pkg (2.2 oz)	260	13	180	39	1
Easter Basket Cakes	1 pkg (2.5 oz)	310	15	180	44	1
Fancy Cakes	1 pkg (2.4 oz)	300	15	160	42	0
Fudge Crispy	1 pkg (1.1 oz)	170	10	50	20	1

FOOD	PORTION	CAL.	FAT	SOD.	CARB.	FIB.
Little Debbie (CONT.)						
Fudge Rounds	1 pkg (3 oz)	350	14	210	59	2
Fudge Rounds	1 pkg (2.5 oz)	290	12	170	49	2
Fudge Rounds	1 pkg (1.2 oz)	140	5	80	23	1
Golden Cremes	1 pkg (1.5 oz)	170	7	180	25	0
Golden Cremes	1 pkg (3 oz)	330	15	350	50	0
Holiday Cake Chocolate	1 pkg (2.4 oz)	290	14	180	43	1
Holiday Cake Vanilla	1 pkg (2.5 oz)	310	15	180	44	1
Honey Bun	1 pkg (3 oz)	380	23	190	39	4
Honey Bun	1 pkg (4 oz)	510	31	250	53	5
Jelly Rolls	1 pkg (2.1 oz)	230	7	160	41	0
Lemon Stix	1 pkg (1.5 oz)	210	10	45	30	1
Marshmallow Supremes	1 pkg (1.1 oz)	130	5	70	22	1
Mint Sprints	1 pkg (1.5 oz)	230	13	70	28	1
Nutty Bar	1 pkg (2 oz)	290	17	115	34	1
Pecan Twins	1 pkg (2 oz)	220	9	200	32	1
Pumpkin Delights	1 pkg (1.1 oz)	130	5	115	21	1
Smiley Faces Cherry	1 pkg (1.2 oz)	140	5	115	23	1
Smiley Faces Pumpkin	1 pkg (1 oz)	130	5	215	20	1
Snack Cake Chocolate	1 pkg (2.5 oz)	300	15	180	43	1
Snack Cake Vanilla	1 pkg (2.6 oz)	320	16	180	45	1
Spice	1 pkg (2.5 oz)	300	15	230	43	1
Star Crunch	1 pkg (1.1 oz)	140	6	85	21	1
Star Crunch	1 pkg (2.6 oz)	330	14	240	51	1
Swiss Rolls	1 pkg (2.1 oz)	250	12	160	36	1
Swiss Rolls	1 pkg (3.2 oz)	380	18	250	57	1
Swiss Rolls	1 pkg (2.7 oz)	320	15	210	47	1
Teddy Berries	1 pkg (1.2 oz)	130	4	105	23	1
Vanilla	1 pkg (3 oz)	370	18	210	53	0
Vanilla Cremes	1 pkg (1.4 oz)	170	7	125	25	0
Zebra Cakes	1 pkg (2.6 oz)	150	16	180	45	1
Nabisco						
Frosted Strawberry	1 (1.7 oz)	190	5	190	35	1
Pepperidge Farm						
Toaster Tart Apple Cinnamon	1	170	7	120	25	—
Toaster Tart Cheese	1	190	10	180	22	—
Toaster Tart Strawberry	1	190	7	120	28	—
Rice Krispies						
Cereal Bar Chocolate Chip	1 (1 oz)	120	4	60	20	1
Sara Lee						
All Butter Pound	1	200	11	190	23	—
Chocolate Fudge Cake	1	190	10	125	24	—

FOOD	PORTION	CAL.	FAT	SOD.	CARB.	FIB.
Sara Lee (CONT.)						
Classic Cheesecake	1	200	14	150	16	—
Coffee Cake Apple Cinnamon	1	290	13	270	40	—
Coffee Cake Butter Streusel	1	230	12	270	27	—
Coffee Cake Pecan	1	280	16	270	30	—
Deluxe Carrot Cake	1	180	7	200	26	—
Sweet Rewards						
Fat Free Brownie	1 bar (1 oz)	90	0	90	21	<1
Tastykake						
Butter Cream Cream Filled Cupcake	1 (32 g)	120	4	120	20	1
Chocolate Cream Filled Cupcake	1 (34 g)	130	5	130	21	1
Chocolate Cupcake	1 (30 g)	100	3	120	19	1
Creamies Banana Treat	1	138	3	—	—	—
Creamies Chocolate	1	174	7	—	—	—
Creamies Vanilla	1	182	8	—	—	—
Honeybun Glazed	1 pkg (92 g)	360	20	220	42	4
Honeybun Iced	1 pkg (92 g)	350	15	250	50	1
Junior Chocolate	1 pkg (94 g)	340	12	220	57	4
Junior Coconut	1 pkg (94 g)	300	6	300	60	3
Junior Lemon	1 pkg (94 g)	310	7	330	75	1
Junior Orange	1 pkg (94 g)	340	9	240	61	1
Kandy Kake Chocolate	1 (19 g)	80	3	35	13	1
Kandy Kake Coconut	1 (19 g)	80	4	40	11	1
Kandy Kake Peanut Butter	1 (19 g)	90	4	40	11	1
Koffee Kake Cream Filled	1 (29 g)	110	4	80	18	0
Koffee Kake Junior	1 pkg (71 g)	260	8	210	44	1
Kreme Kup	1 (25 g)	90	3	115	15	1
Krimpet Butterscotch	1 (28 g)	100	1	85	19	0
Krimpet Jelly	1 (28 g)	90	1	80	19	1
Krimpet Strawberry	1 (28 g)	100	2	85	20	0
Pastry Pocket Apple	1 (85 g)	320	18	220	38	—
Pastry Pocket Cheese	1 (85 g)	330	19	230	38	1
Pastry Pocket Cherry	1 (85 g)	330	17	230	41	1
Pecan Twirls	1 (28 g)	110	1	75	17	—
Royale Chocolate Cupcake	1 (46 g)	170	7	130	28	2
Tasty Too Chocolate Cream Filled Cupcake	1 (32 g)	100	1	115	21	1
Tasty Too Vanilla Cream Filled Cupcake	1 (32 g)	100	1	120	21	1

FOOD	PORTION	CAL.	FAT	SOD.	CARB.	FIB.
Tastykake (CONT.)						
Tasty Twists	1 (4 g)	18	1	—	3	—
Toast-R-Cakes						
Blueberry	1	110	3	158	18	—
Bran	1	103	3	163	18	—
Corn	1	120	4	142	19	—
Toastettes						
Frosted Blueberry	1 (1.7 oz)	190	5	190	45	1
Frosted Brown Sugar Cinnamon	1 (1.7 oz)	190	5	180	35	1
Frosted Cherry	1 (1.7 oz)	190	5	190	35	1
Frosted Fudge	1 (1.7 oz)	190	5	280	34	3
Strawberry	1 (1.7 oz)	190	5	200	35	1
Well-Bred Loaf						
Banana Bread	1 slice (3.5 oz)	330	11	380	52	tr
Banana Nut	1 slice (4.3 oz)	440	19	350	59	2
Blueberry	1 slice (4.3 oz)	440	16	330	69	1
Carrot	1 slice (4.3 oz)	480	24	125	64	2
Carrot Traditional	1 slice (4.3 oz)	440	16	280	71	2
Chocolate Chip	1 slice (4.3 oz)	490	19	320	74	2
Cinnamon Walnut	1 slice (4.3 oz)	480	18	340	72	1
Coconut Rum	1 slice (4.3 oz)	490	23	330	64	tr
Cranberry	1 slice (4.3 oz)	460	15	320	77	1
Marble	1 slice (4.3 oz)	530	18	390	83	1
Pound All Butter	1 slice (4.3 oz)	470	17	360	73	tr
Pound Mandarin Orange	1 slice (4 oz)	460	18	310	68	tr
Raisin	1 slice (4.3 oz)	460	15	310	76	2
devil's food cupcake w/ chocolate frosting	1	120	4	92	20	—
devil's food w/ creme filling	1 (1 oz)	105	4	105	17	—
sponge w/ creme filling	1 (1.5 oz)	155	5	155	27	—
toaster pastry apple	1 (1.75 oz)	204	5	218	37	—
toaster pastry blueberry	1 (1.75 oz)	204	5	218	37	—
toaster pastry brown sugar cinnamon	1 (1.75 oz)	206	7	212	34	—
toaster pastry cherry	1 (1.75 oz)	204	5	218	37	—
toaster pastry strawberry	1 (1.75 oz)	204	5	218	37	—
TAKE-OUT						
baklava	1 oz	126	9	78	10	1
strudel	1 piece (4.1 oz)	272	8	142	50	3
trifle w/ cream	6 oz	291	16	—	34	1

CALZONE
TAKE-OUT

FOOD	PORTION	CAL.	FAT	SOD.	CARB.	FIB.
cheese	1 (12 oz)	1020	54	1760	86	8

FOOD	PORTION	CAL.	FAT	SOD.	CARB.	FIB.
CANADIAN BACON						
Hormel	2 oz	70	3	610	0	0
Jones	1 slice	30	1	160	tr	—
Oscar Mayer						
Canadian Bacon	2 slices (1.6 oz)	50	2	600	0	0
unheated	2 slices (1.9 oz)	89	4	799	1	—
CANDY						
(see also MARSHMALLOW)						
3 Musketeers						
Bar	1 (2.1 oz)	260	8	110	46	1
Bar	2 fun size (1.2 oz)	140	4	60	25	0
5th Avenue	1 (2.1 oz)	290	13	140	39	—
100 Grand						
Bar	1 bar (1.5 oz)	200	8	75	30	tr
After Eight						
Dark Chocolate Wafer Thin Mints	1	35	1	0	6	—
Baby Ruth						
Fun Size	2 pieces	200	9	95	27	1
Bar None						
Candy	1 (1.5 oz)	240	14	50	23	—
Breath Savers						
Sugar Free Mint Cinnamon	1 piece (2 g)	10	0	0	2	—
Sugar Free Peppermint	1 piece (2 g)	10	0	0	2	—
Sugar Free Spearmint	1 piece (2 g)	10	0	0	2	—
Sugar Free Wintergreen	1 piece (2 g)	10	0	0	2	—
Brock						
Butterscotch Discs	3 pieces (0.6 oz)	70	0	80	17	—
Candy Corn	21 pieces (1.4 oz)	150	0	85	37	—
Candy Rolls	2 rolls (0.5 oz)	50	0	0	12	—
Caramel Dots	3 pieces (1.3 oz)	140	3	50	25	tr
Cinnamon Discs	3 pieces (0.6 oz)	70	0	5	17	—
Circus Peanuts	11 pieces (2.5 oz)	260	0	25	65	—
Coconut Mountains	4 pieces (1.4 oz)	170	6	80	29	—
Fruit Basket	3 pieces (0.6 oz)	60	0	0	15	—
Fruit Kisses	3 pieces (0.6 oz)	70	0	5	17	—
Glitters	2 pieces (0.5 oz)	50	0	15	13	—
Gummy Bears	5 pieces (1.4 oz)	130	0	15	30	—
Gummy Squirms	5 pieces (1.3 oz)	120	0	15	28	—
Jelly Beans	12 pieces (1.4 oz)	140	0	15	36	—
Lemon Drops	3 pieces (0.5 oz)	60	0	5	14	—
Orange Slices	4 pieces (1.5 oz)	140	0	20	36	—

FOOD	PORTION	CAL.	FAT	SOD.	CARB.	FIB.
Brock (CONT.)						
Party Mints	9 pieces (0.5 oz)	60	0	0	15	—
Peanut Butter Crunch	3 pieces (0.6 oz)	80	2	45	15	—
Pops Assorted	2 (0.5 oz)	60	0	5	15	—
Sour Balls	3 pieces (0.6 oz)	70	0	5	17	—
Sour Sharks	23 pieces (2.5 oz)	30	3	45	60	—
Spearmint Starlights	3 pieces (0.6 oz)	60	0	5	16	—
Spice Drops	12 pieces (1.4 oz)	130	0	20	33	—
Starlight Mints	3 pieces (0.6 oz)	60	0	5	16	—
Toffee	6 pieces (1.5 oz)	170	5	45	31	—
Butterfinger						
BB's	1 pkg (1.7 oz)	230	10	90	34	1
Fun Size	2 bars (1.6 oz)	200	8	85	30	1
Cellas						
Chocolate Covered Cherries Dark Chocolate	2 pieces (1 oz)	100	4	—	—	—
Chocolate Covered Cherries Milk Chocolate	2 pieces (1 oz)	110	4	15	18	2
Certs						
Mini Sugar Free	1 piece (0.365 g)	1	0	—	tr	—
Sugar Free	1 piece (1.67 g)	7	0	—	2	—
Charleston Chew						
Chocolate	½ bar	120	3	—	—	—
Strawberry	½ bar	120	3	—	—	—
Vanilla	½ bar	120	3	—	—	—
Charms						
Blow Pop	1 (0.7 oz)	80	0	—	—	—
Pop	1 (0.6 oz)	70	0	—	—	—
Clorets						
Mints	1 piece (1.67 g)	6	0	—	2	—
Crunch						
Fun Size	4 bars (1.5 oz)	200	10	55	25	1
Dove						
Dark Chocolate	1 bar (1.3 oz)	200	12	0	22	2
Dark Chocolate Miniatures	7 (1.5 oz)	220	14	0	26	2
Milk Chocolate	1 bar (1.3 oz)	200	12	25	22	1
Milk Chocolate Miniatures	7 (1.5 oz)	230	13	30	25	1
Truffles	3 (1.2 oz)	200	13	15	19	1
Estee						
Caramels Chocolate & Vanilla No Sugar Added	5 (1.3 oz)	150	5	65	26	0

FOOD	PORTION	CAL.	FAT	SOD.	CARB.	FIB.
Estee (CONT.)						
Dark Chocolate	½ bar (1.4 oz)	200	14	10	23	0
Gum Drops Assorted Fruit Sugar Free	23 (1.4 oz)	140	0	0	36	0
Gum Drops Licorice	23 (1.4 oz)	140	0	0	36	—
Gummy Bears Sugar Free	16 (1.4 oz)	140	0	0	31	—
Hard Candies Assorted Fruit Sugar Free	5 (0.5 oz)	60	0	0	16	0
Hard Candies Assorted Mint Sugar Free	5 (0.5 oz)	60	0	0	16	0
Hard Candies Butterscotch Sugar Free	2 (0.4 oz)	50	0	50	12	—
Hard Candies Peppermint Swirls Sugar Free	3 (0.5 oz)	60	0	0	14	—
Hard Candies Tropical Fruit Sugar Free	5 (0.5 oz)	60	0	0	16	0
Lollipops Assorted Fruit Sugar Free	2 (0.5 oz)	60	0	0	16	—
Milk Chocolate	½ bar (1.4 oz)	230	17	65	17	0
Milk Chocolate With Almonds	½ bar (1.4 oz)	230	17	65	16	0
Milk Chocolate With Crisp Rice	1 bar (2.3 oz)	370	26	110	29	0
Milk Chocolate With Fruit & Nuts	½ bar (1.4 oz)	220	16	65	18	0
Mint Chocolate	½ bar (1.4 oz)	200	14	10	23	0
Peanut Brittle No Sugar Added	⅓ box (1.5 oz)	210	9	115	28	1
Peanut Butter Cups	5 (1.3 oz)	200	12	70	19	1
Peanut Butter Cups	1 (0.3 oz)	40	3	0	3	0
Toffee Sugar Free	5 (0.5 oz)	60	0	0	16	—
Ferreo Rocher						
Candy	3 pieces (1.3 oz)	220	15	35	17	1
Candy	2 pieces (0.9 oz)	150	10	24	11	0
Franklin						
Crunch 'N Munch Candied	1.25 oz	170	7	200	28	1
Crunch 'N Munch Caramel	1.25 oz	160	5	130	28	1
Crunch 'N Munch Maple Walnut	1.25 oz	160	6	180	28	1

FOOD	PORTION	CAL.	FAT	SOD.	CARB.	FIB.
Franklin (CONT.)						
Crunch 'N Munch Toffee	1.25 oz	160	5	210	28	1
Glenny's						
Brown Rice Treats Carob & Mint With Oat Bran	1 bar (1.75 oz)	180	2	20	37	2
Brown Rice Treats Cinnamon & Raisin	1 bar (1.75 oz)	170	1	30	38	—
Brown Rice Treats Peanut & Raisin	1 bar (2 oz)	210	5	29	39	—
Brown Rice Treats Plain & Fancy	1 bar (1.25 oz)	120	1	29	28	—
Brown Rice Treats Raisin Bran	1 bar (1.75 oz)	170	1	17	38	—
Brown Rice Treats Toasted Almond With Oat Bran	1 bar (1.75 oz)	200	5	20	34	2
Fruit Drops Black Cherry	1	6	tr	tr	1	—
Fruit Drops Gentle Mint	1	6	tr	tr	1	—
Fruit Drops Mandarin Orange	1	6	tr	tr	1	—
Fruit Drops Mixed Fruit	1	6	tr	tr	1	—
Fruit Drops Twist Of Lemon	1	6	tr	tr	1	—
Hard Candies Fruit	1	19	tr	tr	4	—
Hard Candies Peppermint	1	19	tr	tr	4	—
Lollipops C Pops	1	35	tr	tr	8	—
Lollipops Fruit	1	21	tr	tr	5	—
Moist & Chewy Coconut Almondine Bar	1 bar (1.5 oz)	190	10	20	22	—
Moist & Chewy Oatmeal Raisin Bar	1 bar (1.5 oz)	160	3	25	30	—
Moist & Chewy Peanut Bar	1 bar (1.5 oz)	180	7	20	24	—
Moist & Chewy Sunflower Bar	1 bar (1.5 oz)	180	7	15	24	—
Snack Bar Fat-Free Apple-Cinnamon	1 (1.25 oz)	120	1	15	28	—
Snack Bar Fat-Free Caramel	1 (1.25 oz)	120	tr	70	29	—
Snack Bar Fat-Free Chocolate	1 (1.25 oz)	120	tr	10	28	—
Snack Bar Fat-Free Raspberry	1 (1.25 oz)	120	tr	15	29	—

FOOD	PORTION	CAL.	FAT	SOD.	CARB.	FIB.
Godiva						
Almond Butter Dome	3 pieces (1.5 oz)	240	17	20	19	0
Bouchee Au Chocolat	1 piece (1.5 oz)	210	11	40	25	0
Bouchee Ivory Raspberry	1 piece (1 oz)	160	9	25	17	0
Gold Ballotin	3 pieces (1.5 oz)	210	10	15	27	0
Truffle Amaretto Di Saronno	2 pieces (1.5 oz)	210	12	25	24	0
Truffle Deluxe Liqueur	2 pieces (1.5 oz)	210	13	25	23	0
Goldenberg's						
Peanut Chews	3 pieces (1.3 oz)	180	9	40	22	1
Good & Plenty						
Snacksize	3 boxes (1.5 oz)	140	0	80	34	—
Hershey						
Amazin' Fruit Gummy Candy	2 snack pkg (1.4 oz)	130	0	45	30	—
Bar	1 (1.55 oz)	240	14	40	25	—
Bar With Almonds	1 (1.45 oz)	230	14	55	20	—
Kisses	9 pieces (1.46 oz)	220	13	35	23	—
Special Dark Sweet Chocolate Bar	1 (1.45 oz)	220	12	5	25	—
Joyva						
Halvah	1.5 oz	240	16	80	16	2
Halvah Chocolate Covered	1 bar (2 oz)	380	23	95	20	3
Jells Raspberry	3 pieces (1.6 oz)	200	3	15	25	tr
Joys Raspberry	1 (1.6 oz)	200	3	15	25	1
Marshmallow Twists Chocolate Covered	2 (1.5 oz)	190	4	20	21	0
Rings Orange & Raspberry	3 pieces (1.5 oz)	190	3	15	23	tr
Sesame Crunch	3 pieces (0.5)	80	4	25	7	0
Sticks Orange	3 pieces (1.6 oz)	200	3	15	25	tr
Twists Vanilla & Cherry	2 pieces (1.5 oz)	190	4	20	21	0
Juicefuls						
Candy	3 pieces (0.5 oz)	60	0	0	15	—
Just Born						
Jelly Beans	1 oz	108	tr	—	—	—
Sugar Coated	1½ oz	148	tr	—	—	—
Toasted Coconut	1⅜ oz	140	2	—	—	—
Krackel						
Bar	1 (1.55 oz)	230	13	80	27	—
Kraft						
Butter Mints	7 (0.5 oz)	60	0	25	14	0

FOOD	PORTION	CAL.	FAT	SOD.	CARB.	FIB.
Kraft (CONT.)						
Caramels	5 (1.4 oz)	170	3	110	32	0
Fudgies	5 (1.4 oz)	180	5	90	32	0
Party Mints	7 (0.5 oz)	60	0	35	14	0
Peanut Brittle	5 pieces (1.3 oz)	170	5	310	29	1
Laffy Taffy						
Apple Chews	1 oz	110	1	55	26	—
Banana Chews	1 oz	110	1	55	26	—
Grape Chews	1 oz	110	1	60	26	—
Passion Punch Chews	1 oz	110	1	50	26	—
Strawberry Chews	1 oz	110	1	55	26	—
Sweet & Sour Cherry Chews	1 oz	110	1	55	26	—
Watermelon Chews	1 oz	110	1	55	26	—
Lance						
Chocolaty Peanut Bar	1 (57 g)	320	18	40	29	—
Peanut Bar	1 pkg (50 g)	260	14	80	24	—
Popscotch	1 pkg (35 g)	160	6	120	24	—
Lifesavers						
Big Tablet Candy Cane	4 pieces (0.5 oz)	60	0	0	16	—
Cards 'N Candy	4 pieces (0.4 oz)	40	0	0	10	—
Christmas Tin	4 pieces (0.5 oz)	60	0	20	16	—
Egg-Sortment	1 roll (0.4 oz)	40	0	0	10	—
Fruit Juicers Lollipops	1	40	0	0	10	0
Gummi Bunnies	3 pkg (1.6 oz)	140	0	0	34	—
Gummi Savers Five Flavor	1 roll (1.5 oz)	130	0	0	32	—
Gummi Savers Five Flavor	1 pkg (1.8 oz)	160	0	0	38	—
Gummi Savers Mixed Berry	1 roll (1.5 oz)	130	0	0	32	—
Gummi Savers Mixed Berry	1 pkg (1.8 oz)	160	0	0	38	—
Gummi Savers Tangy Fruits	1 pkg (1.8 oz)	160	0	0	38	—
Gummi Savers Tangy Fruits	1 roll (1.5 oz)	130	0	0	32	—
Gummi Savers Variety	2 pkg (1.3 oz)	120	0	0	27	—
Gummi Savers Wacky Frootz	1 pkg (1.8 oz)	160	0	0	38	—
Gummi Savers Wacky Frootz	1 roll (1.5 oz)	130	0	0	32	—
Holes Five Flavor	20 pieces (5 g)	20	0	0	5	—
Holes Island Fruit	20 pieces (5 g)	20	0	0	5	—

FOOD	PORTION	CAL.	FAT	SOD.	CARB.	FIB.
Lifesavers (CONT.)						
Holes Sour 'N Sweet	16 pieces (5 g)	20	0	0	5	—
Holes Sunshine Fruits	20 pieces (0.2 oz)	20	0	0	5	—
Holes Super Tart	20 pieces (5 g)	20	0	0	5	—
Holes Tangerine	1 candy	2	0	0	1	0
Holes Wild Fruits	20 pieces (5 g)	20	0	0	5	—
Lollipops Candy Cane	1 (0.4 oz)	40	0	0	10	—
Lollipops Christmas	1 (0.4 oz)	40	0	0	10	—
Lollipops Easter	1 (0.4 oz)	40	0	0	10	—
Lollipops Fruit Flavors	1 (0.4 oz)	45	0	0	11	0
Lollipops Swirled Flavors	1 (0.4 oz)	40	0	0	10	—
Lollipops Valentine	1 (0.4 oz)	40	0	0	10	—
Roll Butter Rum	2 pieces (5 g)	20	0	20	5	—
Roll Candy Cane	4 pieces (0.4 oz)	40	0	0	10	—
Roll Cryst-O-Mint	2 pieces (5 g)	20	0	0	5	—
Roll Five Flavor	2 pieces (5 g)	20	0	0	5	—
Roll Fruits On Fire	2 pieces (5 g)	20	0	0	5	—
Roll Pep-O-Mint	3 pieces (5 g)	20	0	0	5	—
Roll Spear-O-Mint	3 pieces (5 g)	20	0	0	5	—
Roll Sunshine Fruits	2 pieces (5 g)	20	0	0	5	—
Roll Tangy Fruit Swirl	2 pieces (5 g)	20	0	0	5	—
Roll Tangy Fruit Watermelon	1 piece (5 g)	20	0	0	5	—
Roll Tangy Fruits	2 pieces (5 g)	20	0	0	5	—
Roll Tropical Fruits	2 pieces (5 g)	20	0	0	5	—
Roll Wild Cherry	1 piece (5 g)	20	0	0	5	—
Roll Wild Flavors	2 pieces (5 g)	20	0	0	5	—
Roll Wild Sour Berries	2 pieces (5 g)	20	0	0	5	—
Roll Wint-O-Green	3 pieces (5 g)	20	0	0	5	—
Sack'it Butter Rum	4 pieces (0.5 oz)	60	0	65	15	—
Sack'it Five Flavor	4 pieces (0.5 oz)	60	0	0	16	—
Sack'it Holiday Tin	4 pieces (0.5 oz)	60	0	65	16	—
Sack'it Pep-O-Mint	4 pieces (0.5 oz)	60	0	0	16	—
Sack'it Tangy Fruits	4 pieces (0.5 oz)	60	0	0	16	—
Sack'it Wild Cherry	4 pieces (0.5 oz)	60	0	0	16	—
Sack'it Wint-O-Green	4 pieces (0.5 oz)	60	0	0	16	—
Sugar Free Iced Mint	1 piece (2 g)	10	0	0	2	—
Sugar Free Vanilla Mint	1 piece (2 g)	10	0	0	2	—
Valentine Book	2 pieces (5 g)	20	0	20	5	—
M&M's						
Almond	1 pkg (1.3 oz)	200	11	20	21	2
Almond	1.5 oz	220	12	20	24	2
Mint	1 pkg (1.7 oz)	230	10	35	34	1

FOOD	PORTION	CAL.	FAT	SOD.	CARB.	FIB.
M&M's (CONT.)						
Mint	1.5 oz	200	9	30	30	1
Peanut	1 pkg (1.7 oz)	250	13	25	30	2
Peanut	1.5 oz	220	11	20	25	2
Peanut	1 fun size (0.7 oz)	110	5	10	13	1
Peanut	½ bag king size (1.6 oz)	240	12	25	28	2
Peanut Butter	1.5 oz	220	12	90	25	2
Peanut Butter	1 pkg (1.6 oz)	240	13	100	27	2
Peanut Butter	1 fun size (0.7 oz)	110	6	45	12	1
Plain	1.5 oz	200	9	30	30	1
Plain	½ pkg king size (1.6 oz)	220	9	30	32	1
Plain	1 pkg (1.7 oz)	230	10	35	34	1
Plain	1 pkg fun size (0.7 oz)	100	4	15	15	0
Mars						
Almond Bar	1 bar (1.8 oz)	240	13	70	31	1
Almond Bar	2 fun size (1.3 oz)	190	10	55	23	1
Mayfair						
Mints	5 pieces (1.3 oz)	180	9	5	26	tr
Milk Duds						
Snack Size	4 boxes (1.3 oz)	160	5	85	26	0
Milky Way						
Bar	2 fun size (1.4 oz)	180	7	60	28	0
Bar	⅓ king size (1.2 oz)	160	6	50	24	0
Dark	1 bar (1.8 oz)	220	8	85	36	1
Dark	1 fun size (0.7 oz)	90	3	35	14	0
Miniature	5 (1.5 oz)	190	7	65	30	0
Mr. Goodbar						
Candy	1 (1.75 oz)	290	19	20	23	—
NECCO						
Mint	1 piece	12	tr	—	—	—
Natural Touch						
Caroby Almond Bar	4 sections (28 g)	150	10	50	12	—
Caroby Milk Bar	4 sections (28 g)	150	9	55	13	—
Caroby Milk Free Bar	4 sections (28 g)	160	11	25	11	—
Caroby Mint Bar	4 sections (28 g)	150	9	55	13	—
Nestle						
Areo Bar	1 bar (1.45 oz)	210	13	20	26	2
Buncha Crunch	1 pkg (1.4 oz)	90	10	95	26	tr
Crunch	1 bar (1.55 oz)	230	12	60	28	1
Milk Chocolate	1 bar (1.45 oz)	220	13	30	23	2
Turtles Pecan Caramel Candy	2 pieces (1.2 oz)	160	9	30	20	1

FOOD	PORTION	CAL.	FAT	SOD.	CARB.	FIB.
Nips						
Butter Rum	2 pieces (0.5 oz)	60	2	35	12	—
Caramel	2 pieces (0.5 oz)	60	2	40	12	—
Chocolate Mint	2 pieces (0.5 oz)	60	2	40	11	—
Chocolate Parfait	2 pieces (0.5 oz)	60	2	35	11	—
Peanut Butter Parfait	2 pieces (0.5 oz)	60	2	40	11	—
Ocean Spray						
Fruit Waves Assorted	3 pieces (0.3 oz)	35	0	0	9	—
Pearson						
Licorice	2 pieces (0.5 oz)	60	2	40	12	—
Planters						
Original Peanut Bar	1 pkg (1.6 oz)	230	14	70	22	2
Reese's						
Peanut Butter Cups	1 (1.8 oz)	280	17	180	26	—
Pieces	1.85 oz	260	11	90	32	—
Rolo						
Carmels In Milk Chocolate	8 pieces (1.93 oz)	270	12	110	37	—
Russell Stover						
Assorted Creams	3 pieces (1.4 oz)	180	7	50	29	0
Skittles						
Original	½ king size (1.3 oz)	150	2	5	34	0
Original	1 pkg (2.8 oz)	250	3	10	55	0
Original	2 pkg fun size (1.6 oz)	180	2	5	41	0
Original	1.5 oz	170	2	5	38	0
Tropical	2 bags fun size (1.4 oz)	160	2	5	36	0
Tropical	1 bag (2.2 oz)	250	3	10	56	0
Tropical	1.5 oz	170	2	5	38	0
Wild Berry	1.5 oz	170	2	5	38	0
Wild Berry	2 bags fun size (1.4 oz)	160	2	5	36	0
Wild Berry	1 bag (2.2 oz)	250	3	10	56	0
Skor						
Toffee Bar	1 (1.4 oz)	220	14	125	22	—
Snickers						
Bar	1 bar (2.1 oz)	280	14	150	36	1
Bar	2 bars fun size (1.4 oz)	190	9	100	24	1
Bar	⅓ king size (1.2 oz)	170	8	85	21	1
Miniatures	4 (1.3 oz)	170	8	90	22	1
Munch Bar	1 (1.4 oz)	230	15	150	17	2
Peanut Butter	1 bar (2 oz)	310	20	150	28	1

FOOD	PORTION	CAL.	FAT	SOD.	CARB.	FIB.
Sour Punch						
Candy Straws Sour Apple	6 pieces (1.4 oz)	130	1	10	31	—
Starburst						
California Fruits	8 pieces (1.4 oz)	160	3	20	33	0
California Fruits	1 stick (2.1 oz)	240	5	35	48	0
Original Fruits	8 pieces (1.4 oz)	160	3	20	33	0
Original Fruits	⅓ king size (1.2 oz)	140	3	20	28	0
Orignal Fruits	1 stick (2.1 oz)	240	5	35	48	0
Strawberry Fruits	1 stick (2.1 oz)	240	5	35	48	0
Strawberry Fruits	8 pieces (1.4 oz)	160	3	20	33	0
Tropical Fruits	8 pieces (1.4 oz)	160	3	20	33	0
Tropical Fruits	1 stick (2.1 oz)	240	5	35	48	0
Sugar Babies						
Tidbits	1 pkg	180	2	—	—	—
Swedish Red Fish						
Candy	19 pieces (1.4 oz)	150	1	20	35	—
Switzer						
Cherry Bites	12 pieces (1.6 oz)	50	0	25	11	—
Licorice Bites	12 pieces (1.6 oz)	46	0	56	11	—
Terry's						
Orange Milk Chocolate	5 pieces (1.5 oz)	240	14	40	26	1
Tootsie Roll						
Dots	12 (1.5 oz)	160	0	—	—	—
Midgees	6 (1.4 oz)	160	3	—	—	—
Pop	1 (0.6 oz)	60	0	—	—	—
Twix						
Caramel	1 king size (0.8 oz)	120	6	45	15	1
Caramel	1 fun size (0.5 oz)	80	4	30	10	0
Caramel	1 (1 oz)	140	7	60	19	0
Caramel	1 pkg (2 oz)	280	14	115	37	0
Peanut Butter	1 (0.9 oz)	130	8	70	13	1
Twizzlers						
Pull-n-Peel Cherry	1 piece (1.1 oz)	110	0	80	23	—
Velamints						
Cocoamint	1 piece (1.7 g)	5	0	0	2	—
Peppermint	1 piece (1.7 g)	5	0	0	2	—
Spearmint	1 piece (1.7 g)	5	0	0	2	—
Wintergreen	1 piece (1.7 g)	5	0	0	2	—
Whatchamacallit						
Bar	1 (1.8 oz)	260	13	130	30	—
Whitman's						
Assorted	3 pieces (1.4 oz)	190	8	50	27	0
Dark Chocolate	3 pieces (1.4 oz)	200	10	55	25	1

FOOD	PORTION	CAL.	FAT	SOD.	CARB.	FIB.
Whitman's (CONT.)						
Little Ambassadors	7 pieces (1.4 oz)	190	9	50	26	1
Pecan Delight	1 bar (2 oz)	310	20	75	27	2
Pecan Roll	1 bar (2 oz)	300	20	95	26	1
Sampler	3 pieces (1.4 oz)	200	11	60	25	1
Y&S						
Bites Cherry	1 oz	100	1	85	23	—
York						
Peppermint Patty	1 snack size (0.5 oz)	57	1	3	11	—
boiled sweets	¼ lb	327	0	—	87	0
butterscotch	1 piece (6 g)	24	tr	3	6	—
butterscotch	1 oz	112	1	12	27	—
candied cherries	1 (4 g)	12	tr	—	3	—
candied citron	1 oz	89	tr	82	23	—
candied lemon peel	1 oz	90	tr	14	23	—
candied orange peel	1 oz	90	tr	14	23	—
candied pineapple slice	1 slice (2 oz)	179	tr	—	45	—
candy corn	1 oz	105	0	57	27	—
caramels	1 piece (8 g)	31	1	20	6	—
caramels	1 pkg (2.5 oz)	271	6	174	55	—
caramels chocolate	1 piece (6 g)	22	tr	—	6	—
caramels chocolate	1 bar (2.3 oz)	231	2	—	56	—
carob bar	1 (3.1 oz)	453	28	—	42	—
crisped rice bar almond	1 bar (1 oz)	130	6	66	18	1
crisped rice bar chocolate chip	1 bar (1 oz)	115	4	79	21	1
dark chocolate	1 oz	150	10	5	16	—
fondant chocolate coated	1 sm (0.4 oz)	40	1	3	9	—
fondant chocolate coated	1 lg (1.2 oz)	128	3	9	28	—
fondant mint	1 oz	105	0	57	27	—
fruit pastilles	1 tube (1.4 oz)	101	0	—	25	—
gumdrops	10 lg (3.8 oz)	420	0	48	108	—
gumdrops	10 sm (0.4 oz)	135	0	15	35	—
hard candy	1 oz	106	0	11	28	—
jelly beans	10 sm (0.4 oz)	40	tr	3	10	—
jelly beans	10 lg (1 oz)	104	tr	7	26	—
lollipop	1 (6 g)	22	0	2	6	—
marzipan	3½ oz	497	25	5	57	—
milk chocolate	1 bar (1.55 oz)	226	14	36	26	—
milk chocolate crisp	1 bar (1.45 oz)	203	11	59	28	—
milk chocolate w/ almonds	1 bar (1.45 oz)	215	14	30	22	—
nougat nut cream	3½ oz	342	31	—	58	—
peanut bar	1 (1.4 oz)	209	14	91	19	—

FOOD	PORTION	CAL.	FAT	SOD.	CARB.	FIB.
peanuts chocolate covered	1 cup (5.2 oz)	773	50	61	74	—
peanuts chocolate covered	10 (1.4 oz)	208	13	16	20	—
pretzels chocolate covered	1 (0.4 oz)	50	2	10	8	—
pretzels chocolate covered	1 oz	130	5	—	20	—
sesame crunch	20 pieces (1.2 oz)	181	12	—	18	—
sesame crunch	1 oz	146	9	—	14	—
sweet chocolate	1 oz	143	10	5	17	—
sweet chocolate	1 bar (1.45 oz)	201	14	7	25	—
HOME RECIPE						
divinity	1 (11 g)	38	0	5	10	—
divinity	1 recipe 48 pieces (19 oz)	1891	tr	247	486	—
fondant	1 recipe 60 pieces (32.6 oz)	3327	tr	374	863	—
fondant	1 piece (0.6 oz)	57	0	6	15	—
fudge brown sugar w/ nuts	1 piece (0.5 oz)	56	1	14	11	—
fudge brown sugar w/ nuts	1 recipe 60 pieces (30.7 oz)	3453	88	852	676	—
fudge chocolate	1 piece (0.6 oz)	65	1	10	14	—
fudge chocolate	1 recipe 48 pieces (29 oz)	3161	70	511	660	—
fudge chocolate marshmallow	1 piece (0.7 oz)	84	3	21	14	—
fudge chocolate marshmallow	1 recipe (43.1 oz)	5182	207	1273	880	—
fudge chocolate marshmallow w/ nuts	1 piece (0.8 oz)	96	4	21	15	—
fudge chocolate marshmallow w/ nuts	1 recipe 60 pieces (43.1 oz)	5182	207	1273	880	—
fudge chocolate marshmallow w/ nuts	1 recipe 60 pieces (46.1 oz)	5742	258	1234	903	—
fudge chocolate w/ nuts	1 piece (0.7 oz)	81	3	11	14	—
fudge chocolate w/ nuts	1 recipe 48 pieces (32.7 oz)	3967	150	562	678	—
fudge peanut butter	1 recipe 36 pieces (20.4 oz)	2161	38	424	456	—
fudge peanut butter	1 piece (0.6 oz)	59	1	12	13	—
fudge vanilla	1 piece (0.6 oz)	59	1	11	13	—
fudge vanilla	1 recipe 48 pieces (27.5 oz)	2893	42	525	644	—
fudge vanilla w/ nuts	1 piece (0.5 oz)	62	2	9	11	—
fudge vanilla w/ nuts	1 recipe 60 pieces (31 oz)	3666	117	538	665	—
peanut brittle	1 recipe (17.6 oz)	2288	95	2269	347	—

FOOD	PORTION	CAL.	FAT	SOD.	CARB.	FIB.
peanut brittle	1 oz	128	5	128	20	—
praline	1 recipe 23 pieces (31.8 oz)	4116	220	559	562	—
praline	1 piece (1.4 oz)	177	10	24	24	—
taffy	1 recipe 48 pieces (25 oz)	2677	24	636	651	—
taffy	1 piece (0.5 oz)	56	1	13	14	—
toffee	1 piece (0.4 oz)	65	4	22	8	—
toffee	1 recipe 48 pieces (19.4 oz)	2997	182	1036	356	—
truffles	1 recipe 49 pieces (21.5 oz)	2985	210	433	275	—
truffles	1 piece (0.4 oz)	59	4	8	5	—

CANTALOUPE
FRESH
Chiquita

Fresh	1 cup	70	0	—	—	—
cubed	1 cup	57	tr	14	13	1
half	½	94	1	23	22	2

FROZEN
Big Valley

Balls	¾ cup (4.9 oz)	40	0	16	10	0

CAPERS

Reese	1 tsp (5 g)	0	0	105	0	—

CARAMBOLA

fresh	1	42	tr	2	10	—

CARAWAY

seed	1 tsp	7	tr	tr	1	—

CARDAMOM

ground	1 tsp	6	tr	tr	1	—

CARDOON

fresh cooked	3½ oz	22	tr	176	5	—
raw shredded	½ cup	36	tr	151	4	—

CARIBOU

roasted	3 oz	142	4	51	0	—

CARISSA

fresh	1	12	tr	1	3	—

CAROB

carob mix	3 tsp	45	0	12	11	—
carob mix as prep w/ whole milk	9 oz	195	8	132	23	—

FOOD	PORTION	CAL.	FAT	SOD.	CARB.	FIB.
flour	1 tbsp	14	tr	3	7	—
flour	1 cup	185	1	36	92	—
CARP						
fresh cooked	3 oz	138	6	54	0	—
fresh cooked	1 fillet (6 oz)	276	12	107	0	—
raw	3 oz	108	5	42	0	—
roe raw	3½ oz	130	2	—	2	—
CARROT JUICE						
Hain	6 fl oz	80	0	170	17	—
Hollywood	6 fl oz	80	0	170	17	2
Odwalla	8 fl oz	70	0	200	18	2
canned	6 oz	73	tr	54	17	—
CARROTS						
CANNED						
Allen						
Sliced	½ cup (4.5 oz)	35	1	230	8	3
Crest Top						
Sliced	½ cup (4.5 oz)	35	1	230	8	3
Del Monte						
Cut	½ cup (4.3 oz)	35	0	300	8	3
Sliced	½ cup (4.3 oz)	35	0	300	8	3
S&W						
Diced Fancy	½ cup	30	0	240	7	—
Julienne French Style Fancy	½ cup	30	0	240	7	—
Sliced Fancy	½ cup	30	0	240	7	—
Sliced Water Pack	½ cup	30	0	50	7	—
Whole Tiny Fancy	½ cup	30	0	240	7	—
Seneca						
Diced	½ cup	30	0	264	6	2
Sliced	½ cup	30	0	264	6	2
slices	½ cup	17	tr	176	4	1
slices low sodium	½ cup	17	tr	31	4	1
FRESH						
Dole	1 med	40	1	40	8	1
baby raw	1 (½ oz)	6	tr	5	1	—
raw	1 (2.5 oz)	31	tr	25	7	2
raw shredded	½ cup	24	tr	19	6	2
slices cooked	½ cup	35	tr	52	8	—
FROZEN						
Big Valley						
Carrots	½ cup (3 oz)	35	0	40	8	2

FOOD	PORTION	CAL.	FAT	SOD.	CARB.	FIB.
Birds Eye						
Baby Whole Deluxe	½ cup	40	0	45	9	2
Polybag Sliced	¾ cup	35	0	40	8	1
Green Giant						
Harvest Fresh Baby	½ cup	18	0	75	5	2
Hanover						
Crinkle Sliced	½ cup	35	0	—	—	—
slices cooked	½ cup	26	tr	43	6	—
CASABA						
cubed	1 cup	45	tr	20	11	—
fresh	¹⁄₁₀	43	tr	20	10	—
CASHEWS						
Beer Nuts						
Cashews	1 pkg (1 oz)	170	13	65	8	—
Eagle						
Honey Roasted	1 oz	170	12	130	9	—
Low Salt	1 oz	170	14	110	7	—
Fisher						
Honey Roasted Halves	1 oz	150	13	—	7	—
Honey Roasted Whole	1 oz	150	13	90	7	—
Oil Roasted Halves	1 oz	170	15	160	8	—
Oil Roasted Whole	1 oz	170	15	140	8	—
Guy's						
Whole Salted	1 oz	170	14	140	5	—
Hain						
Cashew Butter Raw	2 tbsp	190	15	125	8	—
Cashew Butter Raw Unsalted	2 tbsp	210	19	170	8	—
Cashew Butter Toasted	2 tbsp	210	17	190	7	—
Lance						
Cashews	1 pkg (32 g)	190	15	95	8	—
Planters						
Fancy Oil Roasted	1 oz	170	14	120	8	1
Fancy Oil Roasted	1 pkg (2 oz)	340	29	240	16	3
Halves Lightly Salted Oil Roasted	1 oz	160	13	55	9	2
Halves Oil Roasted	1 oz	170	14	120	8	2
Honey Roasted	1 pkg (2 oz)	310	24	240	23	3
Honey Roasted	1 oz	150	12	120	11	1
Munch'N Go Honey Roasted	1 pkg (2 oz)	310	24	240	23	3
Munch'N Go Singles Oil Roasted	1 pkg (2 oz)	330	28	240	16	3

FOOD	PORTION	CAL.	FAT	SOD.	CARB.	FIB.
Planters (CONT.)						
Oil Roasted	1 pkg (1.5 oz)	250	21	240	12	2
Oil Roasted	1 pkg (1 oz)	160	14	120	8	1
cashew butter w/o salt	1 tbsp	94	8	2	4	—
dry roasted	1 oz	163	13	4	9	—
dry roasted salted	1 oz	163	13	213	9	—
oil roasted	1 oz	163	14	5	8	—
oil roasted salted	1 oz	163	14	209	8	—
CASSAVA						
raw	3½ oz	120	tr	8	27	—
CATFISH						
channel breaded & fried	3 oz	194	11	238	7	—
channel raw	3 oz	99	4	54	0	—
CATSUP						
(*see* KETCHUP)						
CAULIFLOWER						
FRESH						
Dole	⅙ med head	18	0	45	3	2
Green	⅕ head	35	0	30	7	—
cooked	½ cup (2.2 oz)	14	tr	9	3	1
flowerets cooked	3 (2 oz)	12	tr	8	2	1
flowerets raw	3 (2 oz)	14	tr	17	3	1
green cooked	½ cup (2.2 oz)	20	tr	14	4	—
green raw	½ cup (1.8 oz)	16	tr	12	3	—
raw	½ cup (1.8 oz)	13	tr	15	3	1
FROZEN						
Big Valley						
Florets	¾ cup (3 oz)	25	0	15	4	1
Birds Eye						
Frzn	⅔ cup	25	0	20	5	2
Polybag	½ cup	20	0	15	4	—
With Cheese Sauce	½ pkg	90	5	480	8	1
Green Giant						
Cuts	½ cup	12	0	25	3	1
In Cheese Sauce	½ cup	60	2	500	10	2
One Serve In Cheese Sauce	1 pkg	80	3	690	14	2
Hanover						
Cauliflower	½ cup	20	0	—	—	—
Florets	½ cup	20	0	—	—	—
cooked	½ cup	17	tr	16	3	—

FOOD	PORTION	CAL.	FAT	SOD.	CARB.	FIB.
JARRED						
Vlasic						
Hot & Spicy	1 oz	4	0	435	1	—
Sweet	1 oz	35	0	225	9	—
CAVIAR						
black granular	1 tbsp	40	3	240	1	—
black granular	1 oz	71	5	420	1	—
red granular	1 oz	71	5	420	1	—
red granular	1 tbsp	40	3	240	1	—
CELERIAC						
fresh cooked	3½ oz	25	tr	61	6	—
raw	½ cup	31	tr	78	7	—
CELERY						
DRIED						
seed	1 tsp	8	tr	3	1	—
FRESH						
Dole	2 med stalks	20	0	140	2	4
diced cooked	½ cup	13	tr	68	3	—
raw	1 stalk (1.3 oz)	6	tr	35	1	1
raw diced	½ cup	10	tr	52	2	1
FROZEN						
Fresh Like	3.5 oz	14	tr	88	3	1
CELTUCE						
raw	3½ oz	22	tr	11	4	—
CEREAL						
COOKED						
Albers						
Hominy Quick Grits uncooked	¼ cup	140	1	0	31	1
Arrowhead						
4 Grain + Flax	¼ cup (1.6 oz)	150	2	0	28	6
7 Grain	⅓ cup (1.4 oz)	140	2	0	25	5
Bear Mush	¼ cup (1.6 oz)	160	1	0	33	2
Oat Flakes Rolled	⅓ cup (1.2 oz)	130	3	0	23	4
Oat Groats	¼ cup (1.5 oz)	160	3	0	29	4
Oatmeal Instant Original	1 oz	100	0	15	22	—
Rice & Shine	¼ cup (1.5 oz)	150	1	0	32	2
Wheat Flakes Rolled	⅓ cup (1.2 oz)	110	1	0	24	5
Aunt Jemima						
Enriched White Hominy Grits Regular	3 tbsp	101	tr	1	22	1

FOOD	PORTION	CAL.	FAT	SOD.	CARB.	FIB.
Erewhon						
Barley Plus	1 oz	110	1	0	22	1
Brown Rice Cream	1 oz	110	1	20	23	—
Oat Bran With Toasted Wheat Germ	1 oz	115	2	15	18	3
Oatmeal Instant Apple Cinnamon	1.25 oz	145	3	100	25	—
Oatmeal Instant Apple Raisin	1.3 oz	150	3	100	27	—
Oatmeal Instant Dates & Walnuts	1.2 oz	130	3	60	24	3
Oatmeal Instant Maple Spice	1.2 oz	140	3	100	24	—
Oatmeal Instant With Added Oat Bran	1.25 oz	125	3	0	23	4
Good Shepherd						
Spelt	1 oz	90	tr	0	20	3
H-O						
Farina Instant	1 pkg	110	0	235	22	3
Farina not prep	3 tbsp	120	0	0	26	3
Oatmeal Instant	1 pkg	110	2	230	18	3
Oatmeal Instant	½ cup	130	2	<5	22	3
Oatmeal Instant Apple Cinnamon	1 pkg	130	2	220	26	3
Oatmeal Instant Maple Brown Sugar	1 pkg	160	2	285	32	3
Oatmeal Instant Raisin & Spice	1 pkg	150	2	140	32	3
Oatmeal Instant Sweet 'n Mellow	1 pkg	150	2	270	30	3
Oats 'n Fiber	⅓ cup	100	2	5	15	3
Oats 'n Fiber	1 pkg	110	2	140	18	3
Oats 'n Fiber Apple & Bran	1 pkg	130	2	140	26	3
Oats 'n Fiber Raisin & Bran	1 pkg	150	2	140	32	3
Oats Gourmet	⅓ cup	100	2	0	18	3
Oats Quick	½ cup	130	2	<5	22	3
Health Valley						
Oat Bran Natural Apples & Cinnamon	¼ cup (1 oz)	100	tr	10	19	4
Oat Bran Natural Raisins & Spice	¼ cup	100	tr	10	19	4
Kashi						
5-Bran	2½ oz	281	6	13	47	16

FOOD	PORTION	CAL.	FAT	SOD.	CARB.	FIB.
Kashi (CONT.)						
Cereal	2 oz	177	1	5	38	5
Little Crow						
Coco Wheat	3 tbsp (36 g)	130	1	12	28	4
Maypo						
30 second	1 oz	100	1	0	19	2
Vermont Style	1 oz	105	1	0	20	2
With Oat Bran	1 oz	130	2	1	26	4
McCann's						
Irish Oatmeal	1 oz	110	2	0	20	3
Mother's						
Oatmeal Instant	½ cup (1.4 oz)	150	3	0	27	4
Whole Wheat Natural	½ cup (1.4 oz)	130	1	0	30	4
Nabisco						
Cream of Rice	1 oz	100	0	0	23	—
Cream of Wheat Instant as prep	1 cup	120	0	0	25	1
Cream of Wheat Quick as prep	1 cup	120	0	—	25	1
Cream of Wheat Regular as prep	1 cup	120	0	0	25	1
Mix'n Eat Cream of Wheat Apple & Cinnamon	1 pkg (1¼ oz)	130	0	250	29	1
Mix'n Eat Cream of Wheat Brown Sugar Cinnamon	1 pkg (1¼ oz)	130	0	230	29	1
Mix'n Eat Cream of Wheat Maple Brown Sugar	1 pkg (1¼ oz)	130	0	180	29	1
Mix'n Eat Cream of Wheat Our Original	1 pkg (1¼ oz)	100	0	170	21	1
Pillsbury						
Farina	⅔ cup	80	tr	170	17	—
Pritikin						
Apple Raisin Spice	1 pkg (1.6 oz)	170	3	5	34	—
Multigrain	1 pkg	160	2	0	33	—
Quaker						
Enriched White Hominy Grits Quick	3 tbsp	101	tr	1	22	1
Instant Grits White Hominy	1 pkg	79	tr	440	18	1
Instant Grits With Imitation Bacon Bits	1 pkg	101	tr	590	22	2

FOOD	PORTION	CAL.	FAT	SOD.	CARB.	FIB.
Quaker (CONT.)						
Instant Grits With Imitation Ham Bits	1 pkg	99	tr	800	21	2
Instant Grits With Real Cheddar Cheese	1 pkg	104	1	497	22	1
Multigrain	½ cup	130	2	10	29	5
Oatmeal Instant	1 pkg (1.2 oz)	130	3	95	22	3
Oatmeal Instant Apples & Cinnamon	1 pkg (1.2 oz)	130	2	105	26	3
Oatmeal Instant Cinnamon Graham Cookie	1 pkg (1.4 oz)	150	3	170	30	3
Oatmeal Instant Cinnamon Spice	1 pkg (1.6 oz)	170	2	290	36	3
Oatmeal Instant Cinnamon Toast	1 pkg (1.2 oz)	130	2	160	27	2
Oatmeal Instant Fruit & Cream Blueberry	1 pkg (1.2 oz)	130	3	140	27	2
Oatmeal Instant Honey Nut	1 pkg (1.2 oz)	130	3	210	25	2
Oatmeal Instant Kids Choice Radical Raspberry	1 pkg (1.4 oz)	150	3	170	29	3
Oatmeal Instant Maple Brown Sugar	1 pkg (1.5 oz)	160	2	240	33	3
Oatmeal Instant Peaches & Cream	1 pkg (1.2 oz)	130	2	150	27	2
Oatmeal Instant Raisin & Walnut	1 pkg (1.3 oz)	140	3	160	27	3
Oatmeal Instant Raisin Date Walnut	1 pkg (1.3 oz)	130	3	240	27	3
Oatmeal Instant Raisin Spice	1 pkg (1.5 oz)	160	2	250	32	3
Oatmeal Instant Strawberries & Cream	1 pkg (1.2 oz)	130	2	160	27	2
Oatmeal Instant Strawberries 'N Stuff	1 pkg (1.4 oz)	150	2	170	30	3
Oats Old Fashion	½ cup	150	3	0	27	4
Oats Quick	½ cup	150	3	0	27	4
Ralston						
Corn Flakes	1¼ cup (1.1 oz)	120	0	280	27	1
Roman Meal						
Apple Cinnamon	1.2 oz	105	2	6	18	6
Cream Of Rye	1.3 oz	111	1	2	20	5

FOOD	PORTION	CAL.	FAT	SOD.	CARB.	FIB.
Roman Meal (CONT.)						
Oats Wheat Dates Raisins Almonds	1.3 oz	129	2	3	24	3
Oats Wheat Honey Coconuts Almonds	1.3 oz	155	5	8	22	3
Original	1 oz	83	1	tr	15	5
Original With Oats	1.2 oz	108	1	1	19	5
Stone-Buhr						
4 Grain	⅓ cup (1.6 oz)	140	2	0	31	5
Cracked Wheat	¼ cup (2.4 oz)	210	1	0	48	6
Manna Golden	6 tsp (1.6 oz)	160	0	0	35	1
Rolled Oats Old Fashion	6 tsp (1.6 oz)	150	3	0	28	5
Scotch Oats	¼ cup (1.6 oz)	150	4	0	28	4
Uncle Roy's						
Muesli Swiss Style	½ cup (1.6 oz)	170	5	20	32	3
corn grits instant	1 pkg (0.8 oz)	82	tr	344	18	—
corn grits quick	1 cup	146	1	0	31	—
corn grits quick not prep	1 cup	579	2	1	124	—
corn grits quick not prep	1 tbsp	36	tr	0	8	—
corn grits regular	1 cup	146	1	0	31	—
corn grits regular not prep	1 cup	579	2	1	124	—
farina	¾ cup	87	tr	1	19	3
farina not prep	1 tbsp	40	0	0	9	tr
oatmeal	1 cup	145	2	1	25	—
oatmeal instant cooked w/o salt	1 cup	145	2	2	25	—
oatmeal not prep	1 cup	311	5	3	54	9
oatmeal quick cooked w/o salt	1 cup	145	2	2	25	—
oatmeal regular cooked w/o salt	1 cup	145	2	2	25	—
READY-TO-EAT						
Arrowhead						
Amaranth Flakes	1 cup (1.2 oz)	130	2	0	25	3
Apple Corns	1 cup (1.5 oz)	150	2	110	35	4
Bran Flakes	1 cup (1 oz)	100	1	80	22	4
Kamut Flakes	1 cup (1.1 oz)	120	1	65	25	3
Maple Corns	1 cup (1.9 oz)	190	3	140	43	6
Multi Grain Flakes	1 cup (1.2 oz)	140	2	130	29	3
Nature O's	1 cup (1.1 oz)	130	2	5	24	3
Oat Bran Flakes	1 cup (1.2 oz)	110	2	60	22	4
Puffed Corn	1 cup (0.8 oz)	80	0	0	16	1
Puffed Kamut	1 cup (0.6 oz)	50	0	0	11	2
Puffed Millet	1 cup (0.9 oz)	90	1	0	19	1

FOOD	PORTION	CAL.	FAT	SOD.	CARB.	FIB.
Arrowhead (CONT.)						
Puffed Rice	1 cup (0.8 oz)	90	0	0	19	1
Puffed Wheat	1 cup (0.9 oz)	90	1	0	20	2
Spelt Flakes	1 cup (1.1 oz)	100	1	60	22	3
Chex						
Corn	1¼ cup (1 oz)	110	0	270	26	1
Double	1¼ cup (1 oz)	120	0	230	27	0
Graham	1 cup (1.8 oz)	210	2	340	45	1
Rice	1 cup (1.1 oz)	120	0	230	27	0
Wheat	¾ cup (1.8 oz)	190	1	390	41	5
Erewhon						
Aztec	1 oz	100	0	85	24	1
Crispy Brown Rice	1 oz	110	1	185	24	4
Fruit 'n Wheat	1 oz	100	1	75	21	3
Raisin Bran	1 oz	100	0	80	22	3
Super-O's	1 oz	110	0	5	24	4
Wheat Flakes	1 oz	100	0	75	22	4
Estee						
Corn Flakes	1 pkg (1 oz)	90	0	310	24	4
Raisin Bran	1 pkg (1 oz)	90	1	100	21	3
General Mills						
Basic 4	¾ cup	130	2	290	28	2
Body Buddies Natural Fruit	1 cup (1 oz)	110	1	280	24	—
Booberry	1 cup (1 oz)	110	1	210	24	—
Cheerios	1¼ cup (1 oz)	110	2	290	20	2
Cheerios Apple Cinnamon	¾ cup (1 oz)	110	2	180	22	2
Cheerios Honey Nut	¾ cup (1 oz)	110	1	250	23	2
Cheerios-to-Go	1 pkg (0.75 oz)	80	2	220	15	2
Cheerios-to-Go Apple Cinnamon	1 pkg (1 oz)	110	2	180	22	2
Cheerios-to-Go Honey Nut	1 pkg (1 oz)	110	1	250	23	2
Cinnamon Toast Crunch	¾ cup (1 oz)	120	3	210	22	1
Clusters	½ cup (1 oz)	110	2	140	22	2
Cocoa Puffs	1 cup (1 oz)	110	1	180	25	—
Count Chocula	1 cup (1 oz)	110	1	210	24	—
Country Corn Flakes	1 cup (1 oz)	110	1	260	24	—
Crispy Wheats 'N Raisins	¾ cup (1 oz)	100	1	140	23	2
Fiber One	½ cup (1 oz)	60	1	140	23	13
Frankenberry	1 cup (1 oz)	110	1	210	24	—
Fruity Yummy Mummy	1 cup (1 oz)	110	1	160	24	—

FOOD	PORTION	CAL.	FAT	SOD.	CARB.	FIB.
General Mills (CONT.)						
Golden Grahams	¾ cup (1 oz)	110	1	280	24	—
Kaboom	1 cup (1 oz)	110	1	270	23	—
Kix	1½ cup (1 oz)	110	1	260	24	—
Lucky Charms	1 cup (1 oz)	110	1	240	24	—
Oatmeal Crisp	½ cup (1 oz)	110	2	180	22	1
Oatmeal Raisin Crisp	½ cup (1.2 oz)	130	2	170	25	2
Raisin Nut Bran	½ cup (1 oz)	110	3	140	20	3
S'Mores Grahams	¾ cup (1 oz)	120	2	250	24	—
Sun Crunchers	1 cup (1.9 oz)	210	3	350	44	3
Total	1 cup (1 oz)	100	1	200	22	3
Total Corn Flakes	1 cup (1 oz)	110	tr	200	24	—
Total Raisin Bran	1 cup (1.5 oz)	140	1	190	33	4
Triples	¾ cup (1 oz)	110	1	250	24	—
Trix	1 cup (1 oz)	110	1	140	25	—
Wheaties	1 cup (1 oz)	100	1	200	23	3
Glenny's						
Maple Frosted Corn	1 oz	109	tr	50	20	—
Oat Mini Puffs	1 oz	108	tr	30	22	—
Oat Mini Puffs No Salt No Sugar	1 oz	108	tr	7	22	—
Rice Mini Puffs	1 oz	109	tr	30	20	—
Good Shepherd						
Millet Rice Flakes Wheat Free	1 oz	95	1	30	19	1
Spelt Flakes	1 oz	100	6	80	21	2
Grist Mill						
Apple Cinnamon Natural	½ cup (1.9 oz)	260	10	20	36	3
Bran	½ cup (1.9 oz)	250	8	40	37	11
Oat & Honey Natural	½ cup (1.9 oz)	270	12	10	34	4
Oat Honey & Raisin Natural	½ cup (1.9 oz)	260	10	10	35	4
Health Valley						
100% Natural Bran With Apples & Cinnamon	¼ cup (1 oz)	100	1	10	22	5
Blue Corn Flakes 100% Organic	½ cup (1 oz)	90	tr	10	19	3
Bran Cereal With Dates 100% Organic	¼ cup (1 oz)	100	1	5	20	5
Bran Cereal With Raisins 100% Organic	¼ cup (1 oz)	100	1	5	20	5
Fiber 7 Flakes 100% Organic	½ cup (1 oz)	90	tr	0	20	5
Fiber 7 Flakes With Raisins 100% Organic	½ cup (1 oz)	90	tr	0	20	5

FOOD	PORTION	CAL.	FAT	SOD.	CARB.	FIB.
Health Valley (CONT.)						
Fruit & Fitness	1 cup (2 oz)	220	4	5	37	11
Fruit Lites Corn	½ cup (0.5 oz)	45	0	2	10	tr
Fruit Lites Rice	½ cup (0.5 oz)	45	1	2	11	tr
Fruit Lites Wheat	½ cup (0.5 oz)	45	1	2	11	2
Healthy Crunch Almond Date	¼ cup (1 oz)	110	3	5	18	4
Healthy Crunch Apple Cinnamon	¼ cup (1 oz)	110	3	10	18	4
Healthy O's 100% Organic	¾ cup (1 oz)	90	1	1	18	3
Lites Puffed Corn	½ cup (1 oz)	50	0	0	11	tr
Lites Puffed Rice	½ cup (1 oz)	50	0	0	12	tr
Lites Puffed Wheat	½ cup (1 oz)	50	0	0	11	1
Oat Bran Flakes 100% Organic	½ cup (1 oz)	100	tr	0	20	4
Oat Bran Flakes Almonds/Dates 100% Organic	½ cup (1 oz)	100	tr	0	20	4
Oat Bran Flakes With Raisins 100% Organic	½ cup (1 oz)	100	tr	0	20	4
Oat Bran O'S 100% Organic	½ cup (1 oz)	110	tr	0	20	3
Oat Bran O'S Fruit & Nuts	½ cup (1 oz)	110	3	0	19	3
Orangeola Almonds & Dates	¼ cup	110	3	5	18	4
Orangeola Bananas & Hawaiian Fruit	¼ cup (1 oz)	120	4	10	20	4
Raisin Bran Flakes 100% Organic	½ cup (1 oz)	100	tr	5	21	6
Real Oat Bran Almond Crunch	¼ cup (1 oz)	110	3	2	17	4
Real Oat Bran Hawaiian Fruit	¼ cup (1 oz)	130	3	2	22	5
Real Oat Bran Raisin Nut	¼ cup (1 oz)	130	3	2	21	5
Rice Bran O's	½ cup	110	1	5	22	2
Rice Bran With Almonds & Dates	½ cup (1 oz)	110	3	2	19	2
Sprouts 7 Bananas & Hawaiian Fruit	¼ cup (1 oz)	90	1	5	16	4
Sprouts 7 Raisin	¼ cup	90	1	5	16	5
Swiss Breakfast Raisin Nut	¼ cup (1 oz)	100	3	10	19	3

FOOD	PORTION	CAL.	FAT	SOD.	CARB.	FIB.
Health Valley (CONT.)						
Swiss Breakfast Tropical Fruit	¼ cup (1 oz)	100	3	10	19	3
Healthy Choice						
Multi-Grain Flakes	1 cup (1.1 oz)	100	0	210	26	3
Mulit-Grain Raisins & Almonds	1¼ cup (2 oz)	200	2	240	44	4
Multi-Grain Squares	1¼ cup (2 oz)	190	1	0	45	6
Heartland						
Coconut	1 oz	130	5	80	18	2
Plain	1 oz	130	4	80	18	2
Raisin	1 oz	130	4	80	18	2
Kashi						
Brittles Sesame/Maple	3½ oz	473	19	85	65	—
Puffed	¾ oz	74	1	2	16	2
Kellogg's						
All-Bran	½ cup (1 oz)	80	1	280	22	10
All-Bran With Extra Fiber	½ cup (1 oz)	50	1	150	22	15
Apple Cinnamon Rice Krispies	¾ cup (1 oz)	110	0	220	27	1
Apple Cinnamon Squares	¾ cup (1.9 oz)	180	1	15	44	0
Apple Jacks	1 cup (1 oz)	110	0	135	26	1
Apple Raisin Crisp	1 cup (1.9 oz)	180	0	340	46	4
Blueberry Squares	¾ cup (1.9 oz)	180	1	15	44	5
Bran Buds	⅓ cup (1 oz)	70	1	210	24	11
Cinnamon Mini Buns	¾ cup (1 oz)	120	1	210	27	1
Cocoa Krispies	¾ cup (1 oz)	120	1	190	27	0
Common Sense Oat Bran	¾ cup (1 oz)	110	1	270	23	4
Complete Bran Flakes	¾ cup (1 oz)	100	1	230	25	5
Corn Flakes	1 cup (1 oz)	110	0	330	26	1
Corn Pops	1 cup (1 oz)	110	0	95	27	1
Cracklin' Oat Bran	¾ cup (1.9 oz)	230	8	180	40	6
Crispix	1 cup (1 oz)	110	0	230	26	1
Double Dip Crunch	¾ cup (1 oz)	110	0	160	27	0
Froot Loops	1 cup (1 oz)	120	1	150	26	1
Frosted Bran	¾ cup (1 oz)	100	0	200	26	3
Frosted Flakes	¾ cup (1 oz)	120	0	200	28	0
Frosted Krispies	¾ cup (1 oz)	110	0	230	27	0
Frosted Mini-Wheats	1 cup (1.9 oz)	190	1	0	45	6
Frosted Mini-Wheats Bite Size	1 cup (1.9 oz)	190	1	0	45	6
Fruitful Bran	1¼ cup (1.9 oz)	170	1	330	44	6

FOOD	PORTION	CAL.	FAT	SOD.	CARB.	FIB.
Kellogg's (CONT.)						
Fruity Marshmallow Krispies	¾ cups (1 oz)	110	0	180	27	0
Just Right Crunchy Nuggets	1 cup (1.9 oz)	200	2	340	46	3
Just Right Fruit & Nut	1 cup (1.9 oz)	210	2	260	46	3
Mueslix Golden Crunch	¾ cup (1.9 oz)	210	5	280	40	6
Nut & Honey Crunch	1¼ cup (1.9 oz)	220	4	370	45	1
Nutri-Grain Almond Raisin	1¼ cup (1.9 oz)	200	2	330	44	4
Nutri-Grain Golden Wheat	¾ cup (1 oz)	100	1	240	23	4
Oatbake Raisin Nut	⅓ cup (1 oz)	110	3	190	21	3
Pop-Tart Crunch Frosted Brown Sugar Cinnamon	¾ cup (1 oz)	120	1	160	26	0
Pop-Tart Crunch Frosted Strawberry	¾ cup (1 oz)	120	1	125	27	0
Product 19	1 cup (1 oz)	110	0	280	25	1
Raisin Bran	1 cup (1.9 oz)	170	1	310	43	7
Raisin Squares	¾ cup (1.9 oz)	180	1	0	44	5
Rice Krispies	1¼ cup (1 oz)	110	0	320	26	1
Special K	1 cup (1 oz)	110	0	250	21	1
Strawberry Squares	¾ cup (1.9 oz)	180	1	10	44	5
Temptations French Vanilla Almond	¾ cup (1 oz)	120	2	210	24	1
Temptations Honey Roasted Pecan	1 cup (1 oz)	120	3	240	24	0
LaLoma						
Ruskets Biscuits	2 biscuits (30 g)	110	0	95	22	—
Mueslix						
Crispy Blend	⅔ cup (1.9 oz)	200	2	190	42	4
Nabisco						
100% Bran	⅓ cup (1 oz)	70	2	130	21	10
Fruit Wheats Apple	1 oz	90	0	15	23	3
Shredded Wheat 'n Bran	⅔ cup (1 oz)	90	1	0	23	4
Shredded Wheat Spoon Size	⅔ cup (1 oz)	90	1	0	23	3
Shredded Wheat With Oat Bran	⅔ cup (1 oz)	100	1	0	22	4
Nut & Honey						
Crunch O's	¾ cup (1 oz)	120	3	200	23	2
Nutri-Grain						
Golden Wheat & Raisin	1¼ cup (1.9 oz)	180	1	310	45	6

FOOD	PORTION	CAL.	FAT	SOD.	CARB.	FIB.
Post						
Alpha-Bits	1 cup (1 oz)	111	1	176	24	1
Alpha-Bits Marshmallow Sweetened Letter Shaped Oats	1 cup	110	1	152	25	1
Cocoa Pebbles	⅞ cup (1 oz)	113	1	160	25	tr
Crispy Critters	1 cup (1 oz)	110	0	232	24	1
Fruit & Fibre Dates Raisins Walnuts With Oat Clusters	⅔ cup	120	2	167	27	5
Fruit & Fibre Tropical Fruit With Oat Clusters	⅔ cup	125	3	167	27	5
Fruity Pebbles	⅞ cup	113	1	156	25	1
Grape-Nuts	¼ cup (1 oz)	105	0	170	23	3
Grape-Nuts Raisin	¼ cup (1 oz)	102	0	141	23	2
Honey Bunches Of Oats Honey Roasted	⅔ cup (1 oz)	111	2	176	23	2
Honey Bunches Of Oats With Almonds	⅔ cup (1 oz)	115	3	157	22	2
Honeycomb	1 ⅓ cups (1 oz)	110	0	172	26	1
Natural Bran Flakes	⅔ cup (1 oz)	88	0	205	23	6
Oat Flakes	⅔ cup (1 oz)	107	1	127	22	2
Post Toasties Corn Flakes	1¼ cup (1 oz)	111	0	310	24	1
Raisin Bran	⅔ cup (40 g)	122	1	198	32	6
Super Golden Crisp	⅞ cup (1 oz)	104	0	44	26	tr
Quaker						
Crunchy Bran	⅔ cup	89	1	316	23	5
Crunchy Not Oh!s	1 cup	127	4	164	22	1
Honey Graham Oh!s	1 cup	122	3	217	23	1
King Vitaman	1½ cup	110	1	280	23	1
Oat Squares	½ cup	105	2	159	21	2
Popeye Sweet Crunch	1 cup	113	2	254	24	1
Puffed Rice	1 cup	54	tr	1	13	tr
Puffed Wheat	1 cup	50	tr	1	11	1
Shredded Wheat	2 biscuits	132	1	1	32	4
Ralston						
Almond Delight	1 cup (1.8 oz)	210	3	410	41	4
Bran Flakes	¾ cup (1.1 oz)	110	1	220	24	5
Chex Multi-Bran	1¼ cup (2 oz)	220	2	320	46	7
Cocoa Crispy Rice	1 cup (1.8 oz)	200	0	340	45	tr
Cocoa Crunchies	¾ cup (1.1 oz)	120	1	170	26	0
Cookie Crisp	1 cup (1 oz)	120	2	110	25	0

FOOD	PORTION	CAL.	FAT	SOD.	CARB.	FIB.
Ralston (CONT.)						
Crisp Crunch	¾ cup (1.1 oz)	120	1	240	26	tr
Crisp Rice	1¼ cup (1.2 oz)	130	0	330	28	0
Frosted Flakes	¾ cup (1.1 oz)	120	0	180	28	1
Fruit Rings	¾ cup (0.9 oz)	100	1	115	23	0
Magic Stair	¾ cup (1.1 oz)	120	1	160	26	tr
Muesli Blueberry	1 cup (1.9 oz)	200	3	170	41	4
Muesli Cranberry	¾ cup (1.9 oz)	200	3	180	40	4
Muesli Peach	¾ cup (1.9 oz)	200	3	170	39	4
Muesli Raspberry	¾ cup (2 oz)	220	3	170	44	4
Muesli Strawberry	1 cup (1.9 oz)	210	3	170	41	4
Multi Vitamin Whole Grain Flakes	1 cup (1.1 oz)	120	1	300	25	3
Nutty Nuggets	½ cup (1.7 oz)	180	2	220	36	5
Raisin Bran	¾ cup (1.9 oz)	190	1	290	41	6
Tasteeos	1¼ cup (1.1 oz)	130	3	260	22	3
Tasteeos Apple Cinnamon	1 cup (1.2 oz)	130	2	150	27	1
Tasteeos Honey Nut	1 cup (1.2 oz)	130	2	250	28	1
Rice Krispies						
Treats	¾ cup (1 oz)	120	1	170	25	0
Stone-Buhr						
7 Grain	⅓ cup (1.6 oz)	140	2	0	31	7
Bran Flakes	¼ cup (0.6 oz)	64	0	160	14	2
Sunbelt						
Muesli	1.9 oz	210	2	70	44	3
US Mills						
Poppets	1 oz	110	1	10	24	1
Uncle Sam	1 oz	110	1	65	20	7
all bran	½ cup (1 oz)	76	1	196	21	—
bran flakes	¾ cup (1 oz)	90	1	264	22	—
corn flakes	1¼ cup (1 oz)	110	tr	351	24	—
corn flakes low sodium	1 cup	100	tr	3	22	—
crispy rice	1 cup	111	tr	205	25	—
fortified oat flakes	1 cup	177	1	429	35	—
puffed rice	1 cup	57	tr	0	13	—
puffed wheat	1 cup	44	tr	0	10	—
shredded wheat	1 biscuit	83	tr	0	19	—
sugar-coated corn flakes	¾ cup (1 oz)	110	1	230	26	—

CHAMPAGNE

Andre

Blush	1 fl oz	22	0	1	1	—
Brut	1 fl oz	21	0	1	1	—

FOOD	PORTION	CAL.	FAT	SOD.	CARB.	FIB.
Andre (CONT.)						
Cold Duck	1 fl oz	25	0	1	2	—
Extra Dry	1 fl oz	23	0	1	1	—
Ballatore						
Spumante	1 fl oz	23	0	2	2	—
Eden Roc						
Brut	1 fl oz	21	0	1	1	—
Brut Rosé	1 fl oz	22	0	1	2	—
Extra Dry	1 fl oz	21	0	1	1	—
Tott's						
Blanc de Noir	1 fl oz	22	0	1	2	—
Brut	1 fl oz	20	0	1	tr	—
Extra Dry	1 fl oz	21	0	1	1	—
sekt german champagne	3.5 fl oz	84	0	—	5	—

CHAYOTE

FOOD	PORTION	CAL.	FAT	SOD.	CARB.	FIB.
fresh cooked	1 cup	38	1	1	8	—
raw	1 (7 oz)	49	1	8	11	—
raw cut up	1 cup	32	tr	198	7	—

CHEESE

(*see also* CHEESE DISHES, CHEESE SUBSTITUTES, COTTAGE CHEESE, CREAM CHEESE)

NATURAL

FOOD	PORTION	CAL.	FAT	SOD.	CARB.	FIB.
Alouette						
Brie Baby	1 oz	110	9	180	2	0
Brie Baby With Herbs	1 oz	110	9	180	2	0
Alpine Lace						
Cheddar Reduced Fat	1 piece (1 oz)	80	5	135	1	0
Colby Reduced Fat	1 piece (1 oz)	80	5	115	1	0
Feta Reduced Fat	1 piece (1 oz)	60	4	370	1	0
Mozzarella Reduced Sodium Part Skim	1 piece (1 oz)	70	5	75	1	0
Muenster Reduced Sodium	1 piece (1 oz)	100	9	85	1	0
Provolone Smoked Reduced Fat	1 piece (1 oz)	70	5	120	1	0
Swiss Reduced Fat	1 piece (1 oz)	90	6	35	1	0
Armour						
Cheddar	1 oz	110	9	—	—	—
Cheddar Lower Salt	1 oz	110	9	106	—	—
Colby Lower Salt	1 oz	110	9	—	—	—
Monterey Jack	1 oz	110	9	—	—	—
Monterey Jack Lower Salt	1 oz	110	9	111	—	—

FOOD	PORTION	CAL.	FAT	SOD.	CARB.	FIB.
BabyBel						
Mini Light	1 (0.7 oz)	45	3	180	0	0
Bongrain						
Chavrie	2 tbsp (0.8 oz)	40	3	110	1	0
Montrachet	1 oz	70	6	135	tr	0
Montrachet Chive	1 oz	70	6	135	tr	0
Montrachet Classic	1 oz	70	6	130	tr	0
Montrachet Classic Herb	1 oz	70	6	150	tr	0
Montrachet Herbs & Garlic	1 oz	70	6	150	tr	0
Montrachet In Oil drained	1 oz	70	6	130	tr	0
Montrachet With Ash	1 oz	70	6	125	tr	0
Breakstone						
Ricotta	¼ cup (2.2 oz)	110	8	90	3	0
Bresse						
Brie	1 oz	110	9	180	2	0
Brie Light	1 oz	70	4	160	1	tr
Brie With Herbs	1 oz	110	9	180	2	0
Creme De Brie	2 tbsp (1 oz)	90	8	220	tr	0
Creme De Brie Herb	2 tbsp (1 oz)	90	8	220	tr	0
Brier Run						
Cherve	1 oz	61	5	70	—	—
Quark	1 oz	34	3	15	—	—
Bristol Gold						
Cheddar Light	1 oz	70	4	150	3	—
French Onion Light	1 oz	70	4	150	3	—
Garlic & Herb Light	1 oz	70	4	150	3	—
Horseradish Light	1 oz	70	4	150	3	—
Smoke Light	1 oz	70	4	150	3	—
Wine Light	1 oz	70	4	150	3	—
Cabot						
Cheddar	1 oz	110	9	175	0	—
Monterey Jack	1 oz	80	5	200	1	—
Vitalait	1 oz	70	4	170	1	—
Vitalait Jalapeno	1 oz	70	4	170	1	—
Churney						
Feta	1 oz	80	6	320	tr	0
Cracker Barrel						
Cheddar Sharp Reduced Fat	1 oz	80	5	220	tr	0
Cheddar Sharp Reduced Fat Shredded	¼ cup (0.9 oz)	80	5	200	tr	0

FOOD	PORTION	CAL.	FAT	SOD.	CARB.	FIB.
Delice De France						
With Herbs	1 oz	110	9	180	2	0
Di Giorno						
Parmesan	2 tsp (5 g)	20	1	55	0	0
Parmesan Grated	2 tsp (5 g)	20	2	85	0	0
Parmesan Shredded	2 tsp (5 g)	20	2	75	0	0
Romano	2 tsp (5 g)	20	2	75	0	0
Romano Grated	2 tsp (5 g)	25	2	90	0	0
Romano Shredded	2 tsp (5 g)	20	2	70	0	0
Dorman						
Cheda-Jack Reduced Fat Low Sodium	1 oz	80	5	140	1	—
Cheddar	1 oz	110	9	200	1	—
Cheddar Reduced Fat Low Sodium	1 oz	80	5	140	1	—
Colby	1 oz	110	9	190	1	—
Edam	1 oz	100	8	200	1	—
Gouda	1 oz	100	8	210	1	—
Monterey Reduced Fat Low Sodium	1 oz	80	5	140	1	—
Monterey Jack	1 oz	100	8	180	1	—
Mozzarella Park Skim	1 oz	90	7	190	1	—
Mozzarella Reduced Fat Low Sodium	1 oz	80	4	140	1	—
Muenster	1 oz	110	9	190	0	—
Muenster Low Sodium	1 oz	110	9	95	0	—
Muenster Reduced Fat Low Sodium	1 oz	80	5	140	tr	—
Parmesan	1 oz	110	7	350	1	—
Provolone	1 oz	90	7	290	1	—
Provolone Reduced Fat Low Sodium	1 oz	80	4	140	1	—
Romano	1 oz	100	7	350	1	—
Swiss	1 oz	100	8	80	0	—
Swiss No Salt Added	1 oz	100	8	10	tr	—
Swiss Reduced Fat Low Sodium	1 oz	90	5	60	tr	—
Father Time						
Cheddar Extra-Sharp Premium	1 oz	110	9	180	1	0
Friendship						
Farmer	2 tbsp (1 oz)	50	3	120	0	0
Farmer No Salt Added	2 tbsp (1 oz)	50	3	10	0	0
Hoop	2 tbsp (1 oz)	20	0	10	0	0

FOOD	PORTION	CAL.	FAT	SOD.	CARB.	FIB.
Frigo						
Asiago	1 oz	110	9	400	1	—
Blue	1 oz	100	8	400	1	—
Cheddar	1 oz	110	9	200	1	—
Cheddar Lite	1 oz	80	5	190	1	—
Feta	1 oz	100	8	400	1	—
Impastata	1 oz	60	5	50	1	—
Mozzarella Lite Whole Milk Low Moisture	1 oz	60	2	140	1	—
Mozzarella Part Skim Low Moisture	1 oz	80	5	190	1	—
Mozzarella Whole Milk Low Moisture	1 oz	90	7	190	1	—
Parmazest	1 oz	120	7	410	5	—
Parmesan & Romano Dry Grated	1 oz	130	9	510	1	—
Parmesan & Romano Grated	1 oz	110	7	350	1	—
Parmesan Dry Grated	1 oz	130	9	510	1	—
Parmesan Grated	1 oz	110	7	350	1	—
Parmesan Whole	1 oz	110	7	350	1	—
Pizza Shredded	1 oz	65	3	150	1	—
Provolone	1 oz	100	7	230	1	—
Provolone Lite	1 oz	70	4	205	1	—
Ricotta Low Fat Low Salt	1 oz	30	1	10	1	—
Ricotta Part Skim	1 oz	40	3	30	1	—
Ricotta Whole Milk	1 oz	60	5	40	1	—
Romano Dry Grated	1 oz	130	9	510	1	—
Romano Grated	1 oz	110	8	350	1	—
Romano Whole	1 oz	110	8	350	1	—
String	1 oz	80	5	190	1	—
String Lite	1 oz	60	2	140	1	—
Swiss	1 oz	110	8	80	1	—
Taco Shredded	1 oz	110	9	200	1	—
Gerard						
Brie	1 oz	90	7	180	2	0
Healthy Choice						
Cheddar Fancy Shreds	¼ cup (1 oz)	45	0	200	2	—
Cheddar Shreds	¼ cup (1 oz)	45	0	200	2	—
Mexican Shreds	¼ cup (1 oz)	45	0	200	2	—
Mozzarella	1 oz	45	0	200	1	—
Mozzarella Fancy Shreds	¼ cup (1 oz)	45	0	200	2	—
Mozzarella Shreds	¼ cup (1 oz)	45	0	200	2	—
Mozzarella String Cheese	1 stick (1 oz)	45	0	200	1	—

FOOD	PORTION	CAL.	FAT	SOD.	CARB.	FIB.
Healthy Choice (cont.)						
Pizza Fancy Shreds	¼ cup (1 oz)	45	0	200	2	—
Pizza String	1 stick (1 oz)	45	0	200	1	—
Heluva Good Cheese						
Cheddar Curds Snack	1 oz	113	9	179	1	0
Cheddar Extra-Sharp	1 oz	110	9	180	1	0
Cheddar Mild	1 oz	110	9	180	1	0
Cheddar Mild Reduced Fat	1 oz	80	6	200	1	0
Cheddar Mild White	1 oz	110	9	180	1	0
Cheddar Sharp	1 oz	110	9	180	1	0
Cheddar Sharp White	1 oz	110	9	180	1	0
Cheddar Shredded	¼ cup (1 oz)	110	9	180	1	0
Cheddar Very Low Sodium	1 oz	110	9	140	0	0
Cheddar White Extra-Sharp	1 oz	110	9	180	1	0
Cheddar White Very Low Sodium	1 oz	110	9	140	0	0
Cheddar White Shredded	¼ cup (1 oz)	110	9	180	1	0
Colby	1 oz	117	9	186	0	0
Colby-Jack	1 oz	110	9	200	0	0
Monterey Jack	1 oz	100	8	180	0	0
Monterey Jack Shredded	¼ cup (1 oz)	100	8	170	1	0
Monterey Jack With Jalapenos	1 oz	100	8	180	0	0
Mozzarella Part Skim Low Moisture Shredded	¼ cup (1 oz)	80	5	170	1	0
Mozzarella Whole Milk	1 oz	80	6	220	tr	0
Muenster	1 oz	100	8	180	0	0
Swiss	1 oz	112	8	62	0	0
Washed Curd Cheese	1 oz	110	9	170	1	0
Holland Farm						
Edam	1 oz	97	8	—	—	—
Farmer	1 oz	102	8	—	—	—
Gouda	1 oz	103	8	—	—	—
Monterey Jack	1 oz	102	9	—	—	—
Muenster	1 oz	102	9	—	—	—
Hollow Road Farms						
Sheep's Milk	1 oz	45	3	65	1	—
Keller's						
Chub	2 tbsp (1 oz)	100	10	120	1	0

FOOD	PORTION	CAL.	FAT	SOD.	CARB.	FIB.
Kraft						
Baby Swiss	1 oz	110	9	110	0	0
Blue	1 oz	100	8	390	tr	0
Blue Crumbles	1 oz	100	8	390	tr	0
Brick	1 oz	110	9	190	0	0
Cheddar	1 oz	110	9	180	tr	0
Cheddar Fat Free Shredded	¼ cup (1 oz)	45	0	220	0	0
Cheddar Mild Reduced Fat	1 oz	80	5	220	0	0
Cheddar Mild Reduced Fat Shredded	¼ cup (1.1 oz)	90	6	230	tr	0
Cheddar Nacho Blend With Peppers	1 oz	110	9	250	0	0
Cheddar Sharp Reduced Fat	1 oz	80	5	220	tr	0
Cheddar Shredded Finely	¼ cup (0.8 oz)	90	8	150	tr	0
Colby	1 oz	110	9	180	tr	0
Colby And Monterey Jack	1 oz	110	9	190	0	0
Colby And Monterey Jack Shredded	¼ cup (1 oz)	120	10	200	tr	0
Colby And Monterey Jack Shredded Reduced Fat Light	1 oz	80	5	220	1	—
Colby Reduced Fat	1 oz	80	5	220	0	0
Farmers	1 oz	100	8	190	tr	0
Gouda	1 oz	110	9	160	tr	0
Havarti	1 oz	120	11	240	0	0
House Italian ⅓ Less Fat Grated	2 tsp (0.2 oz)	25	1	115	1	0
Italian Blend Grated	2 tsp (0.2 oz)	25	2	95	0	0
Limburger	1 oz	90	8	240	0	0
Monterey Jack	1 oz	110	9	190	0	0
Monterey Jack Reduced Fat	1 oz	80	5	220	0	0
Monterey Jack Shredded	¼ cup (1 oz)	110	9	200	tr	0
Monterey Jack With Jalapeno Peppers	1 oz	110	9	190	tr	0
Monterey Jack With Peppers Reduced Fat	1 oz	80	5	220	tr	0
Mozzarella Fat Free Shredded	¼ cup (1 oz)	50	0	280	2	tr

FOOD	PORTION	CAL.	FAT	SOD.	CARB.	FIB.
Kraft (CONT.)						
Mozzarella Low Moisture Part Skim Reduced Fat Shredded	¼ cup (1.1 oz)	80	5	210	tr	0
Mozzarella Low Moisture Part Skim Shredded	¼ cup (1 oz)	90	6	210	tr	0
Mozzarella Low Moisture Part Skim Shredded Finely	¼ cup (0.8 oz)	70	5	160	tr	0
Mozzarella Low Moisture Whole Milk Shredded	¼ cup (1 oz)	90	7	210	tr	0
Mozzarella Part Skim Low Moisture	1 oz	80	5	200	tr	0
Mozzarella String Cheese Low Moisture Part Skim	1 stick (1 oz)	80	6	240	tr	0
Muenster	1 oz	110	9	190	0	0
Parmesan Grated	2 tsp (0.2 oz)	20	2	85	0	0
Parmesan Shredded	2 tsp (0.2 oz)	20	2	75	0	0
Pizza Four Cheeses Shredded	¼ cup (0.9 oz)	90	7	230	tr	0
Pizza Mild Cheddar & Mozzarella Shredded	¼ cup (0.9 oz)	90	7	170	tr	0
Pizza Mozzarella & Cheddar	¼ cup (0.9 oz)	100	8	190	tr	0
Pizza Mozzarella & Provolone	¼ cup (0.9 oz)	90	7	210	tr	0
Provolone Smoke Flavor	1 oz	100	7	240	tr	0
Romano Grated	2 tsp (0.2 oz)	25	2	90	0	0
Shredded	¼ cup (1 oz)	120	10	190	tr	0
String With Jalapeno Peppers	1 oz	80	5	230	1	—
Swiss	1 oz	110	9	50	0	0
Swiss Shredded	¼ cup (1 oz)	80	9	45	0	0
Taco Cheddar & Monterey Jack Shredded	¼ cup (0.9 oz)	100	8	180	tr	0
Land O'Lakes						
Baby Swiss	1 oz	110	8	125	0	0
Brick	1 oz	100	8	160	tr	0
Chedarella	1 oz	100	8	200	0	0
Cheddar Light	1 oz	70	4	230	tr	0
Gouda	1 oz	110	8	230	1	—
Monterey Jack	1 oz	110	9	160	tr	0

FOOD	PORTION	CAL.	FAT	SOD.	CARB.	FIB.
Land O'Lakes (CONT.)						
Mozzarella	1 oz	80	6	190	tr	0
Muenster	1 oz	100	8	220	0	0
Provolone	1 oz	100	8	240	tr	0
Swiss	1 oz	110	8	75	tr	0
Swiss Light	1 oz	80	4	60	tr	0
Laughing Cow						
Babybel	1 oz	90	7	230	0	0
Babybel Mini	1 (0.7 oz)	70	6	170	0	0
Bonbel	1 oz	100	8	230	0	0
Bonbel Mini	1 (0.7 oz)	70	6	170	0	0
Gouda Mini	1 (0.7 oz)	80	6	170	0	0
Marin French Cheese						
Breakfast	1 oz	86	7	—	1	—
Brie	1 oz	86	7	—	1	—
Camembert	1 oz	86	7	—	1	—
Schloss	1 oz	86	7	—	1	—
MayBud						
Edam	1 oz	100	8	210	1	0
Gouda	1 oz	100	8	210	1	0
Gouda Round	1 oz	100	8	210	1	0
New Holland						
Garlic	1 oz	90	7	105	tr	0
Havarti Lower Fat Garden Vegetable	1 oz	80	6	145	0	0
Jalapeno	1 oz	80	6	140	tr	0
Natural Vegetable	1 oz	80	6	110	tr	0
Northfield						
Naturally Slender	1 oz	90	7	—	—	—
Polly-O						
Mozzarella Free	1 oz	35	0	220	tr	—
Mozzarella Lite	1 oz	60	3	230	tr	—
Mozzarella Part Skim	1 oz	70	5	220	tr	—
Mozzarella Part Skim Shredded	¼ cup	80	5	200	tr	—
Mozzarella Shredded Free	¼ cup	45	0	270	1	—
Mozzarella Shredded Lite	¼ cup	60	3	220	1	—
Mozzarella Whole Milk	1 oz	80	6	220	tr	—
Mozzarella Whole Milk Shredded	¼ cup	90	7	200	tr	—
Ricotta Free	¼ cup	50	0	80	2	—
Ricotta Lite	¼ cup	70	3	80	3	—

FOOD	PORTION	CAL.	FAT	SOD.	CARB.	FIB.
Polly-O (CONT.)						
Ricotta Part Skim	¼ cup	90	6	65	2	—
Ricotta Whole Milk	¼ cup	110	8	60	2	—
String	1 oz	80	6	200	1	—
Progresso						
Parmesan Grated	1 tbsp	23	2	95	tr	0
Romano Grated	1 tbsp	23	2	70	tr	0
Quaker						
Chub	2 tbsp (1 oz)	100	10	120	1	0
Sargento						
4 Cheese Mexican Recipe Blend Shredded	¼ cup (1 oz)	110	9	200	tr	0
6 Cheese Italian Recipe Blend Shredded	¼ cup (1 oz)	90	7	180	0	0
Blue Crumbled	¼ cup (1 oz)	100	8	350	1	0
Cheddar	1 slice (1 oz)	110	9	160	1	0
Cheddar Mild Shredded Classic Supreme	¼ cup (1 oz)	110	9	160	1	0
Cheddar Mild Shredded Fancy Supreme	¼ cup (1 oz)	110	9	160	1	0
Cheddar Mild Shredded Preferred Light	¼ cup (1 oz)	70	5	200	tr	0
Cheddar Mild White Shredded Classic Supreme	¼ cup (1 oz)	110	9	160	1	0
Cheddar New York Sharp Shredded Classic Supreme	¼ cup (1 oz)	110	9	160	1	0
Cheddar Sharp Shredded Classic Supreme	¼ cup (1 oz)	110	9	160	1	0
Cheddar Sharp Shredded Fancy Supreme	¼ cup (1 oz)	110	9	160	1	0
Cheese For Nachos & Tacos Shredded	¼ cup (1 oz)	110	9	240	1	0
Cheese For Pizza Shredded	¼ cup (1 oz)	90	6	210	0	0
Cheese For Tacos Shredded	¼ cup (1 oz)	110	9	220	1	0
Cheese For Tacos Shredded Preferred Light	¼ cup (1 oz)	70	5	240	tr	0

FOOD	PORTION	CAL.	FAT	SOD.	CARB.	FIB.
Sargento (CONT.)						
Colby	1 slice (1 oz)	110	9	190	0	0
Colby-Jack Shredded Fancy Supreme	¼ cup (1 oz)	110	9	190	tr	0
Gourmet Parm	1 tbsp	20	1	95	tr	—
Jarlsberg	1 slice (1.2 oz)	120	9	50	1	0
Monterey Jack	1 slice (1 oz)	100	9	190	0	0
MooTown Snackers Cheddar	1 piece (0.8 oz)	100	8	130	1	0
MooTown Snackers Cheddar Mild Light	1 piece (0.8 oz)	60	4	170	tr	0
MooTown Snackers Cheese & Pretzels	1 pkg (1 oz)	90	3	320	12	0
MooTown Snackers Cheese & Sticks	1 pkg (1 oz)	100	4	260	13	0
MooTown Snackers Colby-Jack	1 piece (0.8 oz)	90	8	160	tr	0
MooTown Snackers Pizza Cheese & Sticks	1 pkg (1 oz)	100	4	260	13	0
MooTown Snackers String	1 piece (0.8 oz)	70	5	170	tr	0
MooTown Snackers String Light	1 piece (0.8 oz)	60	3	200	tr	0
Mozzarella	1 slice (1.5 oz)	130	9	230	2	0
Mozzarella Preferred Light	1 slice (1.5 oz)	100	5	210	0	0
Mozzarella Shredded Classic Supreme	¼ cup (1 oz)	80	6	150	1	0
Mozzarella Shredded Fancy Supreme	¼ cup (1 oz)	80	6	150	1	0
Mozzarella Shredded Preferred Light	¼ cup (1 oz)	70	3	140	tr	0
Muenster	1 slice (1 oz)	100	9	200	tr	0
Parmesan & Romano Shredded	¼ cup (1 oz)	110	7	340	1	0
Parmesan Fresh	1 oz	111	7	454	1	—
Parmesan Shredded	¼ cup (1 oz)	110	7	300	1	0
Pizza Double Cheese Shredded	¼ cup (1 oz)	90	6	150	1	0
Provolone	1 slice (1 oz)	100	8	190	0	0
Ricotta Light	¼ cup (2.2 oz)	60	3	55	3	0
Ricotta Old Fashioned	¼ cup (2.2 oz)	90	6	75	3	0
Ricotta Part Skim	¼ cup (2.2 oz)	80	5	75	2	0
Swiss	1 slice (0.7 oz)	80	6	30	0	0

FOOD	PORTION	CAL.	FAT	SOD.	CARB.	FIB.
Sargento (CONT.)						
Swiss Preferred Light	1 slice (1 oz)	80	4	50	tr	0
Swiss Shredded Fancy Supreme	¼ cup (1 oz)	110	8	40	0	0
Swiss Wafer Thin	2 slices (1 oz)	110	9	40	0	0
Treasure Cave						
Blue Crumbled	1 oz	110	9	400	tr	0
Feta Crumbled	1 oz	80	6	370	tr	0
Tree Of Life						
Cheddar 33% Reduced Fat Organic Milk	1 oz	90	6	135	1	—
Cheddar Low Sodium Raw Milk	1 oz	110	9	110	0	—
Cheddar Mild Organic Milk	1 oz	110	9	190	1	—
Cheddar Mild Raw Milk	1 oz	110	9	180	0	—
Cheddar Razor Sharp Raw Milk	1 oz	110	9	180	0	—
Cheddar Sharp Organic Milk	1 oz	110	9	190	0	—
Cheddar Sharp Raw Milk	1 oz	110	9	180	0	—
Colby Organic Milk	1 oz	120	10	190	1	—
Colby Raw Milk	1 oz	110	9	170	1	—
Farmer Part-Skim Organic Milk	1 oz	90	6	110	1	—
Jalapeno Jack Organic Milk	1 oz	110	9	190	1	—
Jalapeno Jack Semi-Soft Organic Milk	1 oz	110	9	150	0	—
Monterey Jack 35% Reduced Fat Organic Milk	1 oz	80	5	190	1	—
Monterey Jack Organic Milk	1 oz	100	8	185	1	—
Monterey Jack Semi-Soft Raw Milk	1 oz	110	9	150	0	—
Mozzarella Low Moisture Part Skim	1 oz	80	5	150	1	—
Mozzarella Low Moisture Part Skim Organic Milk	1 oz	80	5	170	1	—
Muenster Organic Milk	1 oz	100	8	185	1	—
Muenster Semi-Soft Raw Milk	1 oz	100	9	180	0	—

FOOD	PORTION	CAL.	FAT	SOD.	CARB.	FIB.
Tree Of Life (CONT.)						
Provolone	1 oz	100	8	250	1	—
Swiss Raw Milk	1 oz	110	8	75	1	—
Weight Watchers						
Cheddar Mild Shredded	1 oz	80	5	150	1	—
Cheddar Mild White	1 oz	80	5	150	1	—
Cheddar Mild White Low Sodium	1 oz	80	5	70	1	—
Cheddar Mild Yellow	1 oz	80	5	150	1	—
Cheddar Mild Yellow Low Sodium	1 oz	80	5	70	1	—
Cheddar Sharp Cup	1½ tbsp (1 oz)	70	3	190	7	—
Cheddar Sharp White	1 oz	80	5	150	1	—
Cheddar Sharp Yellow	1 oz	80	5	150	1	—
Colby	1 oz	80	5	150	1	—
Monterey Jack	1 oz	80	5	150	1	—
Mozzarella	1 oz	70	4	150	1	—
Mozzarella Shredded	1 oz	80	5	150	1	—
White Clover						
Cheddar Light With Simplesse	1 oz	80	4	160	tr	—
Colby Light With Simplesse	1 oz	80	4	180	tr	—
Monterey Jack Light With Simplesse	1 oz	70	4	190	tr	—
Muenster Light With Simplesse	1 oz	70	4	190	tr	—
bel paese	3½ oz	391	30	—	0	—
blue	1 oz	100	8	396	1	—
blue crumbled	1 cup	477	39	1884	3	—
brick	1 oz	105	8	159	1	—
brie	1 oz	95	8	178	tr	—
cacio di roma sheep's milk cheese	1 oz	130	10	170	0	—
caerphilly	1.4 oz	150	13	—	0	0
camembert	1 wedge (1⅓ oz)	114	9	320	tr	—
camembert	1 oz	85	7	239	tr	—
caraway	1 oz	107	8	196	1	—
cheddar	1 oz	114	9	176	tr	—
cheddar low fat	1 oz	49	2	174	1	—
cheddar low sodium	1 oz	113	9	6	1	—
cheddar reduced fat	1.4 oz	104	6	—	0	0
cheddar shredded	1 cup	455	37	701	1	—
cheshire	1 oz	110	9	198	1	—

FOOD	PORTION	CAL.	FAT	SOD.	CARB.	FIB.
cheshire reduced fat	1.4 oz	108	6	—	tr	0
colby	1 oz	112	9	171	1	—
colby low fat	1 oz	49	2	174	1	—
colby low sodium	1 oz	113	9	6	1	—
derby	1.4 oz	161	14	—	0	0
edam	1 oz	101	8	274	tr	—
edam reduced fat	1.4 oz	92	4	—	tr	0
emmentaler	3½ oz	403	30	450	tr	—
feta	1 oz	75	6	316	1	—
fontina	1 oz	110	9	—	tr	—
fromage frais	1.6 oz	51	3	—	3	0
gjetost	1 oz	132	8	170	12	—
gloucester double	1.4 oz	162	14	—	0	0
goat hard	1 oz	128	10	98	1	—
goat semi-soft	1 oz	103	8	146	1	—
goat soft	1 oz	76	6	104	tr	—
gorgonzola	3½ oz	376	31	—	1	—
gouda	1 oz	101	8	232	1	—
gruyere	1 oz	117	9	95	tr	—
lancashire	1.4 oz	149	12	—	0	0
leicester	1.4 oz	160	14	—	0	0
limburger	1 oz	93	8	227	tr	—
lymeswold	1.4 oz	170	16	—	tr	0
monterey	1 oz	106	9	152	tr	—
mozzarella	1 lb	1276	98	1692	10	—
mozzarella	1 oz	80	6	106	1	—
mozzarella low moisture	1 oz	90	7	118	1	—
mozzarella low moisture part skim	1 oz	79	5	150	1	—
mozzarella part skim	1 oz	72	5	132	1	—
muenster	1 oz	104	9	178	tr	—
parmesan grated	1 oz	129	9	528	1	—
parmesan grated	1 tbsp	23	2	93	tr	—
parmesan hard	1 oz	111	7	454	1	—
port du salut	1 oz	100	8	151	tr	—
provolone	1 oz	100	8	248	1	—
quark 20% fat	3½ oz	116	5	35	3	—
quark 40% fat	3½ oz	167	11	34	3	—
quark made w/ skim milk	3½ oz	78	tr	40	4	—
queso anego	1 oz	106	9	321	1	—
queso asadero	1 oz	101	8	186	1	—
queso chichuahua	1 oz	106	8	175	2	—
ricotta	1 cup	428	32	207	7	—
ricotta	½ cup	216	16	104	4	—

FOOD	PORTION	CAL.	FAT	SOD.	CARB.	FIB.
ricotta part skim	1 cup	340	19	307	13	—
ricotta part skim	½ cup	171	10	155	6	—
romadur 40% fat	3½ oz	289	20	—	tr	—
romano	1 oz	110	8	340	1	—
roquefort	1 oz	105	9	513	1	—
stilton blue	1.4 oz	164	14	—	0	0
stilton white	1.4 oz	145	13	—	0	0
swiss	1 oz	107	8	74	1	—
tilsit	1 oz	96	7	213	1	—
wensleydale	1.4 oz	151	13	—	0	0
whey cheese	3.5 oz	440	27	511	33	0
yogurt cheese	1 oz	20	0	—	—	—
PROCESSED						
Alouette						
French Onion	2 tbsp (0.8 oz)	70	7	160	1	0
Garlic	2 tbsp (0.8 oz)	70	7	135	1	0
Light Dill	2 tbsp (0.8 oz)	50	4	120	2	0
Light Garlic	2 tbsp (0.8 oz)	50	4	120	1	1
Light Herb	2 tbsp (0.8 oz)	50	4	125	2	0
Light Herbs & Garlic	2 tbsp (0.8 oz)	50	4	120	1	0
Light Spring Vegetable	2 tbsp (0.8 oz)	50	4	110	1	0
Salmon	2 tbsp (0.8 oz)	60	5	95	1	0
Scallions	2 tbsp (0.8 oz)	70	7	120	1	0
Spinach	2 tbsp (0.8 oz)	60	6	85	1	0
Alpine Lace						
American	1 slice (0.66 oz)	50	3	260	1	0
American Fat Free	1 piece (1 oz)	45	tr	280	2	0
American Hot Pepper Less Fat Less Sodium	1 piece (1 oz)	80	20	260	2	0
American Less Fat Less Sodium	1 piece (1 oz)	80	6	200	2	0
Cheddar Fat Free	1 piece (1 oz)	45	tr	280	2	0
Fat Free For Parmesan Lovers	2 tsp (5 g)	10	0	65	0	0
Fat Free Mexican Macho	2 tbsp (1 oz)	30	tr	165	1	0
Fat Free Singles	1 slice (0.66 oz)	25	0	280	tr	0
Mozzarella Fat Free	1 piece (1 oz)	45	tr	260	2	0
Borden						
American Slices	1 oz	110	9	490	1	—
American Very Sharp	1 oz	110	9	490	1	—
Lite Line Mozzarella	1 oz	50	2	—	—	—
Lite Line Sharp Cheddar	1 oz	50	2	—	—	—
Lite Line Swiss	1 oz	50	2	—	—	—
Swiss Slices	1 oz	100	8	380	1	—

FOOD	PORTION	CAL.	FAT	SOD.	CARB.	FIB.
Cheez Whiz						
Light	2 tbsp (1.2 oz)	80	3	540	6	0
Spread	2 tbsp (1.2 oz)	90	7	560	2	0
Spread Hot Salsa	2 tbsp (1.2 oz)	90	7	540	2	0
Spread Jalapeno Peppers	2 tbsp (1.2 oz)	90	8	530	2	0
Spread Mild Salsa	2 tbsp (1.2 oz)	90	7	520	2	0
Squeezable	2 tbsp (1.2 oz)	100	8	470	4	0
Zap-A-Pack Cheese Sauce	2 tbsp (1.2 oz)	90	8	580	3	0
Zap-A-Pack Cheese Sauce With Mild Salsa	2 tbsp (1.2 oz)	90	8	580	3	0
Churney						
Diet Snack Cheddar Flavored	1 oz	70	3	—	—	—
Diet Snack Port Wine Flavored	1 oz	70	3	—	—	—
Cracker Barrel						
Cheddar Extra Sharp	2 tbsp (1.1 oz)	100	8	290	3	0
Cheddar Sharp	2 tbsp (1.1 oz)	100	8	290	4	0
Delico						
Alouette Cajun	2 tbsp (0.8 oz)	70	7	120	1	0
Alouette French Onion	2 tbsp (0.8 oz)	70	7	160	1	0
Alouette Garden Vegetable	2 tbsp (0.8 oz)	60	6	130	1	0
Alouette Garlic	2 tbsp (0.8 oz)	70	7	135	1	0
Alouette Horseradish & Chive	2 tbsp (0.8 oz)	60	7	100	1	0
Alouette Spinach	2 tbsp (0.8 oz)	60	6	85	1	0
Dorman's						
Lo-Chol Cheddar	1 oz	100	7	140	1	—
Lo-Chol Colby	1 oz	100	7	140	1	—
Lo-Chol Mozzarella	1 oz	90	6	140	1	—
Lo-Chol Muenster	1 oz	100	7	140	1	—
Lo-Chol Swiss	1 oz	100	7	140	1	—
Easy Cheese						
Spread American	2 tbsp (1.2 oz)	100	7	400	2	0
Spread Cheddar	2 tbsp (1.2 oz)	100	7	410	3	0
Spread Cheddar'n Bacon	2 tbsp (1.2 oz)	100	7	410	3	0
Spread Nacho	2 tbsp (1.2 oz)	100	7	390	3	0
Spread Sharp Cheddar	2 tbsp (1.2 oz)	100	7	440	3	0
Formagg						
Formaggio D'Oro	1 oz	70	5	450	1	0

FOOD	PORTION	CAL.	FAT	SOD.	CARB.	FIB.
Handi-Snacks						
Cheez'n Breadsticks	1 pkg (1.1 oz)	130	7	340	11	0
Cheez'n Crackers	1 pkg (1.1 oz)	130	8	340	10	0
Cheez'n Pretzels	1 pkg (1 oz)	110	6	420	11	tr
Mozzarella String Cheese	1 stick (1 oz)	80	6	240	tr	0
Harvest Moon						
American	0.7 oz	50	3	280	1	0
American	1 slice (0.7 oz)	70	6	320	0	0
Spread American	0.7 oz	60	4	270	2	0
Healthy Choice						
American Singles White	1 slice (0.7 oz)	30	0	290	2	—
American Singles Yellow	1 slice (0.7 oz)	30	0	290	2	—
Loaf	1 in cube (1 oz)	35	0	390	3	—
Heluva Good Cheese						
American	1 slice (0.7)	45	5	390	2	0
Cold Pack Cheddar Sharp	2 tbsp (1 oz)	90	7	210	3	0
Cold Pack Cheddar Sharp With Bacon	2 tbsp (1 oz)	90	7	210	3	0
Cold Pack Cheddar Sharp With Horseradish	2 tbsp (1 oz)	90	7	210	3	0
Cold Pack Cheddar Sharp With Jalapenos	2 tbsp (1 oz)	90	7	210	3	0
Cold Pack Cheddar Sharp With Port Wine	2 tbsp (1 oz)	90	7	210	3	0
Hoffman						
American Yellow	1 oz	110	9	400	1	0
Hot Pepper	1 oz	90	7	460	2	0
Super Sharp	1 oz	110	9	380	1	0
Kraft						
American Grated	1 tbsp (0.2 oz)	25	2	135	1	0
American Shredded	¼ cup (0.9 oz)	110	9	440	tr	0
Cheese With Garlic	1 oz	90	7	370	2	0
Cheese With Jalapeno Peppers	1 oz	60	7	370	2	0
Deluxe 25% Less Fat American	0.7 oz	70	5	350	1	0
Deluxe American	1 slice (0.7 oz)	70	6	310	tr	0
Deluxe American	1 slice (1 oz)	110	9	460	tr	0
Deluxe American	1 oz	100	9	430	tr	0
Deluxe American White	1 slice (1 oz)	110	9	460	tr	0
Deluxe American White	1 slice (0.7 oz)	70	6	310	tr	0

FOOD	PORTION	CAL.	FAT	SOD.	CARB.	FIB.
Kraft (CONT.)						
Deluxe American White	1 oz	100	9	430	tr	0
Deluxe Pimento	1 slice (1 oz)	100	8	430	tr	0
Deluxe Swiss	1 slice (0.7 oz)	70	5	310	0	0
Deluxe Swiss	1 slice (1 oz)	90	7	420	tr	0
Free Singles	1 slice (0.7 oz)	30	0	320	3	0
Free Singles Sharp Cheddar	1 slice (0.7 oz)	30	0	290	3	0
Free Singles Swiss	1 slice (0.7 oz)	30	0	290	3	0
Free Singles White	1 slice (0.7 oz)	30	0	320	3	0
Singles ⅓ Less Fat American	0.7 oz	40	3	330	2	0
Singles ⅓ Less Fat American White	0.7 oz	50	3	330	2	0
Singles ⅓ Less Fat Sharp Cheddar	0.7 oz	50	3	300	2	0
Singles ⅓ Less Fat Swiss	0.7 oz	50	3	270	2	0
Singles American	1 slice (1.2 oz)	110	8	460	3	0
Singles American	1 slice (0.7 oz)	70	5	290	2	0
Singles American White	1 slice (0.7 oz)	70	5	290	2	0
Singles Mild Mexican Jalapeno Peppers	1 slice (0.7 oz)	70	5	330	2	0
Singles Monterey	1 slice (0.7 oz)	70	5	290	2	0
Singles Pimento	1 slice (0.7 oz)	60	5	260	1	0
Singles Sharp	1 slice (0.7 oz)	70	6	300	tr	0
Singles Swiss	1 slice (0.7 oz)	70	5	320	1	0
Spread Jalapeno Pepper	1 oz	80	6	470	2	0
Spread Olive & Pimento	2 tbsp (1.1 oz)	70	6	220	3	0
Spread Pimento	2 tbsp (1.1 oz)	80	6	170	3	0
Spread Pineapple	2 tbsp (1.1 oz)	70	5	120	4	0
Lactaid						
American	3.5 oz	328	25	1189	7	0
Land O'Lakes						
American	1 oz	110	9	430	tr	0
American	2 slices (1 oz)	100	9	460	1	0
American	1 slice (0.75 oz)	80	6	340	tr	0
American Less Salt	1 oz	110	9	270	tr	0
American Light	1 oz	70	5	400	2	0
American Sharp	1 oz	110	9	360	tr	0
American & Swiss	1 oz	100	8	380	0	0
Jalapeno Light	1 oz	70	4	400	1	0
Laughing Cow						
Assorted Wedge	1 (1 oz)	70	6	370	1	0

FOOD	PORTION	CAL.	FAT	SOD.	CARB.	FIB.
Laughing Cow (CONT.)						
Cheesebits	6 pieces (1 oz)	70	6	370	1	0
Original Wedge	1 (1 oz)	70	6	370	1	0
Wedge Light	1 (1 oz)	50	3	370	1	0
Light N'Lively						
Singles 50% Less Fat American	0.7 oz	50	3	260	2	0
Singles 50% Less Fat American White	0.7 oz	50	3	300	2	0
Mohawk Valley						
Spread Limburger	2 tbsp (1.1 oz)	80	7	500	0	0
Old English						
American Sharp	1 oz	100	9	440	tr	0
Spread Sharp	2 tbsp (1.1 oz)	70	8	520	tr	0
Price's						
Cheese & Bacon Spread	2 tbsp (1.1 oz)	90	7	340	2	0
Jalapeno Nacho Dip Hot	2 tbsp (1.1 oz)	80	7	370	2	0
Jalapeno Nacho Dip Mild	2 tbsp (1.1 oz)	80	7	370	2	0
Pimento Cheese Spread	2 tbsp (1.1 oz)	80	7	320	2	0
Pimento Cheese Spread Light	2 tbsp (1.1 oz)	60	4	260	3	0
Vegetable Garden	2 tbsp (1.1 oz)	70	5	290	3	0
Roka						
Spread Blue	2 tbsp (1.1 oz)	80	7	340	2	0
Rondele						
Light Soft Spreadable Garlic & Herb	2 tbsp (0.9 oz)	60	4	190	2	0
Soft Spreadable Garlic & Herb	2 tbsp (1 oz)	100	9	180	1	0
Smart Beat						
American	1 slice (0.6 oz)	35	2	180	2	—
Low Sodium	1 slice (0.6 oz)	35	2	90	2	—
Sharp	1 slice (0.6 oz)	35	2	210	2	—
Spreadery						
Medium Cheddar	2 tbsp (1.1 oz)	80	5	290	3	0
Pimento Spread	2 tbsp (1.1 oz)	100	8	320	3	0
Sharp Cheddar	2 tbsp (1.1 oz)	80	5	290	3	0
Vermont Sharp White Cheddar	2 tbsp (1.1 oz)	80	5	290	3	0
Squeez-A-Snak						
Spread Sharp	2 tbsp (1.1 oz)	90	8	440	tr	0
Velveeta						
Hot Mexican With Jalapeno Peppers Shredded	¼ cup (1.3 oz)	130	9	540	3	0

FOOD	PORTION	CAL.	FAT	SOD.	CARB.	FIB.
Velveeta (CONT.)						
Light	1 oz	60	3	420	3	0
Mild Mexican With Jalapeno Peppers Shredded	¼ cup (1.3 oz)	130	9	520	3	0
Shredded	¼ cup (1.3 oz)	130	9	500	3	0
Spread	1 oz	80	6	420	3	0
Spread Hot Mexican Jalapeno Pepper	1 oz	80	6	520	2	0
Spread Italiana	1 oz	60	6	430	2	0
Spread Mild Mexican With Jalapeno Pepper	1 oz	80	6	440	3	0
Weight Watchers						
American Slices Low Sodium White	2 slices (⅔ oz)	35	1	80	2	—
American Slices Low Sodium Yellow	2 slices (⅔ oz)	35	1	80	2	—
American Slices White	2 slices (⅔ oz)	35	1	270	1	—
American Slices Yellow	2 slices (⅔ oz)	35	1	270	1	—
Port Wine Cup	1½ tbsp (1 oz)	70	3	190	7	—
Sharp Cheddar Slices	2 slices (⅔ oz)	35	1	270	2	—
Swiss Slices	2 slices (⅔ oz)	35	1	270	2	—
WisPride						
Chunk	1 oz	110	8	180	4	0
Garlic & Herb Cup	2 tbsp (1.1 oz)	100	7	270	4	0
Hickory Smoked Cup	2 tbsp (1.1 oz)	100	7	230	4	0
Port Wine Ball	2 tbsp (1.1 oz)	100	8	190	4	0
Port Wine Cup	2 tbsp (1.1 oz)	100	7	230	4	0
Port Wine Light Cup	2 tbsp (1.1 oz)	80	3	200	5	0
Sharp Ball	2 tbsp (1.1 oz)	100	8	190	4	0
Sharp Cheddar Ball	2 tbsp (1.1 oz)	100	8	190	4	0
Sharp Cup	2 tbsp (1.1 oz)	100	7	230	4	0
Sharp Light Cup	2 tbsp (1.1 oz)	80	3	200	5	0
Swiss Ball	2 tbsp (1.1 oz)	110	8	125	5	0
american	1 oz	93	7	337	2	—
american cheese food	1 pkg (8 oz)	745	56	2700	17	—
american cheese spread	1 oz	82	6	381	2	—
american cheese spread	1 jar (5 oz)	412	30	1910	12	—
american cold pack	1 pkg (8 oz)	752	56	2193	19	—
pimento	1 oz	106	9	405	tr	—
swiss	1 oz	95	7	388	1	—
swiss cheese food	1 pkg (8 oz)	734	55	3523	10	—

FOOD	PORTION	CAL.	FAT	SOD.	CARB.	FIB.
CHEESE DISHES						
FROZEN						
Stouffer's						
Welsh Rarebit	¼ cup (1.1 oz)	120	9	280	5	—
HOME RECIPE						
welsh rarebit as prep w/ 1 white toast	1 slice	228	16	—	14	1
TAKE-OUT						
cheese omelette as prep w/ 2 eggs	1 (6.8 oz)	519	44	—	tr	0
fondue	1 cup (7.5 oz)	492	29	283	8	—
fondue	½ cup (3.8 oz)	247	15	142	4	—
macaroni & cheese	6.3 oz	320	19	—	25	1
CHEESE SUBSTITUTES						
Borden						
Taco-Mate	1 oz	100	7	360	2	—
Formagg						
American White	1 slice (0.66 oz)	60	4	260	tr	0
American Yellow	1 slice (0.66 oz)	60	4	260	tr	0
Caesar's Italian Garden American	1 oz	60	3	240	1	0
Cheddar	1 slice (0.66 oz)	60	4	260	tr	0
Cheddar Shredded	1 oz	60	3	190	1	0
Classic American	1 oz	60	3	290	1	0
Macaroni And Cheese Sauce	⅔ cup (5 oz)	190	2	470	35	0
Mozzarella Shredded	1 oz	60	3	140	1	0
Old World Mozzarella	1 oz	60	3	140	1	0
Parmesan Grated	2 tsp (5 g)	15	1	80	tr	tr
Swiss	1 oz	60	3	240	1	0
Swiss White	1 slice (0.66 oz)	60	4	260	tr	0
Vintage Provolone	1 oz	60	3	190	1	0
Zesty Jalapeno American	1 oz	60	3	290	1	0
Frigo						
Imitation Cheddar	1 oz	90	7	280	1	—
Imitation Mozzarella	1 oz	90	7	240	1	—
Georgio's						
Imitation Cheddar Shredded	¼ cup (1 oz)	90	7	450	1	0
Imitation Mozzarella Shredded	¼ cup (1 oz)	90	7	350	1	0
Golden Image						
American	0.7 oz	70	5	270	1	0

FOOD	PORTION	CAL.	FAT	SOD.	CARB.	FIB.
Harvest Moon						
American Shredded	¼ cup (1.3 oz)	120	9	500	3	0
Cheddar Shredded	¼ cup (1.3 oz)	120	9	480	3	0
Mozzarella Shredded	¼ cup (1.3 oz)	110	8	430	1	1
Lunchwagon						
American	1 slice (0.7 oz)	70	5	230	1	0
Sargento						
Classic Supreme Cheddar Shredded	¼ cup (1 oz)	90	6	470	2	0
Classic Supreme Mozzarella Shredded	¼ cup (1 oz)	80	6	320	tr	0
Fancy Supreme Cheddar Shredded	¼ cup (1 oz)	90	6	470	2	0
White Wave						
Soy A Melt Cheddar	1 oz	80	5	170	1	—
Soy A Melt Fat Free Cheddar	1 oz	40	tr	370	3	—
Soy A Melt Fat Free Mozzarella	1 oz	40	tr	370	3	—
Soy A Melt Garlic Herb	1 oz	80	5	170	1	—
Soy A Melt Jalapeno Jack	1 oz	80	5	170	1	—
Soy A Melt Monterey Jack	1 oz	80	5	170	1	—
Soy A Melt Mozzarella	1 oz	80	5	170	1	—
Soy A Melt Singles American	1 slice (¾ oz)	60	4	280	1	—
Soy A Melt Singles Mozzarella	1 slice (¾ oz)	60	4	280	1	—
mozzarella	1 oz	70	3	194	7	—
CHERIMOYA						
fresh	1	515	2	—	131	—
CHERRIES						
CANNED						
Del Monte						
Dark Pitted In Heavy Syrup	½ cup (4.2 oz)	120	0	10	24	tr
Sweet Dark Whole Unpitted In Heavy Syrup	½ cup (4.2 oz)	120	0	10	24	tr
sour in heavy syrup	½ cup	232	tr	18	60	—
sour in light syrup	½ cup	189	tr	18	49	—
sour water packed	1 cup	87	tr	17	22	—

FOOD	PORTION	CAL.	FAT	SOD.	CARB.	FIB.
sweet in heavy syrup	½ cup	107	tr	3	27	—
sweet in light syrup	½ cup	85	tr	3	22	—
sweet juice pack	½ cup	68	tr	3	17	—
sweet water pack	½ cup	57	tr	2	15	—
DRIED						
Chukar						
Bing	2 oz	160	1	3	35	—
Rainer	2 oz	160	1	3	35	—
Tart	2 oz	170	0	10	43	—
Tart 'n Sweet	2 oz	180	0	10	43	—
Sonoma						
Pitted	¼ cup (1.4 oz)	140	0	0	34	2
FRESH						
Dole	1 cup	90	1	0	19	3
sour	1 cup	51	tr	3	13	—
sweet	10	49	1	0	11	—
FROZEN						
Big Valley						
Dark Sweet	¾ cup (4.9 oz)	90	0	0	20	3
sour unsweetened	1 cup	72	1	1	17	—
sweet sweetened	1 cup	232	tr	3	58	—

CHERRY JUICE

FOOD	PORTION	CAL.	FAT	SOD.	CARB.	FIB.
After The Fall						
Black Cherry	1 can (12 oz)	170	0	20	42	0
Hi-C						
Box	8.45 fl oz	140	0	30	35	—
Kool-Aid						
Black Cherry	8 oz	98	0	—	25	—
Drink	8 oz	98	0	—	25	—
Koolers	1 (8.45 oz)	142	0	3	38	—
Sugar Free	8 oz	3	0	3	0	—
Sipps						
Wild Cherry	8.45 oz	130	0	—	—	—
Smucker's						
Black Cherry	8 oz	130	0	10	31	—
Black Cherry Sparkler	10 oz	120	tr	5	30	—
Tang						
Fruit Box	8.45 oz	121	0	2	32	—
Tree Of Life						
Concentrate	8 tsp (1.4 oz)	110	0	0	28	—
Wylers						
Drink Mix Unsweetened Cherry	8 oz	2	0	15	1	—

FOOD	PORTION	CAL.	FAT	SOD.	CARB.	FIB.
Wylers (CONT.)						
Drink Mix Wild Cherry	8 oz	81	0	tr	21	—

CHERVIL

seed	1 tsp	1	tr	tr	tr	—

CHESTNUTS

chinese cooked	1 oz	44	tr	1	10	—
chinese dried	1 oz	103	tr	2	23	—
chinese raw	1 oz	64	tr	1	14	—
chinese roasted	1 oz	68	tr	1	15	—
cooked	1 oz	37	tr	8	8	—
dried peeled	1 oz	105	1	11	22	—
japanese cooked	1 oz	16	tr	1	4	—
japanese dried	1 oz	102	tr	10	23	—
japanese raw	1 oz	44	tr	4	10	—
japanese roasted	1 oz	57	tr	—	13	—
raw peeled	1 oz	56	tr	1	13	—
roasted	1 cup	350	3	3	76	—
roasted	1 oz	70	1	1	15	—

CHEWING GUM

Bazooka						
Fruit Chunk	1 piece (6 g)	25	0	0	5	—
Fruit Soft	1 piece (6 g)	25	0	0	5	—
Gum	1 piece (6 g)	25	0	0	5	—
Gum	1 piece (4 g)	15	0	0	4	—
Beech-Nut						
Peppermint	1 stick (3 g)	10	0	0	2	0
Spearmint	1 stick (3 g)	10	0	0	2	0
Brock						
Bubble Gum	1 piece (0.2 oz)	20	0	0	4	—
Bubble Yum						
Bananaberry Split	1 piece (0.3 oz)	25	0	0	6	—
Cotton Candy	1 piece (0.3 oz)	25	0	0	6	—
Grape	1 piece (0.3 oz)	25	0	0	6	—
Luscious Lime	1 piece (0.3 oz)	25	0	0	6	—
Regular	1 piece (0.3 oz)	25	0	0	6	0
Sour Apple	1 piece (0.3 oz)	25	0	0	6	1
Sour Cherry	1 piece (0.3 oz)	25	0	0	6	0
Sugarless	1 piece (0.2 oz)	15	0	0	3	—
Sugarless Grape	1 piece (0.2 oz)	15	0	0	3	—
Sugarless Peppermint	1 piece (0.2 oz)	15	0	0	3	—
Sugarless Strawberry	1 piece (0.2 oz)	15	0	0	3	—
Sugarless Variety	1 piece (0.2 oz)	15	0	0	3	—

FOOD	PORTION	CAL.	FAT	SOD.	CARB.	FIB.
Bubble Yum (cont.)						
Variety Pack	1 piece (0.3 oz)	25	0	0	6	0
Watermelon	1 piece (0.3 oz)	25	0	0	6	0
Wild Strawberry	1 piece (0.3 oz)	25	0	0	6	0
*Care*Free*						
Sugarless Bubble Gum	1 stick (3 g)	10	0	0	2	—
Sugarless Cinnamon	1 piece (3 g)	5	0	0	2	—
Sugarless Peppermint	1 piece (3 g)	5	0	0	2	—
Sugarless Spearmint	1 piece (3 g)	5	0	0	2	—
Sugarless Wild Cherry	1 stick (3 g)	10	0	0	2	—
Chiclets						
Tiny Size	8 pieces (0.13 g)	tr	0	—	tr	—
Dentyne						
Cinn-A-Burst	1 piece (3.2 g)	9	0	—	2	—
Sugar Free	1 piece (1.88 g)	5	0	—	1	—
Doublemint						
Chewing Gum	1 piece	10	tr	0	2	—
Extra Sugar Free						
Cinnamon	1 piece	8	tr	0	tr	—
Spearmint & Peppermint	1 stick	8	tr	0	tr	—
Winter Fresh	1 piece	8	tr	0	tr	—
Freedent						
Spearmint Peppermint & Cinnamon	1 stick	10	tr	0	3	—
Fruit Stripe						
Bubble Gum Jumbo Pack	1 stick (3 g)	10	0	0	2	0
Variety Pack Chewing & Bubble Gum	1 stick (3 g)	10	0	0	2	0
Hubba Bubba						
Bubble Gum Cola	1 piece	23	tr	0	6	—
Bubble Gum Sugarfree Grape	1 piece	13	tr	0	tr	—
Bubble Gum Sugarfree Original	1 piece	14	tr	0	tr	—
Original	1 piece	23	0	0	6	—
Strawberry Grape Raspberry	1 piece	23	tr	0	6	—
Rain-Blo						
Bubble Gum Balls	1 piece (2 g)	5	0	0	2	—
*Stick*Free*						
Sugarless Peppermint	1 stick (3 g)	10	0	0	2	—
Sugarless Spearmint	1 stick (3 g)	10	0	0	2	—

FOOD	PORTION	CAL.	FAT	SOD.	CARB.	FIB.
Trident						
Soft Bubble Gum	1 piece (3.3 g)	9	0	—	2	—
Wrigley's						
Spearmint	1 stick	10	tr	0	2	—
bubble gum	1 block (8 g)	27	0	0	8	—
stick	1 (3 g)	10	0	0	3	—

CHIA SEEDS

FOOD	PORTION	CAL.	FAT	SOD.	CARB.	FIB.
dried	1 oz	134	7	—	14	—

CHICKEN

(*see also* CHICKEN DISHES, CHICKEN SUBSTITUTES, DINNER, HOT DOGS)

FOOD	PORTION	CAL.	FAT	SOD.	CARB.	FIB.
CANNED						
Hormel						
Chunk	2 oz	70	3	200	0	0
Chunk Breast	2 oz	60	2	100	0	0
No Salt Chunk Breast	2 oz	60	2	20	0	0
Swanson						
Chunk Style Mixin' Chicken	2½ oz	130	8	230	1	—
White	2½ oz	100	4	235	0	—
White & Dark	2½ oz	100	4	240	0	—
Underwood						
Chunky	2.08 oz	150	9	440	2	—
Chunky Light	2.08 oz	80	3	330	2	—
Smoky	2.08 oz	150	8	290	10	—
chicken spread	1 tbsp	25	2	—	1	—
chicken spread	1 oz	55	3	—	2	—
chicken spread barbeque flavored	1 oz	55	3	—	2	—
w/ broth	1 can (5 oz)	234	11	714	0	—
w/ broth	½ can (2.5 oz)	117	6	357	0	—
FRESH						
Perdue						
Breast Oven Stuffer Roaster w/ Skin cooked	1 oz	42	2	11	0	—
Breast Quarters Fresh Young w/ Skin cooked	1 oz	48	3	14	0	—
Breast Skinless & Boneless Oven Stuffer Roaster cooked	1 oz	31	tr	9	0	—
Breast Skinless Boneless cooked	1 oz	30	tr	10	0	—
Breast Split Fresh Young w/ Skin cooked	1 oz	45	3	12	0	—

FOOD	PORTION	CAL.	FAT	SOD.	CARB.	FIB.
Perdue (CONT.)						
Breast Thin-Sliced Skinless & Boneless Oven Stuffer cooked	1 oz	31	tr	9	0	—
Breast Whole Fresh Young w/ Skin cooked	1 oz	45	3	12	0	—
Breast Whole Oven Stuffer Meat Only cooked	3 oz	169	—	—	—	—
Cornish Hen Dark Meat w/ Skin cooked	1 oz	43	3	10	0	—
Cornish Hen White Meat w/ Skin cooked	1 oz	42	3	12	0	—
Drumsticks Fresh Young w/ Skin cooked	1 oz	42	2	21	0	—
Drumsticks Oven Stuffer Roaster w/ Skin cooked	1 oz	41	2	16	0	—
Fresh Young Ground cooked	1 oz	49	3	14	0	—
Fresh Young Legs w/ Skin cooked	1 oz	51	4	16	0	—
Fresh Young Whole Dark Meat w/ Skin cooked	1 oz	47	3	12	0	—
Leg Quarters Fresh Young w/ Skin cooked	1 oz	49	4	15	0	—
Skinless & Boneless Breast Tenders cooked	1 oz	29	tr	14	0	—
Skinless & Boneless Oven Stuffer Roaster Thighs cooked	1 oz	34	2	13	0	—
Soup & Stew Baking Hen Dark Meat w/ Skin cooked	1 oz	41	3	9	0	—
Soup & Stew Baking Hen White Meat w/ Skin cooked	1 oz	41	2	11	0	—
Thighs Fresh Young w/ Skin cooked	1 oz	57	4	15	0	—
Thighs Skinless & Boneless cooked	1 oz	30	2	10	0	—
Whole Fresh Young White Meat w/ Skin cooked	1 oz	43	2	11	0	—

FOOD	PORTION	CAL.	FAT	SOD.	CARB.	FIB.
Perdue (CONT.)						
Whole Oven Stuffer Roaster Dark Meat w/ Skin cooked	1 oz	49	3	16	0	—
Whole Oven Stuffer Roaster White Meat w/ Skin cooked	1 oz	44	2	12	0	—
Wing Drumettes Fresh Young w/ Skin cooked	1 oz	50	3	13	0	—
Wingettes Oven Stuffer Roaster w/ Skin cooked	1 oz	52	3	17	0	—
Wings Fresh Young w/ Skin cooked	1 oz	54	4	19	0	—
Tyson						
Breast	3 oz	116	2	63	0	—
Cornish Hen	3.5 oz	250	15	80	1	—
Drumstick	3 oz	131	4	81	0	—
Thigh	3 oz	152	7	75	0	—
Whole	3 oz	134	4	73	0	—
Wing	3 oz	147	6	78	0	—
Wampler Longacre						
Ground raw	1 oz	50	4	20	0	—
broiler/fryer back w/ skin batter dipped & fried	½ back (2.5 oz)	238	16	228	7	—
broiler/fryer back w/ skin floured & fried	1.5 oz	146	9	40	3	—
broiler/fryer back w/ skin roasted	1 oz	96	7	28	0	—
broiler/fryer back w/ skin stewed	½ back (2.1 oz)	158	11	39	0	—
broiler/fryer back w/o skin fried	½ back (2 oz)	167	9	58	3	—
broiler/fryer breast w/ skin batter dipped & fried	2.9 oz	218	11	231	8	—
broiler/fryer breast w/ skin batter dipped & fried	½ breast (4.9 oz)	364	18	385	13	—
broiler/fryer breast w/ skin roasted	2 oz	115	5	41	0	—
broiler/fryer breast w/ skin roasted	½ breast (3.4 oz)	193	8	69	0	—
broiler/fryer breast w/ skin stewed	½ breast (3.9 oz)	202	8	68	0	—
broiler/fryer breast w/o skin fried	½ breast (3 oz)	161	4	68	tr	—

FOOD	PORTION	CAL.	FAT	SOD.	CARB.	FIB.
broiler/fryer breast w/o skin roasted	½ breast (3 oz)	142	3	63	0	—
broiler/fryer breast w/o skin stewed	2 oz	86	2	36	0	—
broiler/fryer dark meat w/ skin batter dipped & fried	5.9 oz	497	31	493	16	—
broiler/fryer dark meat w/ skin floured & fried	3.9 oz	313	19	98	4	—
broiler/fryer dark meat w/ skin roasted	3.5 oz	256	16	88	0	—
broiler/fryer dark meat w/ skin stewed	3.9 oz	256	16	77	0	—
broiler/fryer dark meat w/o skin fried	1 cup (5 oz)	334	16	136	4	—
broiler/fryer dark meat w/o skin roasted	1 cup (5 oz)	286	14	130	0	—
broiler/fryer dark meat w/o skin stewed	3 oz	165	8	64	0	—
broiler/fryer dark meat w/o skin stewed	1 cup (5 oz)	269	13	104	0	—
broiler/fryer drumstick w/ skin batter dipped & fried	1 (2.6 oz)	193	11	194	6	—
broiler/fryer drumstick w/ skin floured & fried	1 (1.7 oz)	120	7	44	1	—
broiler/fryer drumstick w/ skin roasted	1 (1.8 oz)	112	6	47	0	—
broiler/fryer drumstick w/ skin stewed	1 (2 oz)	116	6	43	0	—
broiler/fryer drumstick w/o skin fried	1 (1.5 oz)	82	3	40	0	—
broiler/fryer drumstick w/o skin roasted	1 (1.5 oz)	76	2	42	0	—
broiler/fryer drumstick w/o skin stewed	1 (1.6 oz)	78	3	37	0	—
broiler/fryer leg w/ skin batter dipped & fried	1 (5.5 oz)	431	26	442	14	—
broiler/fryer leg w/ skin floured & fried	1 (3.9 oz)	285	16	99	3	—
broiler/fryer leg w/ skin roasted	1 (4 oz)	265	15	99	0	—
broiler/fryer leg w/ skin stewed	1 (4.4 oz)	275	16	92	0	—

FOOD	PORTION	CAL.	FAT	SOD.	CARB.	FIB.
broiler/fryer leg w/o skin fried	1 (3.3 oz)	195	9	90	1	—
broiler/fryer leg w/o skin roasted	1 (3.3 oz)	182	8	87	0	—
broiler/fryer leg w/o skin stewed	1 (3.5 oz)	187	8	78	0	—
broiler/fryer light meat w/ skin batter dipped & fried	4 oz	312	17	324	11	—
broiler/fryer light meat w/ skin floured & fried	2.7 oz	192	9	60	1	—
broiler/fryer light meat w/ skin roasted	2.8 oz	175	9	59	0	—
broiler/fryer light meat w/ skin stewed	3.2 oz	181	9	57	0	—
broiler/fryer light meat w/o skin fried	1 cup (5 oz)	268	8	114	1	—
broiler/fryer light meat w/o skin roasted	1 cup (5 oz)	242	6	108	0	—
broiler/fryer light meat w/o skin stewed	1 cup (5 oz)	223	6	91	0	—
broiler/fryer neck w/ skin stewed	1 (1.3 oz)	94	7	20	0	—
broiler/fryer neck w/o skin stewed	1 (.6 oz)	32	1	12	0	—
broiler/fryer skin batter dipped & fried	4 oz	449	33	663	26	—
broiler/fryer skin batter dipped & fried	from ½ chicken (6.7 oz)	748	55	1105	44	—
broiler/fryer skin floured & fried	1 oz	166	14	18	3	—
broiler/fryer skin floured & fried	from ½ chicken (2 oz)	281	24	30	5	—
broiler/fryer skin roasted	from ½ chicken (2 oz)	254	23	36	0	—
broiler/fryer skin stewed	from ½ chicken (2.5 oz)	261	24	40	0	—
broiler/fryer thigh w/ skin batter dipped & fried	1 (3 oz)	238	14	248	8	—
broiler/fryer thigh w/ skin floured & fried	1 (2.2 oz)	162	9	55	2	—
broiler/fryer thigh w/ skin roasted	1 (2.2 oz)	153	10	52	0	—
broiler/fryer thigh w/ skin stewed	1 (2.4 oz)	158	10	49	0	—

FOOD	PORTION	CAL.	FAT	SOD.	CARB.	FIB.
broiler/fryer thigh w/o skin fried	1 (1.8 oz)	113	5	49	1	—
broiler/fryer thigh w/o skin roasted	1 (1.8 oz)	109	6	46	0	—
broiler/fryer thigh w/o skin stewed	1 (1.9 oz)	107	5	41	0	—
broiler/fryer w/ skin floured & fried	½ chicken (11 oz)	844	47	264	10	—
broiler/fryer w/ skin floured & fried	½ breast (3.4 oz)	218	9	75	2	—
broiler/fryer w/ skin fried	½ chicken (16.4 oz)	1347	81	1360	44	—
broiler/fryer w/ skin roasted	½ chicken (10.5 oz)	715	41	244	0	—
broiler/fryer w/ skin stewed	½ chicken (11.7 oz)	730	42	224	0	—
broiler/fryer w/ skin neck & giblets batter dipped & fried	1 chicken (2.3 lbs)	2987	180	2921	93	—
broiler/fryer w/ skin neck & giblets roasted	1 chicken (1.5 lbs)	1598	90	536	tr	—
broiler/fryer w/ skin neck & giblets stewed	1 chicken (1.6 lbs)	1625	93	494	tr	—
broiler/fryer w/o skin fried	1 cup	307	13	127	2	—
broiler/fryer w/o skin roasted	1 cup (5 oz)	266	10	120	0	—
broiler/fryer w/o skin stewed	1 cup (5 oz)	248	9	98	0	—
broiler/fryer w/o skin stewed	1 oz	54	3	18	0	—
broiler/fryer wing w/ skin batter dipped & fried	1 (1.7 oz)	159	11	157	5	—
broiler/fryer wing w/ skin floured & fried	1 (1.1 oz)	103	7	25	1	—
broiler/fryer wing w/ skin roasted	1 (1.2 oz)	99	7	28	0	—
broiler/fryer wing w/ skin stewed	1 (1.4 oz)	100	7	27	0	—
capon w/ skin neck & giblets roasted	1 chicken (3.1 lbs)	3211	165	704	1	—
cornish hen w/o skin & bone roasted	1 hen (3.8 oz)	144	4	67	0	—
cornish hen w/o skin & bone roasted	½ hen (2 oz)	72	2	34	0	—
cornish hen w/skin roasted	½ hen (4 oz)	296	21	73	0	—
cornish hen w/skin roasted	1 hen (8 oz)	595	42	146	0	—

FOOD	PORTION	CAL.	FAT	SOD.	CARB.	FIB.
roaster dark meat w/o skin roasted	1 cup (5 oz)	250	12	133	0	—
roaster light meat w/o skin roasted	1 cup (5 oz)	214	6	71	0	—
roaster w/ skin neck & giblets roasted	1 chicken (2.4 lbs)	2363	140	760	1	—
roaster w/ skin roasted	½ chicken (1.1 lbs)	1071	64	349	0	—
roaster w/o skin roasted	1 cup (5 oz)	469	28	105	0	—
stewing dark meat w/o skin stewed	1 cup (5 oz)	361	21	133	0	—
stewing w/ skin neck & giblets stewed	1 chicken (1.3 lbs)	1636	107	419	tr	—
stewing w/ skin stewed	½ chicken (9.2 oz)	744	49	190	0	—
stewing w/ skin stewed	6.2 oz	507	34	130	0	—
FROZEN						
Tyson						
Boneless Breasts	3.5 oz	210	12	50	0	—
Boneless Skinless Breast	3.5 oz	130	2	50	0	—
Boneless Skinless Thighs	3.5 oz	200	10	70	0	—
Drums & Thighs	3.5 oz	270	17	110	0	—
Skinless Breast Tenders	3.5 oz	120	1	55	0	—
FROZEN PREPARED						
Banquet						
Country Fried	1 serv (3 oz)	270	18	620	13	1
Drum Snackers	2.25 oz	190	13	460	12	1
Fried Breast	1 piece (4.45 oz)	240	26	600	18	4
Fried Chicken Thigh & Drumsticks	1 serv (3 oz)	260	18	540	10	2
Fried Hot & Spicy	1 serv (3 oz)	260	18	590	13	1
Fried Original	1 serv (3 oz)	270	18	620	13	1
Hot & Spicy Nuggets	2.5 oz	230	17	320	11	1
Hot Popcorn Chicken	1 pkg (3 oz)	290	19	790	18	2
Nuggets	3 oz	240	15	540	12	1
Nuggets Chicken & Cheddar	2.7 oz	280	19	560	13	1
Nuggets Chicken & Mozzarella	6 (2.8 oz)	210	11	1060	20	2
Nuggets Southern Fried	6 (4.5 oz)	340	20	840	22	2
Nuggets Sweet & Sour	6 (4.5 oz)	320	18	670	25	2
Patties	1 (2.5 oz)	180	11	360	10	tr
Patties Southern Fried	1 (2.5 oz)	190	12	480	12	tr
Skinless Fried	1 serv (3 oz)	210	13	480	7	2
Skinless Fried Honey BBQ	1 serv (3 oz)	210	13	480	7	2

FOOD	PORTION	CAL.	FAT	SOD.	CARB.	FIB.
Banquet (CONT.)						
Southern Fried	1 serv (3 oz)	270	18	590	13	1
Tenders	3 pieces (3 oz)	260	16	490	16	2
Tenders Southern Fried	3 pieces (3 oz)	260	16	480	16	1
Wings Hot & Spicy	4 pieces (5 oz)	230	16	280	5	1
Country Skillet						
Chicken Chunks	5 (3.1 oz)	270	17	720	18	1
Chicken Nuggets	10 (3.3 oz)	280	18	620	16	1
Chicken Patties	2.5 oz	190	12	500	12	1
Southern Fried Chicken Chunks	5 (3.1 oz)	250	15	550	16	1
Southern Fried Chicken Patties	1 (2.5 oz)	190	12	450	12	1
Empire						
Nuggets	5 (3 oz)	180	9	370	12	1
Stix	4 (3.1 oz)	180	9	420	6	2
Ozark Valley						
Nuggets	4 (2.9 oz)	210	10	590	16	2
Patties	1 (3 oz)	210	11	550	14	1
Sensible Chef						
Fried Breast	1 (3 oz)	200	10	310	8	2
Swanson						
Chicken Nibbles	3¼ oz	300	19	690	19	—
Chicken Nuggets	3 oz	230	14	360	14	—
Fried Chicken Breast Portion	4½ oz	360	20	800	21	—
Pre-Fried Chicken Parts	3¼ oz	270	16	650	16	—
Thighs & Drumsticks	3¼ oz	290	18	610	17	—
Tyson						
BBQ Breast Fillets	3 oz	110	2	200	13	—
Breaded Patties	3 oz	300	20	—	15	—
Breast Chunks	3 oz	240	17	430	10	—
Breast Fillets	3 oz	190	9	400	15	—
Breast Patties	2.6 oz	220	15	640	11	—
Breast Tenders	3 oz	220	12	500	13	—
Chick'n Cheddar	2.6 oz	220	15	310	11	—
Chick'n Chunks	2.6 oz	220	15	500	11	—
Cordon Blue Mini	1	90	4	210	5	—
Diced	3 oz	130	3	40	1	—
Grilled Sandwich	3.5 oz	200	5	470	25	—
Hors D'Oeuvres Mesquite Chunks	3.5 oz	100	1	600	1	—
Hot BBQ Breast Tenders	2.75 oz	110	3	580	4	—
Mesquite Breast Fillets	2.75 oz	100	2	250	3	—

FOOD	PORTION	CAL.	FAT	SOD.	CARB.	FIB.
Tyson (CONT.)						
Mesquite Breast Strips	2.75 oz	100	2	240	2	—
Mesquite Breast Tenders	2.75 oz	110	2	290	2	—
Microwave Chunks	3.5 oz	220	15	—	11	—
Microwave Chunks BBQ Sandwich	4 oz	230	6	600	27	—
Microwave Tenders	3.5 oz	230	11	600	19	—
Roasted Breast Fillets	1 oz	50	2	160	—	—
Roasted Breasts	1 oz	50	3	160	—	—
Roasted Drumsticks	1 oz	50	3	190	—	—
Roasted Half Chicken	1 oz	60	4	150	—	—
Roasted Thighs	1 oz	70	5	180	—	—
Roasted Whole Chicken	1 oz	60	4	150	—	—
Southern Fried Breast Fillets	3 oz	220	11	630	15	—
Southern Fried Breast Patties	2.6 oz	220	15	460	9	—
Southern Fried Chick'n Chunks	2.6 oz	220	15	540	11	—
Thick & Crispy Patties	2.6 oz	220	14	490	13	—
Weaver						
Batter Dipped Breast	4.4 oz	310	20	220	13	—
Batter Dipped Drums & Thighs	3 oz	210	14	220	11	—
Batter Dipped Wings	4 oz	400	28	520	20	—
Breast Fillets	4.5 oz	270	13	520	18	—
Breast Fillets Strips	3.3 oz	200	10	500	14	—
Breast Patties	3 oz	205	11	640	14	—
Chicken Nuggets	2.6 oz	190	12	450	10	—
Crispy Dutch Frye Assorted	3.6 oz	290	18	550	16	—
Crispy Dutch Frye Breasts	4.5 oz	350	22	520	17	—
Crispy Dutch Frye Drums & Thighs	3.5 oz	290	19	640	14	—
Crispy Dutch Frye Wings	4 oz	400	28	520	20	—
Crispy Light Skinless	2.9 oz	170	9	320	9	—
Croquettes	2 pieces	280	16	780	22	—
Croquettes With Gravy	2 pieces + ½ cup gravy	282	18	1040	26	—
Honey Batter Tenders	3 oz	220	12	500	14	—
Hot Wings	2.7 oz	170	11	670	1	—
Mini Drums Crispy	3 oz	210	12	480	13	—
Mini Drums Herbs & Spice	3 oz	200	11	320	13	—

FOOD	PORTION	CAL.	FAT	SOD.	CARB.	FIB.
Weaver (CONT.)						
Premium Tenders	3 oz	170	9	500	11	—
Rondelets Cheese	1 (2.6 oz)	190	11	520	12	—
Rondelets Italian	1 (2.6 oz)	190	11	560	11	—
Rondelets Original	1 (3 oz)	190	10	610	13	—
Weight Watchers						
Chicken Nuggets	5.9 oz	220	7	500	23	—
READY-TO-USE						
Carl Buddig						
Chicken	1 oz	50	3	320	1	0
Chicken By George						
Cajun	1 breast (4 oz)	120	4	650	2	0
Caribbean Grill	1 breast (4 oz)	150	4	550	8	0
Garlic & Herb	1 breast (4 oz)	120	3	800	3	0
Italian Bleu Cheese	1 breast (4 oz)	130	5	790	2	0
Lemon Herb	1 breast (4 oz)	120	3	800	3	0
Lemon Oregano	1 breast (4 oz)	130	4	600	3	0
Mesquite Barbecue	1 breast (4 oz)	120	2	800	5	0
Mustard Dill	1 breast (4 oz)	140	5	650	2	0
Roasted	1 breast (4 oz)	110	3	500	1	0
Teriyaki	1 breast (4 oz)	130	3	650	6	0
Tomato Herb With Basil	1 breast (4 oz)	140	5	630	5	0
Empire						
Barbarcue Whole	5 oz	280	17	460	1	0
Battered & Breaded Cutlets	1 (3.3 oz)	200	9	320	11	2
Battered & Breaded Fried Breasts	3 oz	170	8	440	3	tr
Battered & Breaded Nuggets	5 (3 oz)	200	13	650	9	1
Bologna	3 slices (1.8 oz)	200	7	360	2	0
Fried Drum & Thigh	3 oz	240	16	260	7	2
Falls						
BBQ	3 oz	150	8	310	—	—
Healthy Choice						
Deli-Thin Oven Roasted Breast	6 slices (2 oz)	45	0	410	0	0
Deli-Thin Smoked Breast	6 slices (2 oz)	60	2	420	1	0
Fresh-Trak Oven Roasted Breast	1 slice (1 oz)	30	1	290	0	0
Oven Roasted Breast	1 slice (1 oz)	25	0	220	0	0
Smoked Breast	1 slice (1 oz)	35	1	220	0	0
Hebrew National						
Deli Thin Oven Roasted	1.8 oz	45	1	460	—	—

FOOD	PORTION	CAL.	FAT	SOD.	CARB.	FIB.
Hillshire						
Deli Select Oven Roasted Breast	1 slice	10	tr	115	tr	—
Deli Select Smoked Breast	1 slice	10	tr	95	tr	—
Flavor Pack 90-99% Fat Free Smoked Breast	1 slice (0.75 oz)	20	tr	220	tr	—
Lunch 'N Munch Smoked Chicken/ Monterey Jack	1 pkg (4.5 oz)	350	20	1260	19	—
Lunch 'N Munch Smoked Chicken/ Monterey/ Snickers	1 pkg (4.25 oz)	400	23	1080	31	—
Louis Rich						
Deli-Thin Oven Roasted Breast	4 slices (1.8 oz)	60	2	620	1	0
Deluxe Oven Roasted Breast	1 slice (1 oz)	40	1	330	1	0
Hickory Smoked Breast	1 slice (1 oz)	30	1	360	1	0
Oven Roasted Breast	1 slice (1 oz)	40	3	350	1	0
Mr. Turkey						
Deli Cuts Hardwood Smoked	3 slices	30	tr	305	2	—
Deli Cuts Oven Roasted	3 slices	25	0	220	2	—
Oscar Mayer						
Deli-Thin Honey Glazed Breast	4 slices (1.8 oz)	60	1	740	2	0
Free Oven Roasted Breast	4 slices (1.8 oz)	45	0	650	1	—
Healthy Favorites Oven Roasted Breast	4 slices (1.8 oz)	40	0	620	1	0
Lunchables Chicken/ Monterey Jack	1 pkg (4.5 oz)	350	21	1690	20	1
Lunchables Deluxe Chicken/Turkey	1 pkg (5.1 oz)	380	22	1840	24	1
Lunchables Dessert Chocolate Pudding/ Chicken/ Jack	1 pkg (6.2 oz)	370	18	1490	33	0
Smoked Breast	1 slice (1 oz)	25	tr	397	tr	—
Perdue						
BBQ Breast Half	1 oz	46	2	150	1	—
BBQ Drumsticks	1 oz	53	2	106	2	—
BBQ Half Dark Meat	1 oz	57	4	108	1	—
BBQ Half White Meat	1 oz	40	1	110	1	—

FOOD	PORTION	CAL.	FAT	SOD.	CARB.	FIB.
Perdue (CONT.)						
BBQ Thighs	1 oz	59	3	98	1	—
BBQ Wings	1 oz	62	4	169	1	—
Cornish Hen Roasted Dark Meat	1 oz	45	3	72	tr	—
Cornish Hen Roasted White Meat	1 oz	39	1	93	tr	—
Nuggets Cheese	1 (.67 oz)	54	4	108	3	—
Nuggets Fun Shaped	1 (.73 oz)	54	3	92	4	—
Perdue Done It! Cutlets	3.5 oz	250	14	445	17	—
Perdue Done It! Nuggets Original	1 (.67 oz)	48	3	85	3	—
Perdue Done It! Tenders	1 oz	62	3	116	4	—
Perdue Done It! Wings Hot & Spicy	1 oz	60	4	190	1	—
Roasted Breast	1 oz	45	2	116	1	—
Roasted Drumsticks	1 oz	40	1	115	0	—
Roasted Thighs	1 oz	46	2	114	tr	—
Whole Or Half Roasted Dark Meat	1 oz	51	3	73	tr	—
Whole Or Half Roasted White Meat	1 oz	37	1	85	0	—
Wings Garlic & Herb	1 oz	61	4	172	tr	—
Tyson						
Bologna	1 slice	44	1	185	4	—
Hickory Smoked Breast	1 slice	25	1	195	1	—
Honey Flavored Breast	1 slice	25	1	—	1	—
Oven Roasted Breast	1 slice	25	1	185	1	—
Oven Roasted Mesquite Breast	1 slice	25	1	—	1	—
Roll	1 slice	26	1	153	1	—
Wings Barbecue	6-7 (3.5 oz)	218	14	400	0	—
Wings Hot & Spicy	6-7 (3.5 oz)	218	14	400	0	—
Wings Roasted	6-7 (3.5 oz)	218	14	400	0	—
Wings Teriyaki	6-7 (3.5 oz)	218	14	400	0	—
Wampler Longacre						
Breast	1 oz	35	1	200	1	—
Chef's Select Breast	1 oz	35	1	320	tr	—
Premium Oven Roasted Breast	1 oz	50	3	350	2	—
Roll	1 oz	65	5	240	tr	—
Roll Sliced	1 slice (0.8 oz)	50	4	170	1	—
Weaver						
Roasted Wings	1 oz	70	5	180	—	—

FOOD	PORTION	CAL.	FAT	SOD.	CARB.	FIB.
Weight Watchers						
Roasted & Smoked Breast	2 slices (¾ oz)	25	1	220	tr	—
Roasted Ham	2 slices (¾ oz)	25	1	210	tr	—
chicken roll light meat	1 pkg (6 oz)	271	13	992	4	—
chicken roll light meat	2 oz	90	4	331	1	—
poultry salad sandwich spread	1 oz	238	4	107	2	—
poultry salad sandwich spread	1 tbsp (13 g)	109	2	49	1	—
TAKE-OUT						
boneless breaded & fried w/ barbecue sauce	6 pieces (4.6 oz)	330	18	830	25	—
boneless breaded & fried w/ honey	6 pieces (4 oz)	339	18	537	27	—
boneless breaded & fried w/ mustard sauce	6 pieces (4.6 oz)	323	17	791	21	—
boneless breaded & fried w/ sweet & sour sauce	6 pieces (4.6 oz)	346	18	791	29	—
breast & wing breaded & fried	2 pieces (5.7 oz)	494	30	975	20	—
drumstick breaded & fried	2 pieces (5.2 oz)	430	27	756	16	—
oven roasted breast of chicken	2 oz	60	1	470	0	—
thigh breaded & fried	2 pieces (5.2 oz)	430	27	756	16	—

CHICKEN DISHES

(*see also* CHICKEN SUBSTITUTES, DINNER)

FOOD	PORTION	CAL.	FAT	SOD.	CARB.	FIB.
CANNED						
Dinty Moore						
American Classics Chicken & Noodles	1 bowl (10 oz)	260	8	1150	26	2
American Classics Chicken With Mashed Potatoes	1 bowl (10 oz)	220	4	1080	24	2
Chicken Stew	1 cup (7.5 oz)	180	8	920	18	2
Microwave Cup Chicken & Dumpling	1 cup (7.5 oz)	190	6	670	20	1
Stew	1 cup (8.5 oz)	220	11	960	16	2
Swanson						
Chicken & Dumplings	7½ oz	220	11	980	19	—
Chicken Ala King	5¼ oz	190	12	690	9	—
Chicken Stew	7⅝ oz	160	7	990	15	—
Top Shelf						
Chicken Cacciatore	1 bowl (10 oz)	210	3	850	26	3

FOOD	PORTION	CAL.	FAT	SOD.	CARB.	FIB.
Top Shelf (CONT.)						
Chicken Acapulco Fiesta Chicken	1 bowl (10 oz)	420	16	1070	45	2
Chicken Ala King	1 bowl (10 oz)	380	12	960	47	2
Glazed Breast Of Chicken	1 bowl (10 oz)	200	5	910	17	2
FROZEN						
Croissant Pocket						
Stuffed Sandwich Chicken Broccoli & Cheddar	1 piece (4.5 oz)	300	11	640	37	5
Hot Pocket						
Stuffed Sandwich Chicken & Cheddar With Broccoli	1 (4.5 oz)	300	12	620	37	tr
Jimmy Dean						
Grilled Breast Sandwich	1 (5.5 oz)	330	11	730	27	1
Lean Pockets						
Stuffed Sandwich Chicken Fijita	1 (4.5 oz)	260	8	770	36	3
Stuffed Sandwich Chicken Parmesan	1 (4.5 oz)	260	8	630	34	1
Stuffed Sandwich Glazed Chicken Supreme	1 (4.5 oz)	240	7	600	34	1
Luigino's						
Chicken A La King With Noodles	1 pkg (8 oz)	240	7	660	28	2
Noodles With Chicken Peas & Carrots	1 pkg (8 oz)	300	11	640	38	2
Noodles With Chicken Peas & Carrots	1 cup (6.3 oz)	260	10	560	33	2
Sweet & Sour Chicken With Rice	1 pkg (8 oz)	300	6	480	50	2
MicroMagic						
Chicken Sandwich	1 pkg (4.5 oz)	390	16	650	42	—
Ovenstuffs						
Chicken Turnover	1 (4.75 oz)	350	16	690	36	—
Tyson						
Microwave Breast Sandwich	4.25 oz	328	14	520	33	—
Weight Watchers						
Chicken & Broccoli Pita	1 (5.4 oz)	190	5	420	19	—
Grilled Chicken Sandwich	1 (4 oz)	210	6	420	22	—

FOOD	PORTION	CAL.	FAT	SOD.	CARB.	FIB.
White Castle						
Grilled Chicken Sandwich	2 (4 oz)	250	9	490	24	5
Grilled Chicken Sandwich w/ Sauce	2 (4.8 oz)	290	9	600	33	5
MIX						
Lipton						
Microeasy Barbeque Chicken	¼ pkg	108	1	981	24	—
Microeasy Country Chicken	¼ pkg	78	1	844	15	—
Skillet Chicken Helper						
Cheesy Broccoli as prep	⅕ pkg (7.5 oz)	270	6	790	34	—
Creamy Chicken as prep	⅕ pkg (8.25 oz)	290	10	800	29	—
Creamy Mushroom as prep	⅕ pkg (8 oz)	280	8	800	31	—
Fettucine Alfredo as prep	⅕ pkg (7.5 oz)	270	8	800	29	—
Stir-Fried Chicken as prep	⅕ pkg (7 oz)	330	11	940	36	—
READY-TO-USE						
Spreadables						
Chicken Salad	¼ can	100	6	—	—	—
Wampler Longacre						
Cacciatore	1 serv (4 oz)	118	3	267	5	—
Salad	1 oz	70	3	125	3	—
Salad Lite	1 oz	45	2	95	3	—
Smokey Barbecue	1 serv (4 oz)	175	7	460	11	—
Sweet N Sour	1 serv (4 oz)	106	tr	231	16	—
Szechwan With Peanuts	1 serv (4 oz)	112	4	560	6	—
SHELF-STABLE						
Lunch Bucket						
Dumplings'n Chicken	1 pkg (7.5 oz)	140	2	880	25	—
Light'n Healthy Chicken Fiesta	1 pkg (7.5 oz)	170	3	600	28	—
TAKE-OUT						
chicken cacciatore	¾ cup	394	24	671	9	2
chicken paprikash	1½ cups	296	10	—	—	—
chicken a la king	1 cup	470	34	760	12	—
chicken & dumplings	¾ cup	256	12	1283	12	tr
chicken & noodles	1 cup	365	18	600	26	—
chicken pie w/ top crust	1 slice (5.6 oz)	472	31	—	32	1
fillet sandwich plain	1	515	29	957	39	—
fillet sandwich w/ cheese lettuce mayonnaise & tomato	1	632	39	1238	42	—

FOOD	PORTION	CAL.	FAT	SOD.	CARB.	FIB.

CHICKEN SUBSTITUTES

Harvest Direct

TVP Poultry Chunks	3.5 oz	280	1	15	32	18
TVP Poultry Ground	3.5 oz	280	1	15	32	18

Jaclyn's

Salsa Chicken Style Dinner	11.5 oz	325	9	290	35	—
Sesame Chicken Style Dinner	11.5 oz	345	8	635	40	—

Knox Mountain Farm

Chick'N Wheat Mix	1 serv (⅛ pkg)	110	1	220	3	2

LaLoma

Chicken Supreme not prep	¼ cup (16 g)	50	0	450	4	—
Chik Nuggets	5 nuggets (85 g)	270	20	530	8	—
Fried Chicken	1 piece (57 g)	180	14	570	2	—
Fried Chicken w/ Gravy	2 piece (85 g)	140	10	340	4	—

White Wave

Meatless Sandwich Slices	2 slices (1.6 oz)	80	0	260	8	0

Worthington

Chick-ketts	½ cup (84 g)	160	7	640	6	—
ChickStiks	1 (47 g)	110	7	380	4	—
Chicken Sliced	2 slices (57 g)	130	9	460	3	—
CrispyChik	6 nuggets (85 g)	280	19	500	17	—
CrispyChik	1 patty (71 g)	220	15	620	13	—
Cutlets	1.5 slices (92 g)	100	2	270	4	—
Diced Chik	¼ cup (60 g)	90	8	330	2	—
FriChik	2 pieces (90 g)	180	13	610	13	—
Golden Croquettes	5 pieces (106 g)	280	14	890	20	—
Savory Slices	2 slices (60 g)	90	8	330	2	—
Vegetarian Chicken Pie	1 (227 g)	380	20	1200	43	—

CHICKPEAS

CANNED

Allen

Garbanzo	½ cup (4.4 oz)	120	3	330	19	8

East Texas Fair

Garbanzo	½ cup (4.4 oz)	120	3	330	19	8

Eden

Organic	½ cup (4.1 oz)	110	2	10	17	4

Goya

Spanish Style	7.5 oz	150	2	890	32	9

Green Giant

Garbanzo	½ cup	90	2	320	18	5

FOOD	PORTION	CAL.	FAT	SOD.	CARB.	FIB.
Hanover						
Chickpeas	½ cup	100	1	—	—	—
Old El Paso						
Garbanzo	½ cup	190	tr	250	16	—
S&W						
Garbanzo Lite 50% Less Salt	½ cup	110	0	295	21	—
Garbanzo Premium Large	½ cup	110	1	470	20	—
Garbanzo Water Pack	½ cup	105	1	5	19	—
chickpeas	1 cup	285	3	718	54	—
DRIED						
Bean Cuisine						
Garbanzo	½ cup	115	1	5	—	5
cooked	1 cup	269	4	11	45	—
CHICORY						
greens raw chopped	½ cup	21	tr	41	4	—
root raw	1 (2.1 oz)	44	tr	30	11	—
roots raw cut up	½ cup (1.6 oz)	33	tr	23	8	—
witloof head raw	1 (1.9 oz)	9	tr	1	2	—
witloof raw	½ cup (1.6 oz)	8	tr	1	2	—
CHILI						
CANNED						
Allen						
Mexican Chili Beans	½ cup (4.5 oz)	120	1	300	22	8
Armour						
Chili No Beans	1 cup (8.7 oz)	470	38	1200	18	—
Chili With Beans	1 cup (8.9 oz)	440	28	1270	34	—
Chili With Beans Hot	1 cup (8.9 oz)	440	28	1270	34	—
Chili With Beans Western Style	1 cup (8.8 oz)	460	32	1130	29	—
Brown Beauty						
Mexican Chili Beans	½ cup (4.5 oz)	120	1	300	22	8
Chi-Chi's						
San Antonio	1 cup (8.5 oz)	240	19	900	23	6
Del Monte						
Sauce	1 tbsp (0.6 oz)	20	0	460	0	0
Dennison's						
Chili Beans In Chili Gravy	7.5 oz	180	1	—	—	—
Chili Con Carne w/ Beans	7.5 oz	310	15	—	—	—
Chili Con Carne w/ Beans	7.5 oz	300	19	—	—	—
Chunky Chili w/ Beans	7.5 oz	310	14	—	—	—
Cook-off Chili w/ Beans	7.5 oz	340	19	—	—	—

FOOD	PORTION	CAL.	FAT	SOD.	CARB.	FIB.
Dennison's (cont.)						
Hot Chili Con Carne w/ Beans	7.5 oz	310	16	—	—	—
Gebhardt						
Hot With Beans	1 cup	470	27	1000	47	6
Plain	1 cup	530	43	990	20	1
With Beans	1 cup	495	28	1010	47	6
Hain						
Spicy Tempeh	7½ oz	160	4	1350	24	—
Spicy Vegetarian	7½ oz	160	1	1060	29	—
Spicy Vegetarian Reduced Sodium	7½ oz	170	1	200	31	—
Spicy With Chicken	7½ oz	130	2	1030	19	—
Health Valley						
Mild Vegetarian With Beans	5 oz	160	3	290	21	12
Mild Vegetarian With Beans No Salt Added	5 oz	160	3	30	21	12
Mild Vegetarian With Lentils	5 oz	140	4	290	15	7
Mild Vegetarian With Lentils No Salt Added	5 oz	140	4	50	15	7
Spicy Vegetarian With Beans	5 oz	160	4	280	21	12
Hormel						
Chili Mac	1 can (7.5 oz)	200	9	980	17	2
Chili No Beans	1 cup (8.3 oz)	410	30	950	16	3
Chili With Beans	1 cup (8.7 oz)	340	17	1200	30	9
Chunky Chili With Beans	1 cup (8.7 oz)	330	16	1040	30	8
Hot Chili No Beans	1 cup (8.3 oz)	410	30	950	16	3
Hot Chili With Beans	1 cup (8.7 oz)	340	17	1200	30	9
Hot With Beans	1 can (7.5 oz)	250	11	980	23	6
No Beans	1 can (7.5 oz)	390	30	1030	13	2
Turkey Chili With Beans	1 cup (8.7 oz)	220	3	1280	28	7
Turkey Chili No Beans	1 cup (8.3 oz)	190	3	1210	17	3
With Beans	1 can (7.5 oz)	250	11	1000	23	6
Hunt's						
Chili Beans	4 oz	100	tr	490	18	6
Just Rite						
Hot With Beans	4 oz	195	10	495	16	1
With Beans	4 oz	200	11	500	16	1
Without Beans	4 oz	180	11	515	9	tr
Luck's						
Hot Chili Beans	7.5 oz	200	2	—	—	—

FOOD	PORTION	CAL.	FAT	SOD.	CARB.	FIB.
Manwich						
Chili Fixin's as prep	8 oz	290	14	980	20	5
Micro Cup Meals						
Chili Mac	1 cup (7.5 oz)	200	9	980	17	2
Chili No Beans	1 cup (7.5 oz)	290	17	830	15	3
Chili With Beans	1 cup (10.4 oz)	410	17	1430	41	12
Chili With Beans	1 cup (7.5 oz)	250	11	980	23	6
Hot Chili With Beans	1 cup (7.5 oz)	250	11	980	23	6
Natural Touch						
Vegetarian	⅔ cup (190 g)	230	12	890	19	—
Old El Paso						
Chili With Beans	1 cup	217	10	480	17	6
S&W						
Chili Beans	½ cup	130	1	520	23	—
Chili Makin's Original	½ cup	100	1	782	20	—
Van Camp's						
Chilee Beanee Weenee	1 can (8 oz)	240	12	1090	27	9
Chili With Beans	1 cup (8.9 oz)	350	21	1020	28	7
Wolf Brand						
Chili-Mac	7.5 oz	317	20	854	23	—
Extra Spicy With Beans	7.5 oz	324	21	926	21	—
Extra Spicy Without Beans	7.5 oz	363	25	962	15	—
Plain	7.5 oz	330	22	1165	10	—
With Beans	7.5 oz	345	22	1013	22	—
Without Beans	1 cup	387	27	1042	16	—
chili w/ beans	1 cup	286	14	1330	30	—
DRIED						
Gebhardt						
Chili Powder	1 tsp	15	tr	0	3	tr
Chili Quik Seasoning	1 tsp	10	tr	165	2	tr
Hain						
Hot Chili	¼ pkg	30	1	370	5	—
Medium Chili	¼ pkg	30	1	300	5	—
Mild Chili	¼ pkg	30	1	330	5	—
Nile Spice						
Chili'n Beans Original	1 pkg	150	2	670	25	6
Chili'n Beans Spicy	1 pkg	150	2	720	25	6
Old El Paso						
Chili Seasoning Mix	⅕ pkg	21	1	717	4	1
Watkins						
Chili Seasoning	1¼ tsp (4 g)	15	0	110	2	0
Powder	¼ tsp (0.5 g)	0	0	10	0	0
powder	1 tsp	8	tr	26	1	—

FOOD	PORTION	CAL.	FAT	SOD.	CARB.	FIB.
FROZEN						
Lightlife	4.3 oz	110	3	360	14	—
Lean Cuisine						
Three Bean	1 pkg (9 oz)	210	6	460	32	7
Luigino's						
Chili-Mac	1 pkg (8 oz)	230	7	770	29	3
Stouffer's						
With Beans	1 pkg (8.75 oz)	270	10	1130	29	8
Swanson						
Homestyle Chili Con Carne	8¼ oz	270	10	740	26	—
Tabatchnick						
Vegetarian	7.5 oz	210	6	530	28	10
Tyson						
Chicken Chili	3.5 oz	105	3	420	11	—
SHELF-STABLE						
Lunch Bucket						
Chili With Beans	1 pkg (7.5 oz)	300	14	1120	26	—
Wampler Longacre						
Turkey	1 serv (4 oz)	118	3	850	10	—
TAKE-OUT						
con carne w/ beans	8.9 oz	254	8	1008	22	—

CHINESE CABBAGE
(*see* CABBAGE)

CHINESE FOOD
(*see* ORIENTAL FOOD)

CHINESE PRESERVING MELON

cooked	½ cup	11	tr	93	3	—

CHIPS
(*see also* POPCORN, PRETZELS, SNACKS)

FOOD	PORTION	CAL.	FAT	SOD.	CARB.	FIB.
CORN						
Energy Food Factory						
Corn Pops Fat Free	½ oz	50	0	110	11	1
Corn Pops Nacho	½ oz	50	1	150	12	1
Corn Pops Original	½ oz	50	1	110	11	1
Fritos						
Chili Cheese	34 pieces (1 oz)	160	10	300	15	1
Chips	34 pieces (1 oz)	150	10	220	16	1
Crisp 'N Thin	18 pieces (1 oz)	160	10	240	16	1
Dip Size	13 pieces (1 oz)	150	10	240	16	1
Non-Stop Nacho Cheese	34 pieces (1 oz)	150	9	220	16	1
Rowdy Rustlers Bar-B-Q	34 pieces (1 oz)	150	9	300	17	1

FOOD	PORTION	CAL.	FAT	SOD.	CARB.	FIB.
Fritos (CONT.)						
Wild 'N Mild	32 pieces (1 oz)	160	9	240	16	1
Health Valley						
Chips	1 oz	160	11	90	13	1
No Salt Added	1 oz	160	11	1	13	1
With Cheddar Cheese	1 oz	160	10	120	15	1
Lance						
BBQ	1 pkg (50 g)	260	16	360	25	—
Chips	1 pkg (50 g)	270	17	350	26	—
Planters						
Corn Chips	34 chips (1 oz)	170	10	180	17	2
King Size	17 chips (1 oz)	160	10	180	16	2
Snacks To Go	1 pkg (1.5 oz)	240	15	260	23	3
Snyder's						
BBQ	1 oz	160	11	200	14	2
Weight Watchers						
Corn Snacker	½ oz	60	2	230	10	—
Corn Snackers Nacho Cheese	½ oz	60	2	270	10	—
Wise						
Corn	1 oz	160	10	180	15	—
Corn Crunchies	1 oz	160	10	180	15	—
Crispy Corn	1 oz	160	10	125	15	—
Crispy Corn Nacho Cheese	1 oz	160	10	190	16	—
barbecue	1 bag (7 oz)	1036	65	1511	111	10
barbecue	1 oz	148	9	216	16	1
cones nacho	1 oz	152	9	270	17	—
cones plain	1 oz	145	8	290	18	—
onion	1 oz	142	6	278	19	—
plain	1 bag (7 oz)	1067	66	1248	113	9
plain	1 oz	153	10	179	16	1
puffs cheese	1 bag (8 oz)	1256	78	2383	122	2
puffs cheese	1 oz	157	10	298	15	tr
twists cheese	1 bag (8 oz)	1256	78	2383	122	2
twists cheese	1 oz	157	10	298	15	tr
MULTIGRAIN						
Sunchips						
	12 pieces (1 oz)	150	8	100	18	—
French Onion	12 pieces (1 oz)	140	7	120	18	—
POTATO						
Barrel O' Fun						
Barbeque	1 oz	145	9	250	16	0
Sour Cream & Onion	1 oz	150	9	230	15	0

FOOD	PORTION	CAL.	FAT	SOD.	CARB.	FIB.
Butterfield						
Sticks	⅔ cup (1 oz)	150	9	90	16	2
Sticks	1 pkg (1.7 oz)	250	15	150	26	3
Cottage Fries						
No Salt Added	1 oz	160	11	5	14	—
Eagle						
BBQ Thins	1 oz	150	10	220	15	—
Kettle Fry BBQ Crunchy	1 oz	150	8	140	16	—
Kettle Fry Cape Cod	1 oz	150	8	120	16	—
Kettle Fry Cape Cod No Salt	1 oz	150	8	0	16	—
Kettle Fry Cape Cod Waves	1 oz	150	8	120	16	—
Kettle Fry Cape Cod Waves No Salt	1 oz	150	8	0	16	—
Kettle Fry Dill & Sour Cream	1 oz	150	8	160	16	—
Kettle Fry Dill & Sour Cream No Salt	1 oz	150	8	15	16	—
Kettle Fry Extra Crunchy	1 oz	150	8	180	16	—
Kettle Fry Idaho Russet	1 oz	150	8	180	16	—
Kettle Fry Louisiana BBQ	1 oz	150	8	140	16	—
Ranch Ridged	1 oz	160	10	220	15	—
Ridged	1 oz	150	10	220	15	—
Sour Cream & Onion	1 oz	150	10	240	15	—
Thins	1 oz	150	10	220	15	—
Energy Food Factory						
Potato Pops Au Gratin	½ oz	60	2	110	12	1
Potato Pops Fat Free	½ oz	50	0	110	13	1
Potato Pops Herb & Garlic	½ oz	50	1	110	11	1
Potato Pops Mesquite	½ oz	50	1	110	12	1
Potato Pops Original	½ oz	50	1	110	11	1
Potato Pops Salt N' Vinegar	½ oz	50	1	110	11	1
Health Valley						
Country Ripple	1 oz	160	10	60	15	1
Country Ripple No Salt Added	1 oz	160	10	1	15	1
Dip Chips	1 oz	160	10	60	15	1
Dip Chips No Salt Added	1 oz	160	10	1	15	1
Natural	1 oz	160	10	60	15	1
Natural No Salt Added	1 oz	160	10	1	15	1

FOOD	PORTION	CAL.	FAT	SOD.	CARB.	FIB.
Kelly's						
Bar-B-Q	1 oz	150	9	230	15	1
Chips	1 oz	150	9	160	14	2
Crunchy	1 oz	150	9	140	17	2
Rippled	1 oz	150	9	160	14	2
Sour Cream n' Onion	1 oz	150	9	170	15	1
Unsalted	1 oz	150	10	5	14	—
Lance						
BBQ	1 pkg (32 g)	190	12	270	18	—
Cajun Style	1 pkg (32 g)	160	11	250	16	—
Chips	1 pkg (32 g)	190	15	220	12	—
Hot Fries	1 pkg (28 g)	160	10	220	14	—
Ripple	1 pkg (32 g)	190	15	220	12	—
Sour Cream & Onion	1 pkg (32 g)	190	12	390	18	—
Lay's						
Bar-B-Q	17 pieces (1 oz)	150	9	270	15	1
Cheddar Cheese	17 pieces (1 oz)	150	10	300	14	1
Crunch Tators	16 pieces (1 oz)	150	8	120	17	1
Crunch Tators Amazin' Cajun	16 pieces (1 oz)	150	8	150	17	—
Crunch Tators Hoppin' Jalapeno	16 pieces (1 oz)	140	7	200	18	1
Crunch Tators Mighty Mesquite	16 pieces (1 oz)	150	8	135	17	—
Crunch Tators Supreme Sour Cream	16 pieces (1 oz)	150	8	180	16	—
Flamin' Hot	17 pieces (1 oz)	150	9	190	15	1
Kansas City Style Bar-B-Q	17 pieces (1 oz)	150	9	270	15	1
Salt & Vinegar	17 pieces (1 oz)	150	10	390	14	1
Sour Cream & Onion	17 pieces (1 oz)	160	10	220	15	1
Tangy Ranch	17 pieces (1 oz)	160	10	210	15	1
Unsalted	17 pieces (1 oz)	150	10	10	15	1
Louise's						
"1g" Mesquite BBQ	1 oz	110	1	180	24	2
"1g" Original	1 oz	110	1	180	24	2
70% Less Fat Mesquite BBQ	1 oz	110	3	180	21	2
70% Less Fat Original	1 oz	110	3	200	21	2
Fat-Free Maui Onion	1 oz	110	0	180	23	2
Fat-Free Mesquite BBQ	1 oz	110	0	180	23	2
Fat-Free No Salt	1 oz	110	0	10	24	2
Fat-Free Original	1 oz	110	0	180	23	2
Fat-Free Vinegar & Salt	1 oz	110	0	300	23	2

FOOD	PORTION	CAL.	FAT	SOD.	CARB.	FIB.
Mr. Phipps						
Tater Crisps Bar-B-Que	21 (1 oz)	130	4	270	21	1
Tater Crisps Original	23 (1 oz)	120	7	220	20	1
Tater Crisps Sour Cream 'n Onion	22 (1 oz)	130	4	210	21	1
New York Deli						
Chips	1 oz	160	11	120	14	—
Old Dutch Foods						
Augratin	1 oz	150	8	220	15	—
BBQ	1 oz	140	8	360	16	—
Dill Flavored	1 oz	150	8	340	16	—
Onion & Garlic	1 oz	150	9	420	15	—
Ripple	1 oz	150	9	150	16	—
Sour Cream & Onion	1 oz	150	10	220	15	—
Pringles						
BBQ	14 chips (1 oz)	150	6	200	15	—
Cheez-ums	14 chips (1 oz)	150	10	190	—	—
Original	14 chips (1 oz)	160	11	170	—	—
Ranch	14 chips (1 oz)	150	10	130	—	—
Ridges Cheddar & Sour Cream	12 chips (1 oz)	150	10	200	—	—
Ridges Mesquite BBQ	12 chips (1 oz)	150	10	220	—	—
Ridges Original	12 chips (1 oz)	150	10	150	—	—
Right BBQ	16 chips (1 oz)	140	7	160	18	—
Right Original	16 chips (1 oz)	140	7	135	—	—
Right Ranch	16 chips (1 oz)	140	7	120	18	—
Right Sour Cream 'N Onion	16 chips (1 oz)	140	7	120	18	—
Rippled Original	10 chips (1 oz)	160	11	150	15	—
Sour Cream N'Onion	14 chips (1 oz)	160	10	135	15	—
Ruffles						
Cheddar Cheese & Sour Cream	18 chips (1 oz)	160	10	250	15	1
Chips	18 chips (1 oz)	150	10	135	15	1
Light	18 chips (1 oz)	130	6	140	19	1
Light Sour Cream & Onion	18 chips (1 oz)	130	6	190	18	1
Mesquite Grille B-B-Q	18 chips (1 oz)	160	10	270	15	1
Monterey Jack Cheese Attack	18 chips (1 oz)	160	10	200	15	1
Ranch	18 chips (1 oz)	160	10	220	15	1
Sour Cream & Onion	18 chips (1 oz)	160	10	220	15	1
Snyder's						
BBQ	1 oz	150	10	370	13	1

FOOD	PORTION	CAL.	FAT	SOD.	CARB.	FIB.
Snyder's (CONT.)						
Cheddar Bacon	1 oz	150	10	260	13	1
Coney Island	1 oz	150	10	280	13	1
Grilled Steak & Onion	1 oz	150	10	260	13	1
Hot Buffalo Wings	1 oz	150	10	200	13	1
Kosher Dill	1 oz	150	10	400	13	1
No Salt	1 oz	150	10	0	13	1
Salt & Vinegar	1 oz	150	10	200	13	1
Sausage Pizza	1 oz	150	10	230	13	1
Sour Cream & Onion	1 oz	150	10	190	13	1
Sour Cream & Onion Unsalted	1 oz	150	10	10	13	1
State Line						
Chips	1 pkg (0.5 oz)	80	5	70	7	tr
Suprimos						
Cheddar & Jack	1 oz	140	6	180	17	—
Cool Onion	1 oz	140	6	170	17	—
Weight Watchers						
Great Snackers Barbecue	½ oz	70	3	100	10	—
Great Snackers Cheddar Cheese	½ oz	70	3	130	10	—
Great Snackers Sour Cream & Onion	½ oz	70	3	140	10	—
Wise						
Natural	1 oz	160	11	190	14	—
Ridgies Barbecue	1 oz	150	10	240	14	—
barbecue	1 bag (7 oz)	971	64	1486	105	—
barbecue	1 oz	139	9	213	15	—
cheese	1 bag (6 oz)	842	46	1348	98	—
cheese	1 oz	140	8	225	16	—
light	1 bag (6 oz)	801	35	836	114	—
light	1 oz	134	6	139	19	—
potato	1 bag (8 oz)	1217	79	1347	120	—
potato	1 pkg (8 oz)	1217	79	1347	120	8
potato	1 oz	152	10	168	15	1
sour cream & onion	1 oz	150	10	177	15	—
sour cream & onion	1 bag (7 oz)	1051	67	1237	102	—
sticks	1 oz	148	10	71	15	1
sticks	1 pkg (1 oz)	148	10	71	15	—
sticks	½ cup (0.6 oz)	94	6	45	10	1
TORTILLA						
Barrel O' Fun						
Nacho	1 oz	140	6	160	19	1

FOOD	PORTION	CAL.	FAT	SOD.	CARB.	FIB.
Barrel O' Fun (CONT.)						
Tostada Yellow	1 oz	140	6	40	19	0
White	1 oz	140	6	50	20	0
Doritos						
Lightly Salted	16 chips (1 oz)	150	7	135	18	2
Eagle						
Nacho	1 oz	150	8	200	17	—
Ranch	1 oz	150	8	150	17	—
Restaurant Style	1 oz	150	7	100	18	—
Strips	1 oz	150	8	140	18	—
Frito Lay						
Salsa 'N Cheese	16 (1 oz)	150	8	180	17	2
Guiltless Gourmet						
Baked	22-26 chips (1 oz)	110	1	119	21	1
Hain						
Sesame	1 oz	140	7	190	19	—
Sesame Cheese	1 oz	160	8	270	20	—
Sesame No Salt Added	1 oz	140	7	<5	19	—
Taco Style	1 oz	160	11	320	15	—
La FAMOUS						
No Salt Added	1 oz	140	7	5	18	—
Tortilla	1 oz	140	7	180	18	—
Lance						
Jalapeno Cheese	1 pkg (1⅛ oz)	160	8	—	—	—
Nacho	1 pkg (32 g)	160	8	240	19	—
Louise's						
95% Fat-Free	1 oz	120	2	170	23	1
Mr. Phipps						
Nacho	28 (1 oz)	130	4	150	20	3
Original	28 (1 oz)	130	4	130	21	3
Old El Paso						
NACHIPS	9 chips (1 oz)	150	7	80	18	2
White Corn	12 chips (1 oz)	150	8	60	16	1
Santitas						
Cantina Style	1 oz	140	6	75	19	2
Cantina Style Fajita	1 oz	140	7	95	19	2
Strips	1 oz	140	7	65	19	2
Snyder's						
Enchilada	1 oz	140	7	220	18	2
Nacho Cheese	1 oz	140	7	130	18	2
No Salt	1 oz	140	7	0	18	2
Ranch	1 oz	140	7	150	18	2
Tostitos						
Baked	1 oz	110	1	140	24	2

FOOD	PORTION	CAL.	FAT	SOD.	CARB.	FIB.
Tostitos (CONT.)						
Baked Cool Ranch	1 oz	130	3	170	21	2
Baked Unsalted	1 oz	110	1	0	24	2
Bite Size	16 pieces (1 oz)	150	8	110	18	2
Restaurant Style Lime 'N Chili	7 pieces (1 oz)	150	7	190	18	2
Restaurant Style White Corn	7 pieces (1 oz)	150	6	75	20	2
Tyson						
Nacho Cheese	1 oz	140	7	145	17	—
Ranch Flavor	1 oz	140	2	—	17	—
Traditional	1 oz	140	7	95	17	—
Unsalted	1 oz	140	7	7	17	—
Wise						
Bravos	1 oz	150	8	180	18	—
nacho	1 bag (8 oz)	1131	58	1606	142	12
nacho	1 oz	141	7	201	18	2
nacho light	1 oz	126	4	284	20	—
nacho light	1 bag (6 oz)	757	26	1705	122	—
plain	1 bag (7.5 oz)	1067	56	1124	134	14
plain	1 oz	142	7	150	18	2
ranch	1 bag (7 oz)	969	47	1212	128	—
ranch	1 oz	139	7	174	18	—
taco	1 bag (8 oz)	1089	55	1788	143	—
taco	1 oz	136	7	223	18	—
VEGETABLE						
Eden						
Vegetable Chips	50 (1 oz)	130	4	260	24	0
Wasabi Chip Hot & Spicy	50 (1 oz)	130	4	260	24	0
Hain						
Carrot Chips	1 oz	150	9	160	16	0
Carrot Chips Barbecue	1 oz	140	8	160	16	0
Carrot Chips No Salt Added	1 oz	150	7	30	16	0
Health Valley						
Carrot Lites	0.5 oz	75	4	5	9	tr
Terra Chips						
Sweet Potato	1 oz	140	7	10	18	1
Sweet Potato Spiced	1 oz	140	7	105	16	3
Taro Spiced	1 oz	130	5	170	20	2
Vegetable	1 oz	140	7	70	18	3
Top Banana						
Plantain Chips	1 oz	150	8	85	17	—
taro	10 (0.8 oz)	115	6	79	16	—
taro	1 oz	141	7	97	19	—

FOOD	PORTION	CAL.	FAT	SOD.	CARB.	FIB.
CHITTERLINGS						
pork simmered	3 oz	258	24	33	0	—
CHIVES						
freeze-dried	1 tbsp	1	tr	—	tr	—
fresh chopped	1 tbsp	1	tr	0	tr	—
fresh chopped	1 tsp	0	tr	0	tr	—
CHOCOLATE						
(see also CANDY, CAROB, COCOA, ICE CREAM TOPPINGS, MILK DRINKS)						
BAKING						
Baker's						
German Sweet	1 oz	143	10	1	17	—
German Sweet	¼ cup	200	12	1	27	—
Semi-Sweet	1 oz	135	9	1	17	—
Unsweetened	1 oz	141	15	1	9	—
Hershey						
Premium Semi-Sweet	1 oz	140	8	—	16	—
Premium Unsweetened	1 oz	190	16	5	7	—
Nestle						
Choco Bake	½ oz	80	8	0	5	3
Premier White	½ oz	80	5	15	8	—
Semi-Sweet	½ oz	70	4	0	9	2
Unsweetened	½ oz	80	7	0	5	3
baking	1 oz	145	15	1	8	—
grated unsweetened	1 cup (4.6 oz)	690	73	18	37	18
liquid unsweetened	1 oz	134	14	3	10	—
squares unsweetened	1 square (1 oz)	148	16	4	8	4
CHIPS						
Baker's						
Big Milk Chocolate	¼ cup	239	14	42	30	—
Big Semi-Sweet	¼ cup	220	13	1	31	—
Chips	1 oz	143	8	25	18	—
Real Semi-Sweet	¼ cup	198	12	1	28	—
Semi-Sweet	¼ cup	197	9	29	30	—
Hershey						
Chunks Milk Chocolate	1 oz	160	9	25	16	—
Chunks Semi-Sweet	1 oz	140	8	—	15	—
Milk Chocolate	1 oz	150	12	55	27	—
Mint Chocolate	¼ cup	230	12	—	28	—
Semi-Sweet	¼ cup (1.5 oz)	220	12	5	26	—
Semi-Sweet Miniature	¼ cup (1.5 oz)	220	12	5	26	—
M&M's						
Baking Bits Milk Chocolate	0.5 oz	70	3	0	10	0

FOOD	PORTION	CAL.	FAT	SOD.	CARB.	FIB.
M&M's (CONT.)						
Baking Bits Semi-Sweet	0.5 oz	70	4	0	9	1
Nestle						
Morsels Milk Chocolate	1 tbsp	70	4	0	10	—
Morsels Mint Chocolate	1 tbsp	70	4	0	9	2
Morsels Rainbow	1 tbsp	70	3	0	10	1
Morsels Mini Semi-Sweet	1 tbsp	70	4	0	9	2
Semi-Sweet Morsels	1 tbsp	40	4	0	9	2
milk chocolate	1 cup (6 oz)	862	52	138	100	—
semisweet	60 pieces (1 oz)	136	9	3	18	—
semisweet	1 cup (6 oz)	804	50	19	106	—
MIX						
Hershey						
Chocolate Milk Mix	3 tbsp	90	4	40	22	—
powder	2-3 heaping tsp	75	1	45	20	—
powder as prep w/ whole milk	9 oz	226	9	165	31	—
SYRUP						
Crumpy						
Chocolate Hazelnut Spread	1 tbsp (0.5 oz)	80	5	5	8	0
Estee						
Choco-Syp	2 tbsp (1.2 oz)	50	0	15	11	—
Hershey						
Syrup	2 tbsp	80	1	20	17	—
Marzetti	2 tbsp	40	4	50	21	0
Quik						
Syrup Chocolate	1 ⅔ tbsp	100	1	45	22	—
Red Wing	2 tbsp (1.4 oz)	110	1	10	25	0
chocolate	1 cup	653	3	287	177	—
chocolate	2 tbsp	82	tr	36	22	—
chocolate as prep w/ whole milk	9 oz	232	9	156	34	—
chocolate fudge	1 tbsp (0.7 oz)	73	3	27	12	—
chocolate fudge	1 cup (11.9 oz)	1176	46	442	200	—

CHOCOLATE MILK
(see CHOCOLATE, COCOA, MILK DRINKS)

CHUTNEY
Sonoma

Dried Tomato	1 tbsp (0.7 g)	35	0	0	9	0
apple	1.2 oz	68	0	—	18	1
apple cranberry	1 tbsp	16	0	1	4	—
tomato	1.2 oz	54	0	—	14	1

FOOD	PORTION	CAL.	FAT	SOD.	CARB.	FIB.
CILANTRO						
Watkins						
Dried	¼ tsp (0.5 oz)	0	0	0	0	0
fresh	¼ cup	1	tr	1	tr	—
CINNAMON						
Watkins						
	¼ tsp (0.5 g)	0	0	0	0	0
ground	1 tsp	6	tr	1	2	—
sticks	0.5 oz	39	tr	4	8	3
CISCO						
raw	3 oz	84	2	47	0	—
smoked	3 oz	151	10	409	0	—
smoked	1 oz	50	3	135	0	—
CLAMS						
CANNED						
American Original						
Quahogs	4 oz	66	tr	—	2	—
Doxsee						
Chopped	6.5 oz	90	tr	1020	6	—
Clam Juice	3 fl oz	4	0	110	0	—
Empress						
Whole Baby	4 oz	60	1	540	2	—
Gorton's						
Minced & Chopped	½ can	70	1	640	4	—
Progresso						
Red Clam Sauce	½ cup	70	3	560	7	—
White Clam Sauce	½ cup	110	8	280	1	—
S&W						
Fancy Chopped	2 oz	28	0	280	2	—
Fancy Minced	2 oz	28	0	280	2	—
Whole Baby Chowder Clams	2 oz	33	0	—	1	—
Snow's						
Minced	6.5 oz	90	tr	1020	6	—
liquid only	1 cup	6	tr	516	tr	—
liquid only	3 oz	2	tr	183	tr	—
meat only	1 cup	236	3	179	8	—
meat only	3 oz	126	2	95	4	—
FRESH						
cooked	3 oz	126	2	95	4	—
cooked	20 sm	133	2	100	5	—
raw	20 sm (180 g)	133	2	100	5	—
raw	9 lg (180 g)	133	2	100	5	—
raw	3 oz	63	1	47	2	—

FOOD	PORTION	CAL.	FAT	SOD.	CARB.	FIB.
FROZEN						
Gorton's						
Microwave Crunchy Clam Strips	3.5 oz	330	22	430	24	—
Mrs. Paul's						
Fried	2.5 oz	200	9	450	21	—
Microwave Fried Clams	2.5 oz	260	15	410	23	—
HOME RECIPE						
breaded & fried	3 oz	171	9	309	9	—
breaded & fried	20 sm	379	21	684	19	—
TAKE-OUT						
breaded & fried	¾ cup	451	26	833	39	—

CLOVES

FOOD	PORTION	CAL.	FAT	SOD.	CARB.	FIB.
ground	1 tsp	7	tr	5	1	—

COCOA
(*see also* CHOCOLATE)

FOOD	PORTION	CAL.	FAT	SOD.	CARB.	FIB.
Carnation						
Hot Cocoa 70 Calorie	3 tsp (21 g)	70	tr	—	—	—
Hot Cocoa Milk Chocolate	1 pkg or 4 heaping tsp (1 oz)	110	1	—	—	—
Hot Cocoa Natural Mint	1 pkg or 4 heaping tsp (1 oz)	110	1	—	—	—
Hot Cocoa Rich Chocolate	1 pkg or 4 heaping tsp (1 oz)	110	1	—	—	—
Hot Cocoa Rich Chocolate w/ Marshmallows	1 pkg or 4 heaping tsp (1 oz)	110	1	—	—	—
Hot Cocoa Sugar Free Mint	1 pkg or 4 heaping tsp (15 g)	50	tr	—	—	—
Hot Cocoa Sugar Free Rich Chocolate	1 pkg or 4 heaping tsp (15 g)	50	tr	—	—	—
Hershey						
Cocoa	⅓ cup (1 oz)	120	4	10	13	—
European Cocoa	1 oz	90	3	15	8	—
Hills Bros.						
Hot Cocoa	6 oz	110	2	—	—	—
Hot Cocoa Sugar Free	6 oz	60	2	—	—	—
Nestle						
Hot Cocoa Mix	1 oz	110	1	100	23	—
Hot Cocoa Mix as prep w/ 2% milk	6 oz	210	5	190	32	—
Hot Cocoa Mix as prep w/ skim milk	6 oz	180	1	200	32	—

FOOD	PORTION	CAL.	FAT	SOD.	CARB.	FIB.
Nestle (CONT.)						
Hot Cocoa Mix as prep w/ whole milk	6 oz	230	8	240	32	—
Hot Cocoa Mix With Marshmallows	1 oz	120	1	115	23	—
Hot Cocoa Mix With Marshmallows as prep w/ 2% milk	6 oz	220	5	190	32	—
Hot Cocoa Mix With Marshmallows as prep w/ skim milk	6 oz	190	1	200	32	—
Hot Cocoa Mix With Marshmallows as prep w/ whole milk	6 oz	240	8	240	32	—
Swiss Miss						
Cocoa Diet	6 oz	20	tr	180	3	0
Hot Cocoa Bavarian Chocolate	6 oz	110	3	170	20	0
Hot Cocoa Double Rich	6 oz	110	1	150	22	0
Hot Cocoa Milk Chocolate	6 oz	110	1	125	24	0
Hot Cocoa With Mini Marshmallows	6 oz	110	1	170	23	0
Lite as prep	6 oz	70	tr	160	17	0
Sugar Free With Sugar Free Marshmallows as prep	6 oz	50	tr	120	9	0
Sugar Free as prep	6 oz	60	tr	125	10	0
Ultra Slim-Fast						
Hot Cocoa as prep w/ water	8 oz	190	tr	140	35	5
hot cocoa	1 cup	218	9	123	26	—
mix as prep w/ water	7 oz	103	1	149	23	—
mix w/ Nutrasweet as prep w/ water	7 oz	48	tr	173	9	—
powder unsweetened	1 tbsp (5 g)	11	1	1	3	2
powder unsweetened	1 cup (3 oz)	197	12	18	47	29

COCONUT

FOOD	PORTION	CAL.	FAT	SOD.	CARB.	FIB.
Baker's						
Angel Flake Toasted	⅓ cup	212	17	83	17	—
Premium Shred	⅓ cup	135	9	84	12	—
Coco Lopez						
Cream of Coconut	2 tbsp	120	5	10	20	—

FOOD	PORTION	CAL.	FAT	SOD.	CARB.	FIB.
coconut water	1 tbsp	3	tr	16	1	—
coconut water	1 cup	46	tr	252	9	—
cream canned	1 tbsp	36	3	10	2	—
cream canned	1 cup	568	52	149	25	—
dried sweetened flaked	7 oz pkg	944	64	509	95	—
dried sweetened flaked	1 cup	351	24	189	35	—
dried sweetened flaked canned	1 cup	341	24	15	32	—
dried sweetened shredded	1 cup	466	33	244	44	—
dried sweetened shredded	7 oz pkg	997	71	522	95	—
dried toasted	1 oz	168	13	11	13	—
dried unsweetened	1 oz	187	18	11	7	—
fresh	1 piece (1½ oz)	159	15	9	7	4
fresh shredded	1 cup	283	27	16	12	7
milk canned	1 cup	445	48	29	6	—
milk canned	1 tbsp	30	3	2	tr	—
milk frozen	1 cup	486	50	29	13	—
milk frozen	1 tbsp	30	3	2	1	—

COD

CANNED

FOOD	PORTION	CAL.	FAT	SOD.	CARB.	FIB.
atlantic	3 oz	89	1	185	0	—
atlantic	1 can (11 oz)	327	3	680	0	—
roe	3.5 oz	118	3	—	tr	—

DRIED

FOOD	PORTION	CAL.	FAT	SOD.	CARB.	FIB.
atlantic	3 oz	246	2	5973	0	—

FRESH

FOOD	PORTION	CAL.	FAT	SOD.	CARB.	FIB.
atlantic cooked	1 fillet (6.3 oz)	189	2	141	0	—
atlantic cooked	3 oz	89	1	66	0	—
altantic raw	3 oz	70	1	46	0	—
pacific baked	3 oz	95	1	82	0	—
roe baked w/ butter & lemon juice	3.5 oz	126	3	73	2	—
roe raw	3½ oz	130	2	—	2	—

FROZEN

Gorton's

FOOD	PORTION	CAL.	FAT	SOD.	CARB.	FIB.
Fishmarket Fresh	5 oz	110	1	90	0	—

Mrs. Paul's

FOOD	PORTION	CAL.	FAT	SOD.	CARB.	FIB.
Light Fillets	1 fillet	240	11	430	22	—

Van De Kamp's

FOOD	PORTION	CAL.	FAT	SOD.	CARB.	FIB.
Light Fillets	1 piece	250	11	510	20	—
Natural Fillets	4 oz	90	1	90	0	—

COFFEE

(see also COFFEE BEVERAGES, COFFEE SUBSTITUTES)

INSTANT

Kava

FOOD	PORTION	CAL.	FAT	SOD.	CARB.	FIB.
Kava	1 tsp	2	0	<5	1	—

FOOD	PORTION	CAL.	FAT	SOD.	CARB.	FIB.
cappuccino mix as prep	7 oz	62	2	104	11	—
decaffeinated	1 rounded tsp (1.8 g)	4	0	0	1	—
decaffeinated as prep	6 oz	4	0	6	1	—
french mix as prep	7 oz	57	3	—	7	—
mocha mix as prep	7 oz	51	2	36	8	—
regular	1 rounded tsp	4	0	1	1	—
regular as prep	6 oz	4	0	6	1	—
regular w/ chicory	1 rounded tsp	6	0	5	1	—
regular w/ chicory as prep	6 oz	6	0	10	1	—
REGULAR						
Maryland Club	1 tbsp	16	tr	tr	3	—
Folgers						
Colombian Supreme	1 tbsp	16	tr	tr	3	—
Custom Roast	1 tbsp	16	tr	tr	3	—
Decaffeinated	1 tbsp	17	tr	tr	3	—
French Roast	1 tbsp	16	tr	tr	3	—
Gourmet Supreme	1 tbsp	16	tr	tr	3	—
Instant	1 tsp	8	tr	1	1	—
Instant Decaffeinated	1 tsp	8	tr	2	2	—
Singles	1 bag	21	tr	1	4	—
Singles Decaffeinated	1 bag	21	tr	2	4	—
Special Roast	1 tbsp	16	tr	tr	3	—
Vacuum Pack	1 tbsp	16	tr	tr	3	—
brewed	6 oz	4	0	4	1	—
TAKE-OUT						
cafe au lait	1 cup (8 fl oz)	77	4	62	6	—
cafe brulot	1 cup (4.8 fl oz)	48	0	2	3	—
cappuccino	1 cup (8 fl oz)	77	4	62	6	—
coffee con leche	1 cup (8 fl oz)	77	4	62	6	—
espresso	1 cup (3 fl oz)	2	0	2	tr	—
irish coffee	1 serv (9 fl oz)	107	3	25	3	—
mocha	1 mug (9.6 fl oz)	202	15	28	17	—

COFFEE BEVERAGES

(*see also* COFFEE SUBSTITUTES)

Chock o'ccino

Cinnamon	8 oz	120	2	55	25	—
Coffee	8 oz	120	2	55	25	—
Mocha	8 oz	120	2	55	25	—
General Foods						
International Coffee Cafe Amaretto	6 oz	51	3	—	—	—
International Coffee Cafe Francais	6 oz	55	3	—	—	—

FOOD	PORTION	CAL.	FAT	SOD.	CARB.	FIB.
General Foods (CONT.)						
International Coffee Cafe Irish Creme	6 oz	55	3	—	—	—
International Coffee Cafe Vienna	6 oz	59	2	—	—	—
International Coffee Irish Mocha Mint	6 oz	51	2	—	—	—
International Coffee Orange Cappuccino	6 oz	59	10	—	—	—
International Coffee Sugar Free Cafe Francais	6 oz	35	2	—	—	—
International Coffee Sugar Free Cafe Irish Creme	6 oz	31	3	—	—	—
International Coffee Sugar Free Cafe Vienna	6 oz	29	3	—	—	—
International Coffee Sugar Free Irish Mocha Mint	6 oz	28	2	—	—	—
International Coffee Sugar Free Orange Cappuccino	6 oz	29	2	—	—	—
International Coffee Sugar Free Suisse Mocha	6 oz	29	2	—	—	—
International Coffee Suisse Mocha	6 oz	53	3	—	—	—

COFFEE SUBSTITUTES

FOOD	PORTION	CAL.	FAT	SOD.	CARB.	FIB.
Natural Touch						
Kaffree Roma	1 tsp	6	0	—	1	—
Postum						
Instant	6 oz	11	0	3	3	—
Instant Coffee Flavored	6 oz	11	0	3	3	—
powder	1 tsp	9	tr	2	2	—
powder as prep	6 oz	9	tr	7	2	—
powder as prep w/ milk	6 oz	121	6	91	10	—

COFFEE WHITENERS
(*see also* MILK SUBSTITUTES)
LIQUID
Coffee-Mate

FOOD	PORTION	CAL.	FAT	SOD.	CARB.	FIB.
Liquid	1 tbsp (0.5 fl oz)	16	1	5	2	—

FOOD	PORTION	CAL.	FAT	SOD.	CARB.	FIB.
Coffee Rich	1 tbsp	20	2	—	—	—
Hood						
Non Dairy	1 tbsp (0.5 oz)	20	2	0	2	0
International Delight						
Amaretto	1 tbsp (0.6 fl oz)	45	2	5	7	0
Cinnamon Hazelnut	1 tbsp (0.6 fl oz)	45	2	5	7	0
Irish Creme	1 tbsp (0.6 fl oz)	45	2	5	7	0
No Fat Amaretto	1 tbsp (0.5 fl oz)	30	0	5	7	0
No Fat French Vanilla Royale	1 tbsp (0.5 fl oz)	30	0	5	7	0
No Fat Hawaiian Macadamia	1 tbsp (0.5 fl oz)	30	0	5	7	0
No Fat Irish Creme	1 tbsp (0.5 fl oz)	30	0	5	7	0
Suisse Chocolate Mocha	1 tbsp (0.6 fl oz)	45	2	10	7	0
Mocha Mix						
Fat-Free	1 tbsp (0.5 fl oz)	10	0	0	1	0
Lite	1 tbsp (0.5 fl oz)	10	tr	0	tr	0
Lite	4 fl oz	80	7	24	3	0
Original	1 tbsp (0.5 fl oz)	20	2	5	1	0
Signature Flavors French Vanilla	1 tbsp (0.5 fl oz)	35	0	5	8	—
Signature Flavors Irish Creme	1 tbsp (0.5 fl oz)	35	0	5	8	—
Signature Flavors Kahlua	1 tbsp (0.5 fl oz)	35	0	5	8	—
Signature Flavors Mauna Loa Macadamia Nut	1 tbsp (0.5 fl oz)	35	0	5	8	—
nondairy frzn	1 tbsp	20	2	12	2	—
POWDER						
Coffee-Mate						
Powder	1 tsp (2 g)	10	1	5	1	—
Cremora	1 tsp	12	1	5	1	—
N-Rich Creamer	1 tsp	10	tr	0	1	0
Weight Watchers						
Dairy Creamer Instant Nonfat Dry Milk	1 pkg	10	0	15	1	—
nondairy	1 tsp	11	tr	4	1	—

COLESLAW
(*see* CABBAGE, SALAD DRESSING)

COLLARDS
CANNED

FOOD	PORTION	CAL.	FAT	SOD.	CARB.	FIB.
Allen	½ cup (4.1 oz)	30	1	20	5	3
Sunshine	½ cup (4.1 oz)	30	1	20	5	3

FOOD	PORTION	CAL.	FAT	SOD.	CARB.	FIB.
FRESH						
cooked	½ cup	17	tr	10	4	—
raw chopped	½ cup	6	tr	4	1	—
FROZEN						
chopped cooked	½ cup	31	tr	42	6	—

COOKIES
(see also BROWNIE, CAKE, DOUGHNUT, PIE)

HOME RECIPE

FOOD	PORTION	CAL.	FAT	SOD.	CARB.	FIB.
chocolate chip as prep w/ butter	1 (0.42 oz)	78	5	55	9	—
chocolate chip as prep w/ margarine	1 (0.56 oz)	78	5	58	9	—
macaroons	1 (0.8 oz)	97	3	59	17	—
oatmeal	1 (0.5 oz)	67	3	90	10	—
oatmeal w/ raisins	1 (0.52 oz)	65	2	81	10	—
peanut butter	1 (0.7 oz)	95	5	104	12	—
shortbread as prep w/ butter	1 (0.38 oz)	60	4	51	6	—
shortbread as prep w/ margarine	1 (0.38 oz)	60	4	56	6	—
sugar as prep w/ butter	1 (0.49 oz)	66	3	64	8	—
sugar as prep w/ margarine	1 (0.49 oz)	66	3	69	8	—
MIX						
Betty Crocker						
Chocolate Chip Big Batch	2	120	6	100	16	—
Date Bar Classic Dessert	1	60	2	35	9	—
Estee						
Chocolate Chip	3	130	7	120	17	0
chocolate chip	1 (0.56 oz)	79	4	47	10	—
oatmeal	1 (0.6 oz)	74	3	75	10	tr
oatmeal raisin	1 (0.6 oz)	74	3	75	10	tr
READY-TO-EAT						
Archway						
Almond Crescents	2 (0.8 oz)	100	4	75	17	tr
Apple N'Raisin	1 (1.1 oz)	130	52	105	20	1
Apricot Filled	1 (1 oz)	110	4	90	18	tr
Bells And Stars	3 (1 oz)	150	7	100	19	tr
Blueberry Filled	1 (1 oz)	110	4	115	19	tr
Carrot Cake	1 (1 oz)	120	5	180	18	0
Cherry Filled	1 (1 oz)	110	4	100	19	tr
Cherry Nougat	3 (1 oz)	150	9	40	18	0
Chocolate Chip	1 (1 oz)	130	6	150	19	0

FOOD	PORTION	CAL.	FAT	SOD.	CARB.	FIB.
Archway (CONT.)						
Chocolate Chip & Toffee	1 (1 oz)	140	7	120	19	tr
Chocolate Chip Bag	3 (0.9 oz)	130	7	70	17	0
Chocolate Chip Drop	1 (1 oz)	140	10	105	11	tr
Chocolate Chip Ice Box	1 (1 oz)	140	7	80	19	0
Chocolate Chip Mini	12 (1.1 oz)	150	7	95	20	0
Cinnamon Snaps	12 (1.1 oz)	150	7	115	19	0
Coconut Macaroon	1 (0.8 oz)	90	5	55	14	2
Cookie Jar Hermits	1 (1 oz)	110	3	160	19	tr
Dark Chocolate	1 (1 oz)	110	4	150	20	tr
Dutch Chocolate	1 (1 oz)	120	4	110	19	0
Fig Bars Low Fat	2 (1.1 oz)	100	1	105	23	1
Frosty Lemon	1 (1 oz)	120	5	110	19	0
Frosty Orange	1 (1 oz)	120	4	140	19	1
Fruit And Honey Bar	1 (1 oz)	110	4	120	18	tr
Fruit Bar No Fat	1 (1 oz)	90	0	95	21	0
Fruit Cake	1 (1.1 oz)	140	7	100	20	2
Fudge Nut Bar	1 (1 oz)	110	5	120	17	tr
Fun Chip Mini	12 (1.1 oz)	140	6	100	21	0
Gingersnaps	5 (1.1 oz)	130	5	110	22	0
Granola No Fat	1 (0.5 oz)	50	0	60	11	tr
Holiday Pak	3 (1.1 oz)	150	8	95	19	tr
Iced Gingerbread	3 (1.1 oz)	140	5	130	23	0
Iced Molasses	1 (1 oz)	110	5	170	19	tr
Iced Oatmeal	1 (1 oz)	120	5	85	19	1
Lemon Snaps	12 (1.1 oz)	150	7	120	19	0
New Orleans Cake	1 (1 oz)	110	4	105	18	tr
Nutty Nougat	3 (1.1 oz)	160	10	60	18	0
Oatmeal	1 (0.9 oz)	110	3	95	19	tr
Oatmeal Apple Filled	1 (1 oz)	110	3	105	18	0
Oatmeal Date Filled	1 (1 oz)	110	4	120	18	tr
Oatmeal Mini	12 (1.1 oz)	150	8	130	19	1
Oatmeal Pecan	1 (1 oz)	120	5	100	18	1
Oatmeal Raisin	1 (1 oz)	110	4	115	19	tr
Oatmeal Raisin Bran	1 (1 oz)	110	4	100	19	tr
Old Fashioned Molasses	1 (1 oz)	120	3	150	20	0
Old Fashioned Windmill	1 (0.7 oz)	100	4	95	15	0
Party Treats	3 (1.1 oz)	140	7	105	20	0
Peanut Butter	1 (1 oz)	140	7	125	16	tr
Peanut Butter & Chip	3 (0.9 oz)	130	7	125	16	0
Peanut Butter n' Chips	1 (1 oz)	140	7	115	16	tr
Peanut Butter Nougat	3 (1.1 oz)	160	9	140	18	1
Pecan Crunch	6 (1.1 oz)	150	8	120	18	0
Pecan Ice Box	1 (1 oz)	140	7	100	18	0

FOOD	PORTION	CAL.	FAT	SOD.	CARB.	FIB.
Archway (CONT.)						
Pecan Malted Nougat	3 (1.1 oz)	160	10	60	17	2
Pfeffernusse	2 (1.3 oz)	140	1	100	32	tr
Pineapple Filled	1 (0.9 oz)	100	4	75	16	1
Raisin Oatmeal	1 (1 oz)	130	5	40	19	1
Raisin Oatmeal Bag	3 (1.4 oz)	130	6	55	19	1
Raspberry Filled	1 (1 oz)	110	4	90	18	tr
Rocky Road	1 (1 oz)	130	6	85	18	tr
Ruth's Golden Oatmeal	1 (1 oz)	120	5	135	19	tr
Select Assortment	3 (0.9 oz)	130	6	80	18	0
Soft Molasses Drop	1 (1 oz)	110	4	160	18	1
Soft Sugar	1 (1 oz)	110	4	110	18	0
Strawberry Filled	1 (1 oz)	110	4	90	18	tr
Sugar	1 (1 oz)	120	4	190	20	0
Vanilla Wafer	5 (1.1 oz)	130	4	130	22	0
Wedding Cakes	3 (1.1 oz)	160	8	45	20	0
Bakery Wagon						
Apple Walnut Raisin	1	100	4	130	16	1
Cobbler Apple Cranberry Fat Free	1	70	0	60	16	1
Cobbler Apple Fat Free	1	70	0	55	17	1
Cobbler Mixed Fruit Fat Free	1	70	0	65	16	1
Cobbler Raspberry Fat Free	1	70	0	60	17	1
Ginger Snaps	5	160	7	140	22	1
Honey Fruit Bars	1	100	3	80	17	1
Iced Molasses	1	100	3	120	18	1
Iced Molasses Mini	3	130	3	170	18	1
Oatmeal Apple Filled	1	90	3	65	14	1
Oatmeal Chocolate Chunk	1	100	3	75	16	1
Oatmeal Date Filled	1	90	3	90	17	1
Oatmeal Raspberry Filled	1	100	3	105	16	1
Oatmeal Soft	1	100	4	90	16	1
Oatmeal Walnut Raisin	1	100	4	125	17	1
Vanilla Wafers Cholesterol Free	6	130	6	140	22	1
Barnum's						
Animal Crackers	12 (1.1 oz)	140	4	160	23	1
Biscos						
Sugar Wafers	8 (1 oz)	140	6	40	21	tr
Waffle Cremes	4 (1.2 oz)	180	9	35	24	tr

FOOD	PORTION	CAL.	FAT	SOD.	CARB.	FIB.
Chips Ahoy!						
Bit Size Chocolate Chip	14 (1.1 oz)	170	7	105	21	tr
Chewy Chocolate Chip	3 (1.3 oz)	170	8	125	23	tr
Chunky Chocolate Chip	1 (0.5 oz)	80	4	60	11	tr
Real Chocolate Chip	3 (1.1 oz)	160	8	105	21	1
Reduced Fat	3 (1.1 oz)	150	6	150	23	1
Sprinkled Real Chocolate Chip	3 (1.3 oz)	170	8	120	24	tr
Striped Chocolate Chip	1 (0.5 oz)	80	4	45	10	tr
Cookie Lover's						
Blue Ribbon Brownies	1 (0.8 oz)	90	3	75	14	0
Classic Shortbread	1 (0.8 oz)	110	7	75	12	0
Dutch Chocolate Chip	1 (0.8 oz)	90	4	65	12	0
Fancy Peanut Butter	1 (0.8 oz)	100	6	90	10	0
Grahams Cinnamon Honey	2 (1 oz)	110	1	130	24	1
Grahams Honey	2 (1 oz)	100	2	130	22	1
Old-Time Raisin	1 (0.8 oz)	90	3	60	14	0
Delacre						
Cookie Assortment	4 (1.1 oz)	130	<5	35	18	1
Drake's						
Chocolate Chip	2 (1 oz)	140	6	110	18	—
Chocolate-Chocolate Chip	2 (1 oz)	130	5	85	19	—
Coconut	2 (1 oz)	130	5	95	20	—
Coconut Macaroon	1 (1 oz)	135	7	80	17	—
Hermit	1 (2 oz)	230	7	280	38	—
Oatmeal	2 (1 oz)	120	5	50	19	—
Oatmeal Creme	1 (2 oz)	240	9	250	9	—
Peanut Butter Wafers	1 (2.25 oz)	324	16	135	43	—
Dutch Mill						
Chocolate Chip	3 (1.1 oz)	160	10	85	18	1
Coconut Macaroons	3 (1 oz)	120	7	115	14	0
Oatmeal Raisin	3 (1 oz)	130	6	75	18	1
Entenmann's						
Chocolate Chip	3 (0.9 oz)	140	7	85	19	—
Estee						
Chocolate Chip	4 (1.1 oz)	150	7	30	21	tr
Coconut	4 (1 oz)	140	6	25	19	tr
Creme Wafers Chocolate	7 (1.1 oz)	160	8	0	21	tr
Creme Wafers Lemon	5 (1.2 oz)	170	8	10	23	0
Creme Wafers Peanut Butter	5 (1.2 oz)	170	9	85	21	0
Creme Wafers Triple Decker Banana Split	3 (0.9 oz)	140	7	0	18	0

FOOD	PORTION	CAL.	FAT	SOD.	CARB.	FIB.
Estee (CONT.)						
Creme Wafers Triple Decker Chocolate Caramel & Peanut Butter	3 (0.9 oz)	140	7	45	17	0
Creme Wafers Vanilla	7 (1.1 oz)	160	7	0	22	0
Creme Wafers Vanilla & Strawberry	5 (1.2 oz)	170	8	0	23	0
Fig Bars Apple Low Fat	2 (1 oz)	100	1	25	22	3
Fig Bars Cranberry Low Fat	2 (1 oz)	100	1	20	22	3
Fig Bars Low Fat	2 (1 oz)	100	0	20	23	3
Fudge	4 (1 oz)	150	7	45	19	1
Lemon	4 (1 oz)	140	6	25	19	tr
Oatmeal Raisin	4 (1 oz)	130	5	25	19	1
Sandwich Chocolate	3 (1.2 oz)	160	6	60	24	1
Sandwich Original	3 (1.2 oz)	160	6	45	24	1
Sandwich Peanut Butter	3 (1.2 oz)	160	7	55	22	1
Sandwich Vanilla	3 (1.2 oz)	160	5	35	25	tr
Shortbread Reduced Fat	4 (1 oz)	130	4	150	22	tr
Vanilla	4 (1 oz)	140	6	25	19	tr
FFV						
Animal Crackers	9	110	3	—	—	—
Caramel Patties	2	150	7	—	—	—
Fig Bars Vanilla	1	60	1	—	—	—
Fig Bars Whole Wheat	1	60	1	—	—	—
Ginger Boys Calcium Enriched	6	120	3	—	—	—
Jelly Tarts	2	110	4	—	—	—
Mint Sandwich	2	160	7	—	—	—
Oatmeal Calcium Enriched	5	130	5	—	—	—
Peanut Butter Sandwich	2	170	8	—	—	—
Regal Grahams	2	140	7	—	—	—
Royal Dainty	2	120	6	—	—	—
T.C. Rounds	2	160	8	—	—	—
Tango	2	160	5	—	—	—
Trolley Cakes Devilsfood	2	120	2	—	—	—
Vanilla Wafers	8	120	5	—	—	—
Famous Amos						
Chocolate Chip	3 (1 oz)	140	6	100	20	—
Chocolate Chip Pecan	3 (1 oz)	150	8	98	18	—
Oatmeal Raisin	3 (1 oz)	134	6	137	19	—

FOOD	PORTION	CAL.	FAT	SOD.	CARB.	FIB.
Freihofer's						
Chocolate Chip	2 (0.9 oz)	120	6	75	16	1
Frito Lay						
Peanut Butter Bar	1.75 oz	270	16	65	30	—
Frookie						
7-Grain Oatmeal	1	45	2	35	7	—
Animal Frackers	6	60	2	25	9	—
Apple Cinnamon Oat Bran	1 lg	120	4	100	18	—
Apple Cinnamon Oat Bran	1	45	2	35	7	—
Apple Fruitins	1	60	1	25	12	—
Chocolate Chip	1	45	2	35	7	—
Chocolate Chip	1 lg	120	4	100	18	—
Chocolate Chip Mint	1	45	2	35	7	—
Fig Fruitins	1	60	1	25	12	—
Ginger Spice	1	45	2	35	7	—
Mandarin Chocolate Chip	1	45	2	35	7	—
Oat Bran Muffin	1	45	2	35	7	—
Oat Bran Muffin	1 lg	120	4	100	18	—
Oatmeal Raisin	1	45	2	35	7	—
Oatmeal Raisin	1 lg	120	4	100	18	—
General Mills						
Dunkaroos	1 pkg (1 oz)	130	5	70	19	—
FundaMiddles Vanilla Creme in Chocolate Graham Shells	1 pkg (0.8 oz)	110	4	120	18	—
Glenny's						
Noah'N Friends Animal Peanut Butter	0.5 oz	65	3	35	9	—
Noah'N Friends Animal Vanilla	0.5 oz	65	2	35	10	—
Noah'N Friends Animal Wheat-Free Oatmeal	0.5 oz	65	2	20	10	—
Nookie Bar	1 (1.15 oz)	138	3	—	18	—
Sesame Nookie	1 (0.5 oz)	60	4	8	6	—
Sesame Nookie	1 pkg (1.5 oz)	180	12	24	18	—
Golden Fruit						
Apple	1 (0.7 oz)	80	2	55	15	tr
Cranberry	1 (0.7 oz)	70	1	55	15	tr
Cranberry Low Fat	1 (0.7 oz)	70	1	55	15	tr
Raisin	1 (0.7 oz)	80	2	40	15	tr

FOOD	PORTION	CAL.	FAT	SOD.	CARB.	FIB.
Grandma's						
Animal Cookies Candied	5 (1 oz)	140	6	80	20	—
Chocolate Chip	2 (2.75 oz)	370	17	270	50	—
Chocolate Chip Rich'N Chewy	3 (1 oz)	140	6	80	20	—
Fudge Chocolate Chip	2 (2.75 oz)	350	13	380	54	—
Grab Cookie Bits Chocolate	8 (1 oz)	140	6	180	19	—
Grab Cookie Bits Peanut Butter	8 (1 oz)	140	6	125	19	—
Grab Cookie Bits Vanilla	8 (1 oz)	140	6	75	20	—
Oatmeal Apple Spice	2 (2.75 oz)	330	12	570	51	—
Old Time Molasses	2 (2.75 oz)	320	9	520	58	—
Peanut Butter	2 (2.75 oz)	410	30	410	43	—
Raisin Soft	2 (2.75 oz)	320	10	280	54	—
Health Valley						
Amaranth Cookies	1	70	3	30	12	2
Fancy Fruit Chunks Apricot Almond	2	90	4	45	12	2
Fancy Fruit Chunks Date Pecan	2	90	4	45	13	2
Fancy Fruit Chunks Raisin Oat Bran	2	70	2	95	13	2
Fancy Fruit Chunks Tropical Fruit	2	90	3	45	15	2
Fancy Peanut Chunks	2	90	3	55	12	2
Fat Free Apple Spice	3	75	tr	40	17	3
Fat Free Apricot Delight	3	75	tr	40	16	3
Fat Free Date Delight	3	75	tr	40	17	3
Fat Free Hawaiian Fruit	3	75	tr	40	16	3
Fat Free Jumbos Apple Raisin	1	70	tr	35	16	3
Fat Free Jumbos Raisin	1	70	tr	35	16	3
Fat Free Jumbos Raspberry	1	70	tr	35	16	3
Fat Free Raisin Oatmeal	3	75	tr	40	17	3
Fiber Jumbos Blueberry Nut	1	100	3	45	14	3
Fiber Jumbos Chunky Pecan	1	100	3	45	14	3
Fiber Jumbos Raisin Nut	1	100	3	45	14	3
Fruit & Fitness	5	200	6	115	34	6
Fruit Jumbos Almond Date	1	70	3	30	10	1

FOOD	PORTION	CAL.	FAT	SOD.	CARB.	FIB.
Health Valley (CONT.)						
Fruit Jumbos Oat Bran	1	70	2	35	12	2
Fruit Jumbos Raisin Nut	1	70	3	35	10	1
Fruit Jumbos Tropical Fruit	1	70	3	35	10	2
Graham Amaranth	7	110	3	110	25	3
Graham Honey	7	100	4	125	18	2
Graham Oat Bran	7	120	3	45	20	5
Honey Jumbos Crisp Cinnamon	1	70	4	35	9	1
Honey Jumbos Crisp Peanut Butter	1	70	2	35	11	1
Honey Jumbos Fancy Oat Bran	2	130	4	50	20	4
Oat Bran Animal Cookies	7	110	4	50	17	3
Oat Bran Fruit & Nut	2	110	4	70	17	3
The Great Tofu	2	90	3	30	14	4
The Great Wheat Free	2	80	3	35	14	3
Heyday						
Caramel & Peanut	1 (0.8 oz)	110	5	40	13	tr
Fudge	1 (0.8 oz)	110	5	40	13	tr
Honey Maid						
Cinnamon Grahams	10 (1.1 oz)	140	3	210	26	1
Honey Grahams	8 (1 oz)	120	3	180	22	1
Hydrox						
Reduced Fat	3 (1.1 oz)	130	4	140	24	1
Keebler						
Buttercup	3	70	3	110	11	—
Chocolate Fudge Sandwich	1	80	4	70	12	—
Commodore	1	60	2	65	10	—
Cookies Mates	2	50	2	55	8	—
French Vanilla Creme	1	80	4	80	12	—
Graham Honey Fiber Enriched	2	90	2	110	16	—
Graham Kitchen Rich	2	60	2	55	9	—
Homeplate	1	60	2	130	10	—
Keebies	1	80	4	80	12	—
Krisp Kreem Wafers	2	50	3	20	7	—
Old Fashion Chocolate Chip	1	80	4	75	11	—
Old Fashion Double Fudge	1	80	4	65	11	—
Old Fashion Oatmeal	1	80	4	110	13	—

FOOD	PORTION	CAL.	FAT	SOD.	CARB.	FIB.
Keebler (CONT.)						
Old Fashion Peanut Butter	1	80	4	100	10	—
Old Fashion Sugar	1	80	3	70	13	—
Pitter Patter	1	90	4	115	12	—
Vanilla Wafers	4	80	4	60	10	—
LU						
Chocolatiers	4 (1.1 oz)	170	8	35	20	2
Chocolatiers Dipped	3 (1 oz)	170	11	15	17	1
Little Schoolboy Dark Chocolate	2 (0.9 oz)	130	7	85	15	0
Little Schoolboy Milk Chocolate	2 (0.9 oz)	130	7	85	15	0
Marie Lu	3 (1.2 oz)	170	6	170	25	1
Truffle Lu	4 (1.2 oz)	180	11	410	18	1
La Choy						
Fortune	1	15	tr	1	4	tr
Lance						
Choc-O-Lunch	1 pkg (37 g)	180	7	150	26	—
Choc-O-Mint	1 pkg (35 g)	180	10	90	22	—
Chocolate Chip Fudge	1 (26 g)	130	5	130	20	—
Chocolate Chip Soft	1 (28 g)	130	5	100	19	—
Coated Graham	1 pkg (50 g)	200	10	60	24	—
Fig Bar	1 pkg (42 g)	150	2	85	30	—
Lem-O-Lunch	1 pkg (46 g)	240	11	190	32	—
Lemon Nekot	1 pkg (42 g)	220	11	100	28	—
Malt	1 pkg (35 g)	190	11	125	16	—
Nut-O-Lunch	1 oz	140	5	—	—	—
Oatmeal	1 (57 g)	130	5	70	20	—
Peanut Butter Creme Filled Wafer	1 pkg (50 g)	240	10	80	34	—
Van-O-Lunch	1 pkg (37 g)	180	7	150	26	—
Little Debbie						
Animal	1 pkg (1.5 oz)	190	5	110	33	0
Caramel Cookie Bars	1 pkg (1.2 oz)	160	8	90	23	1
Chocolate Chip Chewy	1 pkg (2 oz)	370	19	280	47	1
Chocolate Chip Crisp	1 pkg (1.5 oz)	210	12	150	26	1
Cookie Wreaths	1 pkg (0.6 oz)	90	5	45	11	0
Creme Filled Chocolate	1 pkg (1.8 oz)	260	11	230	36	1
Creme Filled Chocolate	1 pkg (1.2 oz)	180	8	115	24	1
Easter Puffs	1 pkg (1.2 oz)	140	5	65	25	0
Figaroos	1 pkg (1.5 oz)	160	4	115	31	3
Figaroos	1 pkg (2 oz)	200	5	160	40	2
Fudge Macaroons	1 pkg (1 oz)	140	8	65	18	1

FOOD	PORTION	CAL.	FAT	SOD.	CARB.	FIB.
Little Debbie (CONT.)						
Ginger	1 pkg (0.7 oz)	90	3	55	14	1
Oatmeal Crisp	1 pkg (1.5 oz)	210	11	230	27	1
Oatmeal Lights	1 pkg (1.3 oz)	140	4	190	28	1
Oatmeal Raisin	1 pkg (2.7 oz)	320	13	330	50	2
Peanut Butter	1 pkg (1.5 oz)	210	10	230	27	1
Peanut Butter & Jelly Sandwiches	1 pkg (1.1 oz)	130	5	100	22	1
Peanut Butter Bars	1 pkg (1.9 oz)	270	15	190	33	1
Peanut Clusters	1 pkg (1.4 oz)	190	11	125	23	1
Pecan Spinwheels	1 pkg (1 oz)	110	4	100	16	1
Pecan Shortbread	1 pkg (1.5 oz)	220	13	170	26	0
Manischewitz						
Macaroons Chocolate	2 (0.9 oz)	90	4	80	15	4
Mother's						
Almond Shortbread	3	180	11	115	19	1
Butter	5	140	6	95	21	—
Checkerboard Wafers	8	150	8	40	20	1
Chocolate Chip	2	160	8	105	20	0
Chocolate Chip Angel	3	180	9	70	21	1
Chocolate Chip Bag	4	140	5	85	23	1
Chocolate Chip Parade	4	130	5	100	19	1
Circus Animals	6	140	6	55	20	0
Cocadas	5	150	7	140	20	2
Cookie Parade	4	140	7	95	18	2
Dinosaur Grrrahams	2	130	3	130	24	—
Double Fudge	3	170	8	100	22	2
Duplex Creme	3	170	8	130	23	1
English Tea	2	180	7	100	26	1
Fig Bar	2	130	4	105	24	0
Fig Bar Fat Free	1	70	0	65	16	1
Fig Bar Whole Wheat	2	130	5	140	20	3
Fig Bar Whole Wheat Fat Free	1	70	0	60	17	1
Flaky Flix Fudge	2	140	7	50	17	2
Flaky Flix Vanilla	2	140	8	40	17	1
Frosted Holiday	4	130	6	50	19	0
Fudge Bowl Crowns	2	140	6	55	21	1
Fudge Bowl Nuggets	2	140	6	70	21	1
Gaucho Peanut Butter	2	190	10	200	22	2
Gingerbread Man	6	140	6	160	21	1
Iced Oatmeal	2	120	4	150	20	1
Iced Oatmeal Bag	4	120	4	150	20	1
Iced Raisin	2	180	8	110	24	1

FOOD	PORTION	CAL.	FAT	SOD.	CARB.	FIB.
Mother's (CONT.)						
MLB Double Header Duplex	3	170	8	130	23	1
Macaroon	2	150	8	80	18	2
Marias	3	170	6	150	28	1
North Poles	2	140	7	30	17	0
Oatmeal	2	110	5	150	17	1
Oatmeal Chocolate Chip	2	120	5	140	19	1
Oatmeal Raisin	5	150	7	125	20	2
Oatmeal Walnut Chocolate Chip	2	130	6	135	17	1
Pecan Goldens	2	170	11	110	17	5
Rainbow Wafers	8	150	8	40	20	1
Striped Shortbread	3	170	8	75	22	1
Sugar	2	140	6	75	19	1
Taffy	2	180	8	160	25	2
Triplet Assortment	2	140	7	112	18	1
Vanilla Wafers	6	150	6	85	24	1
Walnut Fudge	2	130	7	90	16	1
Zoo Pals	14	140	5	120	23	1
Nabisco						
Brown Edge Wafers	5 (1 oz)	140	6	80	21	tr
Bugs Bunny Chocolate Graham	13 (1.1 oz)	140	5	180	22	1
Bugs Bunny Cinnamon Graham	13 (1.1 oz)	140	5	160	23	tr
Bugs Bunny Graham	13 (1.1 oz)	140	7	160	23	1
Cameo	2 (1 oz)	130	5	105	21	tr
Chocolate Grahams	3 (1.1 oz)	160	8	90	21	1
Chocolate Chip Snaps	7 (1.1 oz)	150	5	115	24	tr
Chocolate Snaps	7 (1.1 oz)	140	5	180	23	1
Cookie Break	3 (1.1 oz)	160	6	115	23	tr
Danish Imported	5 (1.1 oz)	170	8	80	22	1
Family Favorites Fudge Covered Grahams	3 (1 oz)	140	7	125	19	1
Family Favorites Fudge Striped Shortbread	3 (1.1 oz)	160	8	140	22	1
Family Favorites Oatmeal	1 (0.5 oz)	80	3	65	12	tr
Family Favorites Vanilla Sandwich	3 (1.2 oz)	170	8	120	25	0
Famous Chocolate Wafers	5 (1.1 oz)	140	4	230	24	1
Ginger Snaps Old Fashioned	4 (1 oz)	120	3	170	22	tr

FOOD	PORTION	CAL.	FAT	SOD.	CARB.	FIB.
Nabisco (CONT.)						
Grahams	8 (1 oz)	120	3	180	22	1
Marshmallow Puffs	1 (0.75 oz)	90	4	45	14	0
Marshmallow Twirls	1 (1 oz)	130	6	75	20	tr
Nilla Wafers	8 (1.1 oz)	140	5	105	24	0
Pecan Passion	1 (0.5 oz)	90	5	35	9	0
Pinwheels	1 (1 oz)	130	5	35	21	tr
National						
Arrowroot	1 (5 g)	20	1	15	3	tr
Newtons						
Apple Fat Free	2 (1 oz)	100	0	60	24	1
Cranberry Fat Free	2 (1 oz)	100	0	95	23	1
Fig	2 (1.1 oz)	110	3	120	20	1
Fig Fat Free	1 (1 oz)	100	0	115	22	2
Raspberry Fat Free	2 (1 oz)	100	0	115	23	tr
Strawberry Fat Free	2 (1 oz)	100	0	115	23	tr
Nutra/Balance						
Chocolate Chip	1 (2 oz)	260	14	81	34	8
Oatmeal Raisin	1 (2 oz)	240	9	50	36	8
Nutter Butter						
Bites Peanut Butter Sandwich	10 (1.1 oz)	150	7	125	20	1
Peanut Butter Sandwich	2 (1 oz)	130	6	110	19	1
Peanut Creme Patties	5 (1.1 oz)	160	9	80	17	1
Oreo						
Double Stuf	2 (1 oz)	140	7	150	19	tr
Fudge Covered	1 (0.75 oz)	110	6	85	14	tr
Halloween Treats	2 (1 oz)	140	7	125	19	1
Reduced Fat	3 (1.2 oz)	140	5	190	24	1
White Fudge Covered	1 (0.75 oz)	110	6	70	14	tr
Pally						
Butter	4 (0.88 oz)	100	3	95	17	—
Pepperidge Farm						
Beacon Hill Chocolate Chocolate Walnut	1	120	7	65	14	1
Blondie Chocolate Chip Fat Free	1 (1.4 oz)	120	0	65	29	tr
Bordeaux	2	70	3	40	11	0
Brownie Chocolate Nut	2	110	7	45	11	—
Brownie Nut Large	1	140	8	65	15	—
Brussels	2	110	5	65	13	0
Brussels Mint	2	130	7	40	17	—
Butter Chessman	2	90	4	60	12	—
Cappuccino	1	50	3	20	6	—

FOOD	PORTION	CAL.	FAT	SOD.	CARB.	FIB.
Pepperidge Farm (CONT.)						
Capri	1	80	5	45	10	—
Champagne	2	110	6	—	—	—
Chantilly	1	80	2	35	14	—
Chesapeake Chocolate Chunk Pecan	1	120	7	60	14	1
Cheyenne Peanut Butter Milk Chocolate Chunk	1	110	6	80	13	1
Chocolate Chip	2	100	5	45	12	0
Chocolate Chip Large	1	130	6	60	16	—
Chocolate Chunk Pecan	1	70	4	25	8	—
Dakota Milk Chocolate Oatmeal	1	110	6	70	15	1
Date Pecan	2	110	5	40	15	—
Fruit Filled Apricot-Raspberry	2	100	4	50	15	—
Fruit Filled Strawberry	2	100	5	50	15	—
Geneva	2	130	6	50	14	—
Gingerman	2	70	3	50	10	—
Hazelnut	2	110	6	75	15	—
Irish Oatmeal	2	90	5	80	13	—
Lemon Nut Crunch	2	110	7	50	13	—
Lido	1	90	5	30	10	—
Linzer	1	120	4	55	20	—
Milano	2	120	6	45	15	—
Milk Chocolate Macadamia	2	140	8	—	—	—
Mint Milano	2	150	7	60	17	—
Molasses Crisps	2	70	3	50	8	—
Nantucket Chocolate Chunk	1	120	6	60	15	1
Nassau	1	80	5	45	9	—
Oatmeal Large	1	120	6	105	18	—
Oatmeal Raisin	2	110	5	115	15	—
Old Fashioned Chocolate Chip	2	100	5	45	12	0
Orange Milano	2	150	7	60	17	—
Orleans	3	90	6	30	11	—
Orleans Sandwich	2	120	8	40	14	—
Paris	2	100	5	—	—	—
Pecan Shortbread	1	70	5	15	7	—
Pirouettes Chocolate Laced	2	70	4	20	8	—
Pirouettes Original	2	70	4	35	9	—

FOOD	PORTION	CAL.	FAT	SOD.	CARB.	FIB.
Pepperidge Farm (CONT.)						
Raisin Bran	2	110	5	55	13	—
Ripple Milk Chocolate Fat Free	1 (0.6 oz)	60	0	60	13	tr
Sante Fe Oatmeal Raisin	1	100	4	70	16	1
Sausalito Milk Chocolate Macadamia	1	120	7	65	14	0
Seville	2	100	5	—	—	—
Shortbread	2	150	8	85	17	—
Southport	2	170	10	—	—	—
Sugar	2	100	5	55	13	—
Tahiti	1	90	6	25	9	—
Zurich	1	60	2	30	10	—
Ritz						
Chocolate Covered	3 (1 oz)	150	9	95	17	1
Salerno						
Dinosaur Grrrahams Chocolate	1 pkg (1.25 oz)	167	5	139	25	1
Dinosaur Grrrahams Cinnamon	1 pkg (1.25 oz)	165	5	144	26	1
Dinosaur Grrrahams Original	1 pkg (1.25 oz)	156	3	114	26	1
Sargento						
MooTown Snackers Cookies & Creme Honey Graham Sticks & Vanilla Creme w/ Sprinkle	1 pkg (1.1 oz)	140	7	60	19	0
MooTown Snackers Cookies & Creme Vanilla Sticks & Chocolate Fudge Creme	1 pkg (1.1 oz)	140	7	65	20	0
Snackwell's						
Fat Free Cinnamon Grahams	20 (1 oz)	110	0	90	26	1
Fat Free Devil's Food	1 (0.5 oz)	50	0	25	13	tr
Fat Free Double Fudge	1 (0.5 oz)	50	0	70	12	tr
Reduced Fat Chocolate Chip	13 (1 oz)	130	4	170	22	1
Reduced Fat Chocolate Sandwich With Chocolate Creme	2 (0.9 oz)	100	3	190	20	1
Reduced Fat Oatmeal Raisin	2 (1 oz)	110	3	135	20	1

FOOD	PORTION	CAL.	FAT	SOD.	CARB.	FIB.
Snackwell's (CONT.)						
Reduced Fat Vanilla Sandwich With Vanilla Creme	2 (0.9 oz)	110	3	95	21	1
Stella D'Oro						
Almond Toast Mandel	1	60	1	43	10	—
Angel Bars	1	80	5	15	7	—
Angel Wings	1	70	5	40	7	—
Angelica Goodies	1	110	4	45	16	—
Anginetti	1	30	1	3	5	—
Anisette Sponge	1	50	1	40	10	—
Anisette Toast	1	50	1	50	9	—
Anisette Toast Jumbo	1	110	1	65	23	—
Apple Pastry Low Sodium	1	80	3	5	14	—
Biscottini Cashews	1	110	6	50	14	—
Breakfast Treats	1	100	4	80	15	—
Castelets Chocolate	1	60	3	33	9	—
Chinese Dessert Cookies	1	170	9	90	19	—
Como Delight	1	150	7	60	18	—
Deep Night Fudge	1	65	4	33	8	—
Dutch Apple Bars	1	110	3	35	19	—
Egg Biscuits Low Sodium	3	120	3	15	20	—
Egg Biscuits Sugared	1	80	1	45	14	—
Egg Jumbo	1	50	1	30	9	—
Fruit Delight Apple Cinnamon Fat Free	1	70	0	50	17	—
Fruit Delight Peach Apricot Fat Free	1	70	0	35	17	—
Fruit Delight Raspberry Fat Free	1	70	0	40	17	—
Fruit Slices	1	60	2	45	9	—
Fruit Slices Fat Free	1	50	0	60	12	—
Golden Bars	1	110	4	65	16	—
Holiday Rings & Stars	1	47	1	12	7	—
Holiday Trinkets	1	40	2	31	5	—
Hostess Assortment	1	40	2	20	6	—
Indulgente Cashew Biscottini	1 (1.1 oz)	150	8	70	19	tr
Kichel Low Sodium	21	150	9	25	13	—
Lady Stella Assortment	1	40	2	22	6	—
Margherite Chocolate	1	70	3	40	10	—
Margherite Vanilla	1	70	3	45	11	—

FOOD	PORTION	CAL.	FAT	SOD.	CARB.	FIB.
Stella D'Oro (CONT.)						
Peach Apricot Pastry Sodium Free	1	80	3	0	13	—
Pfeffernusse Spice Drops	1	40	1	18	7	—
Prune Pastry Dietetic	1	90	3	0	14	—
Roman Egg Biscuits	1	140	5	125	20	—
Royal Nuggets	1	2	tr	—	tr	—
Sesame Regina	1	50	2	28	6	—
Swiss Fudge	1	70	3	33	9	—
Sunshine						
Almond Crescents	4 (1.1 oz)	150	6	105	22	tr
Animal Crackers	1 box (2 oz)	260	7	230	43	1
Animal Crackers	14 (1.1 oz)	140	4	125	24	tr
Classics Chocolate Chip With Pecans	1 (0.7 oz)	110	7	45	11	tr
Classics Chocolate Chip With Walnuts	1 (0.7 oz)	100	6	70	11	1
Classics Premier Chocolate Chip	1 (0.7 oz)	100	5	75	13	tr
Dixie Vanilla	2 (0.9 oz)	120	5	105	19	tr
Fig Bars	2 (1 oz)	110	3	60	20	1
Fudge Family Bears Vanilla	2 (1 oz)	140	6	115	20	tr
Fudge Mint Patties	2 (0.8 oz)	130	7	60	16	tr
Fudge Striped Shortbread	3 (1.1 oz)	160	8	85	20	1
Ginger Snaps	7 (1 oz)	130	5	150	22	tr
Grahams Cinnamon	2 (1.1 oz)	140	6	150	22	tr
Grahams Fudge Dipped	4 (1.2 oz)	170	9	75	21	1
Grahams Honey	2 (1 oz)	120	4	130	20	1
Grahamy Bears	1 pkg (2 oz)	260	10	230	41	2
Grahamy Bears	10 (1.1 oz)	140	5	125	22	1
Iced Gingerbread	5 (1 oz)	130	6	135	19	tr
Iced Oatmeal	2 (0.9 oz)	120	6	90	18	tr
Jingles	6 (1.1 oz)	150	5	115	22	tr
Lemon Coolers	5 (1 oz)	140	6	100	21	tr
Mini Chocolate Chip Cookies	5 (1.1 oz)	160	8	120	20	tr
Mini Fudge Royals	15 (1.1 oz)	160	8	90	20	1
Oatmeal Chocolate Chip	3 (1.3 oz)	170	8	130	23	2
Oatmeal Country Style	3 (1.2 oz)	170	7	160	24	1
School House Cookies	20 (1.1 oz)	140	5	115	23	tr
Sugar Wafers Chocolate	3 (0.9 oz)	130	7	30	17	tr

FOOD	PORTION	CAL.	FAT	SOD.	CARB.	FIB.
Sunshine (CONT.)						
Sugar Wafers Peanut Butter	4 (1.1 oz)	170	9	75	19	1
Sugar Wafers Vanilla	3 (0.9 oz)	130	6	20	18	tr
Tru Blu Chocolate	1 (0.6 oz)	80	3	64	11	tr
Tru Blu Lemon	1 (0.6 oz)	80	3	65	11	tr
Tru Blu Vanilla	1 (0.5 oz)	80	3	65	11	tr
Vanilla Wafers	7 (1.1 oz)	150	7	110	20	tr
Vienna Fingers	2 (1 oz)	140	6	105	21	tr
Tastykake						
Chocolate Chip Bar	1 (43 g)	190	8	95	28	1
Chocolate Chunk Macadamia Nut	1 pkg (56 g)	310	14	180	42	2
Fudge Bar	1 (50 g)	200	7	160	35	1
Oatmeal Raisin Bar	1 (50 g)	210	8	250	32	1
Soft'n Chewy Chocolate Chip	1 (39 g)	170	7	170	25	1
Soft'n Chewy Chocolate Chocolate Chip	1 (32 g)	170	7	110	26	1
Soft'n Chewy Oatmeal Raisin	1 (39 g)	160	5	160	27	1
Vanilla Sugar Wafer	1 (6 g)	36	2	10	4	0
Teddy Grahams						
Chocolate	24 (1 oz)	140	5	150	22	1
Cinnamon	24 (1 oz)	140	4	150	23	1
Honey	24 (1 oz)	140	4	150	22	1
Tree Of Life						
Creme Supremes	2 (0.9 oz)	120	5	90	18	1
Creme Supremes Mint	2 (0.9 oz)	120	5	90	18	1
Fat Free Classic Carrot Cake	1 (0.8 oz)	60	0	50	14	1
Fat Free Devil's Food Chocolate	1 (0.8 oz)	70	0	80	15	1
Fat Free Golden Oatmeal Raisin	1 (0.8 oz)	70	0	40	16	1
Fat Free Harvest Fruit & Nut	1 (0.8 oz)	70	0	45	16	1
Fat Free Toasted Almond Butter	1 (0.8 oz)	70	0	35	16	1
Fruit Bars Apple Spice	2 (1.3 oz)	120	3	120	22	2
Fruit Bars Fat Free Fig	1 (0.8 oz)	70	0	100	16	2
Fruit Bars Fat Free Peach Apricot	1 (0.8 oz)	70	0	110	17	1
Fruit Bars Fat Free Wildberry	1 (0.8 oz)	70	0	170	16	2

FOOD	PORTION	CAL.	FAT	SOD.	CARB.	FIB.
Tree Of Life (CONT.)						
Fruit Bars Fig	2 (1.3 oz)	120	3	100	21	3
Fruit Bars Peach Apricot	2 (1.3 oz)	120	3	105	22	2
Honey-Sweet Colossal Carrot Cake	1 (0.8 oz)	110	5	105	16	1
Honey-Sweet Lemon Burst	1 (0.8 oz)	110	5	25	15	1
Honey-Sweet Oh-So-Oatmeal	1 (0.8 oz)	110	5	140	14	1
Honey-Sweet Pecans-A-Plenty	1 (0.8 oz)	125	7	30	14	1
Monster Fat Free Carrot Cake	¼ cookie (0.9 oz)	60	0	30	15	1
Monster Fat Free Devil's Food Chocolate	¼ cookie (0.9 oz)	80	0	45	20	2
Monster Fat Free Gingerbread	¼ cookie (0.9 oz)	80	0	50	19	2
Monster Fat Free Maple Pecan	¼ cookie (0.9 oz)	90	0	50	20	2
Royal Vanilla	2 (0.9 oz)	120	5	115	17	0
Small World Animal Grahams	7 (1 oz)	120	3	60	21	3
Small World Chocolate Chip	7 (1 oz)	120	4	60	20	3
Soft-Bake Chocolate Chip	1 (0.8 oz)	125	7	15	15	1
Soft-Bake Double Fudge	1 (0.8 oz)	110	5	20	16	2
Soft-Bake Maui Macaroon	1 (0.8 oz)	135	10	0	12	2
Soft-Bake Oatmeal	1 (0.8 oz)	115	5	20	16	2
Soft-Bake Peanut Butter	1 (0.8 oz)	125	7	60	13	1
Wheat-Free American Oatmeal	1 (0.8 oz)	90	5	25	11	1
Wheat-Free California Carob	1 (0.8 oz)	105	5	75	14	6
Wheat-Free Georgia Peanut Butter	1 (0.8 oz)	95	6	110	8	1
Wheat-Free Mountain Maple Walnut	1 (0.8 oz)	100	6	50	9	6
Weight Watchers						
Apple Raisin Bar	1	100	3	115	18	—
Chocolate	3	80	3	135	13	—
Chocolate Chip	2	90	2	65	18	—
Chocolate Sandwich	2	90	3	90	15	—

FOOD	PORTION	CAL.	FAT	SOD.	CARB.	FIB.
Weight Watchers (CONT.)						
Fruit Filled Bar Apple	1	80	tr	35	21	—
Fruit Filled Bar Raspberry	1	80	tr	45	22	—
Oatmeal Raisin	2	90	tr	75	20	—
Oatmeal Spice	3	80	2	75	13	—
Shortbread	3	80	2	95	13	—
animal	11 crackers (1 oz)	126	4	112	21	—
animal crackers	1 box (2.4 oz)	299	9	274	51	—
animal crackers	1 (2.5 g)	11	tr	10	2	—
butter	1 (5 g)	23	1	18	3	tr
chocolate chip	1 (0.4 oz)	48	2	32	7	tr
chocolate chip	1 box (1.9 oz)	233	12	188	36	—
chocolate chip low fat	1 (0.25 oz)	45	2	38	7	—
chocolate chip low sugar low sodium	1 (0.24 oz)	31	1	1	5	—
chocolate chip soft-type	1 (0.5 oz)	69	4	49	9	tr
chocolate w/ creme filling	1 (0.35 oz)	47	2	36	7	tr
chocolate w/ creme filling chocolate coated	1 (0.60 oz)	82	5	55	11	—
chocolate w/ creme filling sugar free low sodium	1 (0.35 oz)	46	2	24	7	—
chocolate w/ extra creme filling	1 (0.46 oz)	65	3	64	9	—
chocolate wafer	1 (0.2 oz)	26	1	35	4	—
chocolate wafer cookie crumbs	½ cup (5.9 oz)	728	25	980	120	—
digestive biscuits plain	2	141	7	—	21	1
fig bars	1 (0.56 oz)	56	1	56	11	1
fortune	1 (0.28 oz)	30	tr	22	7	tr
fudge	1 (0.73 oz)	73	1	40	17	tr
gingersnaps	1 (0.24 oz)	29	1	48	5	—
graham	1 square (0.24 oz)	30	1	42	5	—
graham chocolate covered	1 (0.49 oz)	68	3	41	9	—
graham cracker crumbs	½ cup (4.4 oz)	540	13	756	97	3
graham honey	1 (0.24 oz)	30	1	42	5	tr
ladyfingers	1 (0.38 oz)	40	1	16	7	—
marshmallow chocolate coated	1 (0.46 oz)	55	2	22	9	—
marshmallow pie chocolate coated	1 (1.4 oz)	165	7	66	26	—
molasses	1 (0.5 oz)	65	2	69	11	—
oatmeal	1 (0.52 oz)	71	4	62	9	tr
oatmeal	1 (0.6 oz)	81	3	69	12	1

FOOD	PORTION	CAL.	FAT	SOD.	CARB.	FIB.
oatmeal soft-type	1 (0.5 oz)	61	2	52	10	tr
oatmeal raisin	1 (0.6 oz)	81	3	69	12	1
oatmeal raisin low sugar no sodium	1 (0.24 oz)	31	1	1	5	—
oatmeal raisin soft-type	1 (0.5 oz)	61	2	52	10	tr
peanut butter sandwich	1 (0.5 oz)	67	3	52	9	—
peanut butter sandwich sugar free low sodium	1 (0.35 oz)	54	3	41	5	—
peanut butter soft-type	1 (0.5 oz)	69	4	50	9	tr
raisin soft-type	1 (0.5 oz)	60	2	51	10	—
shortbread	1 (0.28 oz)	40	2	36	5	—
shortbread pecan	1 (0.49 oz)	79	5	39	8	tr
sugar	1 (0.52 oz)	72	3	53	10	—
sugar low sugar sodium free	1 (0.24 oz)	30	1	0	5	—
sugar wafers w/ creme filling	1 (0.12 oz)	18	1	5	3	—
sugar wafers w/ creme filling sugar free sodium free	1 (0.14 oz)	20	1	0	3	—
vanilla sandwich	1 (0.35 oz)	48	2	35	7	tr
vanilla wafers	1 (0.21 oz)	28	1	18	4	—
REFRIGERATED						
Pillsbury						
Chocolate Chip	1	70	3	55	9	—
Oatmeal Raisin	1	60	2	55	10	—
Peanut Butter	1	70	3	75	9	—
Sugar	1	70	3	70	9	—
chocolate chip	1 (0.42 oz)	59	3	28	8	—
chocolate chip unbaked	1 oz	126	6	59	17	—
oatmeal	1 (0.4 oz)	56	3	39	8	—
oatmeal raisin	1 (0.4 oz)	56	3	39	8	—
peanut butter	1 (0.4 oz)	60	3	52	7	—
peanut butter dough	1 oz	130	7	112	15	—
sugar	1 (0.42 oz)	58	3	56	8	—
sugar dough	1 oz	124	6	120	17	—
TAKE-OUT						
biscotti with nuts chocolate dipped	1 (1.3 oz)	117	6	33	16	1

CORIANDER

FOOD	PORTION	CAL.	FAT	SOD.	CARB.	FIB.
leaf dried	1 tsp	2	tr	1	tr	—
leaf fresh	¼ cup	1	tr	1	tr	—
seed	1 tsp	5	tr	1	1	—

FOOD	PORTION	CAL.	FAT	SOD.	CARB.	FIB.

CORN
(see also BRAN, CEREAL, CORNMEAL, FLOUR)

CANNED

Del Monte

FOOD	PORTION	CAL.	FAT	SOD.	CARB.	FIB.
Cream Style Golden	½ cup (4.4 oz)	90	1	360	20	2
Cream Style Golden 50% Less Salt	½ cup (4.4 oz)	90	1	180	20	2
Cream Style Golden No Salt Added	½ cup (4.4 oz)	90	1	10	20	2
Cream Style Supersweet Golden	½ cup (4.4 oz)	60	1	360	14	2
Cream Style White	½ cup (4.4 oz)	100	0	360	21	2
Whole Kernel Golden	½ cup (4.4 oz)	90	0	360	18	3
Whole Kernel Golden Supersweet 50% Less Salt	½ cup (4.4 oz)	60	1	130	11	3
Whole Kernel Golden Supersweet No Salt Added	½ cup (4.4 oz)	60	1	10	11	3
Whole Kernel Golden Supersweet No Sugar	½ cup (4.4 oz)	60	0	360	11	3
Whole Kernel Golden Supersweet Vacuum Packed	½ cup (3.7 oz)	70	1	270	13	3
Whole Kernel Golden Supersweet Vacuum Packed No Salt Added	½ cup (3.7 oz)	70	1	10	13	3
Whole Kernel White Sweet	½ cup (4.4 oz)	80	0	360	17	2

Green Giant

FOOD	PORTION	CAL.	FAT	SOD.	CARB.	FIB.
50% Less Salt No Sugar Added	½ cup	50	1	140	11	2
Corn	½ cup	70	0	350	10	2
Cream Style	½ cup	100	tr	390	24	2
Deli Corn	½ cup	80	tr	350	19	2
Golden Kernel 50% Less Salt	½ cup	70	tr	175	16	2
Golden Vacuum Packed	½ cup	80	0	330	20	2
Mexi Corn	½ cup	80	tr	450	19	2
No Salt No Sugar	½ cup	80	tr	0	18	2
Sweet Select	½ cup	60	1	280	12	2
White Vacuum Packed	½ cup	80	0	290	20	2

Ka-Me

FOOD	PORTION	CAL.	FAT	SOD.	CARB.	FIB.
Baby	½ cup (4.5 oz)	20	0	10	3	2

FOOD	PORTION	CAL.	FAT	SOD.	CARB.	FIB.
Ka-Me (CONT.)						
Stir Fry	½ cup (4.5 oz)	20	0	10	3	2
Owatonna						
Cream Style	½ cup	100	1	—	—	—
Whole Kernel In Brine	½ cup	90	1	—	—	—
Whole Kernel Vacuum Pack	½ cup	100	1	—	—	—
S&W						
Cream Style Diet	½ cup	100	1	0	21	—
Cream Style Premium Homestyle	½ cup	105	1	435	25	—
Sweet 'N Natural	½ cup	90	1	180	20	—
Whole Kernel Tender Young	½ cup	90	1	295	20	—
Whole Kernel Water Pack	½ cup	80	1	0	15	—
Seneca						
Cream Style	½ cup	80	0	288	18	1
Whole Kernel	½ cup	90	0	288	21	2
Whole Kernel Natural Pack	½ cup	80	1	0	18	2
cream style	½ cup	93	1	365	23	—
w/ red & green peppers	½ cup	86	1	396	21	—
white	½ cup	66	1	—	15	—
yellow	½ cup	66	1	—	15	1
FRESH						
on-the-cob w/ butter cooked	1 ear	155	3	30	32	—
white cooked	½ cup	89	1	14	21	—
white raw	½ cup	66	1	12	15	—
yellow cooked	1 ear (2.7 oz)	83	1	13	19	—
yellow cooked	½ cup	89	1	14	21	—
yellow raw	½ cup	66	1	12	15	—
yellow raw	1 ear (3 oz)	77	1	14	17	—
FROZEN						
Birds Eye						
Big Ears	1 ear	160	1	0	37	—
In Butter Sauce	½ cup	90	2	170	19	2
Little Ears	2 ears	130	1	0	30	—
On The Cob	1 ear	120	1	0	29	—
Polybag Cut	½ cup	80	1	0	19	2
Polybag Deluxe Tender Sweet	½ cup	80	1	0	20	2
Sweet	½ cup	80	1	0	20	2

FOOD	PORTION	CAL.	FAT	SOD.	CARB.	FIB.
Fresh Like						
Cob Corn	1 ear (5 in)	96	1	4	23	1
Cob Corn	1 ear (3 in)	96	1	4	24	1
Cut	3.5 oz	85	1	5	21	1
Green Giant						
Cream Style	½ cup	110	1	370	25	3
Harvest Fresh Niblets	½ cup	80	1	40	17	2
Harvest Fresh White Shoepeg	½ cup	90	1	60	19	2
In Butter Sauce	½ cup	100	2	310	19	—
Nibblers Corn On The Cob	2 ears	120	1	10	27	2
Niblet Ears	1 ear	120	1	10	27	2
Niblets	½ cup	90	tr	5	19	2
One Serve Niblets In Butter Sauce	1 pkg	120	2	350	24	3
One Serve On The Cob	1 pkg	120	1	10	26	2
Super Sweet Nibblers Corn On The Cob	2 ears	90	2	10	19	2
Super Sweet Niblet Ears	1 ear	90	2	10	19	2
Super Sweet Niblet Select	½ cup	60	1	5	13	2
White In Butter Sauce	½ cup	100	2	280	20	2
White Select	½ cup	90	1	5	19	2
Hanover						
White Shoepeg	½ cup	80	0	—	—	—
White Sweet	½ cup	80	0	—	—	—
Yellow Sweet	½ cup	80	0	—	—	—
Mrs. Paul's						
Fritters	2	240	9	560	35	—
Ore Ida						
Cob Corn	1 ear (6.1 oz)	180	3	5	33	4
Cob Corn Mini-Gold	1 ear (3.1 oz)	90	1	0	16	2
Stouffer's						
Souffle	½ cup (2.4 oz)	170	7	490	21	1
cooked	½ cup	67	tr	4	17	—
on-the-cob cooked	1 ear (2.2 oz)	59	tr	3	14	—
SHELF-STABLE						
Pantry Express						
Golden Whole Kernel	½ cup	60	tr	210	18	1
TAKE-OUT						
fritters	1 (1 oz)	62	2	126	9	1
scalloped	½ cup	258	7	246	43	—

FOOD	PORTION	CAL.	FAT	SOD.	CARB.	FIB.
CORN CHIPS						
(see CHIPS)						
CORNISH HENS						
(see CHICKEN)						
CORNMEAL						
(see also POLENTA)						
Albers						
White	3 tbsp	110	0	0	34	tr
Yellow	3 tbsp	110	0	0	34	tr
Arrowhead						
Yellow	¼ cup (1.2 oz)	120	1	0	27	3
Aunt Jemima						
White	3 tbsp	102	1	1	22	1
Yellow	3 tbsp	102	1	1	22	1
Quaker						
White	3 tbsp	102	1	1	22	1
Yellow	3 tbsp	102	1	1	22	1
corn grits cooked	1 cup	146	tr	0	31	—
corn grits uncooked	1 cup	579	2	1	124	—
degermed	1 cup	506	2	5	107	7
self-rising degermed	1 cup	489	2	1860	103	—
whole grain	1 cup	442	4	43	94	13
HOME RECIPE						
hush puppies	5 (2.7 oz)	256	12	965	35	4
hush puppies	1 (¾ oz)	74	3	147	10	1
MIX						
Arrowhead						
Corn Bread	¼ cup (1.2 oz)	120	1	270	24	4
Aunt Jemima						
Bolded White Mix	3 tbsp	99	1	337	21	—
Buttermilk Self Rising White Mix	3 tbsp	101	1	439	21	—
Self Rising White Mix	3 tbsp	98	1	381	21	1
Self Rising Yellow Mix	3 tbsp	100	1	490	21	—
Golden Dipt						
Corny Dog Batter Mix	1 oz	100	0	490	22	—
Hush Puppy Deluxe Mix	1¼ oz	120	0	520	26	—
Hush Puppy Jalapeno Mix	1¼ oz	120	0	570	27	—
Hush Puppy With Onion	1¼ oz	120	0	520	27	—
Hodgson Mill						
Yellow	¼ cup (1 oz)	100	1	0	22	3
Yelllow Self Rising	¼ cup (1 oz)	90	1	260	21	3

FOOD	PORTION	CAL.	FAT	SOD.	CARB.	FIB.
Kentucky Kernel						
White Corn Meal Mix	¼ cup (1 oz)	100	1	210	22	2
Miracle Maize						
Complete as prep	1 piece (1.5 oz)	193	3	193	34	2
Country Style as prep	1 piece 2 in x 2 in (1.8 oz)	230	5	406	38	2
Sweet as prep	1 piece 2 in x 2 in (1.8 oz)	236	5	260	41	1
Stone-Buhr						
Yellow Corn Meal	¼ cup (1 oz)	100	0	0	23	1
READY-TO-USE						
Aurora						
Polenta	½ cup (5 oz)	110	0	470	24	1
CORNSALAD						
raw	1 cup	12	tr	—	2	—
CORNSTARCH						
Argo						
Cornstarch	1 tbsp (8 g)	30	0	0	7	—
Cornstarch	1 cup (128 g)	460	tr	tr	115	—
Kingsford's						
Cornstarch	1 cup (128 g)	460	tr	tr	115	—
Cornstarch	1 tbsp (8 g)	30	tr	0	7	—
cornstarch	⅓ cup	164	tr	4	39	tr
COTTAGE CHEESE						
Axelrod						
Nonfat	½ cup (4.4 oz)	90	0	500	7	0
Borden						
4%	½ cup	120	5	400	4	—
Dry Curd 0.5%	½ cup	80	1	20	3	—
Unsalted 4%	½ cup	120	5	40	4	—
Breakstone						
2% Fat Large Curd	½ cup (4.2 oz)	90	3	380	4	0
2% Fat Small Curd	½ cup (4.2 oz)	90	3	380	4	0
4% Fat Large Curd	½ cup (4.2 oz)	120	5	400	4	0
4% Fat Small Curd	½ cup (4.2 oz)	120	5	400	4	0
Dry Curd ½% Fat	¼ cup (1.9 oz)	45	0	25	3	0
Cabot						
Light	4 oz	90	1	360	3	—
Friendship						
California Style	½ cup (4 oz)	115	5	380	4	0
Lowfat 1%	½ cup (4 oz)	90	1	360	4	0
Lowfat No Salt Added	½ cup (4 oz)	90	1	40	4	0

FOOD	PORTION	CAL.	FAT	SOD.	CARB.	FIB.
Friendship (CONT.)						
Lowfat Pineapple	½ cup (4 oz)	120	1	300	17	0
Nonfat	½ cup (4 oz)	80	0	380	5	0
Nonfat Plus Peach	½ cup (4 oz)	110	0	300	15	0
Pot Style	½ cup (4 oz)	90	3	430	3	0
With Pineapple	½ cup (4 oz)	140	4	310	15	0
Hood						
1% Fat	½ cup (4 oz)	90	2	390	6	0
1% Fat Chive & Onion	½ cup (4 oz)	90	2	390	6	0
1% Fat No Salt Added	½ cup (4 oz)	90	2	65	6	0
1% Fat Pepper & Herb	½ cup (4 oz)	90	2	450	6	0
1% Fat Pineapple Cherry	½ cup (4 oz)	110	1	290	15	0
4% Fat	½ cup (4 oz)	120	4	390	5	0
4% Fat Chive	½ cup (4 oz)	130	4	380	5	0
4% Fat Pineapple	½ cup (4 oz)	130	4	290	15	0
Nonfat	½ cup (4 oz)	80	0	330	6	0
Nonfat Pineapple	½ cup (4 oz)	110	0	250	16	0
Knudsen						
1.5% Fat Peach	4 oz	110	2	290	12	0
1.5% Fat Pineapple	4 oz	110	2	290	11	0
1.5% Fat Strawberry	4 oz	110	2	280	12	0
1.5% Fat Tropical Fruit	4 oz	120	2	300	15	0
2% Fat Small Curd	½ cup (4.2 oz)	100	3	400	3	0
4% Fat Large Curd	½ cup (4.5 oz)	130	5	340	3	0
4% Fat Small Curd	½ cup (4.3 oz)	120	5	400	2	0
Free	½ cup (4.3 oz)	80	0	370	4	0
Lactaid						
1%	4 oz	72	1	406	3	—
Light N'Lively						
1% Fat	½ cup (4 oz)	80	2	380	4	0
1% Fat Garden Salad	½ cup (4.2 oz)	90	2	410	5	0
1% Fat Peach & Pineapple	½ cup (4.3 oz)	120	1	350	14	0
Free	½ cup (4.4 oz)	80	0	440	5	0
Lite Line						
Lowfat 1½%	½ cup	90	2	400	4	—
Sealtest						
2% Fat Small Curd	½ cup (4.2 oz)	90	3	380	4	0
4% Fat Large Curd	½ cup (4.2 oz)	120	5	400	4	0
4% Fat Small Curd	½ cup (4.2 oz)	120	5	400	4	0
Viva						
Nonfat	½ cup	70	0	430	5	—
Weight Watchers						
1%	½ cup	90	1	460	4	—

FOOD	PORTION	CAL.	FAT	SOD.	CARB.	FIB.
Weight Watchers (cont.)						
2%	½ cup	100	2	460	4	—
creamed	1 cup	217	9	850	6	—
creamed	4 oz	117	5	457	3	—
creamed w/ fruit	4 oz	140	4	457	15	—
dry curd	1 cup	123	1	19	3	—
dry curd	4 oz	96	tr	14	2	—
lowfat 1%	1 cup	164	2	918	6	—
lowfat 1%	4 oz	82	1	459	3	—
lowfat 2%	1 cup	203	4	918	8	—
lowfat 2%	4 oz	101	2	459	4	—

COTTONSEED

FOOD	PORTION	CAL.	FAT	SOD.	CARB.	FIB.
kernels roasted	1 tbsp	51	4	3	2	—

COUGH DROPS

FOOD	PORTION	CAL.	FAT	SOD.	CARB.	FIB.
Halls	1 (3.8 g)	15	0	—	4	—
Halls						
Plus	1 (4.7 g)	18	0	—	5	—
With Vitamin C	1 (3.8 g)	14	0	—	4	—
Lifesavers						
Menthol	2 (0.5 oz)	60	0	0	14	—

COUSCOUS

FOOD	PORTION	CAL.	FAT	SOD.	CARB.	FIB.
Casbah						
Almond Chicken Vegetarian	1 pkg (1.5 oz)	160	2	470	29	tr
Asparagus Au Gratin Organic	1 pkg (1.5 oz)	150	2	400	28	1
Cheddar Broccoli	1 pkg (1.3 oz)	130	2	470	23	tr
Hearty Harvest Zestful Organic as prep	1 pkg (10 fl oz)	180	1	460	36	2
Moroccan Stew	1 pkg (2 oz)	180	1	430	36	1
Pilaf as prep	1 cup	200	tr	480	40	tr
Tomato Parmesan	1 pkg (1.8 oz)	170	2	460	34	2
Kitchen Del Sol						
Moroccan Ginger as prep	½ cup (1.1 oz)	120	3	290	21	1
Spicy Vegetable as prep	½ cup (1.1 oz)	120	3	290	20	1
Tomato & Olive	½ cup (1.1 oz)	120	4	290	19	1
Near East as prep	1¼ cup	260	6	65	46	2
cooked	½ cup	101	tr	4	21	—
dry	½ cup	346	tr	9	71	—

COWPEAS

FOOD	PORTION	CAL.	FAT	SOD.	CARB.	FIB.
catjang dried cooked	1 cup	200	1	32	35	—

FOOD	PORTION	CAL.	FAT	SOD.	CARB.	FIB.
common canned	1 cup	184	1	718	33	—
frozen cooked	½ cup	112	tr	5	20	—
leafy tips chopped cooked	1 cup	12	tr	3	1	—
leafy tips raw chopped	1 cup	10	tr	2	2	—

CRAB
CANNED
S&W
Dungeness Crab	3.25 oz	81	2	920	1	—
blue	3 oz	84	1	283	0	—
blue	1 cup	133	2	5	0	—

FRESH
alaska king cooked	1 leg (4.7 oz)	129	2	1436	0	—
alaska king cooked	3 oz	82	1	911	0	—
alaska king raw	1 leg (6 oz)	144	1	1438	0	—
alaska king raw	3 oz	71	1	711	0	—
blue cooked	3 oz	87	2	237	0	—
blue cooked	1 cup	138	2	376	0	—
blue raw	3 oz	74	1	249	tr	—
blue raw	1 crab (0.7 oz)	18	tr	62	tr	—
dungeness raw	3 oz	73	1	251	1	—
dungeness raw	1 crab (5.7 oz)	140	2	481	1	—
queen steamed	3 oz	98	1	587	0	—

FROZEN
Mrs. Paul's
Deviled Crab	1 cake	180	9	480	18	—
Deviled Crab Miniatures	3½ oz	240	12	540	25	—

READY-TO-USE
crab cakes	1 cake (2.1 oz)	93	5	198	tr	—

TAKE-OUT
baked	1 (3.8 oz)	160	2	550	4	—
cake	1 (2 oz)	160	10	492	5	—
soft-shell fried	1 (4.4 oz)	334	18	1118	31	—

CRACKER CRUMBS
Golden Dipt
Cracker Meal	1 oz	100	0	0	22	—

Honey Maid
Graham Cracker	0.5 oz	70	2	90	13	tr

Keebler
Cracker Meal	1 cup	100	3	5	23	—
Graham Crumbs	1 cup	520	14	630	90	—
Zesty Meal	1 cup	85	10	100	61	—

Kellogg's
Corn Flake Crumbs	2 tbsp (0.4 oz)	40	0	120	9	0

FOOD	PORTION	CAL.	FAT	SOD.	CARB.	FIB.
Lance						
Cracker Meal	1 oz	100	1	1	21	—
Nabisco						
Nilla Cookie Crumbs	2 tbsp (0.5 oz)	70	3	55	13	tr
Oreo						
Cookie Crumbs	2 tbsp (0.5 oz)	80	3	140	13	1
Premium						
Fat Free Cracker Crumbs	¼ cup (1 oz)	100	0	0	23	1
Ritz						
Cracker Crumbs	⅓ cup (1 oz)	140	7	270	17	1
Sunshine						
Graham	3 tbsp (0.6 oz)	80	2	150	13	tr

CRACKERS

(see also CRACKER CRUMBS)

FOOD	PORTION	CAL.	FAT	SOD.	CARB.	FIB.
Adrienne's						
Gourmet Flatbread Caraway & Rye	2	20	tr	45	4	—
Gourmet Flatbread Classic Island	2	20	tr	45	3	—
Gourmet Flatbread Slightly Onion	2	20	tr	45	3	—
Gourmet Flatbread Ten Grain	2	20	tr	45	3	1
American Heritage						
Sesame	9 (1.1 oz)	160	9	300	17	1
Wheat & Bran	9 (1 oz)	140	7	280	17	2
Better Cheddars						
Low Sodium	22 (1 oz)	150	7	75	18	tr
Reduced Fat	24 (1 oz)	140	6	350	19	tr
Burns & Ricker						
Bagel Crisps Garlic	5 (1 oz)	100	0	280	22	1
Cheez-It						
Hot & Spicy	26 (1 oz)	160	8	220	17	1
Hot & Spicy	1 pkg (1.5 oz)	220	12	310	25	1
Low Sodium	27 (1 oz)	160	8	70	16	tr
Party Mix	½ cup (1 oz)	140	5	270	19	1
Reduced Fat	30 (1 oz)	130	5	280	19	tr
White Cheddar	1 pkg (1.5 oz)	220	12	400	24	tr
White Cheddar	26 (1 oz) (1.9 oz)	160	9	280	17	tr
Devonsheer						
Melba Rounds Garlic	½ oz	56	1	132	9	1
Melba Rounds Honey Bran	½ oz	52	1	98	9	1

FOOD	PORTION	CAL.	FAT	SOD.	CARB.	FIB.
Devonsheer (CONT.)						
Melba Rounds Onion	½ oz	51	1	120	10	1
Melba Rounds Plain	½ oz	53	1	111	10	1
Melba Rounds Plain Unsalted	½ oz	52	1	<5	10	1
Melba Rounds Rye	½ oz	53	1	130	10	1
Melba Rounds Sesame	½ oz	57	2	131	8	1
Eagle						
Bacon Cheese	1 oz	140	6	330	18	—
Cheese	1 oz	130	6	330	18	—
Peanut Butter & Cheese	1 oz	280	16	450	26	—
Eden						
Brown Rice	5 (1 oz)	120	2	230	22	2
Estee						
Unsalted	1 (0.5 oz)	70	2	0	10	0
FFV						
Cheddar Thins	7	70	2	—	—	—
Double Cheddar	7	70	2	—	—	—
Ham & Cheese Crispy Wafers	7	70	2	—	—	—
Ocean Crisp	1	60	1	—	—	—
Sesame Crisp	2	120	3	—	—	—
Stoned Wheat	4	60	1	—	—	—
Wheat Crispy Wafers	6	70	3	—	—	—
Frito Lay						
Cheese Filled	6 (1.5 oz)	210	10	470	24	—
Cracker Snacks Cheddar	13-16 (1 oz)	70	4	150	8	—
Cracker Snacks Zesty Italian	13-16 (1 oz)	70	3	115	9	—
Peanut Butter Filled	6 (1.5 oz)	210	10	450	24	—
Goya						
Butter Crackers	1	40	1	60	6	—
Crackers	1	30	0	45	5	—
Hain						
Cheese	1 oz	130	6	180	17	—
Onion	1 oz	130	6	160	17	—
Onion No Salt Added	1 oz	130	6	5	17	—
Rich	1 oz	130	5	160	18	—
Rich No Salt Added	1 oz	130	5	15	18	—
Rye	1 oz	120	4	200	19	—
Rye No Salt Added	1 oz	120	4	10	19	—
Sesame	1 oz	140	7	210	16	—
Sesame No Salt Added	1 oz	140	7	5	16	—
Sour Cream & Chive	1 oz	130	6	150	15	—

FOOD	PORTION	CAL.	FAT	SOD.	CARB.	FIB.
Hain (CONT.)						
Sour Cream & Chive No Salt Added	1 oz	130	6	25	15	—
Sourdough	½ oz	65	3	100	9	—
Sourdough Low Salt	1 oz	130	5	10	18	—
Vegetable	1 oz	130	5	180	10	—
Vegetable No Salt Added	1 oz	130	5	50	10	—
Harvest Crisps						
5 Grain	13 (1.1 oz)	130	4	300	23	1
Oat	13 (1.1 oz)	140	5	300	22	1
Health Valley						
Herb Stoned Wheat	13	55	2	80	9	2
Herb Stoned Wheat No Salt	13	55	2	30	9	2
Rice Bran	7	130	4	65	19	2
Sesame Stoned Wheat	13	55	2	80	9	2
Sesame Stoned Wheat No Salt Added	13	55	2	30	9	2
Seven Grain Vegetable Stoned Wheat	13	55	2	80	9	2
Seven Grain Vegetable Stoned Wheat No Salt Added	13	55	2	30	9	2
Stoned Wheat	13	55	2	80	9	2
Stoned Wheat No Salt Added	13	55	2	30	9	2
Hi Ho						
Butter Flavored	9 (1.1 oz)	160	9	280	19	tr
Cracked Pepper	9 (1.1 oz)	160	9	280	18	tr
Low Salt	9 (1.1 oz)	160	9	135	18	tr
Multi Grain	9 (1.1 oz)	160	9	370	18	1
Reduced Fat	10 (1.1 oz)	140	5	280	21	tr
Whole Wheat	9 (1.1 oz)	150	8	280	18	2
Ideal Crispbread						
Extra Thin	3	48	0	86	9	1
Fiber Thins	2	41	1	81	8	2
Oatbran Thins	2	50	0	80	8	2
J.J. Flats						
Breadflats Caraway	1	52	1	126	10	1
Breadflats Caraway And Salt	1	51	1	213	9	1
Breadflats Cinnamon	1	53	1	126	10	1
Breadflats Flavorall	1	52	1	139	10	1
Breadflats Garlic	1	52	1	127	10	1

FOOD	PORTION	CAL.	FAT	SOD.	CARB.	FIB.
J.J. Flats (CONT.)						
Breadflats Oat Bran	1	49	1	141	8	2
Breadflats Onion	1	53	1	140	10	1
Breadflats Plain	1	53	1	143	10	1
Breadflats Poppy	1	53	1	126	9	1
Breadflats Sesame	1	55	2	124	9	1
Keebler						
Club	2	30	2	75	4	—
Melba Toast Garlic	2	25	tr	35	4	—
Melba Toast Long	2	30	tr	10	7	—
Melba Toast Onion	2	25	tr	35	4	—
Melba Toast Plain	2	25	tr	35	4	—
Melba Toast Sesame	2	25	tr	35	4	—
Oyster Crackers Large	26	80	2	175	13	—
Oyster Crackers Small	50	80	2	175	13	—
Snack Crackers Toasted Rye	2	30	2	70	4	—
Snack Crackers Toasted Sesame	2	30	2	65	4	—
Snack Crackers Toasted Wheat	2	30	2	60	4	—
Toasted Snack Bacon	2	30	2	65	4	—
Toasted Snack Onion	2	30	2	70	4	—
Toasted Snack Pumpernickel	2	30	2	55	4	—
Wholegrain Wheat	2	30	1	70	5	—
Krispy						
Cracked Pepper	5 (0.5 oz)	60	2	180	10	tr
Fat Free	5 (0.5 oz)	60	0	135	12	tr
Mild Cheddar	5 (0.5 oz)	60	2	180	10	tr
Original	5 (0.5 oz)	60	2	180	10	tr
Soup & Oyster Crackers	17 (0.5 oz)	60	2	200	11	tr
Unsalted Tops	5 (0.5 oz)	60	2	120	10	tr
Whole Wheat	5 (0.5 oz)	60	2	130	10	tr
Lance						
Bonnie	1 pkg (34 g)	160	7	170	24	—
Captain Wafers	2	30	1	60	5	—
Captain Wafers Very Low Sodium	2	30	1	25	5	—
Captain Wafers w/ Cream Cheese & Chives	1 pkg (37 g)	170	9	260	23	—
Cheese-On-Wheat	1 pkg (37 g)	180	9	260	22	—
Lanchee	1 pkg (35 g)	180	11	110	19	—

FOOD	PORTION	CAL.	FAT	SOD.	CARB.	FIB.
Lance (CONT.)						
Melba Toast Oblong	2	30	0	50	7	—
Melba Toast Plain	2	20	0	30	4	—
Melba Toast Round Garlic	2	20	0	35	4	—
Melba Toast Round Onion	2	20	0	30	4	—
Melba Toast Sesame	2	25	0	35	4	—
Nekot	1 pkg (42 g)	210	10	95	24	—
Nip-Chee	1 pkg (37 g)	180	8	320	21	—
Oyster Crackers	1 pkg (14 g)	70	2	170	10	—
Peanut Butter Wheat	1 pkg (37 g)	190	11	210	18	—
Rye Twins	2	30	1	65	5	—
Rye-Chee	1 pkg (41 g)	190	9	320	22	—
Saltines	2	25	1	65	4	—
Saltines Slug Pack	4 crackers	50	1	130	8	—
Sesame Twins	2	40	1	65	6	—
Toastchee	1 pkg (39 g)	190	11	310	19	—
Toasty	1 pkg (35 g)	180	10	160	17	—
Wheat Twins	2	30	1	70	5	—
Wheatswafer	2	30	1	50	4	—
Lavash						
Bread Crisp Original	2 (0.5 oz)	60	1	90	11	—
Bread Crisp Sesame	2 (0.5 oz)	60	1	70	10	—
Little Debbie						
Cheese Crackers With Peanut Butter	1 pkg (1.4 oz)	210	10	430	23	1
Cheese Crackers With Peanut Butter	1 pkg (0.9 oz)	140	7	290	16	1
Toasty Crackers With Peanut Butter	1 pkg (0.9 oz)	140	7	290	16	1
Toasty Crackers With Peanut Butter	1 pkg (1.4 oz)	200	10	350	20	1
Wheat Crackers With Cheddar Cheese	1 pkg (0.9 oz)	140	7	270	16	0
Manischewitz						
Tam Tams	10	147	8	171	17	—
Tam Tams No Salt	10	138	7	—	18	—
Tams Garlic	10	153	8	165	19	—
Tams Onion	10	150	8	157	18	—
Tams Wheat	10	150	8	180	18	—
McCrackens						
Cracker Crisp Country Butter	1 oz	140	8	170	18	—

FOOD	PORTION	CAL.	FAT	SOD.	CARB.	FIB.
McCrackens (CONT.)						
Cracker Crisp Sour Cream & Chives	1 oz	140	8	170	18	—
Cracker Crisp Tangy Cheddar	1 oz	140	8	170	18	—
Cracker Crisp Toasted Wheat	1 oz	140	8	170	18	—
Nabisco						
Bacon Flavored	15 (1.1 oz)	160	8	460	19	tr
Chicken In A Biskit	14 (1 oz)	160	9	270	17	tr
Garden Crisps	15 (1 oz)	130	4	290	22	1
Oat Thins	18 (1 oz)	140	1	190	20	2
Royal Lunch	1 (0.4 oz)	50	2	65	8	0
Swiss	15 (1 oz)	140	7	350	18	tr
Tid-Bit Cheese	32 (1 oz)	150	8	420	17	tr
Vegetable Thins	14 (1.1 oz)	160	9	310	19	1
Wheat Thins Original	16 (1 oz)	140	6	170	19	2
Wheat Thins Reduced Fat	18 (1 oz)	120	4	220	21	2
Zings!	1 pkg (1.8 oz)	240	11	420	34	2
NABS						
Cheese Peanut Butter Sandwich	6 (1.4 oz)	190	10	390	24	1
Peanut Butter Toast Sandwich	6 (1.4 oz)	190	10	380	24	1
Nips						
Cheese	29 (1 oz)	150	6	310	18	tr
Old London						
Melba Toast Pumpernickel	½ oz	54	1	156	10	1
Melba Toast Rye	½ oz	52	1	132	10	—
Melba Toast Sesame	½ oz	55	2	148	8	1
Melba Toast Sesame Unsalted	½ oz	55	2	5	8	1
Melba Toast Wheat	½ oz	51	1	121	10	1
Melba Toast White	½ oz	51	1	111	10	1
Melba Toast White Unsalted	½ oz	51	1	4	10	1
Melba Toast Whole Grain	½ oz	52	1	116	9	1
Melba Toast Whole Grain Unsalted	½ oz	53	1	4	10	1
Rounds Bacon	½ oz	53	1	126	9	1
Rounds Garlic	½ oz	56	1	132	9	1
Rounds Onion	½ oz	52	1	121	10	1

FOOD	PORTION	CAL.	FAT	SOD.	CARB.	FIB.
Old London (CONT.)						
Rounds Rye	½ oz	52	1	132	10	—
Rounds Sesame	½ oz	56	2	149	8	1
Rounds White	½ oz	48	1	111	9	1
Rounds Whole Grain	½ oz	54	1	102	9	1
Pepperidge Farm						
Butter Thins	4	70	3	115	10	0
Cracked Wheat	3	100	4	180	14	1
Crispy Graham	4	70	2	115	13	—
English Water Biscuits	4	70	1	100	13	0
Flutters Garden Herb	¾ oz	100	4	190	14	—
Flutters Golden Sesame	¾ oz	110	5	150	13	—
Flutters Original Butter	¾ oz	100	4	150	15	—
Flutters Toasted Wheat	¾ oz	110	5	170	13	—
Garden Vegetable	5	60	2	125	10	—
Goldfish Cheddar Cheese	1 oz	120	4	230	19	1
Goldfish Cheddar Cheese	1 pkg (1½ oz)	190	6	340	28	1
Goldfish Cheese Thins	4	50	2	160	—	0
Goldfish Original	1 oz	130	5	190	18	1
Goldfish Parmesan Cheese	1 oz	120	4	330	19	1
Goldfish Pizza Flavored	1 oz	130	5	220	19	1
Goldfish Pretzel	1 oz	110	3	160	20	1
Hearty Wheat	4	100	5	140	13	1
Multi Grain	4	70	2	115	12	—
Sesame	4	80	4	140	12	2
Snack Mix Classic	1 oz	140	8	360	14	1
Snack Mix Lightly Smoked	1 oz	150	9	350	13	1
Snack Sticks Cheese	8	130	5	400	19	1
Snack Sticks Pretzel	8	120	3	430	23	1
Snack Sticks Pumpernickel	8	140	6	330	20	1
Snack Sticks Sesame	8	140	5	280	19	1
Spicy Lightly Smoked	1 oz	140	8	340	14	1
Toasted Rice	4	60	2	140	10	—
Toasted Wheat With Onion	4	80	3	140	12	0
Planters						
Cheese Peanut Butter Sandwiches	1 pkg (1.4 oz)	190	10	390	24	1
Toast Peanut Butter Sandwiches	1 pkg (1.4 oz)	190	10	380	24	1

FOOD	PORTION	CAL.	FAT	SOD.	CARB.	FIB.
Premium						
Saltine Bits	34 (1 oz)	150	7	340	19	tr
Saltine Fat Free	5 (0.5 oz)	50	0	130	11	0
Saltine Low Sodium	5 (0.5 oz)	60	1	35	10	tr
Saltine Original	5 (0.5 oz)	60	2	180	10	tr
Saltine Unsalted Tops	5 (0.5 oz)	60	2	135	10	tr
Soup & Oyster	23 (0.5 oz)	60	2	230	11	tr
Ralston						
Oat Bran Krisp	2	60	3	140	6	3
Ritz						
Bits	48 (1 oz)	160	9	250	18	1
Bits Sandwiches With Peanut Butter	13 (1 oz)	150	8	130	17	1
Bits Sanwiches With Real Cheese	14 (1.1 oz)	160	10	300	17	1
Crackers	5 (0.5 oz)	80	4	135	10	tr
Low Sodium	5 (0.5 oz)	80	4	35	10	tr
Sandwiches With Real Cheese	1 pkg (1.4 oz)	210	12	450	21	1
Rykrisp						
Natural	2	40	0	75	7	4
Seasoned	2	45	1	105	8	3
Seasoned Twindividuals	2	45	1	105	8	3
Sesame	2	50	2	105	7	3
Ryvita						
Crisp Bread Dark Finn Crisp	2	38	tr	—	—	—
Crisp Bread Dark Rye	1	26	tr	—	—	—
Crisp Bread Dark w/ Caraway Seeds Finn Crisp	2	38	tr	—	—	—
Crisp Bread High Fiber	1	23	tr	—	—	—
Crisp Bread Light Rye	1	26	tr	—	—	—
Crisp Bread Toasted Sesame Rye	1	31	tr	—	—	—
Snackbread High Fiber	1	14	tr	—	—	—
Snackbread Original Wheat	1	20	tr	—	—	—
Sesmark						
Brown Rice	15 (1 oz)	120	2	85	25	tr
Cheese Thins	15 (1 oz)	130	3	110	26	tr
Rice Thins Original	15 (1 oz)	130	3	150	24	tr
Rice Thins Teriyaki Flavored	13 (1 oz)	130	3	170	24	tr

FOOD	PORTION	CAL.	FAT	SOD.	CARB.	FIB.
Sesmark (CONT.)						
Savory Thins Original	15 (1 oz)	125	2	125	25	1
Sesame Thins Cheddar	9 (1 oz)	150	8	400	15	3
Sesame Thins Garlic	9 (1 oz)	150	8	340	16	3
Sesame Thins Original	9 (1 oz)	150	8	380	16	2
Sesame Thins Unsalted	11 (1 oz)	150	8	1	17	3
Snackwell's						
Cracked Pepper	7 (0.5 oz)	60	0	150	13	tr
Fat Free Wheat	5 (0.5 oz)	60	0	170	12	1
Reduced Fat Cheese	38 (1 oz)	130	2	340	23	1
Reduced Fat Classic Golden	6 (0.5 oz)	60	1	140	11	0
Snorkles						
Cheddar	56 (1 oz)	140	5	200	19	1
Sunshine						
Saltines Cracked Pepper	5 (0.5 oz)	60	2	180	10	tr
Tree Of Life						
Bite Size Fat Free Corn & Salsa	12	60	0	90	12	0
Bite Size Fat Free Cracked Pepper	12	55	0	80	12	0
Bite Size Fat Free Garden Vegetable	12	55	0	80	12	0
Bite Size Fat Free Garlic & Herb	12	55	0	80	12	0
Bite Size Fat Free Soya Nut	12	60	0	80	12	0
Bite Size Fat Free Toasted Onion	12	60	0	80	12	0
Bite Size Fat Free Whole Wheat	12	60	0	85	12	2
Fat Free Oyster	40 (0.5 oz)	60	0	130	13	0
Saltine Cracked Pepper Fat Free	4 (0.5 oz)	60	0	130	13	1
Saltine Fat Free	4 (0.5 oz)	50	0	140	11	0
Triscuit						
Crackers	7 (1.1 oz)	140	5	170	21	4
Deli-Style Rye	7 (1.1 oz)	140	5	180	22	4
Garden Herb	6 (1 oz)	130	5	120	20	3
Low Sodium	7 (1.1 oz)	150	6	50	21	3
Reduced Fat	8 (1.1 oz)	130	3	180	24	4
Wheat 'n Bran	7 (1.1 oz)	140	5	170	22	4
Tuscany						
Pita Crisps	1 oz	90	1	—	—	—

FOOD	PORTION	CAL.	FAT	SOD.	CARB.	FIB.
Tuscany (CONT.)						
Pita Crisps Sesame	1 oz	96	2	—	—	—
Toast	1 oz	95	2	—	—	—
Toast Pepato	1 oz	93	2	—	—	—
Toast Pesto	1 oz	96	2	—	—	—
Toast Tomato	1 oz	95	2	—	—	—
Twigs						
Sesame & Cheese Sticks	15 (1 oz)	150	7	300	17	tr
Uneeda Biscuit						
Unsalted Tops	2 (0.5 oz)	60	2	110	11	tr
Venus						
Armenian Thin Bread	2 (0.9 oz)	100	1	165	19	—
Bran Wafers Salt Free	5 (0.5 oz)	60	1	0	11	2
Corn Crackers Salt Free	5 (0.5 oz)	60	1	0	10	2
Cracked Wheat Wafers Salt Free	5 (0.5 oz)	60	1	0	11	—
Cracker Bread	5 (0.5 oz)	60	1	90	11	—
Hors D'oeuvre	3 (0.5 oz)	60	2	20	11	—
Oat Bran Wafers	5 (0.5 oz)	60	1	105	11	2
Oat Bran Wafers Salt Free	5 (0.5 oz)	60	1	0	11	1
Old Brussels Cheddar Waferettes	5 (0.5 oz)	80	5	160	11	—
Old Brussels Jalapeno Waferettes	5 (0.5 oz)	80	5	160	7	1
Rye Wafers Low Salt	5 (0.5 oz)	60	1	110	11	—
Stoned Wheat Wafers Bite Size	7 (0.5 oz)	60	1	180	11	—
Water Crackers Fat Free	5 (0.5 oz)	55	0	70	11	—
Wheat Wafers Low Salt	5 (0.5 oz)	60	2	110	10	1
Wasa Crispbread						
Breakfast	1	50	1	70	9	1
Extra Crisp	1	25	0	40	5	—
Falu Rye	1	30	0	60	6	2
Fiber Plus	1	35	1	60	5	3
Golden Rye	1	30	0	50	7	3
Hearty Rye	1	50	0	75	10	1
Light Rye	1	25	0	40	5	1
Royal	½	26	0	54	6	1
Savory Sesame	1	30	1	45	4	2
Sesame Rye	1	30	1	45	4	2
Sesame Wheat	1	60	2	65	9	1
Toasted Wheat	1	50	1	70	9	1

FOOD	PORTION	CAL.	FAT	SOD.	CARB.	FIB.
Weight Watchers						
Crispbread Garlic	2	30	0	55	7	—
Wheat Thins						
Low Salt	16 (1 oz)	140	6	75	20	2
Multi-Grain	17 (1 oz)	130	4	290	21	2
Wheatworth						
Stone Ground	5 (0.5 oz)	80	4	170	10	1
Zesta						
Saltine	2	25	1	75	4	—
Saltine Unsalted Top	2	25	1	35	4	—
cheese	14 (½ oz)	71	4	141	8	—
cheese	1 (1 in sq) (1 g)	5	tr	10	1	—
cheese low sodium	14 (½ oz)	71	4	68	8	—
cheese low sodium	1 (1 in sq) (1 g)	5	tr	5	1	—
cheese w/ peanut butter filling	1 (0.24 oz)	34	2	69	4	tr
crispbread	3	61	2	—	9	1
crispbread rye	1 (0.35 oz)	37	tr	26	8	2
crispbread rye	3	77	1	—	17	3
melba toast plain	1 (5 g)	19	tr	41	4	tr
melba toast pumpernickel	1 (5 g)	19	tr	45	4	tr
melba toast rye	1 (5 g)	19	tr	45	4	tr
melba toast wheat	1 (5 g)	19	tr	42	4	tr
milk	1 (0.42 oz)	55	2	71	8	—
oyster cracker	1 (1 g)	4	tr	13	1	tr
peanut butter sandwich	1 (7 g)	34	2	66	4	—
rusk toast	1 (0.35 oz)	41	1	25	7	—
rye w/ cheese filling	1 (0.24 oz)	34	2	73	4	—
rye wafers plain	1 (0.9 oz)	84	tr	199	20	—
rye wafers seasoned	1 (0.8 oz)	84	2	195	16	—
saltines	1 (3 g)	13	tr	38	2	tr
saltines fat free low sodium	3 (0.5 oz)	59	tr	95	12	—
saltines fat free low sodium	6 (1 oz)	118	tr	191	25	—
saltines low salt	1 (3 g)	13	tr	19	2	tr
snack cracker	1 (3 g)	15	1	25	2	tr
snack cracker low salt	1 (3 g)	15	1	11	2	tr
snack cracker w/ cheese filling	1 (7 g)	33	2	98	4	—
soup cracker	1 (1 g)	4	tr	13	1	tr
water biscuits	3	92	3	—	16	1
wheat w/ cheese filling	1 (0.24 oz)	35	2	64	4	—
wheat w/ peanut butter filling	1 (0.24 oz)	35	2	57	4	—
wheat thins	1 (2 g)	9	tr	16	1	—

FOOD	PORTION	CAL.	FAT	SOD.	CARB.	FIB.
wheat thins	7 (0.5 oz)	67	3	113	9	1
wheat thins low salt	7 (0.5 oz)	67	3	40	9	1
whole wheat	1 (4 g)	18	1	26	3	—
whole wheat low salt	1 (4 g)	18	1	10	3	—
zwieback	3½ oz	374	4	263	73	4

CRANBERRIES
CANNED
Ocean Spray

Cranberry Sauce Jellied	2 oz	90	0	10	22	—
CranFruit Cranberry Orange Sauce	2 oz	100	0	10	23	—
CranFruit Cranberry Raspberry Sauce	2 oz	100	0	10	23	—
CranFruit Cranberry Strawberry Sauce	2 oz	100	0	10	23	—
Whole Berry Sauce	2 oz	90	0	10	23	—

S&W

Cranberry Sauce Jellied Old Fashioned	½ cup	90	0	20	22	—
Cranberry Sauce Whole Berry Old Fashioned	½ cup	90	0	20	22	—
cranberry sauce sweetened	½ cup	209	tr	40	54	—

FRESH
Ocean Spray

Fresh	½ cup	25	0	0	6	—
chopped	1 cup	54	tr	1	14	—

CRANBERRY BEANS
CANNED

cranberry beans	1 cup	216	1	863	39	—

DRIED
Bean Cuisine

	½ cup	115	1	5	—	5
cooked	1 cup	240	1	1	43	—

CRANBERRY JUICE
After The Fall

Cape Cod Cranberry	1 bottle (10 oz)	130	0	25	30	—
Cranberry Ginger Ale	1 can (12 oz)	140	0	65	35	0

Apple & Eve

Juice	6 fl oz	100	0	10	25	—

Ocean Spray

Cocktail	8 fl oz	140	0	35	34	0
Cocktail Reduced Calorie	8 fl oz	50	0	35	13	0
Lightstyle Low Calorie Cranberry Juice Cocktail	8 fl oz	40	0	35	10	0

FOOD	PORTION	CAL.	FAT	SOD.	CARB.	FIB.
Seneca						
Cocktail frzn as prep	8 fl oz	140	0	0	36	0
Smucker's						
Juice Sparkler	10 oz	140	tr	5	34	—
Snapple						
Cranberry Royal	10 fl oz	150	0	25	37	—
Tree Of Life						
Concentrate	8 tsp (1.4 oz)	110	0	0	28	—
Tropicana						
Twister Ruby Red	1 bottle (10 fl oz)	150	0	30	37	—
Twister Ruby Red	8 fl oz	120	0	25	30	—
cocktail	1 cup	147	tr	10	38	—
cranberry juice cocktail	6 oz	108	tr	4	27	—
cranberry juice cocktail frzn	12 oz can	821	0	13	210	—
cranberry juice cocktail frzn as prep	6 oz	102	0	6	26	—
cranberry juice cocktail low calorie	6 oz	33	0	6	9	—

CRAYFISH
(*see also* LOBSTER)

FOOD	PORTION	CAL.	FAT	SOD.	CARB.	FIB.
cooked	3 oz	97	1	58	0	—
raw	3 oz	76	1	45	0	—
raw	8	24	tr	14	0	—

CREAM
(*see also* SOUR CREAM, SOUR CREAM SUBSTITUTES, WHIPPED TOPPINGS)
LIQUID

FOOD	PORTION	CAL.	FAT	SOD.	CARB.	FIB.
Farmland						
Half & Half	2 tbsp	40	3	15	2	0
Light Cream	2 tbsp	30	3	10	1	0
Hood						
Half & Half	2 tbsp (1 oz)	40	4	15	1	0
Heavy	1 tbsp (0.5 oz)	50	5	0	0	0
Light	1 tbsp (0.5 oz)	30	3	10	tr	0
Whipping Cream	1 tbsp (0.5 oz)	45	5	5	tr	0
Parmalat						
Half & Half	2 tbsp (1 oz)	40	3	20	2	0
half & half	1 tbsp	20	2	6	1	—
half & half	1 cup	315	28	98	10	—
heavy whipping	1 tbsp	52	6	6	tr	—
light coffee	1 tbsp	29	3	6	1	—
light coffee	1 cup	496	46	95	9	—
light whipping	1 tbsp	44	5	5	tr	—

FOOD	PORTION	CAL.	FAT	SOD.	CARB.	FIB.
WHIPPED						
heavy whipping	1 cup	411	44	89	7	—
light whipping	1 cup	345	37	82	7	—
CREAM CHEESE						
Alpine Lace						
Fat Free Garden Vegetable	2 tbsp (1 oz)	30	tr	165	1	0
Fat Free Garlic & Herbs	2 tbsp (1 oz)	30	tr	165	1	0
Breakstone						
Temp-Tee Whipped	3 tbsp (1.2 oz)	110	10	115	1	0
Fleur De Lait						
Bermuda Onion & Chives	2 tbsp (0.9 oz)	90	8	130	2	0
Cinnamon Raisin	2 tbsp (0.9 oz)	90	8	90	6	0
Date Nut Rum	2 tbsp (0.9 oz)	90	8	90	4	0
Fresh Cut Garden Vegetable	2 tbsp (0.9 oz)	80	8	200	1	0
Garden Vegetable	2 tbsp (0.9 oz)	80	8	200	1	0
Garlic & Spice	2 tbsp (0.9 oz)	90	9	160	1	0
Herb & Spice	2 tbsp (0.9 oz)	90	9	190	2	0
Irish Creme	2 tbsp (0.9 oz)	100	9	95	2	0
Lemon	2 tbsp (0.9 oz)	90	7	90	5	0
Lox	2 tbsp (0.9 oz)	90	8	125	1	0
Mandarin Orange	2 tbsp (0.9 oz)	90	7	90	3	0
Peach	2 tbsp (0.9 oz)	90	7	90	3	0
Pineapple	2 tbsp (0.9 oz)	90	8	95	3	0
Strawberry	2 tbsp (0.9 oz)	90	8	90	3	0
Toasted Onion	2 tbsp (0.9 oz)	90	9	190	2	0
Wildberry	2 tbsp (0.9 oz)	90	7	90	4	0
Fresh Cut						
Bac'n & Horseradish	2 tbsp (0.9 oz)	90	9	135	1	0
Bermuda Onion & Chives	2 tbsp (0.9 oz)	90	8	130	2	0
Date Nut & Rum	2 tbsp (0.9 oz)	90	8	90	4	0
Garlic & Spice	2 tbsp (0.9 oz)	90	9	160	1	0
Herb & Spice	2 tbsp (0.9 oz)	90	9	190	2	0
Lox	2 tbsp (0.9 oz)	90	8	125	1	0
Peaches & Cream	2 tbsp (0.9 oz)	90	7	90	3	0
Strawberry	2 tbsp (0.9 oz)	90	8	90	3	0
Friendship						
NY Style Reduced Fat	2 tbsp (1 oz)	50	3	120	0	0
Healthy Choice						
Herbs & Garlic	2 tbsp (1 oz)	25	0	200	2	—

FOOD	PORTION	CAL.	FAT	SOD.	CARB.	FIB.
Healthy Choice (CONT.)						
Plain	2 tbsp (1 oz)	25	0	200	2	—
Strawberry	2 tbsp (1 oz)	30	0	200	5	—
Heluva Good Cheese						
Cream Cheese	1 tbsp (1 oz)	100	10	85	1	0
Philadelphia						
Free	1 oz	25	0	135	2	0
Free Soft	2 tbsp (1.2 oz)	30	0	160	2	0
Light Soft	2 tbsp (1.1 oz)	70	5	150	2	0
Soft	2 tbsp (1 oz)	100	10	100	1	0
Soft Herb & Garlic	2 tbsp (1.1 oz)	110	10	180	2	0
Soft Olive & Pimento	2 tbsp (1.1 oz)	100	9	170	2	0
Soft Pineapple	2 tbsp (1.1 oz)	100	9	100	4	0
Soft Smoked Salmon	2 tbsp (1.1 oz)	100	9	200	1	0
Soft Strawberries	2 tbsp (1.1 oz)	100	9	65	5	0
Soft With Chives & Onions	2 tbsp (1.1 oz)	110	10	110	2	0
Whipped	3 tbsp (1.1 oz)	110	11	95	1	0
Whipped Smoked Salmon	3 tbsp (1.1 oz)	100	9	200	2	0
With Chives	1 oz	90	9	150	tr	0
With Pimentos	1 oz	90	9	150	tr	0
Ultra Delight						
Cheddar Cream Cheese	2 tbsp (0.9 oz)	60	4	150	2	1
Chive	2 tbsp (0.9 oz)	60	4	130	2	1
Garlic	2 tbsp (0.9 oz)	60	4	130	2	1
Mixed Berry	2 tbsp (0.9 oz)	70	4	70	5	1
Nacho	2 tbsp (0.9 oz)	60	4	190	2	1
Salsa	2 tbsp (0.9 oz)	60	4	140	2	1
Shrimp	2 tbsp (0.9 oz)	60	4	130	2	1
Strawberry	2 tbsp (0.9 oz)	60	4	80	4	1
Vegetable	2 tbsp (0.9 oz)	50	4	150	2	1
cream cheese	1 oz	99	10	84	1	—
cream cheese	1 pkg (3 oz)	297	30	251	2	—

CREAM CHEESE SUBSTITUTES

Tofutti						
Better Than Cream Cheese French Onion	1 oz	80	8	135	1	—
Better Than Cream Cheese Herb & Chive	1 oz	80	8	135	1	—
Better Than Cream Cheese Plain	1 oz	80	8	135	1	—

CREAM OF TARTAR

| cream of tartar | 1 tsp | 8 | 0 | 2 | 2 | — |

FOOD	PORTION	CAL.	FAT	SOD.	CARB.	FIB.
CREPES						
basic crepe unfilled	1	75	2	—	—	—
CRESS						
(*see also* WATERCRESS)						
garden cooked	½ cup	16	tr	5	3	—
garden raw	½ cup	8	tr	4	1	—
CROAKER						
atlantic breaded & fried	3 oz	188	11	296	6	—
atlantic raw	3 oz	89	3	47	0	—
CROISSANT						
Pepperidge Farm						
Croissant Sandwich Quartet	1	170	7	250	22	tr
Petite All Butter	1	120	6	170	13	—
Rudy's Farm						
Ham & Swiss Sandwich	1 (3.4 oz)	310	18	830	27	1
Sara Lee						
All Butter	1	170	9	240	19	—
All Butter Petite Size	1	120	6	160	13	—
apple	1 (2 oz)	145	5	156	21	1
cheese	1 (2 oz)	236	12	316	27	2
plain	1 (2 oz)	232	12	424	26	2
plain	1 mini (1 oz)	115	6	211	13	1
TAKE-OUT						
w/ egg & cheese	1	369	25	551	24	—
w/ egg cheese & bacon	1	413	28	889	24	—
w/ egg cheese & ham	1	475	34	1080	24	—
w/ egg cheese & sausage	1	524	38	1115	25	—
CROUTONS						
Arnold						
Crispy Cheddar Romano	½ oz	64	3	154	8	tr
Crispy Cheese Garlic	½ oz	60	2	130	9	tr
Crispy Fine Herbs	½ oz	50	1	150	10	1
Crispy Italian	½ oz	60	3	150	8	tr
Crispy Onion & Garlic	½ oz	60	2	190	9	—
Crispy Seasoned	½ oz	60	3	160	8	—
Brownberry						
Caesar Salad	½ oz	62	3	165	8	1
Cheddar Cheese	½ oz	63	3	155	8	tr
Onion & Garlic	½ oz	60	2	190	9	tr
Seasoned	½ oz	59	2	155	8	1
Toasted	½ oz	56	1	145	10	tr

FOOD	PORTION	CAL.	FAT	SOD.	CARB.	FIB.
Pepperidge Farm						
Cheddar & Romano Cheese	½ oz	60	2	200	10	—
Cheese & Garlic	½ oz	70	3	180	9	—
Onion & Garlic	½ oz	70	3	160	9	—
Seasoned	½ oz	70	3	180	9	—
Sour Cream & Chive	½ oz	70	3	170	9	—
plain	1 cup (1 oz)	122	2	209	22	2
seasoned	1 cup (1.4 oz)	186	7	495	25	2
CUCUMBER						
FRESH						
raw	1 (11 oz)	38	tr	6	8	3
raw sliced	½ cup (1.8 oz)	7	tr	1	1	1
JARRED						
Rosoff's						
Salad	3 slices (1 oz)	12	0	220	3	—
Schorr's						
Cucumber Garden Salad	3 slices (1 oz)	12	0	220	3	—
TAKE-OUT						
cucumber salad	3.5 oz	50	tr	480	11	—
CUMIN						
seed	1 tsp	8	tr	4	1	—
CURRANT JUICE						
black currant nectar	3½ oz	55	0	5	13	—
red currant nectar	3½ oz	54	tr	tr	13	—
CURRANTS						
black fresh	½ cup	36	tr	1	9	—
zante dried	½ cup	204	tr	6	53	—
CUSK						
fillet baked	3 oz	106	1	38	0	—
CUSTARD						
HOME RECIPE						
baked	½ cup (5 oz)	148	7	109	15	—
baked	1 recipe 4 serv (19.8 oz)	549	26	436	60	—
flan	½ cup (5.4 oz)	220	6	86	35	—
flan	1 recipe 10 serv (53.7 oz)	2206	63	864	349	—
MIX						
Jell-O						
Flan	½ cup	151	4	65	26	—

FOOD	PORTION	CAL.	FAT	SOD.	CARB.	FIB.
Jell-O (CONT.)						
Golden Egg Americana as prep	½ cup	160	6	198	23	—
Royal						
Custard	mix for 1 serving	60	0	75	16	—
Flan Caramel Custard	mix for 1 serving	60	0	55	15	—
as prep w/ 2% milk	½ cup (4.7 oz)	148	4	200	24	—
as prep w/ 2% milk	1 recipe 4 serv (18.7 oz)	595	15	801	95	—
as prep w/ whole milk	1 recipe 4 serv (18.7 oz)	652	22	—	94	—
as prep w/ whole milk	½ cup (4.7 oz)	163	5	—	23	—
flan as prep w/ 2% milk	½ cup (4.7 oz)	135	2	68	26	—
flan as prep w/ 2% milk	1 recipe 4 serv (18.7 oz)	542	9	265	102	—
flan as prep w/ whole milk	½ cup (4.7 oz)	150	4	65	25	—
flan as prep w/ whole milk	1 recipe 4 serv (18.7 oz)	600	16	291	102	—
TAKE-OUT						
baked	½ cup (5 oz)	148	7	109	15	—
zabaione	½ cup (57.2 g)	135	5	9	13	0

CUTTLEFISH

| steamed | 3 oz | 134 | 1 | 632 | 1 | — |

DANDELION GREENS

| fresh cooked | ½ cup | 17 | tr | 23 | 3 | — |
| raw chopped | ½ cup | 13 | tr | 21 | 3 | — |

DANISH PASTRY

FROZEN						
Morton						
Honey Buns	1 (2.28 oz)	250	10	160	35	2
Honey Buns Mini	1 (1.23 oz)	160	8	100	19	tr
Pepperidge Farm						
Apple	1	220	8	130	35	—
Cheese	1	240	14	230	25	—
Cinnamon Raisin	1	250	11	170	35	—
Raspberry	1	220	9	140	31	—
Sara Lee						
Apple	1	120	6	120	15	—
Apple Danish Twist	1 slice (1.9 oz)	190	10	200	22	—
Apple Free & Light	1 slice (2 oz)	130	0	120	30	—
Cheese	1	130	8	130	13	—
Cheese Danish Twist	1 slice (1.9 oz)	200	12	270	21	—

FOOD	PORTION	CAL.	FAT	SOD.	CARB.	FIB.
Sara Lee (CONT.)						
Cinnamon Raisin	1	150	8	140	17	—
Raspberry Danish Twist	1 slice (1.9 oz)	200	9	220	25	—
READY-TO-EAT						
Hostess						
Apple	1 (3.8 oz)	400	22	340	47	2
Apple Fruit Roll	1 (2 oz)	180	4	170	33	1
Coffee Cake Raspberry	1 (1.2 oz)	110	3	110	21	tr
plain ring	1 (12 oz)	1305	71	1302	152	—
REFRIGERATED						
Pillsbury						
Caramel Danish w/ Nuts	1	160	8	240	19	—
Cinnamon Raisin Danish w/ Icing	1	150	7	230	20	—
Orange Danish w/ Icing	1	150	7	250	19	—
TAKE-OUT						
almond	1 (4¼ in) (2.3 oz)	280	16	236	30	2
apple	1 (4¼ in) (2.5 oz)	264	13	251	34	1
cheese	1 (3 oz)	353	25	320	29	—
cheese	1 (4¼ in) (2.5 oz)	266	16	319	26	—
cinnamon	1 (3 oz)	349	17	326	47	—
cinnamon	1 (4¼ in) (2.3 oz)	262	15	241	29	1
cinnimon nut	1 (4¼ in) (2.3 oz)	280	16	236	30	2
fruit	1 (3.3 oz)	335	16	333	45	—
lemon	1 (4¼ in) (2.5 oz)	264	13	251	34	1
raisin	1 (4¼ in) (2.5 oz)	264	13	251	34	1
raisin nut	1 (4¼ in) (2.3 oz)	280	16	236	30	2
raspberry	1 (4¼ in) (2.5 oz)	264	13	251	34	1
strawberry	1 (4¼ in) (2.5 oz)	264	13	251	34	1

DATES

FOOD	PORTION	CAL.	FAT	SOD.	CARB.	FIB.
DRIED						
Bordo						
Diced	2 oz	203	1	5	48	—
Dole						
Chopped	½ cup	230	0	5	56	—
Pitted	½ cup	280	0	0	62	—
Dromedary						
Chopped	¼ cup	130	0	0	31	—
Pitted	5	100	0	0	23	—
chopped	1 cup	489	1	5	131	—
whole	10	228	tr	2	61	—

DEER
(see VENISON)

FOOD	PORTION	CAL.	FAT	SOD.	CARB.	FIB.

DELI MEATS/COLD CUTS

(see CHICKEN, HAM, LUNCHEON MEATS/COLD CUTS, MEAT SUBSTITUTES, TURKEY)

DIETING AIDS

(see NUTRITIONAL SUPPLEMENTS)

DILL

Watkins

FOOD	PORTION	CAL.	FAT	SOD.	CARB.	FIB.
Liquid Spice	1 tbsp (0.5 oz)	120	14	0	0	0
seed	1 tsp	6	tr	tr	1	—
sprigs fresh	1 cup	4	tr	5	1	—
sprigs fresh	5	0	tr	1	tr	—
weed dry	1 tsp	3	tr	2	1	—

DINNER

(see also BEEF DISHES, PASTA DINNERS, POT PIES, ORIENTAL FOOD, SPANISH FOODS, VEAL DISHES)

FROZEN

Armour

FOOD	PORTION	CAL.	FAT	SOD.	CARB.	FIB.
Classics Chicken & Noodles	1 meal (11 oz)	280	9	550	30	6
Classics Chicken Mesquite	1 meal (9.5 oz)	280	13	630	39	5
Classics Chicken Parmigiana	1 meal (10.75 oz)	360	18	1020	25	7
Classics Chicken w/ Wine & Mushroom	1 meal (10 oz)	260	11	540	20	4
Classics Glazed Chicken	1 meal (10.75 oz)	280	14	740	20	4
Classics Lite Beef Pepper	1 meal (11 oz)	210	4	870	29	5
Classics Lite Chicken Burgundy	1 meal (10 oz)	210	5	760	20	4
Classics Lite Salisbury Steak	1 meal (11.5 oz)	260	7	860	26	6
Classics Lite Shrimp Creole	1 meal (10 oz)	220	1	720	49	16
Classics Lite Sweet & Sour Chicken	1 meal (11 oz)	220	1	520	38	4
Classics Meatloaf	1 meal (11.25 oz)	300	10	600	33	7
Classics Salisbury Steak	1 meal (11.25 oz)	330	18	1310	20	4
Classics Swedish Meatballs	1 meal (10 oz)	300	17	940	20	4
Classics Turkey and Dressing	1 meal (11.25 oz)	270	7	1020	34	5

FOOD	PORTION	CAL.	FAT	SOD.	CARB.	FIB.
Armour (CONT.)						
Classics Veal Parmigiana	1 meal (11.25 oz)	400	22	1050	35	5
Banquet						
BBQ Style Chicken	1 meal (9 oz)	320	12	800	36	3
Beef	1 meal (9 oz)	240	7	660	19	12
Chicken & Dumplings	1 meal (10 oz)	260	8	780	35	16
Chicken Fried Steak	1 pkg (10 oz)	400	20	1180	39	4
Chicken Nuggets	1 pkg (6.75 oz)	410	21	650	38	11
Chicken Parmigiana	1 pkg (9.5 oz)	290	15	900	27	3
Extra Helping All White Chicken	1 meal (18 oz)	820	41	1890	72	8
Extra Helping Chicken Fried Steak	1 meal (18.5 oz)	800	44	2050	73	6
Extra Helping Chicken Parmigiana	1 meal (19 oz)	650	33	1770	64	9
Extra Helping Fried Chicken	1 meal (18 oz)	790	39	1820	72	8
Extra Helping Meatloaf	1 meal (19 oz)	650	38	2140	49	10
Extra Helping Mexican Style	1 meal (22 oz)	820	34	2060	100	20
Extra Helping Salisbury Steak	1 meal (19 oz)	740	46	1860	52	11
Extra Helping Southern Fried Chicken	1 meal (17.5 oz)	750	37	2140	67	9
Extra Helping Turkey Dinner	1 meal (18.8 oz)	560	20	1910	63	7
Family Entree Beef Stew	1 serv (8.13 oz)	160	4	1120	17	4
Family Entree Chicken & Dumplings	1 serv (7.47 oz)	290	14	1270	30	2
Family Entree Chicken Parmigiana	1 serv (4.67 oz)	240	13	690	18	2
Family Entrees Gravy & Sliced Beef	1 serv (5.6 oz)	100	3	850	7	tr
Family Entree Gravy & Sliced Turkey	1 serv (4.8 oz)	100	5	590	5	tr
Family Entree Gravy w/ Charbroiled Beef	1 serv (4.67 oz)	180	13	640	7	2
Family Entree Onion Gravy w/ Beef	1 serv (4.67 oz)	180	14	630	7	2
Family Entree Salisbury Steak	1 serv (4.67 oz)	200	14	610	7	2
Family Entree Veal Parmigiana	1 serv (4.67 oz)	230	14	740	19	2
Fried Chicken	1 meal (9 oz)	470	27	980	35	6

FOOD	PORTION	CAL.	FAT	SOD.	CARB.	FIB.
Banquet (CONT.)						
Gravy w/ Beef Patty	1 pkg (9.5 oz)	300	20	1060	21	2
Hot Sandwich Toppers Chicken Ala King	1 pkg (4.5 oz)	100	4	480	7	1
Hot Sandwich Toppers Creamed Chipped Beef	1 pkg (4 oz)	100	3	700	8	0
Hot Sandwich Toppers Gravy & Sliced Beef	1 pkg (4 oz)	70	2	440	5	tr
Hot Sandwich Toppers Gravy & Sliced Turkey	1 pkg (5 oz)	90	4	670	7	tr
Hot Sandwich Toppers Salisbury Steak	1 pkg (5 oz)	220	16	790	8	2
Hot Sandwich Toppers Sloppy Joe	1 meal (4 oz)	140	7	530	12	1
Meatloaf	1 meal (9.5 oz)	280	17	1100	23	2
Mexican Style Combo Meal	1 pkg (11 oz)	380	11	1370	55	9
Mexican Style Meal	1 pkg (11 oz)	340	13	1520	56	10
Oriental Style Chicken	1 pkg (9 oz)	260	9	610	34	4
Salisbury Steak	1 meal (9.5 oz)	310	16	910	28	2
Southern Fried Chicken Meal	1 pkg (8.75 oz)	260	30	1610	44	4
Turkey	1 meal (9.25 oz)	270	10	1100	31	3
Veal Parmagiana	1 pkg (9 oz)	530	14	960	35	7
Western Style Meal	1 meal (9.5 oz)	210	20	1400	28	5
White Meat Chicken Meal	1 pkg (8.75 oz)	470	28	1100	33	2
Birds Eye						
Easy Recipe Beef Burgundy not prep	½ pkg	120	5	670	17	4
Easy Recipe Beef Fajitas not prep	½ pkg	80	3	390	14	3
Budget Gourmet						
Beef Cantonese	1 meal (9.1 oz)	270	9	880	31	—
Beef Stroganoff	1 meal (8.75 oz)	260	10	840	27	—
Chicken And Egg Noodles	1 meal (10 oz)	440	26	880	28	—
Chicken Au Gratin	1 meal (9.1 oz)	230	8	820	23	—
Chicken Breast Parmigiana	1 pkg (11 oz)	270	9	530	30	—
Chicken Marsala	1 meal (9 oz)	260	8	730	31	—
Chicken With Fettucini	1 meal (10 oz)	400	21	700	29	—
Chinese Style Vegetables & Chicken	1 meal (10 oz)	280	7	590	47	—

FOOD	PORTION	CAL.	FAT	SOD.	CARB.	FIB.
Budget Gourmet (CONT.)						
French Recipe Chicken	1 meal (10 oz)	220	9	870	21	—
Glazed Turkey	1 meal (9 oz)	260	5	710	38	—
Ham & Asparagus Au Gratin	1 meal (8.7 oz)	300	14	860	26	—
Herbed Chicken Breast With Fettucini	1 pkg (11 oz)	240	6	430	30	—
Italian Style Vegetables & Chicken	1 meal (10.25 oz)	310	8	690	50	—
Mandarin Chicken	1 meal (10 oz)	240	5	710	38	—
Mesquite Chicken Breast	1 pkg (11 oz)	250	6	550	33	—
Orange Glazed Chicken	1 meal (9 oz)	270	3	870	46	—
Oriental Beef	1 meal (10 oz)	290	8	840	36	—
Oriental Chicken With Vegetables	1 meal (9 oz)	280	6	690	44	—
Pepper Steak With Rice	1 meal (10 oz)	300	8	720	40	—
Pot Roast Beef	1 meal (10.5 oz)	230	7	510	19	—
Roast Chicken With Homestyle Gravy	1 meal (11 oz)	280	8	560	36	—
Roast Sirloin Supreme	1 meal (9 oz)	320	15	630	28	—
Sirloin Cheddar Melt	1 meal (9.4 oz)	380	21	950	29	—
Sirloin Of Beef In Herb Sauce	1 meal (9.5 oz)	250	9	860	21	—
Sirloin Of Beef In Wine Sauce	1 pkg (11 oz)	280	8	560	36	—
Sirloin Salisbury Steak	1 meal (9 oz)	220	8	730	24	—
Sirloin Salisbury Steak	1 meal (11 oz)	280	9	530	30	—
Sirloin Tips And Country Vegetables	1 meal (10 oz)	290	17	810	19	—
Special Recipe Sirloin Of Beef	1 pkg (11 oz)	250	9	560	29	—
Stuffed Turkey Breast	1 pkg (11 oz)	250	6	570	31	—
Swedish Meatballs With Noodles	1 meal (10 oz)	590	38	920	37	—
Sweet And Sour Chicken	1 meal (10 oz)	340	5	620	55	—
Teriyaki Beef	1 pkg (10.75 oz)	260	7	530	37	—
Teriyaki Chicken Breast	1 meal (11 oz)	300	8	480	41	—
Healthy Choice						
Beef & Peppers Cantonese	1 meal (11.5 oz)	270	5	560	40	5
Beef Pepper Steak Oriental	1 meal (9.5 oz)	250	4	470	34	3
Beef Tips Francais	1 meal (9.5 oz)	280	5	520	40	4
Beef Tips With Sauce	1 meal (11 oz)	290	6	270	40	5

FOOD	PORTION	CAL.	FAT	SOD.	CARB.	FIB.
Healthy Choice (CONT.)						
Chicken & Vegetables Marsala	1 meal (11.5 oz)	220	1	440	32	3
Chicken Bangkok	1 meal (9.5 oz)	270	4	390	35	5
Chicken Cantonese	1 meal (11.25)	210	1	360	31	5
Chicken Dijon	1 meal (11 oz)	280	4	410	41	9
Chicken Imperial	1 meal (9 oz)	230	4	470	31	3
Chicken Parmigiana	1 meal (11.5 oz)	300	2	490	47	6
Chicken Picante	1 meal (11.25 oz)	220	2	330	30	6
Chicken Teriyaki	1 meal (12.25 oz)	270	2	420	42	5
Classics Beef Broccoli Beijing	1 meal (12 oz)	330	3	500	55	5
Classics Cacciatore Chicken	1 meal (12.5 oz)	260	3	510	36	6
Classics Chicken Fransesca	1 meal (12.5 oz)	360	5	500	51	5
Classics Country Inn Roast Turkey	1 meal (10 oz)	250	4	530	29	6
Classics Ginger Chicken Hunan	1 meal (12.6 oz)	350	3	430	59	5
Classics Mesquite Beef Barbecue	1 meal (11 oz)	310	4	490	45	6
Classics Salisbury Steak	1 meal (11 oz)	260	6	500	32	5
Classics Sesame Chicken Shanghai	1 meal (12 oz)	310	5	460	42	5
Classics Shrimp & Vegetables Maria	1 meal (12.5 oz)	260	2	540	46	5
Country Glazed Chicken	1 meal (8.5 oz)	200	2	480	30	3
Country Herb Chicken	1 meal (11.5 oz)	270	4	340	40	6
Country Roast Turkey With Mushroom	1 meal (8.5 oz)	220	4	440	28	3
Country Turkey & Pasta	1 meal (12.6 oz)	300	4	450	42	6
Homestyle Turkey With Vegetables	1 meal (9.5 oz)	260	2	490	34	3
Honey Mustard Chicken	1 meal (9.5 oz)	260	2	550	40	4
Lemon Pepper Fish	1 meal (10.7 oz)	290	5	360	47	7
Mandarin Chicken	1 meal (10 oz)	280	3	520	44	4
Mesquite Chicken Barbecue	1 meal (10.5 oz)	320	2	290	55	6
Shrimp Marinara	1 meal (10.5 oz)	220	1	220	44	5
Smoky Chicken Barbecue	1 meal (12.75 oz)	380	5	450	57	7
Southwestern Glazed Chicken	1 meal (12.5 oz)	300	3	430	48	6

FOOD	PORTION	CAL.	FAT	SOD.	CARB.	FIB.
Healthy Choice (CONT.)						
Sweet & Sour Chicken	1 meal (11.5 oz)	310	5	250	42	5
Traditional Beef Tips	1 meal (11.25 oz)	260	5	390	32	6
Traditional Breast Of Turkey	1 meal (10.5 oz)	280	3	460	40	7
Traditional Meat Loaf	1 meal (12 oz)	320	8	460	46	7
Tradtional Salisbury Steak	1 meal (11.5 oz)	320	6	470	48	7
Yankee Pot Roast	1 meal (11 oz)	280	5	460	38	5
Kid Cuisine						
Chicken Sandwiche	1 pkg (9.43 oz)	480	15	770	71	4
Chicken Nuggets	1 pkg (9.1 oz)	440	16	1070	54	5
Fish Sticks	1 pkg (8.25 oz)	370	12	550	55	4
Fried Chicken	1 pkg (10.1 oz)	440	19	940	49	5
Hot Dogs w/ Buns	6.7 oz	450	19	880	57	—
Macaroni & Beef	1 pkg (9.6 oz)	370	9	900	58	5
Le Menu						
Beef Sirlion Tips	11½ oz	400	18	760	29	—
Beef Stroganoff	10 oz	430	24	980	28	—
Chicken A La King	10¼ oz	330	13	830	29	—
Chicken Cordon Bleu	11 oz	460	20	850	47	—
Chicken In Wine Sauce	10 oz	280	7	680	27	—
Chicken Parmigiana	11¾ oz	410	20	1030	31	—
Chopped Sirloin Beef	12¼ oz	430	24	1010	28	—
Entree LightStyle Chicken A La King	8¼ oz	240	5	670	29	—
Entree LightStyle Chicken Dijon	8 oz	240	7	590	21	—
Entree LightStyle Empress Chicken	8¼ oz	210	5	690	26	—
Entree LightStyle Glazed Turkey	8¼ oz	260	6	720	34	—
Entree LightStyle Herb Roast Chicken	7¾ oz	260	6	500	29	—
Entree LightStyle Swedish Meatballs	8 oz	260	8	700	30	—
Entree LightStyle Traditional Turkey	8 oz	200	5	610	19	—
Ham Steak	10 oz	300	11	1500	31	—
LightStyle Glazed Chicken Breast	10 oz	230	3	480	25	—
LightStyle Herb Roasted Chicken	10 oz	240	7	400	18	—
LightStyle Salisbury Steak	10 oz	280	9	400	31	—

FOOD	PORTION	CAL.	FAT	SOD.	CARB.	FIB.
Le Menu (CONT.)						
LightStyle Sliced Turkey	10 oz	210	5	540	21	—
LightStyle Sweet & Sour Chicken	10 oz	250	7	530	29	—
LightStyle Turkey Divan	10 oz	260	7	420	23	—
LightStyle Veal Marsala	10 oz	230	3	700	28	—
Pepper Steak	11½ oz	370	13	1020	36	—
Salisbury Steak	10½ oz	370	20	880	28	—
Sliced Breast Of Turkey w/ Mushroom Gravy	10½ oz	300	7	1020	38	—
Sweet & Sour Chicken	11¼ oz	400	18	1020	41	—
Veal Parmigiana	11½ oz	390	17	840	36	—
Yankee Pot Roast	10 oz	330	13	700	27	—
Lean Cuisine						
Baked Chicken	1 meal (8 oz)	240	5	480	31	3
Beef Pot Roast	1 meal (9 oz)	210	7	570	21	3
Chicken A L'Orange	1 meal (8 oz)	260	3	260	40	1
Chicken & Vegetables	1 meal (10.5 oz)	240	5	520	30	5
Chicken In Honey Barbecue Sauce	1 pkg (8.75 oz)	250	5	560	35	6
Chicken In Peanut Sauce	1 pkg (9 oz)	280	6	590	33	3
Chicken Italiano	1 pkg (9 oz)	270	6	560	31	3
Chicken Marsala	1 meal (8.1 oz)	180	4	470	13	5
Chicken Oriental	1 pkg (9 oz)	260	6	530	30	3
Chicken Parmesan	1 meal (10.9 oz)	220	5	530	22	5
Chicken Pie	1 meal (9.5 oz)	320	10	590	39	3
Fiesta Chicken	1 pkg (8.5 oz)	240	5	590	31	3
Fish Divan	1 pkg (10.4 oz)	210	6	490	15	3
Glazed Chicken	1 meal (8.5 oz)	240	6	460	24	2
Homestyle Turkey	1 pkg (9.4 oz)	230	5	590	26	3
Honey Mustard Chicken	1 pkg (7.5 oz)	250	5	460	32	4
Meatloaf	1 pkg (9.4 oz)	270	10	530	24	4
Oriental Beef	1 meal (9 oz)	250	8	480	30	4
Roasted Turkey Breast	1 pkg (9.75 oz)	290	40	530	48	3
Salisbury Steak With Macaroni & Cheese	1 meal (9.5 oz)	200	10	590	22	2
Stuffed Cabbage	1 meal (9.5 oz)	220	7	460	27	5
Swedish Meatballs	1 pkg (9.1 oz)	290	8	590	32	3
Sweet & Sour Chicken	1 pkg (10.4 oz)	260	3	440	43	3
Turkey Pie	1 pkg (9.5 oz)	300	9	590	34	3
Life Choice						
Garden Potato Casser	1 meal (13.4 oz)	160	1	590	37	9
Morton						
Breaded Chicken Pattie	1 meal (6.75 oz)	280	15	840	24	4

FOOD	PORTION	CAL.	FAT	SOD.	CARB.	FIB.
Morton (CONT.)						
Chicken Nugget	1 meal (7 oz)	320	17	460	30	3
Fried Chicken	1 meal (9 oz)	420	25	1000	30	4
Meatloaf	1 meal (9 oz)	250	13	1110	24	5
Mexican	1 meal (10 oz)	260	7	1000	40	8
Salisbury Steak	1 meal (9 oz)	210	9	950	23	3
Turkey	1 meal (9 oz)	230	8	1090	27	5
Veal Parmagiana	1 meal (8.75 oz)	280	13	950	30	4
Western	1 meal (9 oz)	290	16	1210	26	6
Patio						
Chili	1 cup (8 oz)	260	13	1010	13	4
Ranchera	1 pkg (13 oz)	410	15	2400	14	14
Stouffer's						
Chicken A La King	1 pkg (9.5 oz)	320	10	750	43	3
Chicken Divan	1 pkg (8 oz)	210	10	570	10	1
Creamed Chicken	1 pkg (6.5 oz)	280	20	720	8	1
Creamed Chipped Beef	½ cup (4.5 oz)	150	11	690	6	1
Creamed Chipped Beef Over Country Biscuit	1 pkg (9 oz)	460	28	1650	40	3
Escalloped Chicken & Noodles	1 pkg (10 oz)	440	29	880	28	2
Green Pepper Steak	1 pkg (10.5 oz)	330	9	650	45	3
Ham & Asparagus Bake	1 pkg (9.5 oz)	520	36	1040	32	2
Homestyle Baked Chicken	1 pkg (8.9 oz)	270	12	750	19	2
Homestyle Beef Pot Roast	1 pkg (8.9 oz)	270	10	640	25	4
Homestyle Breaded Chicken Tenders	1 pkg (6.6 oz)	380	18	1060	33	4
Homestyle Chicken & Noodles	1 pkg (10 oz)	310	14	1030	23	2
Homestyle Chicken Monterey	1 pkg (9.4 oz)	410	20	700	35	4
Homestyle Chicken Parmigiana	1 pkg (10.9 oz)	320	10	890	30	4
Homestyle Fish Filet With Macaroni & Cheese	1 pkg (9 oz)	430	21	930	37	2
Homestyle Fried Chicken	1 pkg (7.1 oz)	330	16	780	29	3
Homestyle Meatloaf	1 pkg (9.9 oz)	380	24	910	24	3
Homestyle Roast Turkey	1 pkg (7.9 oz)	280	11	950	25	1
Homestyle Salisbury Steak	1 pkg (9.6 oz)	370	19	1220	26	—
Homestyle Sliced Beef & Potatoes	1 pkg (8.1 oz)	270	10	900	25	2

FOOD	PORTION	CAL.	FAT	SOD.	CARB.	FIB.
Stouffer's (CONT.)						
Homestyle Veal Parmigiana	1 pkg (11.9 oz)	420	19	1200	43	6
Lunch Express Chicken With Garden Vegetables	1 pkg (9.9 oz)	340	11	750	45	2
Lunch Express Mandarin Chicken	1 pkg (9.75 oz)	270	6	520	41	2
Lunch Express Mexican Style Rice With Chicken	1 pkg (9 oz)	270	8	390	39	3
Lunch Express Oriental Beef	1 pkg (6.2 oz)	260	8	1220	34	4
Lunch Express Stir-Fry Rice & Chicken	1 pkg (9 oz)	280	9	590	39	3
Stuffed Pepper	1 pkg (10 oz)	200	8	900	24	1
Swedish Meatballs	1 pkg (9.25 oz)	440	23	840	36	3
Swanson						
Beans & Franks	10½ oz	440	19	900	53	—
Beef	11¼ oz	310	6	770	38	—
Beef In Barbecue Sauce	11 oz	460	17	860	51	—
Chicken Duet Gourmet Nuggets Pizza Style	3 oz	210	12	—	—	—
Chopped Sirloin Beef	10¾ oz	340	16	790	28	—
Fish 'n' Chips	10 oz	500	21	960	60	—
Fried Chicken Dark Meat	9¾ oz	560	28	1130	55	—
Fried Chicken White Meat	10¼ oz	550	25	1460	60	—
Homestyle Chicken Cacciatore	10.95 oz	260	8	1030	33	—
Homestyle Chicken Nibbles	4¼ oz	340	20	730	29	—
Homestyle Fish & Fries	6½ oz	340	16	670	37	—
Homestyle Fried Chicken	7 oz	390	21	1100	33	—
Homestyle Salisbury Steak	10 oz	320	16	980	22	—
Homestyle Scalloped Potatoes & Ham	9 oz	300	13	1080	26	—
Homestyle Seafood Creole With Rice	9 oz	240	6	810	40	—
Homestyle Sirloin Tips In Burgundy Sauce	7 oz	160	5	550	16	—
Homestyle Turkey With Dressing & Potatoes	9 oz	290	11	1010	30	—

FOOD	PORTION	CAL.	FAT	SOD.	CARB.	FIB.
Swanson (CONT.)						
Homestyle Veal Parmigiana	10 oz	330	13	960	33	—
Hungry-Man Boneless Chicken	17¾ oz	700	28	1530	65	—
Hungry-Man Chopped Beef Steak	16¾ oz	640	37	1600	41	—
Hungry-Man Fried Chicken Dark Meat	14¼ oz	860	45	1660	77	—
Hungry-Man Fried Chicken White Meat	14¼ oz	870	46	2150	80	—
Hungry-Man Salisbury Steak	16½ oz	680	41	1730	37	—
Hungry-Man Sliced Beef	15¼ oz	450	12	1060	49	—
Hungry-Man Turkey	17 oz	550	18	1810	61	—
Hungry-Man Veal Parmigiana	18¼ oz	590	26	1840	57	—
Loin Of Pork	10¾ oz	280	12	790	27	—
Macaroni & Beef	12 oz	370	15	930	48	—
Meatloaf	10¾ oz	360	15	960	41	—
Noodles & Chicken	10½ oz	280	8	740	45	—
Salisbury Steak	10¾ oz	400	17	880	43	—
Swedish Meatballs	8½ oz	360	20	790	26	—
Swiss Steak	10 oz	350	11	700	37	—
Turkey	11½ oz	350	11	1090	42	—
Turkey	8¾ oz	270	11	—		—
Veal Parmigiana	12¼ oz	430	20	1010	42	—
Western Style	11½ oz	430	19	1060	43	—
Tyson						
Beef Champignon	1 pkg (10.5 oz)	370	15	830	31	—
Chicken Picante	1 pkg (9 oz)	250	4	390	26	—
Chicken Supreme	1 pkg (9 oz)	230	6	480	23	—
Francais	1 pkg (9.5 oz)	280	14	1130	20	—
Glazed Chicken With Sauce	1 pkg (9.25 oz)	240	4	930	29	—
Grilled Chicken	1 pkg (7.75 oz)	220	3	520	22	—
Grilled Italian Chicken	1 pkg (9 oz)	210	3	420	19	—
Healthy Portions BBQ Chicken	1 pkg (12.5 oz)	400	8	600	56	—
Healthy Portions Chicken Marinara	1 pkg (13.75 oz)	340	7	590	37	—
Healthy Portions Herb Chicken	1 pkg (13.75 oz)	340	4	550	43	—
Healthy Portions Honey Mustard Chicken	1 pkg (13.75 oz)	390	6	520	52	—

FOOD	PORTION	CAL.	FAT	SOD.	CARB.	FIB.
Tyson (CONT.)						
Healthy Portions Italian Style Chicken	1 pkg (13.75 oz)	310	4	600	38	—
Healthy Portions Mesquite Chicken	1 pkg (13.25 oz)	330	5	600	38	—
Healthy Portions Salsa Chicken	1 pkg (13.75 oz)	370	6	470	52	—
Healthy Portions Sesame Chicken	1 pkg (13.5 oz)	400	6	400	59	—
Honey Roasted Chicken	1 pkg (9 oz)	220	4	500	23	—
Kiev	1 pkg (9.25 oz)	450	25	950	39	—
Marsala	1 pkg (9 oz)	200	4	670	19	—
Mexquite	1 pkg (9 oz)	320	8	660	39	—
Picatta	1 pkg (9 oz)	200	4	550	18	—
Roasted Chicken	1 pkg (9 oz)	200	2	430	21	—
Sweet & Sour	1 pkg (11 oz)	420	15	850	50	—
Turkey With Gravy	1 pkg (9.5 oz)	320	12	900	34	—
Ultra Slim-Fast						
Beef Pepper Steak	12 oz	270	4	590	36	0
Chicken & Vegetable	12 oz	290	3	850	45	4
Chicken Fettucini	12 oz	380	12	980	38	1
Country Style Vegetable & Beef Tips	12 oz	230	5	960	26	4
Mesquite Chicken	12 oz	360	1	300	61	5
Roasted Chicken In Mushroom Sauce	12 oz	280	6	830	30	0
Shrimp Creole	12 oz	240	4	730	45	5
Shrimp Marinara	12 oz	290	3	880	53	0
Sweet & Sour Chicken	12 oz	330	2	340	57	0
Turkey Medallions In Herb Sauce	12 oz	280	6	950	33	0
Weight Watchers						
Barbecue Glazed Chicken	7 oz	200	6	450	22	—
Beef Sirloin Tips	7.5 oz	210	6	560	20	—
Beef Stroganoff	8.5 oz	280	9	590	29	—
Chicken Ala King	9 oz	230	4	460	30	—
Chicken Cordon Bleu	7.7 oz	170	5	560	15	—
Chicken Kiev	7 oz	190	5	470	22	—
Homestyle Chicken & Noodles	9 oz	240	7	450	25	—
Imperial Chicken	8.5 oz	210	4	420	26	—
London Broil	7.5 oz	110	3	320	4	—
Oven Baked Fish	7 oz	150	4	260	6	—

FOOD	PORTION	CAL.	FAT	SOD.	CARB.	FIB.
Weight Watchers (CONT.)						
Southern Baked Chicken	6.3 oz	170	7	520	10	—
Stuffed Turkey Breast	8.5 oz	270	8	520	31	—
Veal Patty Parmigiana	8.2 oz	150	4	550	5	—
SHELF-STABLE						
My Own Meal						
Beef Stew	1 pkg (10 oz)	260	11	480	22	4
Chicken & Black Beans	1 pkg (10 oz)	240	5	460	30	6
Chicken Mediterranean	1 pkg (10 oz)	270	9	320	28	4
Chicken Noodles	1 pkg (10 oz)	270	8	900	29	3
Old World Stew	1 pkg (10 oz)	310	12	510	31	3
DIP						
Breakstone						
Sour Cream Bacon & Onion	2 tbsp (1.1 oz)	60	5	170	2	0
Sour Cream Chesapeake Clam	2 tbsp (1.1 oz)	50	4	190	2	0
Sour Cream French Onion	2 tbsp (1.1 oz)	50	4	160	2	0
Sour Cream Jalapeno Cheddar	2 tbsp (1.1 oz)	60	4	170	2	0
Sour Cream Toasted Onion	2 tbsp (1.1 oz)	50	4	180	2	0
Chi-Chi's						
Fiesta Bean	2 tbsp (0.9 oz)	35	2	140	4	1
Fiesta Cheese	2 tbsp (0.9 oz)	40	3	270	3	0
Eagle						
Bean	1 oz	35	2	140	4	—
Frito Lay						
Cheddar Cheese	1 oz	45	3	180	3	—
French Onion	1 oz	50	4	180	3	—
Jalapeno Bean	1 oz	30	1	115	4	—
Picante Sauce	1 oz	10	0	160	3	—
Guiltless Gourmet						
Black Bean Mild	1 oz	25	0	80	5	1
Black Bean Spicy	1 oz	25	0	80	5	1
Pinto Bean	1 oz	25	0	80	5	1
Hain						
Hot Bean	4 tbsp	70	1	250	10	—
Mexican Bean	4 tbsp	60	1	260	9	—
Onion Bean	4 tbsp	70	1	270	10	—
Taco Dip & Sauce	4 tbsp	25	1	350	1	—
Heluva Good Cheese						
Bacon Horseradish	2 tbsp (1.1 oz)	60	5	200	2	0

FOOD	PORTION	CAL.	FAT	SOD.	CARB.	FIB.
Heluva Good Cheese (CONT.)						
Clam	2 tbsp (1.1 oz)	50	5	130	2	0
French Onion	2 tbsp (1.1 oz)	50	5	160	2	0
Homestyle Onion	2 tbsp (1.1 oz)	60	5	290	3	0
Light French Onion	2 tbsp (1.1 oz)	35	2	180	3	0
Light Jalapeno Cheddar	2 tbsp (1.1 oz)	40	2	160	3	0
Ranch	2 tbsp (1.1 oz)	60	5	180	2	0
Knudsen						
Nacho Cheese	2 tbsp (1.1 oz)	60	4	200	3	0
Sour Cream Bacon & Onion	2 tbsp (1.1 oz)	60	5	170	2	0
Sour Cream French Onion	2 tbsp (1.1 oz)	50	4	160	2	0
Kraft						
Avocado	2 tbsp (1.1 oz)	60	4	240	4	0
Bacon & Horseradish	2 tbsp (1.1 oz)	60	5	220	3	0
Clam	2 tbsp (1.1 oz)	60	4	250	3	0
French Onion	2 tbsp (1.1 oz)	60	4	230	4	0
Green Onion	2 tbsp (1.1 oz)	60	4	190	4	0
Jalapeno	2 tbsp (1.1 oz)	60	4	260	3	0
Jalapeno Cheese	2 tbsp (1.1 oz)	60	5	250	1	0
Premium Bacon & Horseradish	2 tbsp (1.1 oz)	50	5	200	2	0
Premium Bacon & Onion	2 tbsp (1.1 oz)	60	5	160	2	0
Premium Blue Cheese	2 tbsp (1.1 oz)	45	4	200	2	0
Premium Clam	2 tbsp (1.1 oz)	45	4	210	2	0
Premium Creamy Cucumber	2 tbsp (1.1 oz)	50	4	140	2	0
Premium Creamy Onion	2 tbsp (1.1 oz)	45	4	160	2	0
Premium French Onion	2 tbsp (1.1 oz)	50	4	160	2	0
Premium Nacho Cheese	2 tbsp (1.1 oz)	60	5	270	2	0
Ranch	2 tbsp (1.1 oz)	60	4	210	2	0
Louise's						
Fat Free Honey Mustard	1 oz	40	0	170	9	0
Fat Free Sour Cream & Onion	1 oz	25	0	195	4	0
Fat Free White Cheese Peppercorn	1 oz	25	0	195	4	0
Marzetti						
Blue Cheese Veggie	2 tbsp	200	21	230	1	0
Lemon Dill Veggie	2 tbsp	140	14	190	2	0
Light Ranch Veggie	2 tbsp	60	7	290	5	1
Ranch Veggie	2 tbsp	140	14	200	1	0
Sour Cream & Onion	2 tbsp	130	14	200	2	0

FOOD	PORTION	CAL.	FAT	SOD.	CARB.	FIB.
Marzetti (CONT.)						
Southwestern Veggie	2 tbsp	130	14	170	1	0
Spinach Veggie	2 tbsp	130	13	220	1	0
Old El Paso						
Chunky Salsa Medium	2 tbsp	10	0	230	1	1
Chunky Salsa Mild	2 tbsp	10	0	230	1	1
Jalapeno Bean Mild	1 tbsp	14	0	53	2	1
Sealtest						
French Onion	2 tbsp (1.1 oz)	50	4	160	2	0
Snyder's						
Mustard Pretzel	2 tbsp (1.2 oz)	90	4	20	13	1
Wise						
Jalapeno Bean	2 tbsp	25	0	100	5	—
Taco	2 tbsp	12	0	115	3	—
DOCK						
fresh cooked	3½ oz	20	1	3	3	—
raw chopped	½ cup	15	tr	3	2	—
DOGFISH						
raw	3½ oz	193	15	14	0	—
DOLPHINFISH						
fresh baked	3 oz	93	1	96	0	—
fresh fillet baked	5.6 oz	174	1	179	0	—
DOUGHNUTS						
Drake's						
Old Fashion Donuts	1 (1.7 oz)	182	8	238	25	—
Powdered Sugar Donut Delites	7 (2.5 oz)	300	15	316	38	—
Dutch Mill						
Cider	1 (2.1 oz)	240	10	220	35	1
Cinnamon	1 (1.8 oz)	210	11	250	26	1
Donut Holes Double-Dipped Chocolate	3 (1.4 oz)	220	16	140	19	0
Donut Holes Shootin' Stars	3 (1.4 oz)	190	10	110	23	0
Double-Dipped Chocolate	1 (2.1 oz)	280	17	360	31	1
Glazed	1 (2.1 oz)	250	12	220	34	1
Glazed Chocolate	1 (2.4 oz)	270	11	380	40	1
Plain	1 (1.8 oz)	210	12	270	25	1
Sugared	1 (1.8 oz)	220	11	260	27	1
Earth Grains						
Cinnamon Apple	1	310	17	—	—	—

FOOD	PORTION	CAL.	FAT	SOD.	CARB.	FIB.
Earth Grains (CONT.)						
Devil's Food	1	330	21	—	—	—
Glazed Old Fashioned	1	310	18	—	—	—
Powdered Old Fashioned	1	290	19	—	—	—
Entenmann's						
Crumb Topped	1 (2.1 oz)	260	12	220	34	—
Devil's Food Crumb	1 (2.1 oz)	250	12	200	34	—
Rich Frosted	1 (2 oz)	280	18	210	27	—
Freihofer's						
Assorted	1 (2 oz)	270	17	170	26	0
Hostess						
Assorted Regular	1 (1.6 oz)	200	11	230	23	tr
Cinnamon Family Pack	1 (1 oz)	110	5	140	15	tr
Cinnamon Swirl	1 (1.6 oz)	180	7	220	28	tr
Crumb Regular	1 (1 oz)	130	8	115	14	tr
Frosted Regular	1 (1.4 oz)	180	11	170	20	1
Gem Donettes Cinnamon	6 (3 oz)	320	11	390	53	1
Gem Donettes Frosted	6 (3 oz)	390	23	360	42	2
Gem Donettes Frosted Strawberry Filled	3 (3 oz)	240	13	210	29	1
Gem Donettes Powdered	6 (3 oz)	350	16	380	47	1
Gem Donettes Powdered Strawberry Filled	3 (3 oz)	210	9	210	31	tr
Glazed Party	1 (2.3 oz)	260	10	310	39	1
Jumbo Frosted	1 (2 oz)	260	16	240	28	1
Jumbo Plain	1 (1.1 oz)	140	7	190	16	tr
Jumbo Powdered	1 (1.3 oz)	160	9	170	19	tr
Mini Chocolate	5 (2 oz)	220	9	220	33	1
O's Raspberry Filled Powdered	1 (2.2 oz)	230	10	230	35	tr
Old Fashioned Glazed	1 (2.1 oz)	250	12	230	33	tr
Old Fashioned Glazed Honey Wheat	1 (2.1 oz)	250	12	270	33	1
Old Fashioned Plain	1 (1.5 oz)	170	9	230	21	tr
Plain Regular	1 (1 oz)	120	6	160	13	tr
Powdered Family Pack	1 (1 oz)	110	6	135	15	1
Little Debbie						
Donut Sticks	1 pkg (3 oz)	390	23	370	45	1
Donut Sticks	1 pkg (2 oz)	250	15	250	30	1
Donut Sticks	1 pkg (2.5 oz)	320	19	310	37	1
Donut Sticks	1 pkg (1.6 oz)	210	13	210	25	1
Tastykake						
Cinnamon	1 (47 g)	180	8	210	26	1
Frosted Rich	1 (57 g)	260	16	200	28	3

FOOD	PORTION	CAL.	FAT	SOD.	CARB.	FIB.
Tastykake (CONT.)						
Frosted Rich Mini	1 (14 g)	44	3	60	8	1
Honey Wheat	1 (57 g)	210	8	200	32	1
Honey Wheat Mini	1 (12 g)	40	1	50	7	0
Orange Glazed	1 (57 g)	210	9	180	32	1
Plain	1 (47 g)	190	10	170	22	1
Powdered Sugar	1 (46 g)	180	9	220	24	1
Powdered Sugar Mini	1 (12 g)	40	1	70	7	0
cake type unsugared	1 (1.6 oz)	198	11	257	23	1
chocolate glazed	1 (1.5 oz)	175	8	143	24	1
chocolate sugared	1 (1.5 oz)	175	8	143	24	1
chocolate coated	1 (1.5 oz)	204	13	185	21	1
creme filled	1 (3 oz)	307	21	262	26	—
french cruller glazed	1 (1.4 oz)	169	8	142	24	—
frosted	1 (1.5 oz)	204	13	185	21	1
honey bun	1 (2.1 oz)	242	14	205	27	1
jelly	1 (3 oz)	289	16	249	33	—
old fashioned	1 (1.6 oz)	198	11	257	23	1
sugared	1 (1.6 oz)	192	10	181	23	1
wheat glazed	1 (1.6 oz)	162	9	160	19	—
wheat sugared	1 (1.6 oz)	162	9	160	19	—
yeast glazed	1 (2.1 oz)	242	14	205	27	1

DRESSING

(*see* STUFFING/DRESSING)

DRINK MIXERS

(*see also* SODA, MINERAL/BOTTLED WATER)

FOOD	PORTION	CAL.	FAT	SOD.	CARB.	FIB.
Bacardi						
Margarita Mix w/ rum	8 fl oz	160	0	0	24	—
Margarita Mix w/o liquor	8 fl oz	100	0	0	25	—
Pina Colada	8 fl oz	140	0	10	34	—
Rum Runner	8 fl oz	140	0	10	35	—
Strawberry Daiquiri w/o liquor	8 fl oz	140	0	0	35	—
Canada Dry						
Collins Mixer	8 fl oz	120	0	20	25	0
Sour Mixer	8 fl oz	90	0	25	22	0
Libby						
Bloody Mary Mix	6 oz	40	0	1120	8	—
McIlhenny						
Tabasco Bloody Mary Mix	8 fl oz	56	tr	1548	11	1
Schweppes						
Collins Mixer	8 fl oz	100	0	55	24	0

FOOD	PORTION	CAL.	FAT	SOD.	CARB.	FIB.
Tabasco						
Bloody Mary Mix Extra Spicy	8 fl oz	58	tr	1645	11	2
whiskey sour mix	2 oz	55	0	66	14	—
whiskey sour mix as prep	3.6 oz	169	0	48	16	—
DRUM						
freshwater fillet baked	5.4 oz	236	10	148	0	—
freshwater baked	3 oz	130	5	82	0	—
DUCK						
FRESH						
w/ skin roasted	½ duck (13.4 oz)	1287	108	227	0	—
w/ skin roasted	6 oz	583	49	103	0	—
w/o skin roasted	3.5 oz	201	11	65	0	—
w/o skin roasted	½ duck (7.8 oz)	445	25	143	0	—
wild breast w/o skin raw	½ breast (2.9 oz)	102	4	47	0	—
wild w/ skin raw	½ duck (9.5 oz)	571	41	152	0	—
DUMPLING						
FROZEN						
Pepperidge Farm						
Apple Dumpling	1 (3 oz)	260	13	230	33	—
DURIAN						
fresh	3½ oz	141	2	1	29	—
EEL						
fresh cooked	1 fillet (5.6 oz)	375	24	104	0	—
fresh cooked	3 oz	200	13	55	0	—
raw	3 oz	156	10	43	0	—
smoked	3.5 oz	330	28	—	0	0
EGG						
(see also EGG DISHES, EGG SUBSTITUTES*)*						
CHICKEN						
fried w/ margarine	1	91	7	162	1	—
frozen	1 cup	363	24	307	3	—
frozen	1	75	5	63	1	—
hard cooked	1	77	5	62	1	—
hard cooked chopped	1 cup	210	14	169	2	—
poached	1	74	5	140	1	—
raw	1	75	5	63	1	—
scrambled plain	2	200	15	211	2	—
scrambled w/ whole milk & margarine	1 cup	365	27	616	5	—
scrambled w/ whole milk & margarine	1	101	7	171	1	—

FOOD	PORTION	CAL.	FAT	SOD.	CARB.	FIB.
white only	1 cup	121	0	399	2	—
white only	1	17	0	55	tr	—
OTHER POULTRY						
duck raw	1	130	10	102	1	—
goose raw	1	267	19	—	2	—
quail raw	1	14	1	—	tr	—
turkey raw	1	135	9	—	1	—

EGG DISHES

FROZEN

Chefwich

Cheese Omelet	5 oz	380	17	—	—	—
Ham & Cheese Omelet	5 oz	340	14	—	—	—
Sausage & Cheese Omelet	5 oz	400	19	—	—	—
Western Style Omelet	5 oz	350	13	—	—	—

Downyflake

Scrambled Eggs With Ham & Hash Browns	1 pkg (6.25 oz)	360	26	730	17	—
Scrambled Eggs With Ham & Pecan Twirl	1 pkg (6.25 oz)	470	28	670	40	—
Scrambled Eggs With Hash Browns & Sausage	1 pkg (6.25 oz)	420	34	790	17	—
Scrambled Eggs With Sausage & Pecan Twirl	1 pkg (6.25 oz)	510	33	710	39	—

Great Starts

Egg Sausage & Cheese	5½ oz	460	28	1310	35	—
Omelets With Cheese & Ham	7 oz	390	29	1220	15	—
Reduced Cholesterol Eggs With Mini Oatbran Muffins	4¾ oz	250	12	400	27	—
Scrambled Eggs & Bacon With Home Fries	5.6 oz	340	26	690	16	—
Scrambled Eggs & Home Fries	4.6 oz	260	19	380	14	—
Scrambled Eggs & Sausage With Hash Browns	6½ oz	430	34	760	19	—
Scrambled Eggs With Cheese & Cinnamon Pancakes	3.4 oz	290	23	380	14	—

FOOD	PORTION	CAL.	FAT	SOD.	CARB.	FIB.
Quaker						
Scrambled Eggs & Sausage With Hash Browns	1 pkg (5.7 oz)	290	20	810	14	—
Scrambled Eggs & Sausage With Pancakes	1 pkg (5.2 oz)	270	14	880	21	—
Scrambled Eggs Cheddar Cheese & Fried Potatoes	1 pkg (5.9 oz)	250	13	910	22	—
Weight Watchers						
Garden Vegetable Omelet Sandwich	1 (3.6 oz)	210	6	—	28	—
Ham & Cheese Handy Omelet	4 oz	180	5	—	18	—
TAKE-OUT						
deviled	2 halves	145	13	180	1	—
salad	½ cup	307	28	565	2	—
sandwich w/ cheese	1	340	19	804	26	—
sandwich w/ cheese & ham	1	348	16	1005	31	—
scotch egg	1 (4.2 oz)	301	21	—	16	2

EGG SUBSTITUTES

FOOD	PORTION	CAL.	FAT	SOD.	CARB.	FIB.
Egg Beaters						
Eggs Substitute	¼ cup	25	0	80	1	0
Omelette Cheese	½ cup	110	5	480	2	—
Omelette Vegetable	½ cup	50	0	170	5	—
Healthy Choice						
Cholesterol Free	¼ cup (2 oz)	25	0	95	tr	0
LaLoma						
Scramblers Links Muffins	1 pkg (4 oz)	220	10	400	22	—
Morningstar Farms						
Better'n Eggs	¼ cup (57 g)	30	0	100	1	—
Scramblers	¼ cup (57 g)	60	3	125	3	—
Scramblers Cheese Home Fries	1 pkg (5 oz)	210	9	310	20	—
Scramblers Links Hash Browns	1 pkg (5 oz)	240	13	580	20	—
Scramblers Sandwich w/ Cheese	1 (3.5 oz)	220	7	420	29	—
Scramblers Sandwich w/ Pattie	1 (4.5 oz)	300	12	590	29	—
Scramblers Sandwich w/ Pattie Cheese	1 (5 oz)	350	15	780	33	—

FOOD	PORTION	CAL.	FAT	SOD.	CARB.	FIB.
Second Nature						
No Cholesterol	2 fl oz	60	2	90	3	—
No Fat	2 fl oz	40	0	100	3	—
No Fat With Garden Vegetables	2.5 fl oz	40	0	100	4	—
frozen	¼ cup	96	7	120	2	—
frozen	1 cup	384	27	479	8	—
liquid	1 cup	211	8	444	2	—
liquid	1½ oz	40	2	83	tr	—
powder	0.7 oz	88	3	158	4	—
powder	0.35 oz	44	1	79	2	—

EGGNOG

FOOD	PORTION	CAL.	FAT	SOD.	CARB.	FIB.
Borden						
	4 fl oz	160	9	80	16	—
Light	½ cup	130	2	80	23	—
Hood						
Fat Free	4 fl oz	100	0	100	21	0
Golden	4 fl oz	180	8	100	22	0
Light	4 fl oz	120	2	105	23	0
Select	4 fl oz	210	12	100	22	0
eggnog	1 qt	1368	76	553	138	—
eggnog	1 cup	342	19	138	34	—
eggnog flavor mix as prep w/ milk	9 oz	260	8	163	39	—

EGGPLANT

CANNED

FOOD	PORTION	CAL.	FAT	SOD.	CARB.	FIB.
Progresso						
Caponata	2 tbsp (1 oz)	30	2	130	2	2
FRESH						
cubed cooked	½ cup	13	tr	2	3	—
raw cut up	½ cup (1.4 oz)	11	tr	1	2	—
slices cooked	4 (7 oz)	38	0	—	0	—
whole peeled raw	1 (1 lb)	117	1	14	28	—
FROZEN						
Mrs. Paul's						
Parmigiana	5 oz	240	16	600	18	—
TAKE-OUT						
baba ghannouj	¼ cup	55	4	95	5	—

ELDERBERRIES

FOOD	PORTION	CAL.	FAT	SOD.	CARB.	FIB.
fresh	1 cup	105	1	—	27	—

ELDERBERRY JUICE

FOOD	PORTION	CAL.	FAT	SOD.	CARB.	FIB.
elderberry	3½ oz	38	0	1	8	—

FOOD	PORTION	CAL.	FAT	SOD.	CARB.	FIB.
ELK						
roasted	3 oz	124	2	52	0	—
ENDIVE						
fresh	3½ oz	9	tr	53	tr	2
raw chopped	½ cup	4	tr	6	1	—
ENGLISH MUFFIN						
FROZEN						
Great Starts						
Egg Beefsteak & Cheese	5.9 oz	360	20	730	27	—
Egg Canadian Bacon & Cheese	4.1 oz	290	15	770	25	—
Weight Watchers						
Sandwich With Egg Ham & Cheese	1 (4 oz)	230	8	590	25	—
HOME RECIPE						
cinnamon raisin	1	186	3	123	38	—
english muffin	1	158	2	122	30	—
honey bran	1	153	3	154	30	—
whole wheat	1	167	tr	135	34	—
READY-TO-EAT						
Arnold						
Extra Crisp	1	130	1	230	26	1
Sourdough	1	130	1	250	25	1
Matthew's						
9 Grain & Nut	1	140	4	220	26	5
Cinnamon Raisin	1	160	2	290	33	4
Golden White	1	140	4	340	23	1
Whole Wheat	1	150	2	340	31	4
Pepperidge Farm						
Cinnamon Apple	1	140	1	210	27	—
Cinnamon Chip	1	160	3	180	28	—
Cinnamon Raisin	1	150	2	200	29	—
Plain	1	140	1	220	27	—
Sourdough	1	135	1	260	27	—
Roman Meal						
English Muffin	1 (2.2 oz)	135	1	332	25	3
Tastykake						
Cinnamon Raisin	1 (64 g)	150	1	150	31	—
Sourdough	1 (57 g)	130	1	210	25	—
Thomas'						
Honey Wheat	1	128	1	199	24	—
Oat Bran	1	116	1	192	26	3
Raisin Cinnamon	1	151	1	183	31	—

FOOD	PORTION	CAL.	FAT	SOD.	CARB.	FIB.
Thomas' (CONT.)						
Regular	1	130	1	206	25	—
Sandwich Size	1 (92 g)	210	2	330	42	2
Sour Dough	1	131	1	210	25	—
Wonder						
Raisin Rounds	1 (2.1 oz)	150	2	240	30	2
Sourdough	1 (2 oz)	120	1	290	25	1
apple cinnamon	1	138	2	255	28	—
granola	1	155	1	275	31	—
mixed grain	1	155	1	275	31	—
plain	1	134	1	265	26	—
plain toasted	1	133	1	262	26	—
raisin cinnamon	1	138	2	255	28	—
sourdough	1	134	1	265	26	—
wheat	1	127	1	218	26	—
whole wheat	1	134	1	420	27	4
REFRIGERATED						
Roman Meal	½ muffin (1.1 oz)	66	tr	95	14	1
Honey Nut Oat Bran	½ muffin (1.1 oz)	81	1	114	16	1
TAKE-OUT						
w/ butter	1	189	6	386	30	—
w/ cheese & sausage	1	394	24	1036	29	—
w/ egg cheese & bacon	1	487	31	1135	31	—
w/ egg cheese & canadian bacon	1	383	20	785	31	—

EPPAW

FOOD	PORTION	CAL.	FAT	SOD.	CARB.	FIB.
raw	½ cup	75	1	6	16	—

FALAFEL

FOOD	PORTION	CAL.	FAT	SOD.	CARB.	FIB.
MIX						
Near East as prep	2½ patties	230	15	560	18	5
TAKE-OUT						
falafel	3 (1.8 oz)	170	9	150	16	—
falafel	1 (1.2 oz)	57	3	50	5	—

FAT

(*see also* BUTTER, BUTTER BLENDS, BUTTER SUBSTITUTES, MARGARINE, OIL)

FOOD	PORTION	CAL.	FAT	SOD.	CARB.	FIB.
Crisco	1 tbsp (0.4 oz)	110	12	0	0	—
Butter Flavor	1 tbsp	110	12	0	0	—
Sticks	1 tbsp (0.4 oz)	110	12	0	0	0
Sticks Butter Flavor	1 tbsp (0.4 oz)	110	12	0	0	0
Empire						
Chicken Fat Rendered	1 tbsp (0.5 oz)	120	13	0	tr	0

FOOD	PORTION	CAL.	FAT	SOD.	CARB.	FIB.
Wesson						
Shortening	1 tbsp	100	12	0	0	0
beef cooked	1 oz	193	20	12	0	—
beef suet	1 oz	242	27	—	0	—
beef tallow	1 tbsp (13 g)	115	13	0	0	—
chicken	1 cup	1846	205	—	0	—
chicken	1 tbsp	115	13	—	0	—
cocoa butter	1 tbsp	120	14	—	0	—
duck	1 tbsp	115	13	—	0	—
goose	3.5 oz	900	100	—	0	—
goose	1 tbsp	115	13	—	0	—
lamb new zealand raw	1 oz	182	19	6	0	—
lard	1 tbsp (13 g)	115	13	0	0	—
lard	1 cup (205 g)	1849	205	tr	0	—
nutmeg butter	1 tbsp	120	14	—	0	—
pork backfat	1 oz	230	25	—	—	—
pork cooked	1 oz	200	21	9	0	—
pork cured	1 oz	164	17	—	—	—
pork cured roasted	1 oz	167	18	—	—	—
salt pork	1 oz	212	23	404	0	—
shortening	1 tbsp	113	13	—	0	—
shortening	1 cup	1812	205	—	0	—
turkey	1 tbsp	115	13	—	0	—
ucuhuba butter	1 tbsp	120	14	—	0	—
FAVA BEANS						
CANNED						
Progresso	½ cup	90	tr	420	15	12
FEIJOA						
fresh	1 (1.75 oz)	25	tr	2	5	—
puree	1 cup	119	2	7	26	—
FENNEL						
fresh bulb	1 (8.2 oz)	72	tr	122	17	—
fresh sliced	1 cup	27	tr	45	6	—
leaves	3.5 oz	24	tr	86	3	4
seed	1 tsp	7	tr	2	1	—
FENUGREEK						
seed	1 tsp	12	tr	2	2	—
FIBER						
Delta						
Natural Fiber	½ cup (1 oz)	20	tr	20	2	20
FIGS						
CANNED						
S&W						
Kadota Figs Whole Fancy	½ cup	100	0	—	28	—

FOOD	PORTION	CAL.	FAT	SOD.	CARB.	FIB.
in heavy syrup	3	75	tr	1	19	—
in light syrup	3	58	tr	1	15	—
water pack	3	42	tr	1	11	—
DRIED						
Sonoma						
White Misson	3-4 (1.4 oz)	110	0	0	26	5
cooked	½ cup	140	1	6	16	—
whole	10	477	2	20	122	17
FRESH						
fig	1 med	50	tr	1	10	—

FISH

(*see also* FISH SUBSTITUTES, INDIVIDUAL NAMES, SUSHI)

FOOD	PORTION	CAL.	FAT	SOD.	CARB.	FIB.
CANNED						
Holmes						
Finest Kippered Snacks drained	1 can (3.2 oz)	135	8	470	0	0
Port Clyde						
Fish Steaks In Louisiana Hot Sauce	1 can (3.75 oz)	150	9	960	2	0
Fish Steaks In Mustard Sauce	1 can (3.75 oz)	140	7	540	1	0
Fish Steaks In Soybean Oil drained	1 can (3.3 oz)	220	17	360	0	0
Fish Steaks In Soybean Oil With Hot Chilies drained	1 can (3.3 oz)	155	8	420	0	0
Progresso						
Mixed Seafood Sauce	½ cup	110	6	445	12	—
Seafood	½ cup	190	15	570	5	tr
FROZEN						
Cajun Cookin'						
Seafood Gumbo	17 oz	330	7	1330	51	—
Gorton's						
Crispy Batter Dipped Fillets	2	290	19	550	18	—
Crispy Batter Sticks	4	260	18	480	16	—
Crunch Fillets	2	230	13	420	16	—
Crunchy Sticks	4	210	13	240	15	—
Light Recipe Lightly Breaded Fish Fillets	1 fillet	180	8	380	16	—
Light Recipe Tempura Fillets	1 fillet	200	14	400	8	—
Microwave Crispy Batter Large Cut Fillets	1	320	21	680	20	—

FOOD	PORTION	CAL.	FAT	SOD.	CARB.	FIB.
Gorton's (CONT.)						
Microwave Entree Fillets In Herb Butter	1 pkg	190	8	450	3	—
Microwave Fillets	2	340	26	400	17	—
Microwave Larger Cut Fillets	1	320	22	500	20	—
Microwave Larger Cut Ranch Fillet	1	330	21	520	24	—
Microwave Sticks	6	340	22	420	24	—
Potato Crisp Fillets	2	300	20	360	18	—
Potato Crisp Sticks	4	260	16	390	21	—
Value Pack Portions	1 portion	180	11	490	13	—
Value Pack Sticks	4	190	9	420	17	—
Kineret						
Fish Sticks	5 pieces (4 oz)	280	14	430	27	1
Mrs. Paul's						
Buttered Fillet Microwave	1 fillet	80	4	130	10	—
Entree Light Seafood Dijon	8¾ oz	200	5	650	17	—
Entree Light Seafood Florentine	8 oz	220	8	820	10	—
Entree Light Seafood Mornay	9 oz	230	10	670	12	—
Fillet Sandwich Microwave	1	280	15	460	27	—
Fillets Microwave	1 fillet	280	19	390	16	—
Fish Cakes	2	190	7	690	24	—
Fish Fillets Batter Dipped	2 fillets	330	17	650	28	—
Fish Fillets Crispy Crunchy	2 fillets	220	9	380	23	—
Fish Fillets Crunchy Batter	2 fillets	280	14	730	26	—
Fish Sticks 40 Crunchy	4 (2.75 oz)	200	10	340	18	—
Fish Sticks Crispy Crunchy	4 sticks	190	8	560	18	—
Fish Sticks Microwave	5	290	20	330	18	—
In Butter Sauce Light Fillets	1 fillet	140	6	520	1	—
Portions Battered Fish	2 portions	300	19	540	21	—
Portions Crispy Crunchy Breaded Fish	2 portions	230	15	300	14	—
Seafood Platter Combination	9 oz	600	33	408	55	—

FOOD	PORTION	CAL.	FAT	SOD.	CARB.	FIB.
Mrs. Paul's (CONT.)						
Sticks Battered Fish	4 sticks	210	12	590	15	—
Sticks Crispy Crunchy Breaded Fish	4 sticks	140	6	340	14	—
Van De Kamp's						
Crispy Microwave Fillets	1 piece	140	9	210	9	—
Crispy Microwave Fish Sticks	3 pieces	130	7	280	11	—
Crispy Microwave Large Fillets	1 piece	290	17	640	21	—
Fish Fillets Battered	1	170	10	350	13	—
Fish Fillets Breaded	2	280	18	280	18	—
Fish Sticks Battered	4	160	9	350	12	—
Fish Sticks Breaded	4	200	12	290	15	—
Fish Sticks Breaded Value Pack	4	170	10	270	13	—
breaded fillet	1 (2 oz)	155	7	332	14	—
sticks	1 stick (1 oz)	76	3	163	7	—
MIX						
Golden Dipt						
Beer Batter Fry	1 oz	100	0	650	22	—
Cajun Style Fish Fry	⅔ oz	60	0	470	14	—
Fish & Chips Batter Mix	1¼ oz	120	0	910	27	—
Fish Fry	⅔ oz	60	0	430	14	—
Seafood Frying Mix	⅔ oz	60	0	600	14	—
Tempura Batter Mix	1 oz	100	0	130	22	—
TAKE-OUT						
fish cake	1 (4.7 oz)	166	7	—	6	—
kedgeree	5.6 oz	242	11	—	15	1
sandwich w/ tartar sauce	1	431	55	615	41	—
sandwich w/ tartar sauce & cheese	1	524	29	939	48	—
stew	1 cup (7.9 oz)	157	4	—	10	—
taramasalata	3.5 oz	446	46	—	4	—

FISH PASTE

FOOD	PORTION	CAL.	FAT	SOD.	CARB.	FIB.
fish paste	2 tsp	15	1	—	tr	0

FISH SUBSTITUTES

FOOD	PORTION	CAL.	FAT	SOD.	CARB.	FIB.
LaLoma						
Ocean Platter mix not prep	¼ cup (16 g)	50	0	260	5	—
Worthington						
Fillets	2 (85 g)	180	9	910	9	—
Tuno	2 oz (57 g)	100	7	310	3	—

FOOD	PORTION	CAL.	FAT	SOD.	CARB.	FIB.
FLAXSEED						
Arrowhead	3 tbsp (1 oz)	140	10	0	11	6
Stone-Buhr	1 tsp (1 oz)	150	10	20	11	5
FLOUNDER						
FRESH						
cooked	1 fillet (4.5 oz)	148	2	133	0	—
cooked	3 oz	99	1	89	0	—
FROZEN						
Gorton's						
Fishmarket Fresh	5 oz	110	1	170	1	—
Microwave Entree Stuffed	1 pkg	350	18	850	21	—
Mrs. Paul's						
Crunchy Batter Fillets	2 fillets	220	9	560	23	—
Light Fillets	1 fillet	240	10	450	20	—
Van De Kamp's						
Light Fillets	1 piece	260	12	480	21	—
Natural Fillets	4 oz	100	2	100	0	—
TAKE-OUT						
battered & fried	3.2 oz	211	11	484	15	—
breaded & fried	3.2 oz	211	11	484	15	—
FLOUR						
Arrowhead						
Kamut	¼ cup (1.2 oz)	110	1	0	25	4
Pastry	⅓ cup (1.1 oz)	100	1	0	22	3
Rye Whole Grain	¼ cup (1.6 oz)	160	1	0	34	6
Spelt	¼ cup (1.2 oz)	100	1	0	24	5
Teff	¼ cup (1.4 oz)	140	1	5	29	5
Unbleached White	⅓ cup (1.6 oz)	160	1	0	33	0
Whole Grain Wheat	¼ cup (1.6 oz)	160	1	0	34	7
Whole Wheat	¼ cup (1.2 oz)	130	1	0	25	4
Aunt Jemima						
Self-Rising	3 tbsp	90	0	310	20	1
Ballard						
All Purpose	1 cup	400	1	0	87	—
Self-Rising	1 cup	380	1	1290	84	—
Ceresota						
All Purpose	1 cup	390	1	0	83	—
Whole Wheat	1 cup	400	2	0	80	—
General Mills						
Drifted Snow	1 cup	400	1	—	—	—
Softasilk	¼ cup	100	0	—	—	—

FOOD	PORTION	CAL.	FAT	SOD.	CARB.	FIB.
Gold Medal						
All Purpose	1 cup	400	1	0	87	—
La Pina	1 cup	390	1	—	—	—
Oat Blend	1 cup	390	3	0	81	—
Self-Rising	1 cup	380	1	1520	83	—
Unbleached	1 cup	400	1	0	87	—
Whole Wheat	1 cup	350	2	0	78	10
Whole Wheat Blend	1 cup	380	2	0	84	8
Heckers						
All Purpose	1 cup	390	1	0	83	—
Whole Wheat	1 cup	400	2	0	80	—
Hodgson Mill						
50/50 Flour	¼ cup (1 oz)	100	1	0	21	2
Best For Bread	¼ cup (1 oz)	100	0	0	22	1
Buckwheat	⅓ cup (1.6 oz)	160	1	10	33	2
Oat Bran Blend	¼ cup (1 oz)	110	1	120	24	3
Oat Bran Flour	¼ cup (1 oz)	110	2	4	23	3
Rye	¼ cup (1 oz)	90	1	0	22	5
Seasoned Flour	¼ cup (1 oz)	90	0	1360	20	0
White	¼ cup (1 oz)	100	0	0	23	3
Whole Wheat	¼ cup (1 oz)	100	1	0	22	3
King Arthur						
All Purpose Unbleached	¼ cup (1 oz)	100	0	0	22	tr
Pillsbury						
All Purpose Best	1 cup	400	1	0	87	—
Bohemian Style Rye and Wheat Best	1 cup	400	1	0	86	—
Bread Best	1 cup	400	2	0	83	—
Rye Medium Best	1 cup	400	2	0	83	—
Self-Rising Best	1 cup	380	1	1290	84	—
Shake & Blend Best	2 tbsp	50	0	0	11	—
Unbleached Best	1 cup	400	1	0	86	—
Whole Wheat Best	1 cup	400	2	10	80	—
Red Band						
All-Purpose	1 cup	390	1	—	—	—
Self-Rising	1 cup	380	1	—	—	—
Robin Hood						
All Purpose	1 cup	400	1	0	85	—
Rye Stone Ground	1 cup	360	2	10	86	13
Self-Rising	1 cup	380	1	1520	83	—
Unbleached	1 cup	400	1	0	85	—
Stone Ground Mills						
White Unbleached Organic	¼ cup (1.4 oz)	130	0	0	25	1

FOOD	PORTION	CAL.	FAT	SOD.	CARB.	FIB.
Stone Ground Mills (CONT.)						
Whole Wheat 100% Stone Ground	3 tbsp (1 oz)	90	1	0	20	3
White Deer						
All-Purpose	1 cup	400	1	—	—	—
corn masa	1 cup	416	4	6	87	—
corn whole grain	1 cup	422	5	6	90	8
cottonseed lowfat	1 oz	94	tr	10	10	—
peanut defatted	1 cup	196	tr	108	21	—
peanut defatted	1 oz	92	tr	50	10	—
peanut lowfat	1 cup	257	13	0	19	—
potato	1 cup (6.3 oz)	628	1	61	143	—
rice brown	1 cup	574	4	12	121	4
rice white	1 cup	578	2	1	127	2
rye dark	1 cup	415	3	2	88	—
rye light	1 cup	374	1	2	82	7
rye medium	1 cup	361	2	3	79	7
sesame lowfat	1 oz	95	tr	11	10	—
triticale whole grain	1 cup	440	2	3	95	9
white all-purpose	1 cup	455	1	2	95	2
white bread	1 cup	495	2	2	99	—
white cake	1 cup	395	tr	2	85	—
white self-rising	1 cup	442	1	1587	93	—
whole wheat	1 cup	407	2	6	87	8

FRANKFURTER
(see HOT DOG)

FRENCH BEANS

FOOD	PORTION	CAL.	FAT	SOD.	CARB.	FIB.
dried cooked	1 cup	228	1	11	43	—

FRENCH FRIES
(see POTATOES)

FRENCH TOAST
FROZEN

FOOD	PORTION	CAL.	FAT	SOD.	CARB.	FIB.
Aunt Jemima						
Cinnamon Swirl	2 pieces (4.1 oz)	240	6	330	37	2
Slices	2 pieces (4.1 oz)	240	6	360	38	1
Downyflake						
Extra Thick	1	150	9	340	11	—
Texas Style & Sausage	1 pkg (4.25 oz)	400	24	550	37	—
Great Starts						
Cinnamon Swirl With Sausage	5½ oz	390	21	530	37	—
French Toast With Sausage	5½ oz	380	21	550	35	—

FOOD	PORTION	CAL.	FAT	SOD.	CARB.	FIB.
Great Starts (CONT.)						
Mini French Toast With Sausage	2½ oz	190	9	320	22	—
Oatmeal French Toast With Lite Links	4.65 oz	310	13	500	35	—
Healthy Starts						
French Toast With LeanLinks	6.5 oz	400	13	595	51	—
Quaker						
French Toast Sticks & Syrup	1 pkg (5.2 oz)	400	20	640	48	—
French Toast Wedges & Sausage	1 pkg (5.3 oz)	360	17	780	40	—
Weight Watchers						
French Toast With Cinnamon	2 slices (3 oz)	160	5	280	24	—
French Toast With Links	4.5 oz	270	11	—	24	—
french toast	1 slice (2 oz)	126	4	292	19	2
HOME RECIPE						
as prep w/ 2% milk	1 slice	149	7	311	16	—
as prep w/ whole milk	1 slice	151	7	311	16	—
TAKE-OUT						
w/ butter	2 slices	356	19	513	36	—

FROG'S LEGS

frog leg as prep w/ seasoned flour & fried	1 (0.8)	70	5	—	15	—

FROSTING
(*see* CAKE)

FRUCTOSE

Estee	1 pkg (3 g)	10	0	0	3	—
Estee	1 tsp (4 g)	15	0	0	4	—

FRUIT DRINKS
(*see also* LEMONADE)
FROZEN

Bright & Early						
Fruit Punch	8 fl oz	130	0	5	31	—
Dole						
100% Juice Blend Country Raspberry as prep	8 fl oz	140	0	30	34	0
100% Juice Blend Orchard Peach as prep	8 fl oz	140	0	30	34	0

FOOD	PORTION	CAL.	FAT	SOD.	CARB.	FIB.
Dole (CONT.)						
Mountain Cherry 100% Juice Blend as prep	8 fl oz	120	0	30	30	0
Pineapple Grapefruit as prep	8 fl oz	130	0	20	29	0
Pineapple Orange as prep	8 fl oz	120	0	20	29	0
Pineapple Orange Banana as prep	8 fl oz	130	0	20	32	0
Pineapple Orange Guava as prep	8 fl oz	120	0	20	30	0
Pineapple Passion Banana as prep	8 fl oz	120	0	20	30	0
Tropical Fruit as prep	8 fl oz	140	0	30	34	0
Five Alive						
Berry Citrus	8 fl oz	120	0	0	30	—
Citrus	8 fl oz	120	0	0	30	—
Tropical Citrus	8 fl oz	120	0	25	29	—
Minute Maid						
Berry Punch	8 fl oz	130	0	5	31	—
Citrus Punch	8 fl oz	120	0	5	31	—
Fruit Punch	8 fl oz	120	0	5	31	—
Limeade	8 fl oz	100	0	0	26	—
Pineapple Orange	8 fl oz	120	0	0	31	—
Tropical Punch	8 fl oz	120	0	5	31	—
Seneca						
Cranberry-Apple Juice Cocktail frzn as prep	8 fl oz	140	0	0	33	0
Raspberry-Cranberry Juice Cocktail frzn as prep	8 fl oz	140	0	35	36	0
Tree Top						
Apple Citrus as prep	6 oz	90	0	10	22	—
Apple Cranberry as prep	6 oz	100	0	10	25	—
Apple Grape as prep	6 oz	100	0	10	25	—
Apple Pear as prep	6 oz	90	0	10	22	—
Apple Raspberry as prep	6 oz	80	0	10	21	—
citrus juice drink as prep	1 cup	114	0	7	28	—
citrus juice drink not prep	1 can (12 fl oz)	684	tr	12	171	—
fruit punch as prep w/ water	1 cup	113	tr	11	29	—
fruit punch not prep	1 can (12 fl oz)	678	tr	34	173	—
limeade	1 can (6 oz)	408	tr	—	108	—
limeade as prep w/ water	1 cup	102	tr	6	27	—

FOOD	PORTION	CAL.	FAT	SOD.	CARB.	FIB.
MIX						
Crystal Light						
Berry Blend Sugar Free	8 oz	3	0	—	0	—
Fruit Punch Sugar Free	8 oz	3	0	—	0	—
Lemon-Lime	8 oz	4	0	—	0	—
Tropic Quencher	8 oz	5	0	—	0	—
Kool-Aid						
Lemon-Lime	8 oz	98	0	—	25	—
Purplesaurus Rex	8 oz	98	0	6	25	—
Rainbow Punch	8 oz	98	0	—	25	—
Sharkleberry Fin	8 oz	98	0	—	25	—
Sugar Free Berry Blue	8 oz	3	0	6	0	—
Sugar Free Berry Punch	8 oz	3	0	33	0	—
Sugar Free Purplesaurus Rex	8 oz	3	0	6	0	—
Sugar Free Rainbow Punch	8 oz	4	0	—	0	—
Sugar Free Sharkleberry Fin	8 oz	3	0	—	0	—
Sugar Free Tropical Punch	8 oz	3	0	8	0	—
Sugar Sweetened Mountain Berry Punch	8 oz	98	0	15	25	—
Sugar Sweetened Purplesaurus Rex	8 oz	84	0	6	21	—
Sugar Sweetened Rainbow Punch	8 oz	84	0	20	21	—
Sugar Sweetened Sharkleberry Fin	8 oz	84	0	—	21	—
Sugar Sweetened Sunshine Punch	8 oz	83	0	—	21	—
Sugar Sweetened Surfin' Berry Punch	8 oz	79	0	27	20	—
Sugar Sweetened Tropical Punch	8 oz	84	0	—	21	—
Tropical Punch	8 oz	98	0	—	25	—
Unsweetened Berry Blue	8 oz	98	0	6	25	—
Wylers						
Drink Mix Unsweetened Bunch O' Berries	8 oz	2	0	28	1	—
Drink Mix Unsweetened Pink	8 oz	3	0	19	1	—
Drink Mix Unsweetened Tropical Punch	8 oz	2	0	tr	1	—

FOOD	PORTION	CAL.	FAT	SOD.	CARB.	FIB.
fruit punch as prep w/ water	9 oz	97	0	38	25	—
READY-TO-DRINK						
After The Fall						
Amaretto Almond	1 can (12 oz)	170	0	25	42	0
American Pie Cherry	1 can (12 oz)	190	0	20	35	0
Apple Apricot	1 cup (8 oz)	100	0	20	26	0
Apple Raspberry	1 bottle (10 oz)	110	0	25	29	—
Apple Strawberry	1 bottle (10 oz)	120	0	23	30	—
Banana Casablanca	1 bottle (10 oz)	120	0	13	24	—
Berrymeister	1 can (12 oz)	160	0	25	40	0
Cranberry Meets Raspberry	1 bottle (10 oz)	120	0	25	29	—
Georgia Peach Blend	1 bottle (10 oz)	130	0	23	33	—
Mango Montage	1 bottle (10 oz)	140	0	15	33	—
Maui Grove	1 bottle (10 oz)	120	0	20	29	—
Orange Icicle Cream	1 can (12 oz)	170	0	25	42	0
Oregon Berry	1 bottle (10 oz)	130	0	30	31	—
Passion Of The Islands	1 bottle (10 oz)	125	0	15	32	—
Peach Vanilla	1 can (12 oz)	170	0	35	42	0
Strawberry Vanilla	1 can (12 oz)	160	0	25	42	0
Twist O' Strawberry	1 can (12 oz)	190	0	25	37	0
Vanilla Bean Cream	1 can (12 oz)	170	0	25	42	0
Apple & Eve						
Apple Cranberry	6 fl oz	80	0	5	19	—
Apple Grape	6 fl oz	120	0	0	29	—
Cranberry Grape	6 fl oz	100	0	5	23	—
Fruit Punch	6 fl oz	78	0	0	18	—
Raspberry Cranberry	6 fl oz	90	0	10	21	—
BAMA						
Fruit Punch	8.45 fl oz	130	0	15	32	—
Boku						
White Grape Raspberry	16 fl oz	120	0	75	29	—
Chiquita						
Orange Banana	6 fl oz	90	0	—	—	—
Crystal Geyser						
Juice Squeeze Citrus Grape	1 bottle (12 fl oz)	145	0	20	35	—
Juice Squeeze Orange & Passion Fruit	1 bottle (12 fl oz)	130	0	20	31	—
Juice Squeeze Passion Fruit & Mango	1 bottle (12 fl oz)	125	0	20	31	—
Juice Squeeze Wild Berry	1 bottle (12 fl oz)	130	0	20	31	—

FOOD	PORTION	CAL.	FAT	SOD.	CARB.	FIB.
Dole						
Pineapple Orange	6 fl oz	90	0	10	22	—
Pineapple Orange Banana	6 fl oz	100	0	10	23	—
Pineapple Orange Guava	6 fl oz	100	0	10	21	—
Pineapple Passion Banana	6 fl oz	100	0	10	21	—
Five Alive						
Citrus	1 can (11.5 fl oz)	170	0	35	43	—
Citrus	6 fl oz	90	0	20	22	—
Citrus	1 bottle (16 fl oz)	120	0	25	31	—
Citrus Chilled	8 fl oz	120	0	25	30	—
Hawaiian Punch						
Fruit Juicy Red	6 fl oz	90	0	—	—	—
Island Fruit Cocktail	6 fl oz	90	0	—	—	—
Lite Fruit Juicy Red	6 fl oz	60	0	—	—	—
Tropical Fruits	6 fl oz	90	0	—	—	—
Very Berry	6 fl oz	90	0	—	—	—
Wild Fruit	6 fl oz	90	0	—	—	—
Hi-C						
Boppin' Berry Box	8.45 fl oz	140	0	30	33	—
Boppin' Berry	8 fl oz	130	0	30	32	—
Double Fruit Box	8.45 fl oz	130	0	35	32	—
Double Fruit Cooler	8 fl oz	130	0	30	31	—
Ecto Cooler	1 can (11.5 fl oz)	180	0	40	45	—
Ecto Cooler	8 fl oz	130	0	25	32	—
Ecto Cooler Box	8.45 fl oz	130	0	35	32	—
Fruit Punch	1 can (11.5 fl oz)	190	0	40	46	—
Fruit Punch	8 fl oz	130	0	30	32	—
Fruit Punch Box	8.45 fl oz	140	0	30	32	—
Fruity Bubble Gum	8 fl oz	120	0	25	30	—
Fruity Bubble Gum Box	8.45 fl oz	130	0	30	32	—
Hula Punch	8 fl oz	120	0	30	29	—
Hula Punch	1 can (11.5 fl oz)	170	0	40	42	—
Hula Punch Box	8.45 fl oz	120	0	30	30	—
Jammin' Apple Box	8.45 fl oz	130	0	30	33	—
Stompin' Banana Berry	8 fl oz	130	0	30	31	—
Stompin' Banana Berry Box	8.45 fl oz	130	0	30	32	—
Wild Berry	8 fl oz	120	0	30	30	—
Wild Berry Box	8.45 fl oz	130	0	30	32	—
Hood						
Natural Blenders Apple Cranberry Raspberry	1 cup (8 oz)	130	0	5	32	—

FOOD	PORTION	CAL.	FAT	SOD.	CARB.	FIB.
Hood (CONT.)						
Natural Blenders Apple Grape Cherry	1 cup (8 oz)	130	0	5	32	—
Natural Blenders Apple Peach Pear	1 cup (8 oz)	120	0	5	30	—
Natural Blenders Apple Wild Blueberry Strawberry	1 cup (8 oz)	120	0	5	30	—
Natural Blenders Pineapple Orange Kiwi	1 cup (8 oz)	120	0	5	30	—
Juice Works						
Appleberry	6 fl oz	100	0	—	—	—
Juicy Juice						
Apple Grape	1 box (8.45 fl oz)	120	0	10	29	—
Berry	1 box (8.45 fl oz)	130	0	15	30	—
Berry	1 bottle (6 fl oz)	90	0	10	22	—
Punch	1 bottle (6 fl oz)	100	0	10	23	—
Punch	1 box (8.45 fl oz)	140	0	10	33	—
Tropical	1 box (8.45 fl oz)	150	0	10	36	—
Tropical	1 bottle (6 fl oz)	110	0	10	26	—
Kern's						
Apple Strawberry Nectar	6 fl oz	110	0	0	26	—
Apricot Pineapple Nectar	6 fl oz	110	0	5	27	—
Banana Pineapple Nectar	6 fl oz	110	0	0	27	—
Coconut Pineapple Nectar	6 fl oz	140	0	25	26	—
Orange Banana Nectar	6 fl oz	110	0	0	25	—
Strawberry Banana Nectar	6 fl oz	110	0	0	28	—
Tropical Nectar	6 fl oz	110	0	5	27	—
Kool-Aid						
Koolers Mountainberry Punch	1 pkg (8.45 fl oz)	142	0	3	37	—
Koolers Rainbown Punch	1 pkg (8.45 fl oz)	135	0	3	36	—
Koolers Sharkleberry Fin	1 pkg (8.45 fl oz)	140	0	3	37	—
Koolers Tropical Punch	1 pkg (8.45 fl oz)	132	0	3	35	—
Libby						
Strawberry Banana Nectar	1 can (11.5 fl oz)	220	0	10	51	—
Lifesavers						
Fruit Punch	8 fl oz	140	0	25	34	—
Lime Punch	8 fl oz	140	0	25	34	—

FOOD	PORTION	CAL.	FAT	SOD.	CARB.	FIB.
Mauna La'i						
Island Guava Hawaiian Guava Fruit Juice Drink	8 fl oz	130	0	35	32	0
Mango & Hawaiian Guava Fruit Juice Drink	8 fl oz	130	0	35	33	0
Paradise Guava Hawaiian Guava & Passion Fruit Juice Drink	8 fl oz	130	0	35	32	0
Minute Maid						
Berry Punch Box	8.45 fl oz	130	0	25	31	—
Berry Punch Chilled	8 fl oz	130	0	25	31	—
Citrus Punch Chilled	8 fl oz	130	0	25	31	—
Fruit Punch Box	8.45 fl oz	120	0	25	31	—
Fruit Punch Chilled	8 fl oz	120	0	25	31	—
Juices To Go Citrus Punch	1 bottle (10 fl oz)	160	0	35	39	—
Juices To Go Citrus Punch	1 can (11.5 fl oz)	180	0	40	45	—
Juices To Go Concord Punch	1 bottle (10 fl oz)	160	0	35	40	—
Juices To Go Concord Punch	1 can (11.5 fl oz)	180	0	40	46	—
Juices To Go Concord Punch	1 bottle (16 fl oz)	130	0	25	32	—
Juices To Go Fruit Punch	1 can (11.5 fl oz)	180	0	40	44	—
Juices To Go Fruit Punch	1 bottle (10 fl oz)	160	0	35	39	—
Juices To Go Fruit Punch	1 bottle (16 fl oz)	120	0	25	31	—
Juices To Go Orange Blend	1 can (11.5 fl oz)	170	0	40	43	—
Juices To Go Orange Blend	1 bottle (10 fl oz)	150	0	35	37	—
Naturals Apple Cranberry	8 fl oz	170	0	25	42	—
Naturals Concord Medley	8 fl oz	130	0	25	32	—
Naturals Fruit Medley	8 fl oz	120	0	25	31	—
Naturals Orange Grape Medley	8 fl oz	120	0	25	30	—
Naturals Tropical Medley	8 fl oz	120	0	25	31	—
Tropical Punch Box	8.45 fl oz	130	0	25	32	—
Tropical Punch Chilled	8 fl oz	120	0	25	31	—

FOOD	PORTION	CAL.	FAT	SOD.	CARB.	FIB.
Mott's						
Apple Cranberry Blend	10 fl oz	180	0	15	44	0
Apple Cranberry From Concentrate as prep	8 fl oz	120	0	20	30	0
Apple Grape From Concentrate as prep	8 fl oz	120	0	20	30	0
Apple Raspberry Blend	10 fl oz	140	0	10	33	0
Apple Raspberry From Concentrate	8.45 fl oz	120	0	25	30	0
Fruit Basket Apple Raspberry Juice Cocktail as prep	8 fl oz	130	0	5	30	0
Fruit Basket Tropical Blend Juice Cocktail as prep	8 fl oz	120	0	5	30	0
Fruit Punch From Concentrate	8.45 fl oz	120	0	20	29	0
Fruit Punch From Concentrate	10 fl oz	170	0	0	42	0
Grape Apple	10 fl oz	170	0	10	41	0
Pineapple Orange	10 fl oz	170	0	15	42	0
Ocean Spray						
Cran.Blueberry	8 fl oz	160	0	35	41	0
Cran.Cherry	6 fl oz	160	0	35	39	0
Cran.Grape	8 fl oz	170	0	35	41	0
Cran.Raspberry	8 fl oz	140	0	35	36	0
Cran.Raspberry Reduced Calorie	8 fl oz	50	0	35	13	0
Cran.Strawberry	8 fl oz	140	0	35	36	tr
Cranapple	8 fl oz	160	0	35	41	tr
Cranapple Reduced Calorie	8 fl oz	50	0	35	13	0
Cranicot	8 fl oz	160	0	35	40	0
Crantastic	8 fl oz	150	0	35	37	0
Fruit Punch	8 fl oz	130	0	35	32	0
Lightstyle Low Calorie Cran.Grape	8 fl oz	40	0	35	9	0
Lightstyle Low Calorie Cran.Raspberry	8 fl oz	40	0	35	10	0
Refreshers Juice Drink Citrus Cranberry	8 fl oz	140	0	35	35	0
Refreshers Juice Drink Citrus Peach	8 fl oz	120	0	35	30	0
Refreshers Juice Drink Orange Cranberry	8 fl oz	130	0	35	33	0

FOOD	PORTION	CAL.	FAT	SOD.	CARB.	FIB.
Ocean Spray (CONT.)						
Ruby Red & Tangerine Grapefruit Juice Cocktail	8 fl oz	130	0	35	32	0
Odwalla						
Boyzenberry Mango	8 fl oz	140	0	20	34	2
C Monster	16 fl oz	300	0	110	72	4
Fruitshake Blackberry	8 fl oz	160	0	50	39	3
Guanaba Dabba Doo!	8 fl oz	130	0	35	29	0
Lotta Colada	8 fl oz	160	3	45	33	2
Mango Tango	8 fl oz	150	3	55	37	6
Mo Beta	16 fl oz	280	1	290	69	3
Raspberry Smoothie	8 fl oz	140	0	25	35	2
Strawberry Banana Smoothie	8 fl oz	100	0	10	26	2
Strawberry Go Man Go	8 fl oz	100	1	25	26	2
Super Protein	16 fl oz	400	6	250	40	5
Pek						
Mango Guava Ecstasy	1 bottle (20 fl oz)	110	0	20	27	0
Passionate Peach Grapefruit	8 fl oz	110	0	20	27	0
S&W						
Apricot Pineapple Nectar	6 fl oz	120	0	10	29	—
Apricot Pineapple Nectar Diet	6 fl oz	80	0	10	20	—
Sipps						
Fruit Punch	8.45 oz	130	0	—	—	—
Lemon Lime Cooler	8.45 oz	130	0	—	—	—
Mixed Berry	8.45 oz	130	0	—	—	—
Sunshine Punch	8.45 oz	130	0	—	—	—
Smucker's						
Apple Cranberry	8 oz	120	0	10	32	—
Orange Banana	8 oz	120	0	10	30	—
Snapple						
Diet Kiwi Strawberry	8 fl oz	13	0	10	3	—
Fruit Punch	8 fl oz	120	0	5	29	—
Kiwi Strawberry Cocktail	8 fl oz	130	0	10	33	—
Melonberry Cocktail	8 fl oz	120	0	10	29	—
Vitamin Supreme	10 fl oz	150	0	20	38	—
Squeezit						
Berry B. Wild	1 (6.75 fl oz)	90	0	0	22	—
Chucklin' Cherry	1 (6.75 fl oz)	90	0	5	23	—
Grumpy Grape	1 (6.75 fl oz)	90	0	0	23	—
Mean Green Puncher	1 (6.75 fl oz)	90	0	0	23	—

FOOD	PORTION	CAL.	FAT	SOD.	CARB.	FIB.
Squeezit (CONT.)						
Silly Billy Strawberry	1 (6.75 fl oz)	90	0	0	23	—
Smarty Arty Orange	1 (6.75 fl oz)	90	0	50	23	—
Sunny Delight						
Drink	6 fl oz	90	0	—	—	—
Tang						
Mixed Fruit	8.45 fl oz	137	0	2	36	—
Tree Top						
Apple Citrus	6 fl oz	90	0	10	22	—
Apple Cranberry	6 fl oz	100	0	10	25	—
Apple Grape	6 fl oz	100	0	10	25	—
Apple Pear	6 fl oz	90	0	10	22	—
Apple Raspberry	6 fl oz	80	0	10	21	—
Tropicana						
Berry Punch	8 fl oz	120	0	25	29	—
Citrus Punch	1 bottle (10 fl oz)	180	0	15	45	—
Citrus Punch	8 fl oz	140	0	20	36	—
Cranberry Punch	1 can (11.5 fl oz)	200	0	15	49	—
Cranberry Punch	1 bottle (10 fl oz)	170	0	10	43	—
Cranberry Punch	8 fl oz	140	0	10	34	—
Fruit Punch	1 bottle (10 fl oz)	150	0	25	39	—
Fruit Punch	1 can (11.5 fl oz)	170	0	30	42	—
Fruit Punch	8 fl oz	130	0	25	31	—
Fruit Punch	1 container (10 fl oz)	160	0	25	39	—
Orange Pineapple	8 fl oz	110	0	15	27	—
Orange Pineapple	1 bottle (10 fl oz)	130	0	15	32	—
Pineapple Punch	8 fl oz	120	0	15	31	—
Pineapple Punch	1 bottle (10 fl oz)	160	0	20	39	—
Season's Best Cranberry Medley	8 fl oz	120	0	20	29	—
Tropics Apple Cranberry Kiwi	8 fl oz	120	0	15	30	—
Tropics Orange Strawberry Banana	8 fl oz	110	0	5	27	—
Tropics Orange Kiwi Passion	8 fl oz	100	0	15	26	—
Tropics Orange Peach Mango	8 fl oz	110	0	15	28	—
Tropics Orange Pineapple	8 fl oz	110	0	15	27	—
Tropics Pineapple Passion	8 fl oz	120	0	25	30	—
Twister Apple Raspberry Blackberry	8 fl oz	120	0	20	31	—

FOOD	PORTION	CAL.	FAT	SOD.	CARB.	FIB.
Tropicana (CONT.)						
Twister Apple Raspberry Blackberry	1 bottle (10 fl oz)	150	0	25	38	—
Twister Apple Raspberry Blackberry	1 can (11.5 fl oz)	180	0	25	44	—
Twister Cranberry Raspberry Strawberry	8 fl oz	120	0	5	31	—
Twister Cranberry Raspberry Strawberry	1 bottle (10 fl oz)	160	0	5	39	—
Twister Light Cranberry Raspberry Strawberry	8 fl oz	45	0	10	11	—
Twister Light Cranberry Raspberry Strawberry	1 container (10 fl oz)	50	0	15	13	—
Twister Light Orange Cranberry	8 fl oz	30	0	20	7	—
Twister Light Orange Cranberry	1 container (10 fl oz)	35	0	25	9	—
Twister Light Orange Raspberry	8 fl oz	35	0	20	9	—
Twister Light Orange Raspberry	1 container (10 fl oz)	45	0	25	11	—
Twister Light Orange Strawberry Banana	8 fl oz	35	0	20	9	—
Twister Light Orange Strawberry Banana	1 container (10 fl oz)	45	0	25	11	—
Twister Orange Cranberry	1 container (10 fl oz)	140	0	20	35	—
Twister Orange Cranberry	1 bottle (10 fl oz)	140	0	20	36	—
Twister Orange Cranberry	8 fl oz	120	0	15	29	—
Twister Orange Peach	1 can (11.5 fl oz)	160	0	20	41	—
Twister Orange Peach	1 bottle (10 fl oz)	140	0	25	36	—
Twister Orange Peach	8 fl oz	120	0	20	29	—
Twister Orange Raspberry	1 bottle (10 fl oz)	140	0	20	36	—
Twister Orange Raspberry	8 fl oz	120	0	20	29	—
Twister Orange Strawberry Banana	1 container (10 fl oz)	140	0	20	35	—
Twister Strawberry Banana	1 bottle (10 fl oz)	140	0	20	35	—
Twister Strawberry Banana	8 fl oz	120	0	20	29	—

FOOD	PORTION	CAL.	FAT	SOD.	CARB.	FIB.
Tropicana (CONT.)						
Twister Strawberry Banana	1 can (11.5 fl oz)	160	0	30	41	—
Twister Strawberry Guava	1 bottle (10 fl oz)	140	0	25	35	—
Twister Strawberry Guava	8 fl oz	110	0	20	28	—
Veryfine						
Apple Cherryberry	8 fl oz	130	0	<25	33	—
Apple Cranberry	8 fl oz	130	0	<10	33	—
Apple Raspberry	8 fl oz	110	0	<15	27	—
Fruit Punch	8 fl oz	130	0	<35	33	—
Guava Strawberry	8 fl oz	120	0	<25	30	—
Lemon & Lime	8 fl oz	120	0	<10	30	—
Papaya Punch	8 fl oz	120	0	<10	30	—
Passionfruit Orange	8 fl oz	110	0	<25	26	—
Pineapple Orange	8 fl oz	130	0	<10	32	—
White House						
Apple Cherry	6 fl oz	90	0	10	22	0
cranberry apple drink	6 fl oz	123	0	4	32	—
cranberry apricot drink	6 fl oz	118	0	4	30	—
fruit punch	6 fl oz	87	tr	41	22	—
orange & apricot	8 fl oz	128	tr	—	32	—
orange grapefruit juice	8 fl oz	107	tr	8	25	—
pineapple & grapefruit	8 fl oz	117	tr	14	29	—
pineapple & orange drink	8 fl oz	125	0	9	29	—

FRUIT MIXED
(*see also individual names*)

CANNED

FOOD	PORTION	CAL.	FAT	SOD.	CARB.	FIB.
Del Monte						
Fruit Cocktail Fruit Naturals	½ cup (4.4 oz)	60	0	10	15	1
Fruit Cocktail In Heavy Syrup	½ cup (4.5 oz)	100	0	10	24	1
Fruit Cocktail Lite	½ cup (4.4 oz)	60	0	10	15	1
Lite Mixed Fruits Chunky	½ cup (4.4 oz)	60	0	10	15	1
Mixed Fruits Chunky Fruit Naturals	½ cup (4.4 oz)	60	0	10	15	1
Mixed Fruits Chunky In Heavy Syrup	½ cup (4.5 oz)	100	0	10	24	1
Snack Cups Mixed Fruit Fruit Naturals	1 serv (4.5 oz)	60	0	10	16	1
Snack Cups Mixed Fruit Fruit Naturals EZ-Open Lid	1 serv (4.5 oz)	60	0	10	15	1

FOOD	PORTION	CAL.	FAT	SOD.	CARB.	FIB.
Del Monte (CONT.)						
Snack Cups Mixed Fruit In Heavy Syrup	1 serv (4.5 oz)	100	0	10	24	1
Snack Cups Mixed Fruit In Heavy Syrup EZ-Open Lid	1 serv (4.2 oz)	90	0	10	23	1
Snack Cups Mixed Fruit Lite	1 serv (4.5 oz)	60	0	10	16	1
Snack Cups Mixed Fruit Lite EZ-Open Lid	1 serv (4.5 oz)	60	0	10	15	1
Dole						
Tropical Fruit Salad	½ cup	70	0	10	17	—
Hunt's						
Fruit Cocktail	4 oz	90	tr	7	23	tr
Libby						
Chunky Mixed Lite	½ cup (4.3 oz)	60	0	5	14	1
Fruit Cocktail Lite	½ cup (4.3 oz)	60	0	10	15	1
S&W						
Chunky Mixed Diet	½ cup	40	0	5	10	—
Chunky Mixed Natural Style	½ cup	90	0	5	21	—
Chunky Mixed Unsweetened	½ cup	40	0	5	10	—
Fruit Cocktail Diet	½ cup	40	0	5	10	—
Fruit Cocktail Heavy Syrup	½ cup	90	0	15	24	—
Fruit Cocktail Natural Lite	½ cup	60	0	5	15	—
Fruit Cocktail Natural Style	½ cup	90	0	5	21	—
Fruit Cocktail Unsweetened	½ cup	40	0	5	10	—
fruit cocktail in heavy syrup	½ cup	93	tr	7	24	—
fruit cocktail juice pack	½ cup	56	tr	4	15	—
fruit cocktail water pack	½ cup	40	tr	5	10	—
fruit salad in heavy syrup	½ cup	94	tr	7	24	—
fruit salad in light syrup	½ cup	73	tr	7	19	—
fruit salad juice pack	½ cup	62	tr	7	16	—
fruit salad water pack	½ cup	37	tr	4	10	—
mixed fruit in heavy syrup	½ cup	92	tr	5	24	—
tropical fruit salad in heavy syrup	½ cup	110	tr	3	29	—
DRIED						
Del Monte						
Mixed	⅓ cup (1.4 oz)	110	0	50	30	5

FOOD	PORTION	CAL.	FAT	SOD.	CARB.	FIB.
Planters						
Fruit'n Nut Mix	1 oz	140	9	105	13	2
Sonoma						
Diced	⅓ cup (1.4 oz)	120	0	0	31	3
Trail Mix	¼ cup (1.4 oz)	160	7	5	24	2
mixed	11 oz pkg	712	1	52	188	—
FROZEN						
Big Valley						
Burst O' Berries	⅔ cup (4.9 oz)	70	0	0	16	3
California Tropics	⅔ cup (4.9 oz)	60	0	0	15	2
Cup A Fruit	1 pkg (4 oz)	50	0	0	7	2
Mixed	4.9 oz	60	0	0	14	2
Birds Eye						
Mixed Fruit	½ cup	120	0	5	31	1
Dole						
Applesauce Strawberry	1 pkg (4 oz)	60	0	0	15	1
mixed fruit sweetened	1 cup	245	tr	8	61	—
FRUIT SNACKS						
Betty Crocker						
String Thing Berry 'N Blue	1 pkg (0.7 oz)	80	1	40	17	—
String Thing Cherry	1 pkg (0.7 oz)	80	1	40	17	—
String Thing Strawberry	1 pkg (0.7 oz)	80	1	40	17	—
Brock						
Beauty & The Beast	1 pkg (0.9 oz)	90	0	25	21	—
Cinderella	1 pkg (0.9 oz)	90	0	25	21	—
Dinosaurs	1 pkg (0.9 oz)	90	0	25	21	—
Ninja Trolls	1 pkg (0.9 oz)	90	0	25	21	—
Sharks	1 pkg (0.9 oz)	90	0	25	21	—
Del Monte						
Sierra Trail Mix	1 pkg (1 oz)	120	6	50	16	2
Sierra Trail Mix	1 pkg (0.9 oz)	110	6	45	15	2
Sierra Trail Mix	¼ cup (1.2 oz)	150	8	65	20	3
Fruit By The Foot						
Cherry	1	80	2	45	18	—
Grape	1	80	2	45	18	—
Strawberry	1	80	2	45	18	—
Fruit Roll-Ups						
Cherry	1 (½ oz)	50	tr	40	12	—
Crazy Colors	1 (½ oz)	50	tr	40	12	—
Fruit Punch	1 (½ oz)	50	tr	40	12	—
Grape	1 (½ oz)	50	tr	40	12	—
Raspberry	1 (½ oz)	50	tr	40	12	—

FOOD	PORTION	CAL.	FAT	SOD.	CARB.	FIB.
Fruit Roll-Ups (CONT.)						
Strawberry	1 (½ oz)	50	tr	40	12	—
General Mills						
Garfield And Friends 1-2 Punch	1 pkg	100	1	60	22	—
Garfield And Friends Cat Cooler	1 pkg	100	1	60	22	—
Garfield And Friends Fat Cat Funnies	1 (½ oz)	50	tr	20	12	—
Garfield And Friends Fruit Party	1 (½ oz)	50	tr	40	12	—
Garfield And Friends Very Strawberry	1 pkg	100	1	60	22	—
Shark Bites & Berry Bears Assorted Fruit	1 pkg	100	tr	20	22	—
Shark Bites & Berry Bears Fruit Punch	1 pkg	100	tr	20	22	—
Surf's Up! Sun Splash	1 pkg	100	1	30	22	—
Surf's Up! Tutti Frutti	1 pkg	100	1	20	22	—
Thunder Jets Assorted Fruit Squadron	1 pkg	100	1	30	24	—
Thunder Jets Mach 1 Fruit Mix	1 pkg	100	1	30	24	—
Health Valley						
Bakes Apple	1 bar	100	3	25	16	3
Bakes Date	1 bar	100	3	25	16	3
Bakes Raisin	1 bar	100	3	20	16	3
Fat Free Fruit Bars 100% Organic Apple	1 bar	140	tr	10	33	4
Fat Free Fruit Bars 100% Organic Apricot	1 bar	140	tr	10	33	4
Fat Free Fruit Bars 100% Organic Date	1 bar	140	tr	10	33	4
Fat Free Fruit Bars 100% Organic Raisin	1 bar	140	tr	10	33	4
Fruit & Fitness Bars	2 bars	200	5	75	35	5
Oat Bran Bakes Apricot	1 bar	100	3	15	16	2
Oat Bran Bakes Fig & Nut	1 bar	110	3	10	16	2
Oat Bran Jumbo Fruit Bar Almond & Date	1 bar	170	5	10	28	7
Oat Bran Jumbo Fruit Bar Raisin & Cinnamon	1 bar	160	2	10	32	6

FOOD	PORTION	CAL.	FAT	SOD.	CARB.	FIB.
Health Valley (CONT.)						
Rice Bran Jumbo Fruit Bar Almond & Date	1 bar	160	5	5	27	4
Lipton						
Hanna Barbera Flintstones	1 pkg (1 oz)	100	0	15	22	—
Hanna Barbera Jetsons	1 pkg (1 oz)	100	0	15	22	—
Hanna Barbera Yo Yogi!	1 pkg (1 oz)	100	0	15	22	—
Tiny Toons Bunch Of Berries	1 pkg (0.9 oz)	100	1	10	22	—
Tiny Toons Fruit Assortment	1 pkg (0.9 oz)	100	1	10	22	—
Tiny Toons Paaaarrrty Punch	1 pkg (0.9 oz)	100	1	10	22	—
Sovex						
Fruit Bites Jungle Pals	1 pkg (0.9 oz)	90	1	15	21	—
Stretch Island						
Fruit Leather Berry Blackberry	2 pieces (1 oz)	90	0	0	24	3
Fruit Leather Chunky Cherry	2 pieces (1 oz)	90	0	0	24	2
Fruit Leather Great Grape	2 pieces (1 oz)	90	0	0	24	2
Fruit Leather Organic Apple	2 pieces (1 oz)	90	0	10	24	2
Fruit Leather Organic Grape	2 pieces (1 oz)	90	0	5	24	2
Fruit Leather Organic Raspberry	2 pieces (1 oz)	90	0	10	25	2
Fruit Leather Rare Raspberry	2 pieces (1 oz)	90	0	0	24	2
Fruit Leather Snappy Apple	2 pieces (1 oz)	90	0	0	25	3
Fruit Leather Tangy Apricot	2 pieces (1 oz)	90	0	0	23	2
Fruit Leather Truly Tropical	2 pieces (1 oz)	90	0	0	22	1
Sunbelt						
Fruit Boosters Apple	1 (1.3 oz)	130	2	60	27	0
Fruit Boosters Blueberry	1 (1.3 oz)	130	2	60	27	1
Fruit Boosters Strawberry	1 (1.3 oz)	130	2	65	27	0
Fruit Jammers	1 (1 oz)	100	1	20	23	0

FOOD	PORTION	CAL.	FAT	SOD.	CARB.	FIB.
Sunkist						
Fruit Flippits Cherry	0.8 oz	107	4	18	18	—
Fruit Flippits Strawberry	0.8 oz	107	4	18	18	—
Fruit Roll Apricot	1	76	1	17	18	0
Fruit Roll Cherry	1	75	tr	18	18	0
Fruit Roll Grape	1	76	tr	13	19	0
Fruit Roll Raspberry	1	75	tr	20	18	0
Fruit Roll Strawberry	1	74	tr	11	18	0
Fun Fruit Animals	0.9 oz	100	1	10	22	0
Fun Fruit Dinosaurs Strawberry	0.9 oz	100	1	10	22	0
Fun Fruit Galactic Gems	0.9 oz	100	1	10	22	—
Fun Fruit Mario Nintendo	0.9 oz	100	tr	10	22	—
Fun Fruit Meteorites	0.9 oz	100	1	10	22	—
Fun Fruit Spooky Fruit	1 pkg	100	1	10	22	0
Fun Fruit Strawberry	0.9 oz	100	1	10	22	—
Fun Fruit Wacky Players	0.9 oz	100	1	10	22	—
Weight Watchers						
Apple	½ oz	50	tr	140	13	—
Apple Chips	¾ oz	70	0	110	19	—
Cinnamon	½ oz	50	tr	140	13	—
Peach	½ oz	50	tr	140	13	—
Strawberry	½ oz	50	tr	140	13	—
fruit leather	1 bar (0.8 oz)	81	1	18	18	—
fruit leather pieces	1 oz	97	2	114	22	—
fruit leather pieces	1 pkg (0.9 oz)	92	2	109	21	—
fruit leather rolls	1 sm (0.5 oz)	49	tr	8	12	—
fruit leather rolls	1 lg (0.7 oz)	73	1	13	18	—

GARBANZO
(*see* CHICKPEAS)

GARLIC
Watkins						
Garlic & Chive Seasoning	1 tbsp (7 g)	25	2	280	2	0
Garlic Lover's Herb Blend	¼ tsp (0.5 oz)	0	0	0	0	0
Liquid Spice	1 tbsp (0.5 oz)	120	14	0	0	0
clove	1	4	tr	1	1	—
powder	1 tsp	9	tr	1	2	—

GEFILTE FISH
READY-TO-USE
| *Manischewitz* | 1 piece | 107 | 4 | — | 4 | — |

FOOD	PORTION	CAL.	FAT	SOD.	CARB.	FIB.
Manischewitz (CONT.)						
Gefiltefish & Pike	1 piece	99	4	—	5	—
Gefiltefish & Pike Sweet	1 piece	129	4	—	9	—
Homestyle	1 piece	111	4	—	6	—
Sweet	1 piece	132	4	—	9	—
sweet	1 piece (1.5 oz)	35	1	220	3	—

GELATIN

DRINKS
Knox
Orange Flavored Drinking Gelatin w/ Nutrasweet	1 pkg	39	tr	17	4	0

MIX
D-Zerta
Cherry	½ cup	8	0	4	0	—
Lemon	½ cup	8	0	4	0	—
Lime	½ cup	9	0	4	0	—
Orange	½ cup	8	0	4	0	—
Raspberry	½ cup	8	0	4	0	—
Strawberry	½ cup	8	0	4	0	—

Emes
Kosher-Jel	½ cup (4 fl oz)	60	0	7	15	—
Kosher-Jel Plain	1 tbsp (7 g)	21	0	tr	5	1

Jell-O
Apricot	½ cup	82	tr	51	19	0
Black Cherry	½ cup	82	tr	51	19	tr
Black Raspberry	½ cup	82	tr	37	19	tr
Blackberry	½ cup	82	tr	51	19	tr
Cherry Sugar Free	½ cup	9	0	81	0	—
Concord Grape	½ cup	82	tr	37	19	0
Hawaiian Pineapple Sugar Free	½ cup	8	tr	50	0	—
Lemon	½ cup	82	tr	75	19	0
Lemon Sugar Free	½ cup	8	0	60	0	—
Lime	½ cup	82	tr	58	19	tr
Lime Sugar Free	½ cup	9	0	63	0	—
Mixed Fruit	½ cup	82	tr	51	19	tr
Mixed Fruit Sugar Free	½ cup	8	0	50	0	—
Orange	½ cup	82	tr	51	19	tr
Orange Sugar Free	½ cup	8	0	53	0	—
Peach Sugar Free	½ cup	8	tr	49	0	—
Raspberry Sugar Free	½ cup	8	0	57	0	—
Strawberry Banana Sugar Free	½ cup	9	0	55	0	—

FOOD	PORTION	CAL.	FAT	SOD.	CARB.	FIB.
Jell-O (CONT.)						
Strawberry Sugar Free	½ cup	9	0	64	0	—
Triple Berry Sugar Free	½ cup	8	tr	50	0	—
Wild Strawberry	½ cup	81	tr	75	19	tr
Kojel						
Diet	1 serv	10	tr	16	4	—
Royal						
Apple	½ cup	80	0	95	19	—
Blackberry	½ cup	80	0	95	19	—
Cherry	½ cup	80	0	95	19	—
Cherry Sugar Free	½ cup	8	0	90	1	—
Concord Grape	½ cup	80	0	130	19	—
Fruit Punch	½ cup	80	0	90	19	—
Lemon	½ cup	80	0	250	19	—
Lemon-Lime	½ cup	80	0	95	19	—
Lime	½ cup	80	0	125	19	—
Lime Sugar Free	½ cup	8	0	100	1	—
Mixed Berry	½ cup	80	0	90	19	—
Orange	½ cup	80	0	95	19	—
Orange Sugar Free	½ cup	10	0	90	1	—
Peach	½ cup	80	0	95	19	—
Pineapple	½ cup	80	0	95	19	—
Raspberry	½ cup	80	0	125	19	—
Raspberry Sugar Free	½ cup	8	0	90	1	—
Strawberry	½ cup	80	0	105	19	—
Strawberry Banana Sugar Free	½ cup	8	0	85	1	—
Strawberry Orange	½ cup	80	0	110	19	—
Strawberry Sugar Free	½ cup	8	0	90	1	—
Tropical Fruit	½ cup	80	0	110	19	—
low calorie	½ cup	8	0	9	0	0
mix artificially sweetened as prep	½ cup (4.1 oz)	8	0	56	1	—
mix artificially sweetened as prep	1 pkg 4 serv (16.5 oz)	33	0	224	3	—
mix as prep	½ cup (4.7 oz)	80	0	57	19	—
mix as prep	1 pkg 4 serv (19 oz)	319	0	227	76	—
mix not prep	1 pkg (3 oz)	324	0	216	77	—
mix w/ fruit as prep	½ cup (3.7 oz)	73	tr	30	18	—
mix w/ fruit as prep	1 pkg 8 serv (19 oz)	588	2	242	144	—
powder unsweetened	1 oz	94	0	55	0	—
powder unsweetened	1 pkg (7 g)	23	0	14	0	—

FOOD	PORTION	CAL.	FAT	SOD.	CARB.	FIB.
READY-TO-USE						
Del Monte						
Gel Snack Cups Blue Berry	1 serv (3.5 oz)	70	0	40	19	tr
Gel Snack Cups Cherry	1 serv (3.5 oz)	70	0	40	19	tr
Gel Snack Cups Orange	1 serv (3.5 oz)	70	0	40	19	tr
Gel Snack Cups Strawberry	1 serv (3.5 oz)	70	0	40	19	tr
GIBLETS						
capon simmered	1 cup (5 oz)	238	8	80	0	—
chicken floured & fried	1 cup (5 oz)	402	19	164	6	—
chicken simmered	1 cup (5 oz)	228	7	85	1	—
turkey simmered	1 cup (5 oz)	243	7	85	3	—
GINGER						
Ka-Me						
Crystallized Slices	5 pieces (1 oz)	100	0	23	25	1
Sliced	20 pieces (0.5 oz)	0	0	70	0	0
ground	1 tsp (1.8 g)	6	tr	1	1	—
root fresh	5 slices	8	tr	1	2	—
root fresh	¼ cup	17	tr	3	4	—
root fresh sliced	¼ cup	17	tr	3	4	—
GINKGO NUTS						
canned	1 oz	32	tr	87	6	—
dried	1 oz	99	tr	4	21	—
raw	1 oz	52	tr	1	11	—
GIZZARDS						
chicken simmered	1 cup (5 oz)	222	5	97	2	—
turkey simmered	1 cup (5 oz)	236	6	79	1	—
GOAT						
roasted	3 oz	122	3	73	0	—
GOOSE						
w/ skin roasted	6.6 oz	574	41	132	0	—
w/ skin roasted	½ goose (1.7 lbs)	2362	170	543	0	—
w/o skin roasted	5 oz	340	18	108	0	—
w/o skin roasted	½ goose (1.3 lbs)	1406	75	447	0	—
GOOSEBERRIES						
fresh	1 cup	67	1	1	15	—
CANNED						
in light syrup	½ cup	93	tr	3	24	—

FOOD	PORTION	CAL.	FAT	SOD.	CARB.	FIB.

GRANOLA

BARS

Carnation

FOOD	PORTION	CAL.	FAT	SOD.	CARB.	FIB.
Chocolate Chunk	1 (1.26 oz)	140	5	65	23	1
Honey & Oats	1 (1.26 oz)	130	4	60	23	1
Fi-Bar						
Coconut	1	120	4	30	20	6
Peanut Butter	1	130	4	30	20	6
General Mills						
Nature Valley Cinnamon	1	120	5	70	17	1
Nature Valley Oat Bran Honey Graham	1	110	4	90	16	1
Nature Valley Oats N'Honey	1	120	5	65	17	1
Nature Valley Peanut Butter	1	120	6	70	15	1
Nature Valley Rice Bran Cinnamon Graham	1	90	4	75	13	1
Grist Mill						
Chewy Apple Cinnamon	1 (1 oz)	120	4	35	21	1
Chewy Chocolate Chip	1 (1 oz)	130	4	30	21	1
Chewy Chunky Nut & Raisin	1 (1 oz)	130	6	35	18	1
Chewy Peanut Butter	1 (1 oz)	130	5	45	20	1
Chewy Peanut Butter Chocolate	1 (1 oz)	130	4	40	20	2
Chocolate Snack Chocolate Chip	1 (1.2 oz)	180	10	60	21	1
Chocolate Snack Nutty Fudge	1 (1.3 oz)	190	11	90	19	2
Crunchy Cinnamon	1 (0.8 oz)	110	5	60	16	1
Crunchy Oats 'N Honey	1 (0.8 oz)	110	5	60	15	1
Hershey						
Chocolate Covered Chocolate Chip	1 (1.2 oz)	170	8	50	22	—
Chocolate Covered Cocoa Creme	1 (1.2 oz)	180	9	50	22	—
Chocolate Covered Cookies & Creme	1 (1.2 oz)	170	8	50	22	—
Chocolate Covered Peanut Butter	1 (1.2 oz)	180	10	65	19	—
Kellogg's						
Low Fat Crunchy	1 (0.7 oz)	80	2	60	16	1

FOOD	PORTION	CAL.	FAT	SOD.	CARB.	FIB.
Kellogg's (CONT.)						
Almond & Brown Sugar						
Low Fat Crunchy Apple Spice	1 (0.7 oz)	80	2	60	16	1
Low Fat Crunchy Cinnamon Raisin	1 (0.7 oz)	80	2	60	16	1
Kudos						
Chocolate Chunk	1 (0.7 oz)	90	3	60	13	1
Chocolate Coated Chocolate Chip	1 (1 oz)	120	5	75	18	1
Chocolate Coated Milk & Cookies	1 (1 oz)	130	5	70	18	1
Chocolate Coated Nutty Fudge	1 (1 oz)	130	5	65	18	1
Chocolate Coated Peanut Butter	1 (1 oz)	130	5	85	18	1
Low Fat Blueberry	1 (0.7 oz)	90	2	90	15	1
Low Fat Strawberry	1 (0.7 oz)	80	2	90	15	1
New Country						
Chocolate Covered Cookies & Creme	1	200	11	85	23	—
Quaker						
Chewy Chocolate Chip	1	128	5	90	19	1
Chewy Chunky Nut & Raisin	1	131	6	86	17	2
Chewy Cinnamon Raisin	1	128	5	92	19	1
Chewy Honey & Oats	1	125	4	95	19	1
Chewy Peanut Butter	1	128	5	116	18	1
Chewy Peanut Butter Chocolate Chip	1	131	6	112	17	1
Dipps Caramel Nut	1	148	6	81	21	1
Dipps Chocolate Chip	1	139	6	78	19	1
Dipps Chocolate Fudge	1	160	8	74	20	—
Dipps Peanut Butter	1	170	9	74	9	1
Dipps Peanut Butter Chocolate Chip	1	174	10	102	10	—
Dipps Rocky Road	1	140	7	—	—	—
Sunbelt						
Chewy Chocolate Chip	1 (1.8 oz)	220	10	95	32	2
Chewy Chocolate Chip	1 (1.25 oz)	160	7	65	23	2
Chewy Oats & Honey	1 (1 oz)	130	5	65	19	1
Chewy Oats & Honey	1 (1.7 oz)	210	9	105	32	2
Chewy With Almonds	1 (1 oz)	130	7	60	17	2

FOOD	PORTION	CAL.	FAT	SOD.	CARB.	FIB.
Sunbelt (CONT.)						
Chewy With Almonds	1 (1.5 oz)	190	10	95	25	2
Chewy With Raisins	1 (1.2 oz)	150	6	65	25	2
Fudge Dipped Chewy Chocolate Chip	1 (1.5 oz)	190	8	80	28	2
Fudge Dipped Chewy Macaroon	1 bar (2 oz)	280	17	90	32	3
Fudge Dipped Chewy Macaroon	1 (1.4 oz)	200	13	60	22	2
Fudge Dipped Chewy With Peanuts	1 bar (1.5 oz)	210	12	65	24	2
Fudge Dipped Chewy With Peanuts	1 (2 oz)	270	15	95	32	2
almond	1 (0.8 oz)	117	6	60	15	—
almond	1 (1 oz)	140	7	73	18	—
chewy chocolate coated chococate chip	1 (1 oz)	132	7	57	18	1
chewy chocolate coated chocolate chip	1 (1.25 oz)	165	9	71	23	1
chewy chocolate coated peanut butter	1 (1 oz)	144	9	55	15	—
chewy chocolate coated peanut butter	1 (1.3 oz)	187	11	71	20	—
chewy raisin	1 (1.5 oz)	191	8	120	28	2
chewy raisin	1 (1 oz)	127	5	80	19	1
chocolate chip	1 (0.8 oz)	103	4	81	17	1
chocolate chip	1 (1 oz)	124	5	97	20	1
chocolate chip chewy	1 (1.5 oz)	178	7	116	29	2
chocolate chip chewy	1 (1 oz)	119	5	77	10	1
chocolate chip graham & marshmallow chewy	1 (1 oz)	121	4	90	20	1
nut & raisin chewy	1 (1 oz)	129	6	72	18	2
peanut	1 (1 oz)	136	6	79	18	—
peanut	1 (0.8 oz)	113	5	66	15	1
peanut butter	1 (1 oz)	137	7	80	18	—
peanut butter	1 (0.8 oz)	114	6	67	15	—
peanut butter & chocolate chip chewy	1 (1 oz)	122	6	93	18	1
peanut butter chewy	1 (1 oz)	121	5	116	18	1
plain	1 (1 oz)	134	7	83	18	2
plain	1 (0.9 oz)	115	4	72	19	1
plain chewy	1 (1 oz)	126	5	79	19	1
CEREAL						
Erewhon						
Date Nut	1 oz	130	6	45	17	—

FOOD	PORTION	CAL.	FAT	SOD.	CARB.	FIB.
Erewhon (CONT.)						
Honey Almond	1 oz	130	6	65	17	—
Maple	1 oz	130	5	55	17	—
Spiced Apple	1 oz	130	6	55	17	—
Sunflower Crunch	1 oz	130	4	60	18	—
With Bran	1 oz	130	6	10	17	4
General Mills						
Nature Valley Cinnamon & Raisin	⅓ cup (1 oz)	120	4	90	20	1
Nature Valley Fruit & Nut	⅓ cup (1 oz)	130	5	75	19	1
Nature Valley Toasted Oat	⅓ cup (1 oz)	130	5	90	20	1
Good Shepherd						
Crunchy	1 oz	130	5	15	19	2
Honey Almond	1 oz	120	4	10	20	2
Organic 5 Grain Muesli	1 oz	160	3	55	27	3
Organic Brown Rice	1 oz	130	4	35	16	4
Organic Wheat Free	1 oz	90	3	3	39	2
Organic Wheat Free Apple Cinnamon	1 oz	125	4	35	20	3
Organic Wheat Free Blueberry Amaranth	1 oz	110	1	10	22	2
Organic Wheat Free Strawberry Amaranth	1 oz	110	1	12	22	2
Grist Mill						
Low-Fat With Raisins	⅔ cup (1.9 oz)	220	3	100	42	3
Kellogg's						
Low Fat	½ cup (1.9 oz)	210	3	120	43	3
Low Fat With Raisins	⅔ cup (1.9 oz)	210	3	135	43	3
Post						
Post Hearty	¼ cup (1 oz)	128	4	78	21	1
Stone-Buhr						
Hot Apple	⅓ cup (1.6 oz)	153	1	0	31	5
Sun Country						
100% Natural With Almonds	¼ cup	130	5	11	19	1
100% Natural With Raisins & Dates	¼ cup	123	5	9	20	2
With Raisins	¼ cup	125	5	10	19	2
Sunbelt						
Banana Nut	1.9 oz	250	9	60	37	4
Fruit & Nut	1.9 oz	230	7	100	38	4
Low Fat	1.9 oz	200	3	80	42	4

FOOD	PORTION	CAL.	FAT	SOD.	CARB.	FIB.
Uncle Roy's						
Cashew Raisin	½ cup (1.6 oz)	180	6	20	32	3
Fat Free Apple Cinnamon	½ cup (1.6 oz)	175	1	20	38	3
Fat Free Wild Cherry	½ cup (1.6 oz)	175	1	20	38	3
Fruit & Nut	½ cup (1.6 oz)	175	5	20	30	3
Low Fat Berries Jubilee	½ cup (1.6 oz)	175	3	20	34	3
Low Fat Crispy	½ cup (1.4 oz)	160	3	20	31	3
Low Fat Luscious Raspberry	½ cup (1.6 oz)	175	3	20	34	3
Low Fat True Blueberry	½ cup (1.6 oz)	175	3	20	34	3
Maple Date Nut	½ cup (1.6 oz)	180	6	20	29	3
Nut Butter & Almonds	½ cup (1.6 oz)	195	8	20	29	3
Organic Golden Honey	½ cup (1.6 oz)	190	6	20	30	3
Organic Maple Nut'N Rice	½ cup (1.4 oz)	170	6	20	27	3
Organic Maple Raisin	½ cup (1.6 oz)	190	6	20	30	3
granola	¼ cup	138	8	3	16	—
GRAPE JUICE						
BAMA	8.45 fl oz	120	0	25	29	—
Bright & Early						
Frozen	8 fl oz	140	0	5	34	—
Hi-C						
Box	8.45 fl oz	130	0	30	33	—
Kool-Aid						
Drink	8 oz	98	0	—	25	—
Sugar Free	8 oz	3	0	—	0	—
Sugar Sweetened	8 oz	80	0	24	21	—
Lifesavers						
Grape Punch	8 fl oz	150	0	25	36	—
Minute Maid						
Chilled	8 fl oz	130	0	5	33	—
Grape Punch frzn	8 fl oz	130	0	5	32	—
Punch Chilled	8 fl oz	130	0	25	32	—
Mott's						
Drink	10 fl oz	170	0	50	42	0
Fruit Basket Cocktail as prep	8 fl oz	130	0	5	32	0
S&W						
Concord Unsweetened	6 oz	100	0	9	25	—
Seneca						
Blush Grape Juice frzn as prep	8 fl oz	170	0	0	39	0
Fortified With Vitamin C frzn as prep	8 fl oz	170	0	24	39	0

FOOD	PORTION	CAL.	FAT	SOD.	CARB.	FIB.
Seneca (CONT.)						
Sweetened frzn as prep	8 fl oz	140	0	24	39	0
White Grape Juice frzn as prep	8 fl oz	140	0	0	33	0
Sippin' Pak						
100% Pure	8.45 fl oz	130	0	25	32	—
Sipps						
Juice	8.45 oz	130	0	—	—	—
Snapple						
Grapeade	8 fl oz	120	0	5	30	—
Tang						
Fruit Box	8.45 oz	131	0	2	34	—
Tree Top						
Juice	6 oz	120	0	10	30	—
Sparkling Juice	6 oz	120	0	—	29	—
Tropicana						
Season's Best	8 fl oz	160	0	25	39	—
Veryfine						
100%	8 oz	153	0	<20	37	—
Grape Drink	8 oz	130	0	<10	34	—
Wylers						
Drink Mix Unsweetened	8 oz	2	0	12	1	—
bottled	1 cup	155	tr	7	38	—
frzn sweetened as prep	1 cup	128	tr	5	32	—
frzn sweetened not prep	6 oz	386	1	15	96	—
grape drink	6 oz	84	0	12	22	—

GRAPE LEAVES
Cedar's

FOOD	PORTION	CAL.	FAT	SOD.	CARB.	FIB.
Grape Leaves Stuffed With Rice	6 pieces (4.9 oz)	180	8	870	22	8

GRAPEFRUIT
CANNED
S&W

FOOD	PORTION	CAL.	FAT	SOD.	CARB.	FIB.
Sections In Light Syrup	½ cup	80	0	0	14	—
Sections Natural Style	½ cup	40	0	—	9	—
Sections Unsweetened	½ cup	40	0	0	9	—
juice pack	½ cup	46	tr	9	11	—
unsweetened	1 cup	93	tr	3	22	—
water pack	½ cup	44	tr	2	11	—
FRESH						
Chiquita						
Ruby Red	½ fruit	40	0	—	—	—

FOOD	PORTION	CAL.	FAT	SOD.	CARB.	FIB.
Ocean Spray						
Pink	½ med	50	0	0	13	—
White	½ med	45	0	0	12	—
pink	½	37	tr	0	9	1
pink sections	1 cup	69	tr	1	18	1
red	½	37	tr	0	9	—
red sections	1 cup	69	tr	1	18	—
white	½	39	tr	0	10	1
white sections	1 cup	76	tr	0	19	1

GRAPEFRUIT JUICE

FOOD	PORTION	CAL.	FAT	SOD.	CARB.	FIB.
After The Fall						
Pink	1 bottle (10 oz)	100	0	10	23	—
Crystal Geyser						
Juice Squeeze	1 bottle (12 fl oz)	150	0	20	36	—
Hood						
Select	1 cup (8 oz)	100	0	1	23	—
Minute Maid						
Frozen	8 fl oz	100	0	25	23	—
Juices To Go	1 bottle (16 fl oz)	100	0	25	23	—
Juices To Go	1 bottle (10 fl oz)	120	0	35	29	—
Juices To Go	1 can (11.5 fl oz)	140	0	40	33	—
Juices To Go Pink Cocktail	1 bottle (16 fl oz)	110	0	25	27	—
Juices To Go Pink Cocktail	1 bottle (10 fl oz)	140	0	35	34	—
Juices to Go Pink Cocktail	8 fl oz	160	0	40	39	—
Mott's						
From Concentrate as prep	8 fl oz	120	0	10	27	0
Ocean Spray						
100% Juice	8 oz	100	0	35	24	tr
Lightstyle Low Calorie Pink Cocktail	8 fl oz	40	0	35	9	0
Pink Juice Cocktail	8 oz	110	0	35	28	0
Ruby Red Drink	8 oz	130	0	35	33	0
S&W						
Unsweetened	6 oz	80	0	—	18	—
Snapple						
Pink Grapefruit Cocktail	8 fl oz	120	0	5	31	—
Tropicana						
Ruby Red	1 container (10 fl oz)	120	0	0	30	—

FOOD	PORTION	CAL.	FAT	SOD.	CARB.	FIB.
Tropicana (CONT.)						
Ruby Red	8 fl oz	100	0	0	25	—
Season's Best	1 bottle (10 fl oz)	110	0	5	27	—
Season's Best	1 bottle (7 fl oz)	80	0	5	19	—
Season's Best	8 fl oz	90	0	5	22	—
Season's Best	1 can (11.5 fl oz)	120	0	5	31	—
Twister Light Pink	1 container (10 fl oz)	50	0	25	12	—
Twister Light Pink	8 fl oz	40	0	20	10	—
Twister Pink	1 container (10 fl oz)	140	0	25	35	—
Twister Pink	1 can (11.5 fl oz)	160	0	30	40	—
Twister Pink	8 fl oz	110	0	20	28	—
Veryfine						
100%	8 oz	101	0	<10	23	—
Pink	8 oz	120	0	<20	29	—
fresh	1 cup	96	tr	2	23	—
frzn as prep	1 cup	102	tr	2	24	—
frzn not prep	6 oz	302	1	6	72	—
sweetened	1 cup	116	tr	4	28	—

GRAPES
CANNED
S&W

FOOD	PORTION	CAL.	FAT	SOD.	CARB.	FIB.
Thompson Seedless Premium	½ cup	100	0	5	25	—
thompson seedless in heavy syrup	½ cup	94	tr	7	25	—
thompson seedless water pack	½ cup	48	tr	7	13	—
FRESH						
Dole	1½ cup	85	0	3	24	2
grapes	10	36	tr	1	9	tr

GRAVY
(*see also* SAUCE)
CANNED
Franco-American

FOOD	PORTION	CAL.	FAT	SOD.	CARB.	FIB.
Au Jus	2 oz	10	0	330	2	—
Beef	2 oz	25	1	340	4	—
Chicken	2 oz	45	4	240	3	—
Chicken Giblet	2 oz	30	2	310	3	—
Cream	2 oz	35	2	220	3	—
Mushroom	2 oz	25	1	290	3	—
Pork	2 oz	40	3	330	3	—

FOOD	PORTION	CAL.	FAT	SOD.	CARB.	FIB.
Franco-American (CONT.)						
Turkey	2 oz	30	2	290	3	—
Rudy's Farm						
Sausage Gravy	¼ cup (2 oz)	50	1	330	7	0
au jus	1 cup	38	tr	—	6	—
beef	1 cup	124	6	1305	11	—
beef	1 can (10 oz)	155	7	1630	14	—
chicken	1 cup	189	14	1375	13	—
mushroom	1 cup	120	6	1259	13	—
turkey	1 cup	122	5	—	12	—
DRY						
Bournvita	2 heaping tsp	34	1	—	7	—
Bovril	1 heaping tsp	9	0	—	tr	0
Cajun King						
Oil-Less Roux And Gravy Mix	3.5 oz	394	4	348	78	—
Hain						
Brown	¼ pkg	16	0	600	3	—
LaLoma						
Brown Gravy Quik as prep	2 tsp	45	4	150	2	—
Chicken Gravy Quik as prep	2 tsp	45	4	180	2	—
Country Quik Gravy as prep	2 tsp	10	tr	200	2	—
Mushroom Quik Gravy as prep	2 tsp	10	tr	160	2	—
Onion Quik Gravy as prep	2 tsp	10	tr	120	2	—
Pillsbury						
Brown	¼ cup	15	0	300	3	—
Chicken	¼ cup	25	1	230	4	—
Home Style	¼ cup	15	0	300	3	—
au jus as prep w/ water	1 cup	32	1	964	4	—
brown as prep w/ water	1 cup	75	2	1076	13	—
chicken as prep	1 cup	83	2	1133	14	—
mushroom as prep	1 cup	70	1	1402	14	—
onion as prep w/ water	1 cup	77	2	1013	16	—
pork as prep	1 cup	76	2	1235	13	—
turkey as prep	1 cup	87	2	1498	15	—

GREAT NORTHERN BEANS
CANNED

Allen	½ cup (4.5 oz)	100	1	310	19	7

FOOD	PORTION	CAL.	FAT	SOD.	CARB.	FIB.
Green Giant	½ cup	80	1	290	18	5
Hanover						
Great Northern	½ cup	110	0	—	—	—
Trappey						
With Sausage	½ cup (4.5 oz)	100	1	460	18	7
great northern	1 cup	300	1	11	55	14
DRIED						
Bean Cuisine	½ cup	115	1	5	—	5
cooked	1 cup	210	1	4	37	—
GREEN BEANS						
CANNED						
Allen						
Cut	½ cup (4.2 oz)	30	1	320	6	3
Cut No Added Salt	½ cup (4.2 oz)	15	0	10	3	2
French Style	½ cup (4.2 oz)	25	0	300	4	2
Italian	½ cup (4.2 oz)	35	1	320	7	3
Shell Outs	½ cup (4.5 oz)	30	0	460	6	2
Alma						
Cut	½ cup (4.2 oz)	30	1	320	6	3
Crest Top						
Cut	½ cup (4.2 oz)	30	1	320	6	3
Del Monte						
Cut	½ cup (4.3 oz)	20	0	360	4	2
Cut 50% Less Salt	½ cup (4.3 oz)	20	0	180	4	2
Cut Italian	½ cup (4.3 oz)	30	0	360	6	3
Cut No Salt Added	½ cup (4.3 oz)	20	0	10	4	2
French Style	½ cup (4.3 oz)	20	0	360	4	2
French Style 50% Less Salt	½ cup (4.3 oz)	20	0	180	4	2
French Style No Salt Added	½ cup (4.3 oz)	20	0	10	4	2
French Style Seasoned	½ cup (4.3 oz)	20	0	360	4	2
Whole	½ cup (4.3 oz)	20	0	360	4	2
GaBelle						
Cut	½ cup (4.2 oz)	30	1	320	6	3
Green Giant						
Almondine	½ cup	45	3	300	5	2
Cut	½ cup	16	0	300	4	1
French	½ cup	16	0	330	4	1
Kitchen Sliced	½ cup	16	0	280	4	1
Hanover						
Cut	½ cup	20	0	—	—	—
Owatonna						
Cut	½ cup	20	0	—	—	—

FOOD	PORTION	CAL.	FAT	SOD.	CARB.	FIB.
Owatonna (CONT.)						
French	½ cup	20	0	—	—	—
S&W						
Cut Water Pack	½ cup	20	0	5	4	—
Cut Premium Blue Lake	½ cup	20	0	385	4	—
Dilled	½ cup	60	0	385	15	—
French Style Premium Blue Lake	½ cup	20	0	385	4	—
Green Beans & Wax Beans	½ cup	20	0	385	5	—
Whole Fancy Stringless	½ cup	20	0	385	4	—
Whole Vertical Pack	½ cup	20	0	385	4	—
Seneca						
Cut	½ cup	20	0	360	6	2
Cuts Natural Pack	½ cup	25	0	0	6	2
French	½ cup	20	0	360	6	2
French Natural Pack	½ cup	25	0	0	6	2
Whole	½ cup	20	0	360	6	2
Sunshine						
Cut	½ cup (4.2 oz)	30	1	320	6	3
Italian	½ cup (4.2 oz)	35	1	320	7	3
FROZEN						
Birds Eye						
Cut	½ cup	25	0	0	6	2
Farm Fresh Whole	¾ cup	30	0	0	7	2
French Cut	½ cup	25	0	0	6	2
In Sauce French Green Beans With Toasted Almonds	½ cup	50	2	340	8	2
Italian	½ cup	30	0	0	7	3
Polybag Cut	½ cup	25	0	0	6	2
Polybag Deluxe Whole	½ cup	20	0	0	4	2
Polybag French Cut	½ cup	25	0	0	6	2
Whole Deluxe	½ cup	45	0	0	5	2
Fresh Like						
Cut	3.5 oz	29	tr	6	7	1
French	3.5 oz	29	tr	6	7	1
Italian	3.5 oz	35	tr	6	8	1
Whole	3.5 oz	29	tr	6	6	1
Green Giant						
Cut	½ cup	16	0	95	4	1
Cut In Butter Sauce	½ cup	30	1	230	4	2
One Serve In Butter Sauce	1 pkg	60	2	370	8	3

FOOD	PORTION	CAL.	FAT	SOD.	CARB.	FIB.
Hanover						
Cut	½ cup	20	0	—	—	—
French Style Blue Lake	½ cup	25	0	—	—	—
Italian Cut	½ cup	35	0	—	—	—
Whole Blue Lake	½ cup	30	0	—	—	—
Southland						
Cut Beans	3 oz	25	0	—	—	—
French	3 oz	25	0	—	—	—
Stouffer's						
Green Bean Mushroom Casserole	½ cup (1.9 oz)	130	8	530	13	2
SHELF-STABLE						
Pantry Express						
Cut	½ cup	12	0	20	3	1

GREENS
CANNED
Allen

Mixed	½ cup (4.2 oz)	30	1	10	8	4
Sunshine						
Mixed	½ cup (4.2 oz)	30	1	10	8	4

GROUNDCHERRIES

fresh	½ cup	37	tr	—	8	—

GROUPER

cooked	3 oz	100	1	45	0	—
cooked	1 fillet (7.1 oz)	238	3	107	0	—
raw	3 oz	78	1	45	0	—

GUANABANA JUICE
Libby

Nectar	1 can (11.5 fl oz)	210	0	25	50	—

GUAVA

fresh	1	45	1	2	11	—
guava sauce	½ cup	43	tr	4	11	—

GUAVA JUICE
Kern's

Nectar	6 fl oz	110	0	0	28	—
Libby						
Nectar	6 oz	110	0	15	26	—
Nectar	1 can (11.5 fl oz)	220	0	10	54	—
Snapple						
Guava Mania	8 fl oz	110	0	0	29	—

FOOD	PORTION	CAL.	FAT	SOD.	CARB.	FIB.
GUINEA HEN						
w/ skin raw	½ hen (12.1 oz)	545	22	—	0	—
w/o skin raw	½ hen (9.3 oz)	292	7	—	0	—
HADDOCK						
FRESH						
cooked	1 fillet (5.3 oz)	168	1	131	0	—
cooked	3 oz	95	1	74	0	—
raw	3 oz	74	1	58	0	—
roe raw	3½ oz	130	2	—	2	—
FROZEN						
Gorton's						
Fishmarket Fresh	5 oz	110	1	120	0	—
Microwave Entree	1 pkg	360	21	730	19	—
Haddock In Lemon						
Butter						
Mrs. Paul's						
Crunchy Batter Fillets	2 fillets	190	5	580	22	—
Light Fillets	1 fillet	220	9	350	15	—
Van De Kamp's						
Battered	2 pieces	250	15	580	19	—
Breaded Fillets	2 pieces	270	16	290	19	—
Light Fillets	1 piece	240	11	590	21	—
Natural Fillets	4 oz	90	1	125	0	—
SMOKED						
smoked	1 oz	33	tr	214	0	—
smoked	3 oz	99	1	649	0	—
HAKE						
raw	3½ oz	84	1	101	0	—
HALIBUT						
FRESH						
atlantic & pacific cooked	3 oz	119	2	59	0	—
atlantic & pacific cooked	½ fillet (5.6 oz)	223	5	110	0	—
atlantic & pacific raw	3 oz	93	2	46	0	—
greenland baked	3 oz	203	15	87	0	—
greenland baked	5.6 oz	380	28	163	0	—
FROZEN						
Van De Kamp's						
Battered	2 pieces	150	6	400	16	—
HALVA						
(*see* SESAME)						
HAM						
(*see also* HAM DISHES, PORK, TURKEY)						
Alpine Lace						
Boneless Cooked	2 oz	60	2	440	1	0

FOOD	PORTION	CAL.	FAT	SOD.	CARB.	FIB.
Armour						
1877 Boneless	1 oz	42	2	—	—	—
Chopped Ham Canned	2 oz	120	9	880	2	—
Deviled Ham Canned	1 pkg (3 oz)	200	16	800	0	—
Golden Star Boneless	1 oz	33	1	—	—	—
Golden Star Canned	1 oz	32	tr	—	—	—
Lower Salt 93% Fat Free	1 oz	35	1	221	—	—
Lower Salt Boneless	1 oz	34	1	—	—	—
Star Boneless	1 oz	41	2	—	—	—
Star Canned	1 oz	34	1	—	—	—
Star Speedy Cut	1 oz	44	3	—	—	—
Black Label						
Chopped	2 oz	140	11	650	3	0
Carl Buddig						
Ham	1 oz	50	3	400	1	0
Honey Ham	1 oz	50	3	400	1	—
Hansel n'Gretel						
Baked Virginia	1 oz	34	1	245	2	—
Black Forest	1 oz	32	1	—	tr	—
Cappy	1 oz	31	1	—	1	—
Cooked Fresh	1 oz	33	1	120	tr	—
Deluxe	1 oz	31	1	245	1	—
Honey Valley	1 oz	31	1	260	1	—
Jalapeno	1 oz	25	1	260	1	—
Lessalt	1 oz	30	1	200	1	—
Lessalt Virginia	1 oz	32	1	190	1	—
Light AM	1 oz	27	1	200	1	—
Travane	1 oz	31	1	210	tr	—
Healthy Choice						
Baked Cooked	3 slices (2.2 oz)	70	2	560	1	0
Cooked	3 slices (2.2 oz)	70	2	580	1	0
Deli-Thin Baked Cooked With Natural Juices	6 slices (2 oz)	60	2	500	2	0
Deli-Thin Cooked	6 slices (2 oz)	60	2	510	1	0
Deli-Thin Honey With Natural Juices	6 slices (2 oz)	60	2	540	2	0
Deli-Thin Smoked With Natural Juices	6 slices (2 oz)	60	2	530	1	0
Fresh-Trak Cooked	1 slice (1 oz)	30	1	250	1	0
Fresh-Trak Honey	1 slice (1 oz)	30	1	250	1	0
Honey Boneless	3 oz	100	3	580	5	0
Smoked	3 slices (2.2 oz)	70	2	560	1	0
Variety Pack Regular	3 slices (2.2 oz)	70	2	570	1	0

FOOD	PORTION	CAL.	FAT	SOD.	CARB.	FIB.
Hillshire						
Brown Sugar	1 oz	40	2	440	2	—
Cooked Ham	1 oz	30	1	470	tr	—
Deli Select Baked Ham	1 slice	10	tr	95	tr	—
Deli Select Brown Sugar Baked	1 slice	10	tr	90	tr	—
Deli Select Cajun Ham	1 slice	10	tr	120	tr	—
Deli Select Honey Ham	1 slice	10	tr	100	tr	—
Deli Select Lower Salt	1 slice	10	tr	80	tr	—
Deli Select Smoked Ham	1 slice	10	tr	95	tr	—
Flavor Pack 90-99% Fat Free Brown Sugar Baked	1 slice (0.6 oz)	20	tr	170	1	—
Flavor Pack 90-99% Fat Free Honey Ham	1 slice (0.6 oz)	20	tr	180	1	—
Flavor Pack 90-99% Fat Free Smoked	1 slice (0.6 oz)	20	tr	170	tr	—
Genuine Baked	1 oz	35	1	290	1	—
Honey Ham	1 oz	40	2	440	2	—
Lower Salt	1 oz	30	1	300	1	—
Lunch 'N Munch Cooked Ham/Swiss	1 pkg (4.5 oz)	360	22	1380	19	—
Lunch 'N Munch Cooked Ham/Swiss Oreo	1 pkg (4.125 oz)	370	21	1160	30	—
Lunch 'N Munch Cooked Ham/Swiss Snickers/Hi-C	1 pkg (4.25 oz + 6 fl oz)	470	21	1180	54	—
Lunch 'N Munch Honey Ham/ Cheddar/ Snickers/Hi-C	1 pkg (4.25 oz + 6 fl oz)	500	23	1030	56	—
Hormel						
Black Label Canned (refrigerated)	3 oz	100	5	960	0	0
Black Label Canned (self stable)	3 oz	110	5	900	0	0
Canned Chunk	2 oz	90	6	600	0	0
Cure 81 Half Ham	3 oz	100	5	890	0	0
Curemaster	3 oz	80	3	940	0	0
Deli Cooked	1 oz	29	1	344	1	—
Deviled Ham	4 tbsp (2 oz)	150	12	430	1	0
Ham & Cheese Patties	1 patty (2 oz)	190	17	470	0	0
Light & Lean	3 oz	90	3	950	2	0
Light & Lean 97	3 oz	90	3	950	2	0
Light & Lean 97 Cuts	16 pieces (1 oz)	35	1	420	0	0

FOOD	PORTION	CAL.	FAT	SOD.	CARB.	FIB.
Hormel (CONT.)						
Light & Lean 97 Sliced	1 slice (1 oz)	25	1	340	0	0
Patties	1 patty (2 oz)	180	17	550	1	0
Primissimo Proscuitti	1 oz	70	5	540	0	0
Spread	4 tbsp (2 oz)	100	11	580	1	0
Supreme Cut Canned	1 oz	31	1	299	tr	—
Jones						
Family Ham	1 slice	40	2	290	tr	—
Ham Slices	1 slice	30	1	200	tr	—
Louis Rich						
Carving Board Baked With Natural Juices	2 slices (1.6 oz)	45	1	510	1	0
Carving Board Carved Thin Honey With Natural Juices	6 slices (2.1 oz)	70	2	760	2	0
Carving Board Honey With Natural Juices	2 slices (1.6 oz)	50	2	530	1	0
Carving Board Smoked Cooked With Natural Juices	1 slice (1.6 oz)	50	2	560	0	0
Dinner Slices Baked	1 slice (3.3 oz)	80	2	1150	1	0
Mr. Turkey						
Deli Cuts Honey Cured	3 slices	35	1	300	1	—
Oscar Mayer						
Baked	3 slices (2.2 oz)	60	1	720	2	0
Boiled	3 slices (2.2 oz)	60	3	820	0	0
Chopped	1 slice (1 oz)	50	4	320	1	0
Deli-Thin Boiled	4 slices (1.8 oz)	50	2	680	0	0
Deli-Thin Honey Ham	4 slices (1.8 oz)	60	2	630	2	0
Deli-Thin Smoked	4 slices (1.8 oz)	50	2	620	0	0
Dinner Slices	3 oz	90	3	1030	0	0
Dinner Steaks	1 (2 oz)	60	2	750	0	0
Ham & Cheese Loaf	1 slice (1 oz)	70	5	350	1	0
Healthy Favorites Baked	4 slices (1.8 oz)	50	1	600	1	0
Healthy Favorites Honey Ham	4 slices (1.8 oz)	50	2	630	2	0
Healthy Favorites Smoked Cooked	4 slices (1.8 oz)	50	2	620	0	0
Honey Ham	3 slices (2.2 oz)	70	3	760	2	0
Lower Sodium	3 slices (2.2 oz)	70	3	520	2	0
Lunchables Cookies/ Ham/ Swiss	1 pkg (4.2 oz)	360	19	1420	29	tr
Lunchables Dessert Chocolate Pudding/ Ham/ American	1 pkg (6.2 oz)	390	20	1540	34	tr

FOOD	PORTION	CAL.	FAT	SOD.	CARB.	FIB.
Oscar Mayer (CONT.)						
Lunchables Ham/ Cheddar	1 pkg (4.5 oz)	340	20	1830	19	0
Lunchables Ham/Garden Vegetable Cheese	1 pkg (4.5 oz)	380	21	1240	36	1
Lunchables Honey Ham/ Herb & Chive Cheese	1 pkg (4.5 oz)	390	21	1270	37	1
Smoked Cooked	3 slices (2.2 oz)	60	3	750	0	0
Russer						
Baked	2 oz	70	3	750	4	—
Canadian Brand Maple	2 oz	70	2	750	4	—
Chopped	2 oz	130	9	540	5	—
Cooked Ham	2 oz	60	2	650	2	—
Ham & Cheese Loaf	2 oz	120	8	600	5	—
Honey & Maple Cured	2 oz	70	2	550	3	—
Honey Cured	2 oz	60	3	600	2	—
Hot	2 oz	70	2	750	3	—
Light Cooked	2 oz	60	2	400	2	—
Light Smoked	2 oz	60	2	400	2	—
Smoked Virginia	2 oz	70	3	750	3	—
Spiced	2 oz	160	12	540	5	—
Sara Lee						
Bavarian Brand Baked	2 oz	80	4	610	1	—
Bavarian Brand Baked Honey	2 oz	80	4	490	2	—
Honey Roasted	2 oz	90	5	590	3	—
Spreadables						
Ham Salad	¼ can	100	6	—	—	—
Underwood						
Deviled	2.08 oz	220	19	430	tr	—
Deviled Light	2.08 oz	120	8	250	1	—
Deviled Smoked	2.08 oz	190	18	260	tr	—
Weight Watchers						
Deli Thin Oven Roasted	5 slices (⅓ oz)	12	tr	95	tr	—
Deli Thin Oven Roasted Honey Ham	5 slices (⅓ oz)	12	tr	95	tr	—
Deli Thin Premium Smoked	5 slices (⅓ oz)	12	tr	85	tr	—
Oven Roasted Honey Ham	2 slices (¾ oz)	25	1	220	tr	—
Oven Roasted Smoked	2 slices (¾ oz)	25	1	220	tr	—
Premium Cooked	2 slices (¾ oz)	25	1	220	tr	—
boneless 11% fat	3 oz	151	8	—	—	—
boneless extra lean roasted	3 oz	140	7	—	—	—

FOOD	PORTION	CAL.	FAT	SOD.	CARB.	FIB.
canned 13% fat	1 oz	54	4	—	—	—
canned 13% fat	3 oz	192	13	800	tr	—
canned extra lean	3 oz	142	7	—	—	—
canned extra lean	1 oz	41	2	—	—	—
canned extra lean 4% fat	3 oz	116	4	965	tr	—
center slice lean & fat	4 oz	229	15	1566	tr	—
center slice lean only	4 oz	220	9	—	—	—
chopped	1 oz	65	5	389	0	—
chopped canned	1 oz	68	5	387	tr	—
ham & cheese loaf	1 oz	73	6	762	1	—
ham & cheese spread	1 oz	69	5	339	1	—
ham & cheese spread	1 tbsp	37	3	179	tr	—
ham salad spread	1 oz	61	4	259	3	—
ham salad spread	1 tbsp	32	2	137	2	—
minced	1 oz	75	6	353	1	—
patties grilled	1 patty (2 oz)	203	18	—	—	—
patties uncooked	1 (2.3 oz)	206	18	—	—	—
sliced extra lean 5% fat	1 oz	37	1	405	tr	—
sliced regular 11% fat	1 oz	52	3	373	1	—
steak boneless extra lean	1 oz	35	1	360	0	—
whole lean & fat roasted	3 oz	207	14	—	—	—
whole lean only roasted	3 oz	133	5	—	—	—

HAM DISHES
FROZEN
Croissant Pocket

Stuffed Sandwich Ham & Cheddar	1 piece (4.5 oz)	360	17	710	39	5

Hot Pocket

Stuffed Sandwich Ham & Cheese	1 (4.5 ox)	340	15	840	37	4

Ovenstuffs

Ham/Turkey Deli Melt	1 (4.75 oz)	360	15	1050	35	—

Weight Watchers

Handy Pocket Cheese Sauce & Ham	1 (4 oz)	200	6	490	24	—

TAKE-OUT

croquettes	1 (3.1 oz)	217	14	475	11	tr
salad	½ cup	287	23	671	5	tr
sandwich w/ cheese	1	353	15	772	33	—

HAMBURGER
(*see also* BEEF)
FROZEN
Jimmy Dean

Burger	1 (2 oz)	220	21	380	0	0

FOOD	PORTION	CAL.	FAT	SOD.	CARB.	FIB.
Jimmy Dean (CONT.)						
Flamed Broiled Cheeseburger	1 (6.3 oz)	540	34	760	34	1
Mini Cheeseburger	2 (3 oz)	270	14	530	23	1
Kid Cuisine						
Beef Patty Sandwich w/ Cheese	1 (8.5 oz)	410	15	540	58	4
MicroMagic						
Cheeseburger	1 pkg (4.75 oz)	450	25	790	29	—
Hamburger	1 pkg (4 oz)	350	18	500	26	—
Rudy's Farm						
Mild Burger	1 (3 oz)	360	35	730	0	0
White Castle						
Cheeseburger	2 (3.6 oz)	310	17	480	23	6
Hamburger	2 (3.2 oz)	270	14	270	23	5
TAKE-OUT						
double patty w/ bun	1 reg	544	28	554	43	—
double patty w/ catsup mayonnaise onion pickle tomato & bun	1 reg	649	35	920	53	—
double patty w/ catsup cheese mayonnaise mustard pickle tomato & bun	1 lg	706	44	1149	40	—
double patty w/ catsup mustard mayonnaise onion pickle tomato & bun	1 lg	540	27	791	40	—
double patty w/ catsup mustard onion pickle & bun	1 reg	576	32	742	39	—
double patty w/ cheese & bun	1 reg	457	28	635	22	—
double patty w/ cheese & double bun	1 reg	461	22	892	44	—
double patty w/ cheese catsup mayonnaise onion pickle tomato & bun	1 reg	416	21	1051	35	—
single patty w/ bacon catsup cheese mustard onion pickle & bun	1 lg	609	37	1044	37	—
single patty w/ bun	1 lg	400	23	474	25	—
single patty w/ bun	1 reg	275	12	387	31	—

FOOD	PORTION	CAL.	FAT	SOD.	CARB.	FIB.
single patty w/ catsup cheese ham mayonnaise pickle tomato & bun	1 lg	745	48	1713	38	—
single patty w/ catsup mustard mayonnaise onion pickle tomato & bun	1 reg	279	13	504	27	—
single patty w/ cheese & bun	1 lg	608	33	1589	47	—
single patty w/ cheese & bun	1 reg	320	15	500	32	—
triple patty w/ catsup mustard pickle & bun	1 lg	693	41	713	29	—
triple patty w/ cheese & bun	1 lg	769	51	1211	27	—

HAZELNUTS
Crumpy

FOOD	PORTION	CAL.	FAT	SOD.	CARB.	FIB.
Chocolate Hazelnut Spread	1 tbsp (0.5 oz)	80	5	5	8	0
dried blanched	1 oz	191	19	1	5	—
dried unblanched	1 oz	179	18	1	4	—
dry roasted unblanched	1 oz	188	19	1	5	—
oil roasted unblanched	1 oz	187	18	1	5	2

HEART

FOOD	PORTION	CAL.	FAT	SOD.	CARB.	FIB.
beef simmered	3 oz	148	5	54	tr	—
chicken simmered	1 cup (5 oz)	268	11	69	tr	—
lamb braised	3 oz	158	7	54	2	—
pork braised	1 heart (4.3 oz)	191	7	—	—	—
turkey simmered	1 cup (5 oz)	257	9	79	3	—
veal braised	3 oz	158	6	50	tr	—

HEARTS OF PALM

FOOD	PORTION	CAL.	FAT	SOD.	CARB.	FIB.
canned	1 (1.2 oz)	9	tr	141	2	—
canned	1 cup (5.1 oz)	41	1	622	7	—

HERBAL TEA
(*see* TEA/HERBAL TEA)

HERBS/SPICES
(*see also individual names*)
Ac'cent

FOOD	PORTION	CAL.	FAT	SOD.	CARB.	FIB.
Flavor Enhancer	½ tsp	5	0	300	0	0
Herbal All Purpose Seasoning	½ tsp	0	0	0	0	0

FOOD	PORTION	CAL.	FAT	SOD.	CARB.	FIB.
Golden Dipt						
All Purpose Seafood	¼ tsp	2	0	85	0	—
Blackened Redfish	¼ tsp	2	0	140	0	—
Broiled Fish	¼ tsp	2	0	125	0	—
Cajun Style Shrimp & Crab	¼ tsp	2	0	200	0	—
Lemon Pepper Seafood	¼ tsp	8	0	115	1	—
Ka-Me						
Five Spice Powder	¼ tsp (1 g)	0	0	0	1	0
Lawry's						
Seasoning Blend Sloppy Joe	1 pkg	126	tr	3442	28	1
McIlhenny						
Crab Boil	3 oz	378	17	95	40	32
Mrs. Dash						
Extra Spicy	1 tsp (3.4 g)	12	tr	4	3	—
Garlic & Herb	1 tsp (3.4 g)	12	tr	2	2	—
Lemon & Herb	1 tsp (3.4 g)	12	tr	4	3	—
Low Pepper Blend	1 tsp (3.4 g)	12	tr	4	3	—
Original	1 tsp (3.4 g)	12	tr	4	2	—
Table Blend	1 tsp (3.4 g)	12	tr	4	2	—
Watkins						
Apple Bake Seasoning	¼ tsp (0.5 g)	0	0	0	0	0
Barbecue Spice	¼ tsp (0.5 g)	0	0	30	0	0
Bean Soup Seasoning	¾ tsp (2 g)	5	0	150	1	0
Beef Jerky Seasoning	2 tsp (6 g)	15	0	600	3	0
Chicken Seasoning	½ tsp (1 g)	0	0	110	0	0
Cole Slaw Seasoning	½ tsp (1.5 g)	5	0	190	1	0
Egg Sensations	1 tsp (3 g)	10	0	180	1	0
Fajita Seasoning	½ tsp (3 g)	10	0	0	2	0
Grill Seasoning	¼ tsp (1 g)	0	0	210	0	0
Ground Beef Seasoning	⅛ tsp (0.5 g)	0	0	70	0	0
Italian Blend	1 tsp (3 g)	1	0	120	2	0
Meat Tenderizer	⅛ tsp (0.5 g)	0	0	140	0	0
Meatloaf Seasoning	½ tbsp (5 g)	15	0	270	4	0
Mexican Blend	½ tbsp (4 g)	15	0	90	3	0
Omelet & Souffle Seasoning	¾ tsp (2 g)	5	0	110	1	0
Oriental Ginger Garlic Liquid Spice Blend	1 tbsp (0.5 oz)	120	14	0	0	0
Potato Salad Seasoning	¼ tsp (1 g)	0	0	135	0	0
Pumpkin Pie Spice	¼ tsp (0.5 g)	0	0	0	0	0
Smokehouse Liquid Blend	1 tbsp (0.5 oz)	120	14	0	0	0

FOOD	PORTION	CAL.	FAT	SOD.	CARB.	FIB.
Watkins (CONT.)						
Soup & Vegetable Seasoning	¼ tsp (0.5 g)	0	0	70	0	0
Spanish Seasoning Blend	¼ tsp (0.5 oz)	0	0	0	0	0
curry powder	1 tsp	6	tr	1	1	—
poultry seasoning	1 tsp	5	tr	tr	1	—
pumpkin pie spice	1 tsp	6	tr	1	1	—
HERRING						
CANNED						
roe	3.5 oz	118	3	—	tr	—
FRESH						
atlantic cooked	3 oz	172	10	98	0	—
atlantic cooked	1 fillet (5 oz)	290	17	165	0	—
atlantic raw	3 oz	134	8	76	0	—
pacific baked	3 oz	213	15	81	0	—
pacific fillet baked	5.1 oz	360	26	137	0	—
roe raw	3½ oz	130	2	—	2	—
READY-TO-USE						
atlantic kippered	1 fillet (1.4 oz)	87	5	367	0	—
atlantic pickled	½ oz	39	3	131	1	—
HICKORY NUTS						
dried	1 oz	187	18	0	5	—
HOMINY						
CANNED						
Allen						
Golden	½ cup (4.5 oz)	120	1	340	27	4
Mexican	½ cup (4.5 oz)	120	1	340	25	3
White	½ cup (4.5 oz)	100	1	340	22	4
Uncle William						
Golden	½ cup (4.5 oz)	120	1	340	27	4
Mexican	½ cup (4.5 oz)	120	1	340	25	3
White	½ cup (4.5 oz)	100	1	340	22	4
Van Camp's						
Golden	½ cup (4.3 oz)	80	1	540	17	1
White	½ cup (4.3 oz)	80	1	530	15	1
canned	½ cup	57	tr	168	11	—
HONEY						
Burleson's						
Clover	1 tbsp	60	0	1	16	0
Creamed	1 tbsp	60	0	1	16	0
Natural	1 tbsp	60	0	1	16	0

FOOD	PORTION	CAL.	FAT	SOD.	CARB.	FIB.
Burleson's (CONT.)						
Pure	1 tbsp	60	0	1	16	0
Raw	1 tbsp	60	0	1	16	0
Rocky Mountain Clover	1 tbsp	60	0	1	16	0
Smucker's						
Single Serving	½ oz	45	0	—	11	—
Tree Of Life						
Alfalfa	1 tbsp (0.7 oz)	60	0	0	17	—
Avocado	1 tbsp (0.7 oz)	60	0	0	17	—
Buckwheat	1 tbsp (0.7 oz)	60	0	0	17	—
Clover	1 tbsp (0.7 oz)	60	0	0	17	—
Honeybear Wildflower	1 tbsp (0.7 oz)	60	0	0	17	—
Orange	1 tbsp (0.7 oz)	60	0	0	17	—
Tupelo	1 tbsp (0.7 oz)	60	0	0	17	—
Wildflower	1 tbsp (0.7 oz)	60	0	0	17	—
honey	1 cup (11.9 oz)	1031	0	12	279	—
honey	1 tbsp (0.7 oz)	64	0	1	17	—

HONEYDEW
FRESH
Chiquita

Fresh	1 cup	70	0	—	—	—
cubed	1 cup	60	tr	17	16	—
wedge	⅒	46	tr	13	12	—

FROZEN
Big Valley

Balls	¾ cup (4.9 oz)	45	0	16	11	1

HORSE

roasted	3 oz	149	5	47	0	—

HORSERADISH
Gold's

Hot	1 tsp	4	tr	60	tr	—
Red	1 tsp	4	0	75	tr	—
White	1 tsp	4	tr	55	tr	—
Hebrew National						
White	1 tbsp	7	0	160	1	—
Heluva Good Cheese						
Horseradish	1 tsp (5 g)	0	0	6	0	—
Ka-Me						
Wasabi Powder	¼ tsp (1 g)	0	0	0	1	0
Kraft						
Cream Style	1 tsp (0.2 oz)	0	0	50	0	0
Horseradish Mustard	1 tsp (0.2 oz)	0	0	55	0	0

FOOD	PORTION	CAL.	FAT	SOD.	CARB.	FIB.
Kraft (CONT.)						
Prepared	1 tsp (0.2 oz)	0	0	50	0	0
Rosoff's						
Red	1 tbsp (0.5 oz)	8	0	160	2	—
White	1 tbsp (0.5 oz)	7	0	160	1	—
Sauceworks						
Horseradish	1 tsp (0.2 oz)	20	2	35	tr	0
Schorr's						
Red	1 tbsp (0.5 oz)	8	0	160	2	—
White	1 tbsp (0.5 oz)	7	0	160	1	—

HOT CAKES
(see PANCAKES)

HOT DOG
(see also MEAT SUBSTITUTES, SAUSAGE, SAUSAGE SUBSTITUTES)

FOOD	PORTION	CAL.	FAT	SOD.	CARB.	FIB.
CHICKEN						
Empire	1 (2 oz)	100	7	465	1	0
Health Valley						
Weiners	1	96	8	90	1	0
Tyson						
Cheese	1	145	11	680	1	—
Wampler Longacre						
Chicken	1 (2 oz)	130	11	440	0	—
Chicken	1 (1.6 oz)	110	9	400	0	—
chicken	1 (1.5 oz)	116	9	617	3	—
MEAT						
Armour						
Lower Salt Jumbo	1	170	15	450	—	—
Lower Salt Jumbo Beef	1	170	15	460	—	—
Star Jumbo	1	190	18	590	—	—
Star Jumbo Beef	1	190	18	590	—	—
Chefwich						
Chili Dog	5 oz	380	15	—	—	—
Healthy Choice						
Beef	1 (1.8 oz)	60	2	480	5	0
Bunsize	1 (2 oz)	70	2	590	5	0
Franks	1 (1.6 oz)	50	2	450	4	0
Jumbo	1 (2 oz)	70	2	570	5	0
Hebrew National						
Beef	1 (1.7 oz)	150	14	370	—	—
Cocktail Beef	6 (1.8 oz)	160	15	410	—	—
Dinner Beef	1 (4 oz)	350	34	890	—	—
Reduced Fat Beef	1 (1.7 oz)	120	10	350	—	—

FOOD	PORTION	CAL.	FAT	SOD.	CARB.	FIB.
Hillshire						
Franks Bun Size Beef	2 oz	180	16	560	2	—
Light & Mild Franks Jumbo	1 link	110	8	570	2	—
Light & Mild Wieners	1 link	90	7	580	2	—
Lit'l Franks Beef	2 oz	180	16	580	1	—
Lit'l Wieners	2 oz	180	16	560	2	—
Wieners Bun Size	2 oz	180	16	550	2	—
Wieners Natural Casing	2 oz	180	17	470	2	—
Hormel						
Big 8	1 (2 oz)	170	15	480	1	0
Light & Lean 97	1 (1.6 oz)	45	1	490	4	0
Light & Lean 97 Beef	1 (1.6 oz)	45	1	490	4	0
Jimmy Dean						
Mini	1 (2 oz)	110	6	370	6	0
Nathan's						
Natural Casing Franks	1	158	14	422	1	—
Skinless Franks	1	176	16	463	1	—
Oscar Mayer						
Beef	1 (1.6 oz)	150	13	450	1	0
Big & Juicy Deli Style Beef	1 (2.7 oz)	250	23	680	1	0
Big & Juicy Hot 'N Spicy	1 (2.7 oz)	220	20	770	1	0
Big & Juicy Original	1 (2.7 oz)	240	23	690	0	0
Big & Juicy Original Beef	1 (2.7 oz)	230	21	700	1	0
Big & Juicy Quarter Pound Beef	1 (4 oz)	350	32	1050	2	0
Big & Juicy Smokie Links	1 (2.7 oz)	200	18	770	1	0
Bun-Length Beef	1 (2 oz)	180	17	570	1	0
Cheese	1 (1.6 oz)	150	14	450	1	0
Free	1 (1.8 oz)	40	0	460	2	—
Healthy Favorites Turkey & Beef	1 (2 oz)	60	2	570	2	0
Light Beef	1 (2 oz)	110	8	620	2	0
Weiners Bun-Length Pork & Turkey	1 (2 oz)	180	17	570	1	0
Wieners Light Pork Turkey Beef	1 (2 oz)	110	8	580	2	0
Wieners Little	6 (2 oz)	170	16	540	1	0
Wieners Pork & Turkey	1 (1.6 oz)	150	13	450	1	0
Russer						
Lil'Salt Deli Franks	1 (2.67 oz)	160	11	640	3	—

FOOD	PORTION	CAL.	FAT	SOD.	CARB.	FIB.
Shofar						
Kosher Beef	1 (1.8 oz)	150	14	370	0	0
Kosher Beef Reduced Fat Reduced Sodium	1 (1.8 oz)	120	10	360	0	0
Wrangler						
Beef	1 (2 oz)	170	15	530	1	0
Cheese	1 (2 oz)	170	15	550	1	0
Smoked	1 (2 oz)	170	15	530	1	0
beef	1 (1.5)	142	13	462	1	—
beef	1 (2 oz)	180	16	585	1	—
beef & pork	1 (2 oz)	183	17	639	1	—
beef & pork	1 (1.5 oz)	144	13	504	1	—
pork cheesefurter smokie	1 (1.5 oz)	141	12	465	1	—
TAKE-OUT						
corndog	1	460	19	972	56	—
w/ bun chili	1	297	13	480	31	—
w/ bun plain	1	242	15	671	18	—
TURKEY						
Empire						
	1 (2 oz)	90	6	410	1	0
Louis Rich						
Bun Length	1 (2 oz)	110	8	630	2	0
Turkey	1 (1.5 oz)	80	6	480	1	0
Turkey	1 (1.6 oz)	90	7	500	1	0
Turkey Cheese	1 (1.6 oz)	90	7	490	2	0
Mr. Turkey						
Bun Size	1	130	11	670	2	—
Cheese	1	140	12	670	2	—
Wampler Longacre						
Turkey	1 (2 oz)	130	11	440	0	0
Turkey	1 (1.6 oz)	110	9	400	0	0
turkey	1 (1.5 oz)	102	8	642	1	—
HUMMUS						
Casbah						
Mix as prep	¼ cup	120	5	180	15	1
Cedar's						
No Salt Added Hummus Tahini	2 tbsp (1 oz)	50	2	70	5	3
hummus	1 cup	420	21	599	50	—
hummus	⅓ cup	140	7	200	17	—
HYACINTH BEANS						
DRIED						
cooked	1 cup	228	1	13	40	—

FOOD	PORTION	CAL.	FAT	SOD.	CARB.	FIB.

ICE CREAM AND FROZEN DESSERTS

(*see also* ICES AND ICE POPS, PUDDING POPS, SHERBET, YOGURT FROZEN)

3 Musketeers

FOOD	PORTION	CAL.	FAT	SOD.	CARB.	FIB.
Single Chocolate	1 (2 fl oz)	160	10	30	16	0
Single Vanilla	1 (2 fl oz)	160	10	30	16	0
Snack Chocolate	1 (0.72 fl oz)	60	4	10	6	0
Snack Vanilla	1 (0.72 fl oz)	60	4	10	6	0
Avari						
Creme Glace All Flavors	1 oz	10	0	35	3	—
Ben & Jerry's						
Banana Walnut	½ cup (3.9 oz)	290	21	50	26	1
Butter Pecan	½ cup (3.9 oz)	310	26	160	20	1
Cherry Garcia	½ cup (3.7 oz)	240	16	60	25	0
Cherry Vanilla	½ cup (3.9 oz)	240	15	60	26	0
Chocolate Chip Cookie Dough	½ cup (3.7 oz)	270	17	95	30	0
Chocolate Fudge Brownie	½ cup (3.7 oz)	250	14	100	31	2
Chunky Monkey	½ cup (3.7 oz)	280	19	50	29	1
Coconut Almond	½ cup (3.7 oz)	260	20	80	19	1
Coconut Almond Fudge Chip	½ cup (3.8 oz)	320	25	85	24	2
Coffee Almond Fudge	½ cup (3.7 oz)	290	20	85	24	2
Coffee Toffee Crunch	½ cup (3.7 oz)	280	19	120	28	0
English Toffee Crunch	½ cup (4 oz)	310	21	130	30	0
Mint Chocolate Cookie	½ cup (3.8 oz)	260	17	120	27	1
New York Super Fudge Chunk	½ cup (3.7 oz)	290	20	55	28	2
No Fat Strawberry	½ cup (3.3 oz)	140	0	60	31	0
No Fat Vanilla Fudge Swirl	½ cup (3.1 oz)	150	0	80	32	0
Peanut Butter Cup	½ cup (4.1 oz)	370	26	140	30	2
Pop Chocolate Chip Cookie Dough	1 (4.1 oz)	450	28	150	48	1
Pop English Toffee Crunch	1 (3.7 oz)	340	23	55	35	0
Pop Vanilla	1 (3.9 oz)	360	28	75	30	0
Rain Forest Crunch	½ cup (3.7 oz)	300	23	140	24	0
Smooth Aztec Harvest Coffee	½ cup (3.8 oz)	230	16	55	22	0
Smooth Deep Dark Chocolate	½ cup (3.9 oz)	260	15	55	32	2
Smooth Double Chocolate Fudge	½ cup (4.1 oz)	280	16	60	35	3

FOOD	PORTION	CAL.	FAT	SOD.	CARB.	FIB.
Ben & Jerry's (CONT.)						
Smooth Mocho Fudge	½ cup (4 oz)	270	18	65	30	1
Smooth Vanilla	½ cup (3.8 oz)	230	17	55	21	0
Smooth Vanilla Bean	½ cup (3.8 oz)	230	17	55	21	0
Smooth Vanilla Caramel Fudge	½ cup (4.1 oz)	280	17	75	33	1
Smooth White Russian	½ cup (3.8 oz)	240	16	55	23	0
Vanilla	½ cup (3.7 oz)	230	17	55	21	0
Wavy Gravy	½ cup (4.1 oz)	330	24	95	29	2
Bon Bons						
Vanilla With Milk Chocolate Coating	8 pieces	330	23	60	27	0
Vanilla With Milk Chocolate Coating	5 pieces	200	14	35	17	0
Borden						
Buttered Pecan	½ cup	180	12	65	16	—
Chocolate Swirl	½ cup	130	6	65	18	—
Dutch Chocolate Olde Fashioned Recipe	½ cup	130	6	65	16	—
Fat Free Black Cherry	½ cup	90	tr	40	21	—
Fat Free Chocolate	½ cup	100	tr	50	21	—
Fat Free Peach	½ cup	90	tr	40	21	—
Fat Free Strawberry	½ cup	90	tr	40	21	—
Fat Free Vanilla	½ cup	90	tr	50	20	—
Ice Milk Chocolate	½ cup	100	2	80	18	—
Ice Milk Strawberry	½ cup	90	2	65	17	—
Ice Milk Vanilla	½ cup	90	2	65	17	—
Strawberries 'N Cream Olde Fashioned Recipe	½ cup	130	5	55	19	—
Strawberry	½ cup	130	6	55	18	—
Sundae Cone	1	210	12	110	23	—
Vanilla Olde Fashioned Recipe	½ cup	130	7	55	15	—
Bounty						
Cherry/Dark	1 (0.84 fl oz)	70	5	20	8	0
Coconut/Dark	1 (0.84 fl oz)	70	5	20	7	0
Coconut/Milk	1 (0.84 fl oz)	70	5	20	7	0
Bresler's						
All Flavors Ice Cream	3.5 oz	230	12	—	23	—
All Flavors Royale Cremes	4 oz	260	16	—	24	—
All Flavors Royale Lites	4 oz	217	0	—	49	—

FOOD	PORTION	CAL.	FAT	SOD.	CARB.	FIB.
Breyers						
Bar Vanilla	1 (2.7 oz)	250	17	45	21	tr
Bar Vanilla Caramel w/ Chocolate Brittle Coating	1 (2.7 oz)	260	15	65	26	0
Bar Vanilla With Chocolate Coating	1 (2.6 oz)	230	15	45	20	0
Butter Almond	½ cup	170	11	120	15	0
Butter Pecan	½ cup (2.6 oz)	180	12	125	15	0
Cherry Vanilla	½ cup	150	7	40	17	0
Chocolate	½ cup (2.6 oz)	160	8	30	19	1
Chocolate Chip	½ cup (2.5 oz)	170	10	40	18	0
Chocolate Chip Cookie Dough	½ cup (2.5 oz)	190	10	45	20	0
Chocolate Chocolate Chip	½ cup (2.5 oz)	180	10	30	21	1
Chocolate Peanut Butter Twirl	½ cup (2.6 oz)	220	13	75	20	1
Coffee	½ cup (2.6 oz)	150	8	45	15	0
Cookies n'Cream	½ cup (2.6 oz)	170	9	55	19	0
Deluxe Rocky Road	½ cup (2.5 oz)	190	9	30	24	1
French Vanilla	½ cup (2.5 oz)	170	10	45	15	0
Light Brownie Marble Fudge	½ cup (2.6 oz)	150	5	55	23	tr
Light Chocolate	½ cup (2.4 oz)	130	4	55	19	tr
Light Chocolate Fudge Twirl	½ cup (2.6 oz)	140	4	55	22	1
Light Heavenly Hash	½ cup (2.4 oz)	150	5	55	22	tr
Light Rocky Road Deluxe	½ cup (2.4 oz)	150	5	50	22	tr
Light Strawberry	½ cup (2.4 oz)	120	4	45	18	0
Light Toffee Fudge Parfait	½ cup (2.6 oz)	150	5	55	23	tr
Light Vanilla	½ cup (2.4 oz)	130	5	55	18	0
Light Vanilla Chocolate Strawberry	½ cup (2.4 oz)	120	4	50	18	0
Mint Chocolate Chip	½ cup (2.6 oz)	170	10	40	18	0
Mocha Almond Fudge	½ cup (2.7 oz)	190	10	45	20	1
Peach	½ cup (2.6 oz)	130	6	30	18	0
Reduced Fat Chocolate Chocolate Chip	½ cup (2.4 oz)	150	5	50	21	tr
Reduced Fat Heavenly Hash	½ cup (2.4 oz)	150	5	55	22	tr
Reduced Fat Mocha Almond Fudge	½ cup (2.5 oz)	160	6	55	20	tr

FOOD	PORTION	CAL.	FAT	SOD.	CARB.	FIB.
Breyers (CONT.)						
Reduced Fat Praline Almond Crunch	½ cup (2.4 oz)	140	5	70	20	tr
Reduced Fat Swiss Almond Fudge Twirl	½ cup (2.5 oz)	160	6	55	22	tr
Sandwich Vanilla	1 (2.8 oz)	250	11	160	32	1
Strawberry	½ cup (2.6 oz)	130	6	35	15	0
Toffee Bar Crunch	½ cup (2.5 oz)	180	11	65	18	0
Vanilla	½ cup (2.6 oz)	150	8	45	15	0
Vanilla Caramel Praline	½ cup (2.6 oz)	190	10	90	23	0
Vanilla Chocolate	½ cup (2.5 oz)	160	8	35	17	0
Vanilla Chocolate Strawberry	½ cup (2.5 oz)	150	8	35	16	0
Vanilla Fudge Twirl	½ cup (2.6 oz)	160	8	50	19	tr
Vanilla Peanut Butter Fudge Sundae	½ cup (2.5 oz)	170	9	65	18	0
Carnation						
Berry Swirl Bar Raspberry	1 bar	70	3	—	—	—
Berry Swirl Bar Strawberry	1 bar	70	3	—	—	—
Cheesecake Bar Original	1 bar	120	6	—	—	—
Cheesecake Bar Strawberry	1 bar	125	6	—	—	—
Chocolate Malted Bar	1 bar	70	3	—	—	—
Creamy Lites Bar Chocolate	1 bar	50	2	—	—	—
Creamy Lites Bar Strawberry	1 bar	50	2	—	—	—
Sundae Cup Strawberry	1 (3.3 oz)	200	8	55	29	0
Chiquita						
Cherry & Ice Cream Swirl	1 bar	80	3	—	—	—
Mixed Berry & Ice Cream Swirl	1 bar	80	3	—	—	—
Orange & Ice Cream Swirl	1 bar	80	3	—	—	—
Raspberry & Ice Cream Swirl	1 bar	80	3	—	—	—
Strawberry & Ice Cream Swirl	1 bar	80	3	—	—	—
Cool Creations						
Cookies & Cream Sandwich	1 (3.5 oz)	240	11	250	34	1

FOOD	PORTION	CAL.	FAT	SOD.	CARB.	FIB.
Cool Creations (CONT.)						
Mini Sandwich	1 (2.3 oz)	110	5	70	16	0
Cool 'N Creamy						
Amarello With Chocolate Swirl	1 bar	62	2	50	10	—
Chocolate Vanilla	1 bar	54	2	51	7	—
Double Chocolate Fudge	1 bar	55	2	57	7	—
Orange Vanilla	1 bar	31	1	18	5	—
Cyrk						
Chocolate	3 oz	209	16	32	18	0
Maple Walnut	3 oz	299	22	34	25	1
Mint Chocolate Chip	3 oz	258	18	40	22	0
Strawberry	3 oz	208	15	31	17	tr
Vanilla	3 oz	209	16	30	16	0
DoveBar						
Almond	1 (3.67 fl oz)	335	22	75	30	0
Bite Size Almond Praline	1 (0.75 fl oz)	80	5	15	8	0
Bite Size Cherry Royale	1 (0.75 fl oz)	70	5	10	8	0
Bite Size Classic Vanilla	1 (0.75 fl oz)	70	5	10	7	0
Bite Size French Vanilla	1 (0.75 fl oz)	70	5	10	7	0
Bite Size Mint Supreme	1 (0.75 fl oz)	80	5	5	8	0
Caramel Pecan	1 (3.67 fl oz)	350	35	85	35	0
Chocolate Milk Chocolate	1 (3.8 fl oz)	340	21	80	35	0
Coffee Cashew	1 (3.67 fl oz)	335	22	55	31	0
Crunchy Cookie	1 (3.8 fl oz)	340	21	65	35	0
Peanut	1 (3.8 fl oz)	380	25	100	35	0
Single Vanilla/Dark	1 (2 fl oz)	200	12	50	24	0
Vanilla Dark Chocolate	1 (3.8 fl oz)	340	22	65	34	0
Vanilla Milk Chocolate	1 (3.8 fl oz)	340	21	60	34	0
Drumstick						
Cone Chocolate	1 (4.6 oz)	340	19	95	37	2
Cone Chocolate Dipped	1 (4.6 oz)	340	17	95	41	1
Cone Vanilla	1 (4.6 oz)	350	20	95	36	2
Cone Vanilla Caramel	1 (4.6 oz)	360	20	100	39	6
Cone Vanilla Fudge	1 (4.6 oz)	370	21	105	40	2
Eagle Brand						
Vanilla	½ cup	150	9	55	16	—
Edy's						
American Dream Chocolate	3 oz	90	1	45	20	—
American Dream Chocolate Chip	3 oz	100	1	45	22	—
American Dream Cookies'N'Cream	3 oz	100	1	45	22	—

FOOD	PORTION	CAL.	FAT	SOD.	CARB.	FIB.
Edy's (CONT.)						
American Dream Mocha Almond Fudge	3 oz	110	1	45	24	—
American Dream Rocky Road	3 oz	110	1	45	24	—
American Dream Strawberry	3 oz	70	tr	40	16	—
American Dream Toasted Almond	3 oz	110	1	45	24	—
American Dream Vanilla	3 oz	80	tr	45	18	—
American Dream Vanilla Chocolate Strawberry	3 oz	80	1	45	18	—
Light Almond Praline	4 oz	140	5	50	18	—
Light Banana-Politan	4 oz	110	4	50	15	—
Light Butter Pecan	4 oz	140	5	50	18	—
Light Cafe Au Lait	4 oz	110	4	50	13	—
Light Candy Bar	4 oz	140	5	50	20	—
Light Chocolate Chip	4 oz	120	4	50	16	—
Light Chocolate Fudge Mousse	4 oz	130	5	50	18	—
Light Cookies'N'Cream	4 oz	120	5	50	18	—
Light Dreamy Caramel Cream	4 oz	140	4	50	16	—
Light Malt Ball 'N' Fudge	4 oz	140	5	50	20	—
Light Marble Fudge	4 oz	120	4	50	15	—
Light Mocha Almond Fudge	4 oz	140	5	50	19	—
Light Peanut Butter & Chocolate	4 oz	130	5	50	19	—
Light Raspberry Truffle	4 oz	110	5	50	19	—
Light Rocky Road	4 oz	130	5	50	17	—
Light Strawberry	4 oz	110	4	50	15	—
Light Vanilla	4 oz	100	4	50	13	—
Vanilla Chocolate Strawberry	4 oz	110	4	50	14	—
Fi-Bar						
Banana Cream	1 bar	93	tr	—	21	—
Cocoa-Fudge 'N Cream	1 bar	93	tr	—	21	—
Raspberries 'N Cream	1 bar	93	tr	—	21	—
Wildberry Cream	1 bar	93	tr	—	21	—
Flintstones						
Cool Cream	1 (2.75 oz)	90	2	30	18	0
Push-Up	1 (2.75 oz)	100	2	25	20	0
Friendly's						
Black Raspberry	½ cup	150	7	35	17	0

FOOD	PORTION	CAL.	FAT	SOD.	CARB.	FIB.
Friendly's (CONT.)						
Chocolate Almond Chip	½ cup	170	10	45	18	0
Forbidden Chocolate	½ cup	150	9	40	14	0
Fudge Nut Brownie	½ cup	200	11	60	23	0
Heath English Toffee	½ cup (2.7 oz)	190	10	240	24	0
Purely Pistachio	½ cup	160	10	50	16	0
Vanilla	½ cup	150	8	40	16	0
Vanilla Chocolate Strawberry	½ cup	150	8	35	16	tr
Vienna Mocha Chunk	½ cup	180	11	50	19	0
Frusen Gladje						
Butter Pecan	½ cup	280	21	160	16	—
Chocolate	½ cup	240	17	65	17	—
Chocolate Chocolate Chip	½ cup	270	18	60	21	—
Strawberry	½ cup	230	15	60	20	—
Swiss Chocolate Candy Almond	½ cup	270	19	60	18	—
Vanilla	½ cup	230	17	70	16	—
Vanilla Swiss Almond	½ cup	270	19	65	18	—
Good Humor						
Banana Bob	1 (3 fl oz)	155	7	55	22	0
Bar Classic Almond	1 (3.1 fl oz)	210	12	50	21	1
Bar Classic Toasted Almond	1 (3.1 fl oz)	170	9	40	22	1
Bar Classic Vanilla	1 (3.1 fl oz)	190	10	35	22	0
Bar Sidewalk Sundae	1	280	20	65	21	2
Bubble O'Bill	1 (3.6 fl oz)	170	10	45	20	1
Bubble Play	1	110	1	5	25	—
Chip Burrrger	1 (4.7 oz)	320	15	190	44	1
Chip Sandwich	1 (4.7 oz)	320	15	190	44	1
Choco Taco	1 (4.4 fl oz)	320	17	100	38	1
Chocolate Eclair Classic	1 (3.1 fl oz)	170	9	60	21	1
Classic Candy Center Crunch Vanilla	1	280	21	75	21	0
Colonel Crunch Chocolate	1 (3.1 oz)	160	7	60	21	1
Colonel Crunch Strawberry	1 (3.1 oz)	170	8	45	22	0
Combo Cup	1 (6.2 fl oz)	200	10	65	25	1
Cone Olde Nut Sundae	1 (3.9 oz)	230	9	100	32	2
Cone Sidewalk Sundae	1 (4.2 oz)	270	14	125	31	1
Creamee Burrrger	1 (4.7 oz)	310	17	150	40	1
Crunch Classic Candy Center	1 (3.1 fl oz)	260	19	60	21	1

FOOD	PORTION	CAL.	FAT	SOD.	CARB.	FIB.
Good Humor (CONT.)						
Dinosaur Bar	1	110	2	5	25	—
Far Frog	1 (3.6 oz)	150	8	45	19	1
Fun Box Ice Cream Sandwich	1 (3.1 fl oz)	160	5	140	27	1
King Cone	1 (5.7 fl oz)	300	14	110	38	2
King Cone Classic Vanilla	1 (4.8 oz)	300	10	110	48	1
King Cone Strawberry	1 (5.7 oz)	250	10	105	38	1
Light Chocolate Chip	½ cup (2.4 oz)	130	4	45	20	0
Light Chocolate Chocolate Chip	½ cup (2.4 oz)	130	4	40	20	tr
Light Coffee	½ cup (2.4 oz)	110	3	45	18	0
Light Cookies N'Cream	½ cup (2.4 oz)	130	3	70	21	0
Light Heavenly Hash	½ cup (2.4 oz)	140	4	45	23	tr
Light Praline Almond Crunch	½ cup (2.4 oz)	130	3	65	20	0
Light Toffee Bar Crunch	½ cup (2.4 oz)	130	4	55	20	0
Light Vanilla	½ cup (2.4 oz)	110	3	50	19	0
Light Vanilla Chocolate Strawberry	½ cup (2.4 oz)	110	3	45	19	0
Light Vanilla Fudge	½ cup (2.6 oz)	120	3	50	21	0
Magnum Almond	1 (4.2 fl oz)	270	12	50	35	5
Magnum Chocolate	1 (4.2 fl oz)	260	12	60	38	2
Number One Bar	1 (4.1 fl oz)	190	11	45	22	1
Popsicle Ice Cream Bar	1 (3.1 fl oz)	160	11	35	15	1
Popsicle Ice Cream Sandwich	1 (3.6 fl oz)	190	8	120	28	1
Sandwich Classic Chip Cookie	1 (4.1 fl oz)	300	13	215	43	1
Sandwich Giant Neapolitan	1 (5.2 fl oz)	260	10	150	39	1
Sandwich Giant Vanilla	1 (5.2 fl oz)	240	10	160	35	1
Sandwich Ice Cream	1	190	8	120	28	1
Sandwich Sidewalk Sundae	1 (3.1 oz)	160	5	140	27	1
Sandwich Sprinkle	1 (3.1 fl oz)	180	6	65	28	1
Strawberry Shortcake Bar Classic	1 (3.1 fl oz)	160	8	60	20	1
Sundae Twist Cup	1	160	3	100	33	0
Toffee Taco	1 (4.4 fl oz)	300	16	120	35	1
Viennetta Chocolate	1 (4.2 fl oz)	160	9	80	19	1
Viennetta Vanilla	1 (4.2 fl oz)	160	10	80	15	0
WWF Bar	1 (3.7 fl oz)	200	10	100	24	1

FOOD	PORTION	CAL.	FAT	SOD.	CARB.	FIB.
Good Humor (CONT.)						
X-Men Bar	1 (3 fl oz)	150	6	90	23	0
Haagen-Dazs						
Baileys Original Irish Cream	½ cup (3.6 oz)	280	18	100	23	0
Brownies A La Mode	½ cup (3.7 oz)	280	18	130	25	0
Butter Pecan	½ cup (3.7 oz)	320	24	140	20	tr
Cappuccino Commotion	½ cup (3.6 oz)	310	21	105	25	1
Caramel Cone Explosion	½ cup (3.6 oz)	310	20	130	27	tr
Chocolate	½ cup (3.7 oz)	270	18	75	22	1
Chocolate Chocolate Chip	½ cup (3.7 oz)	300	20	70	26	2
Coffee	½ cup (3.7 oz)	270	18	85	21	0
Cookie Dough Dynamo	½ cup (3.6 oz)	300	19	140	29	0
Cookies & Cream	½ cup (3.6 oz)	270	17	115	23	0
DiSaronno Amaretto	½ cup (3.6 oz)	260	15	80	26	0
Macadamia Brittle	½ cup (3.7 oz)	300	20	120	25	0
Multi Pack Bars Caramel Cone Explosion	1 (3.1 oz)	330	22	150	30	tr
Multi Pack Bars Chocolate & Dark Chocolate	1 (3.2 oz)	320	22	70	27	3
Multi Pack Bars Coffee & Almond Crunch	1 (3 oz)	290	21	70	22	tr
Multi Pack Bars Iced Cappuccino Explosion	1 (2.9 oz)	290	21	60	21	tr
Multi Pack Bars Triple Brownie Overload	1 (3 oz)	320	23	95	23	1
Multi Pack Bars Vanilla & Almonds	1 (3 oz)	300	22	65	21	1
Multi Pack Bars Vanilla & Dark Chocolate	1 (3.2 oz)	320	22	50	27	4
Multi Pack Bars Vanilla & Milk Chocolate	1 (3 oz)	280	20	65	20	0
Peanut Butter Burst	½ cup (3.6 oz)	330	22	150	26	1
Rum Raisin	½ cup (3.7 oz)	270	17	75	22	0
Single Pack Bars Caramel Cone Explosion	1 (3.3 oz)	350	23	160	32	tr
Single Pack Bars Chocolate & Dark Chocolate	1 (3.9 oz)	400	27	90	33	4

FOOD	PORTION	CAL.	FAT	SOD.	CARB.	FIB.
Haagen-Dazs (CONT.)						
Single Pack Bars Coffee & Almond Crunch	1 (3.7 oz)	360	26	85	27	1
Single Pack Bars Cookie Dough Dynamo	1 (3.5 oz)	380	25	125	34	1
Single Pack Bars Iced Cappuccino	1 (3.4 oz)	330	24	70	24	tr
Single Pack Bars Triple Brownie Overload	1 (3.5 oz)	380	27	110	28	1
Single Pack Bars Vanilla & Almonds	1 (3.7 oz)	370	27	80	26	1
Single Pack Bars Vanilla & Dark Chocolate	1 (3.9 oz)	400	27	65	33	4
Single Pack Bars Vanilla & Milk Chocolate	1 (3.5 oz)	330	25	75	24	tr
Strawberry	½ cup (3.7 oz)	250	16	80	23	tr
Strawberry Cheesecake Craze	½ cup (3.7 oz)	290	18	160	28	tr
Triple Brownie Overload	½ cup (3.5 oz)	300	20	100	26	0
Vanilla	½ cup (3.7 oz)	270	18	85	21	0
Vanilla Fudge	½ cup (3.7 oz)	280	18	105	25	0
Vanilla Swiss Almond	½ cup (3.7 oz)	310	21	80	23	1
Healthy Choice						
Black Forest	½ cup (2.5 oz)	120	2	50	23	1
Bordeaux Cherry Chocolate Chip	½ cup (2.5 oz)	110	2	55	19	tr
Butter Pecan Crunch	½ cup (2.5 oz)	120	2	60	22	1
Cappuccino Chocolate Chunk	½ cup (2.5 oz)	120	2	60	32	1
Cookies 'N Cream	½ cup (2.5 oz)	120	2	90	21	tr
Double Fudge Swirl	½ cup (2.5 oz)	120	2	50	21	1
Fudge Brownie	½ cup (2.5 oz)	120	2	55	22	2
Malt Caramel Cone	½ cup (2.5 oz)	120	2	60	22	1
Mint Chocolate Chip	½ cup (2.5 oz)	120	2	50	21	tr
Peanut Butter Cookie Dough 'N Fudge	½ cup (2.5 oz)	120	2	60	22	tr
Praline & Caramel	½ cup (2.5 oz)	130	2	70	25	tr
Rocky Road	½ cup (2.5 oz)	140	2	60	28	2
Vanilla	½ cup	100	2	50	18	1
Heaven						
Sundae Bars Chocolate Fudge	1 bar	150	9	—	—	—

FOOD	PORTION	CAL.	FAT	SOD.	CARB.	FIB.
Heaven (CONT.)						
Sundae Bars Vanilla Fudge	1 bar	150	9	—	—	—
Vanilla Caramel Nut	1 bar	225	15	—	—	—
Vanilla Nut Fudge	1 bar	222	15	—	—	—
Hood						
Bar Orange Cream	1 bar (1.8 oz)	90	2	30	18	0
Bar Vanilla	1 bar (1.6 oz)	160	12	45	11	0
Caramel Butterscotch Blast	½ cup (2.3 oz)	160	8	70	20	0
Chocolate	½ cup (2.3 oz)	140	7	40	17	0
Chocolate Chip	½ cup (2.3 oz)	160	9	55	18	0
Chocolate Eclair	1 bar (1.6 oz)	150	10	45	14	0
Christmas Tree	½ cup (2.3 oz)	140	7	45	18	0
Coffee	½ cup (2.3 oz)	140	7	50	16	0
Cookie Dough Delight	½ cup (2.3 oz)	160	8	70	21	0
Cookies N Cream	½ cup (2.3 oz)	160	8	75	19	0
Cooler Cups	1 (2.1 oz)	80	1	25	18	0
Crispy Bar	1 (1.9 oz)	180	13	40	15	0
Egg Nog	½ cup (2.3 oz)	130	6	45	17	0
Fabulous Fudge & Peanut Butter Swirled Fudge Bars	1 bar (2.1 oz)	110	4	45	17	0
Fabulous Fudgies Assorted Bars	1 bar (2.1 oz)	100	3	50	19	0
Fat Free Chocolate Passion	½ cup (2.5 oz)	100	0	50	23	0
Fat Free Classic Harlequin	½ cup (2.5 oz)	100	0	50	23	0
Fat Free Double Brownie Sundae	½ cup (2.5 oz)	120	0	60	27	0
Fat Free Heavenly Hash	½ cup (2.5 oz)	120	0	75	27	0
Fat Free Mississippi Mud Pie	½ cup (2.5 oz)	130	0	75	29	0
Fat Free Praline Pecan Delight	½ cup (2.5 oz)	120	0	55	27	0
Fat Free Raspberry Blush	½ cup (2.5 oz)	120	0	55	26	0
Fat Free Super Strawberry Swirl	½ cup (2.5 oz)	100	0	40	23	0
Fat Free Vanilla Fudge Twist	½ cup (2.5 oz)	120	0	50	26	0
Fat Free Very Vanilla	½ cup (2.5 oz)	100	0	50	23	0
Fudge Bars	1 bar (2.7 oz)	100	1	80	21	0
Grasshopper Pie	½ cup (2.3 oz)	160	7	70	22	0

FOOD	PORTION	CAL.	FAT	SOD.	CARB.	FIB.
Hood (CONT.)						
Heavenly Hash	½ cup (2.3 oz)	140	6	55	21	0
Hendrie's Cherry Chocolate Dips	1 bar (1.3 oz)	120	9	30	11	0
Hoodsie Cup Vanilla & Chocolate	1 (1.7 oz)	100	5	35	12	0
Light Almond Praline Delight	½ cup (2.4 oz)	110	5	75	23	0
Light Brownie Nut Sundae	½ cup (2.4 oz)	140	5	55	22	0
Light Caribbean Coffee Royale	½ cup (2.4 oz)	110	4	50	18	0
Light Chocolate Almond Chip Sundae	½ cup (2.4 oz)	140	5	60	22	0
Light Chocolate Chocolate Chip Cookie Dough	½ cup (2.4 oz)	140	5	70	21	0
Light Cookies N Cream	½ cup (2.4 oz)	130	4	70	21	0
Light Heath Toffee Chunk Swirl	½ cup (2.4 oz)	140	5	95	23	0
Light Heavenly Hash	½ cup (2.4 oz)	130	4	55	22	0
Light Maple Sugar Shack	⅓ cup (2.4 oz)	130	4	65	23	0
Light Massachusetts Mud Pie	½ cup (2.4 oz)	140	5	60	20	0
Light Raspberry Swirl	½ cup (2.4 oz)	120	3	55	22	0
Light Strawberry Supreme	½ cup (2.4 oz)	110	3	45	19	0
Light Triple Nut Cluster Sundae	½ cup (2.4 oz)	140	5	50	22	0
Light Vanilla	½ cup (2.4 oz)	110	4	50	18	0
Light Vanilla Chocolate Strawberry	½ cup (2.4 oz)	110	4	45	18	0
Low Fat No Sugar Added Caramel Swirl	½ cup (2.4 oz)	120	3	80	18	0
Low Fat No Sugar Added Chocolate Supreme	½ cup (2.4 oz)	120	3	60	19	0
Low Fat No Sugar Added Mocha Fudge	½ cup (2.4 oz)	110	3	45	18	0
Low Fat No Sugar Added Raspberry Swirl	½ cup (2.4 oz)	110	3	45	17	0
Low Fat No Sugar Added Vanilla	½ cup (2.4 oz)	100	3	50	14	0
Maple Walnut	½ cup (2.3 oz)	160	9	45	16	0
Rockets	1 (2 oz)	120	5	50	18	1

FOOD	PORTION	CAL.	FAT	SOD.	CARB.	FIB.
Hood (CONT.)						
Sandwich Light	1 (2.2 oz)	160	4	160	29	1
Sandwich Vanilla	1 (2.2 oz)	180	7	170	27	1
Sports Bar	1 (2.9 oz)	250	17	55	23	0
Spumoni	½ cup (2.3 oz)	140	9	45	17	0
Strawberry	½ cup (2.3 oz)	130	7	45	16	0
Super Sortment Chocolate & Banana Fudge Bar	1 bar (2.1 oz)	100	3	30	18	0
Super Sortment Root Beer Float & Orange Cream Bar	1 bar (1.5 oz)	70	3	25	12	0
Vanilla	½ cup (2.3 oz)	140	7	50	16	0
Vanilla Chocolate Patchwork	½ cup (2.3 oz)	140	7	45	17	0
Vanilla Chocolate Strawberry	½ cup (2.3 oz)	140	7	45	16	0
Vanilla Fudge	½ cup (2.3 oz)	140	6	55	20	0
Klondike						
Almond Bar	1 (5.2 fl oz)	310	21	90	26	3
Caramel Crunch	1 (5.2 fl oz)	300	18	95	31	tr
Chocolate Chocolate Bar	1 (5.2 fl oz)	280	20	60	22	tr
Coffee Bar	1 (5.2 fl oz)	290	20	65	25	0
Dark Chocolate Bar	1 (5.2 fl oz)	290	20	75	24	tr
Gold Bar	1 (5.2 fl oz)	340	23	60	30	1
Krispy Bar	1 (5.2 fl oz)	300	20	85	28	0
Krunch	1 (3.1 fl oz)	200	13	160	17	1
Lite Bar	1 (2.3 fl oz)	110	6	55	14	1
Lite Bar Caramel	1 (2.4 fl oz)	120	6	65	18	1
Movie Bites Chocolate	8 pieces (4.6 fl oz)	340	26	50	22	1
Movie Bites Vanilla	8 pieces (4.6 fl oz)	320	22	60	27	1
Original Bar	1 (5.2 fl oz)	290	20	65	24	0
Sandwich Chocolate	1 (5.2 fl oz)	270	10	200	41	2
Sandwich Lite	1 (2.9 fl oz)	100	2	105	18	1
Sandwich Vanilla	1 (5.2 fl oz)	250	9	230	37	1
Mars						
Almond Bar	1 (1.85 fl oz)	210	14	45	20	0
Meadow Gold						
Sundae Cone	1	210	12	110	23	—
Milky Way						
Single Chocolate/Milk	1 (2 fl oz)	210	11	60	24	0
Snack Chocolate/Milk	1 (0.72 fl oz)	70	4	25	9	0
Snack Vanilla/Dark	1 (0.72 fl oz)	70	4	25	9	0

FOOD	PORTION	CAL.	FAT	SOD.	CARB.	FIB.
Mocha Mix						
Berry Berry Berry	½ cup	140	6	60	20	0
Dutch Chocolate	½ cup (2.3 oz)	140	8	80	16	0
Mocha Almond Fudge	½ cup (2.3 oz)	150	8	65	19	0
Neapolitan	½ cup (2.3 oz)	140	7	70	18	0
Strawberry Swirl	½ cup (2.3 oz)	140	6	55	20	0
Vanilla	½ cup (2.3 oz)	140	7	70	18	0
Nestle Crunch						
Chocolate	1 bar (3 oz)	200	14	40	18	0
Cones	1 (4.6 oz)	300	16	95	36	2
Crunch King	1 (4 oz)	270	19	45	21	0
Nuggets	8 pieces	140	9	30	12	0
Reduced Fat	1 (2.5 oz)	130	7	40	14	0
Vanilla	1 bar (3 oz)	200	14	40	17	0
Rice Dream						
Bar Chocolate	1	270	16	115	33	—
Bar Chocolate Nutty	1	330	23	110	29	—
Bar Strawberry	1	260	15	110	31	—
Bar Vanilla	1	275	16	120	33	—
Bar Vanilla Nutty	1	330	23	100	29	—
Cappuccino	½ cup	130	5	80	17	—
Carob	½ cup	130	5	80	20	—
Carob Almond	½ cup	140	6	80	20	—
Carob Chip	½ cup	140	6	80	20	—
Carob Chip Mint	½ cup	140	6	80	20	—
Cocoa Marble Fudge	½ cup	140	6	80	19	—
Dream Pie Chocolate	1	380	19	225	47	—
Dream Pie Mint	1	380	19	225	47	—
Dream Pie Mocha	1	380	19	225	47	—
Dream Pie Vanilla	1	380	19	225	47	—
Lemon	½ cup	130	5	80	17	—
Peanut Butter Fudge	½ cup	160	7	100	19	—
Strawberry	½ cup	130	5	80	17	—
Vanilla	½ cup	130	5	80	17	—
Vanilla Fudge	½ cup	140	6	80	21	—
Vanilla Swiss Almond	½ cup	140	6	80	20	—
Wildberry	½ cup	130	5	80	17	—
Sealtest						
American Glory	½ cup (2.4 oz)	130	6	45	17	0
Butter Pecan	½ cup (2.4 oz)	160	9	115	16	0
Candy Cane Crunch	½ cup (2.4 oz)	150	6	50	21	0
Chocolate	½ cup (2.4 oz)	140	7	50	19	tr
Chocolate Butter Pecan	½ cup (2.4 oz)	150	8	85	17	0
Chocolate Chip	½ cup (2.4 oz)	150	8	50	18	0

FOOD	PORTION	CAL.	FAT	SOD.	CARB.	FIB.
Sealtest (CONT.)						
Coconut Chocolate	½ cup (2.4 oz)	160	8	55	18	tr
Coffee	½ cup (2.4 oz)	140	7	55	16	0
Cupid's Scoops	½ cup (2.5 oz)	140	6	55	20	0
Dessert Bar Free Chocolate Fudge	1	90	0	30	19	—
Dessert Bar Free Vanilla Fudge	1	80	0	30	18	—
Dessert Bar Free Vanilla Strawberry Swirl	1	80	0	40	17	—
Free Black Cherry	½ cup	100	0	45	25	—
Free Chocolate	½ cup	100	0	50	23	—
Free Peach	½ cup	100	0	45	23	—
Free Strawberry	½ cup	100	0	40	23	—
Free Vanilla	½ cup	100	0	45	24	—
Free Vanilla Fudge Royale	½ cup	100	0	50	24	—
Free Vanilla Strawberry Royale	½ cup	100	0	35	25	—
French Vanilla	½ cup (2.4 oz)	140	8	50	16	0
Fudge Royale	½ cup (2.5 oz)	150	7	55	19	0
Heavenly Hash	½ cup (2.4 oz)	150	7	50	20	tr
Maple Walnut	½ cup (2.4 oz)	160	9	50	16	0
Strawberry	½ cup (2.4 oz)	130	6	45	19	0
Triple Chocolate Passion	½ cup (2.5 oz)	160	7	50	21	tr
Vanilla	½ cup (2.4 oz)	140	7	55	16	0
Vanilla Chocolate Strawberry	½ cup (2.4 oz)	140	6	50	18	0
Vanilla With Orange Sherbet	½ cup (2.7 oz)	130	4	45	22	0
Simple Pleasures						
Chocolate	4 oz	140	tr	—	25	—
Chocolate Caramel Sundae Light	4 oz	90	tr	—	20	—
Chocolate Chip	4 oz	150	3	—	25	—
Chocolate Light	4 oz	80	tr	—	16	—
Coffee	4 oz	120	tr	—	22	—
Cookies n' Cream	4 oz	150	2	—	25	—
Mint Chocolate Chip	4 oz	150	2	—	26	—
Peach	4 oz	120	tr	—	21	—
Pecan Praline	4 oz	140	2	—	25	—
Rum Raisin	4 oz	130	tr	—	35	—
Strawberry	4 oz	120	tr	—	22	—
Toffee Crunch	4 oz	130	tr	—	22	—

FOOD	PORTION	CAL.	FAT	SOD.	CARB.	FIB.
Simple Pleasures (CONT.)						
Vanilla	4 oz	120	tr	—	22	—
Vanilla Fudge Swirl Light	4 oz	90	tr	—	20	—
Vanilla Light	4 oz	80	tr	—	16	—
Snickers						
Single	1 (2 fl oz)	220	13	65	22	0
Snack	1 (1 fl oz)	110	7	35	11	0
Tofu Ice Creme						
Carob	4 fl oz	190	8	55	28	—
Vanilla	4 fl oz	190	8	55	28	—
Tofutti						
Frutti Vanilla Apple Orchard	4 fl oz	100	0	90	20	—
Turkey Hill						
Black Cherry	½ cup (2.3 oz)	140	7	30	18	0
Butter Pecan	½ cup (2.3 oz)	170	11	50	16	0
Choco Mint Chip	½ cup (2.3 oz)	160	10	45	17	0
Cookies 'N Cream	½ cup (2.3 oz)	160	9	60	19	0
Lite Butter Pecan	½ cup (2.3 oz)	130	6	80	17	0
Lite Choco Mint Chip	½ cup (2.3 oz)	140	5	75	19	0
Lite Cookies 'N Cream	½ cup (2.3 oz)	130	5	90	21	0
Lite Vanilla & Chocolate	½ cup (2.3 oz)	110	3	60	18	0
Lite Vanilla Bean	½ cup (2.3 oz)	110	3	65	18	0
Neapolitan	½ cup (2.3 oz)	150	8	30	18	0
Rocky Road	½ cup (2.3 oz)	170	8	40	23	0
Tin Roof Sundae	½ cup (2.3 oz)	160	9	70	19	0
Vanilla	½ cup (2.3 oz)	140	8	35	16	0
Vanilla & Chocolate	½ cup (2.3 oz)	150	8	35	17	0
Vanilla Bean	½ cup (2.3 oz)	140	8	35	16	0
Ultra Slim-Fast						
Bar Fudge	1	90	tr	50	17	2
Bar Vanilla Cookie Crunch	1	90	4	70	14	1
Chocolate	4 oz	100	tr	45	19	2
Chocolate Fudge	4 oz	120	tr	65	24	2
Peach	4 oz	100	tr	55	22	2
Pralines & Caramel	4 oz	120	tr	95	25	2
Sandwich Vanilla	1	140	2	220	28	1
Sandwich Vanilla Chocolate	1	140	2	220	28	1
Sandwich Vanilla Oatmeal	1	150	3	160	26	3
Vanilla	4 oz	90	tr	55	19	2
Vanilla Fudge Cookie	4 oz	110	tr	90	24	2

FOOD	PORTION	CAL.	FAT	SOD.	CARB.	FIB.
Weight Watchers						
Bar Chocolate Dip	1 (2 oz)	110	7	45	10	—
Bar Double Fudge	1 (1.75 oz)	60	1	50	12	—
Bar English Toffee Crunch	1 (2 oz)	120	11	60	11	—
Bar Fat Free Vanilla Sandwich	1 (2.5 oz)	130	0	170	30	—
Bar Sugar Free Chocolate Mousse	1 (1.75 oz)	35	tr	30	9	—
Bar Sugar Free Chocolate Treat	1 (2.75 oz)	90	0	75	18	—
Bar Sugar Free Fat Free Orange Vanilla Treat	1 (1.75 oz)	30	0	40	9	—
Fat Free Frozen Dessert Chocolate	½ cup	80	0	75	19	—
Fat Free Frozen Dessert Chocolate Swirl	½ cup	90	0	75	22	—
Fat Free Frozen Dessert Neapolitan	½ cup	80	0	75	19	—
Fat Free Frozen Dessert Vanilla	½ cup	80	0	75	20	—
Ice Milk Chocolate Chip	½ cup	120	4	80	18	—
Ice Milk Pecan Pralines 'n Cream	½ cup	130	4	90	20	—
ONE-ders Brownies'n Creme	4 oz	130	4	115	20	—
ONE-ders Chocolate Chip	4 oz	120	4	80	18	—
ONE-ders Heavenly Hash	4 oz	130	3	90	22	—
ONE-ders Pralines'n Creme	4 oz	130	4	90	19	—
ONE-ders Strawberry	4 oz	110	3	75	17	—
chocolate	½ cup (4 fl oz)	143	7	50	19	—
dixie cup chocolate	1 (3.5 fl oz)	125	6	44	16	—
dixie cup strawberry	1 (3.5 fl oz)	112	5	35	16	—
dixie cup vanilla	1 (3.5 fl oz)	116	6	46	14	—
french vanilla soft serve	½ cup (4 fl oz)	185	11	52	19	—
french vanilla soft serve	½ gal	3014	180	1228	306	—
strawberry	½ cup (4 fl oz)	127	6	40	18	—
vanilla	½ cup (4 fl oz)	132	7	53	16	—
vanilla light	½ cup	92	3	56	15	—
vanilla rich	½ cup	178	12	41	17	—
vanilla soft serve	½ cup	111	2	62	19	—
vanilla 10% fat	½ gal	2153	115	929	254	—

FOOD	PORTION	CAL.	FAT	SOD.	CARB.	FIB.
vanilla 16% fat	½ gal	2805	190	868	256	—
vanilla light	1 cup	184	6	105	29	—
vanilla light	½ gal	1469	45	836	232	—
vanilla light soft serve	1 cup	223	5	163	38	—
vanilla light soft serve	½ gal	1787	37	1303	307	—
TAKE-OUT						
cone vanilla light soft serve	1 (4.6 oz)	164	6	92	24	—
gelato chocolate hazelnut	½ cup (5.3 oz)	370	29	49	26	2
gelato vanilla	½ cup (3 oz)	211	15	78	18	0
sundae caramel	1 (5.4 oz)	303	9	195	49	—
sundae hot fudge	1 (5.4 oz)	284	9	182	48	—
sundae strawberry	1 (5.4 oz)	269	8	92	45	—

ICE CREAM CONES AND CUPS
Comet

Cups	1 (5 g)	20	0	20	1	tr
Sugar Cones	1 (12 g)	50	0	40	11	tr
Waffle Cone	1 (17 g)	70	1	30	14	1
Dutch Mill						
Chocolate Covered Wafer Cups	1 (0.5 oz)	80	5	—	8	0
Keebler						
Sugar Cones	1	45	tr	35	11	—
Vanilla Cups	1	15	tr	20	4	—
Oreo						
Chocolate Cones	1 (13 g)	50	1	110	10	tr
Teddy Grahams						
Cinnamon Cones	1 (0.5 oz)	60	1	55	13	tr
sugar cone	1	40	tr	32	8	tr
wafer cone	1	17	tr	6	3	tr

ICE CREAM TOPPINGS
(*see also* SYRUP)
Hershey

Chocolate Fudge	2 tbsp	100	4	30	14	—
Chocolate Shoppe Candy Bar Sprinkles York	2 tbsp (1.1 oz)	170	8	0	22	2
Kraft						
Butterscotch	2 tbsp (1.4 oz)	130	2	150	28	0
Caramel	2 tbsp (1.4 oz)	120	0	90	28	0
Chocolate	2 tbsp (1.4 oz)	110	0	30	26	1
Hot Fudge	2 tbsp (1.4 oz)	140	4	100	24	tr
Pineapple	2 tbsp (1.4 oz)	110	0	15	28	0
Strawberry	2 tbsp (1.4 oz)	110	0	15	29	0

FOOD	PORTION	CAL.	FAT	SOD.	CARB.	FIB.
Marzetti						
Caramel Apple	2 tbsp	60	7	95	23	0
Caramel Apple Reduced Fat	2 tbsp	30	3	100	26	0
Peanut Butter Caramel	2 tbsp	60	6	135	21	1
Planters						
Nut	2 tbsp (0.5 oz)	100	9	0	3	1
Smucker's						
Butterscotch	2 tbsp	140	1	75	33	—
Butterscotch Special Recipe	2 tbsp	160	3	40	33	—
Caramel	2 tbsp	140	1	110	33	—
Chocolate	2 tbsp	130	0	35	27	—
Chocolate Fudge	2 tbsp	130	1	50	31	—
Dark Chocolate Special Recipe	2 tbsp	130	1	45	31	—
Hot Caramel	2 tbsp	150	4	75	28	—
Hot Fudge	2 tbsp	110	4	55	18	—
Hot Fudge Light	2 tbsp	70	tr	35	19	—
Hot Fudge Special Recipe	2 tbsp	150	5	60	23	—
Hot Toffee Fudge	2 tbsp	110	4	55	18	—
Magic Shell Chocolate	2 tbsp	190	15	25	16	—
Magic Shell Chocolate Fudge	2 tbsp	190	15	50	16	—
Magic Shell Chocolate Nut	2 tbsp	200	16	40	25	—
Marshmallow	2 tbsp	120	0	0	29	—
Peanut Butter Caramel	2 tbsp	150	2	120	29	—
Pecans in Syrup	2 tbsp	130	1	0	28	—
Pineapple	2 tbsp	130	0	0	32	—
Strawberry	2 tbsp	120	0	0	30	—
Swiss Milk Chocolate Fudge	2 tbsp	140	1	70	31	—
Walnuts in Syrup	2 tbsp	130	1	0	27	—
butterscotch	2 tbsp (1.4 oz)	103	tr	143	27	—
caramel	2 tbsp (1.4 oz)	103	tr	143	27	—
marshmallow cream	1 oz	88	tr	13	23	—
marshmallow cream	1 jar (7 oz)	615	tr	90	157	—
pineapple	1 cup (11.5 oz)	861	—	214	226	—
pineapple	2 tbsp (1.5 oz)	106	0	26	28	—
strawberry	2 tbsp (1.5 oz)	107	tr	9	28	—
strawberry	1 cup (11.5 oz)	863	1	73	225	—
walnuts in syrup	2 tbsp (1.4 oz)	167	9	—	22	—

FOOD	PORTION	CAL.	FAT	SOD.	CARB.	FIB.

ICED TEA
(see also TEA/HERBAL TEA*)*

MIX

4C

Instant	8 oz	90	0	0	22	—
Bigelow						
Nice Over Ice	5 fl oz	1	tr	1	tr	—
Celestial Seasonings						
Iced Delight	8 fl oz	4	tr	14	1	—
Crystal Light						
Decaffeinated Sugar Free	8 oz	2	0	—	0	—
Sugar Free	8 oz	3	0	1	0	—
Lipton						
Instant	6 oz	0	0	0	0	—
Instant Decaffeinated	6 oz	0	0	0	0	—
Instant Lemon	8 oz	3	0	1	1	—
Instant Raspberry	8 oz	3	0	1	1	—
Lemon	6 oz	55	0	1	14	—
Lemon w/ Vitamin C	6 oz	58	0	6	15	0
Sugar Free	8 oz	1	0	6	tr	—
Sugar Free Peach	8 oz	5	0	1	1	—
Sugar Free Raspberry	8 oz	5	0	1	1	—
With Nutrasweet	8 oz	3	0	1	1	—
With Nutrasweet Decaffeinated	8 oz	3	0	1	1	—
Nestea						
100% Instant Tea as prep	8 oz	2	0	0	0	—
Ice Teasers Citrus	8 oz	6	0	0	1	—
Ice Teasers Lemon	8 oz	6	0	0	1	—
Ice Teasers Orange	8 oz	6	0	0	1	—
Ice Teasers Tropical	8 oz	6	0	0	1	—
Ice Teasers Wild Cherry	8 oz	6	0	0	1	—
Lemon	8 oz	6	0	0	1	—
Peach	8 fl oz	88	tr	25	22	—
Raspberry	8 fl oz	88	tr	25	22	—
Sugarfree	8 oz	4	0	0	1	—
With Sugar & Lemon	1 bottle (16 fl oz)	176	0	50	44	—
With Sugar & Lemon	1 can (11.5 fl oz)	127	0	36	32	—
With Sugar & Lemon as prep	8 oz	70	0	0	19	—
instant artificially sweetened lemon flavored as prep w/ water	8 oz	5	0	24	1	—

FOOD	PORTION	CAL.	FAT	SOD.	CARB.	FIB.
instant sweetened lemon flavor as prep w/ water	9 oz	87	tr	—	22	—
instant unsweetened lemon flavor as prep w/ water	8 oz	4	0	14	0	—
READY-TO-DRINK						
Schweppes	8 fl oz	90	0	60	22	0
Arizona						
Raspberry	8 fl oz	95	0	20	25	—
Clearly Canadian						
Clearly Tea Original	8 fl oz	80	0	9	19	—
Clearly Tea Tangy Lemon	8 fl oz	80	0	9	19	—
Royal Mistic						
Diet	12 fl oz	8	0	34	2	—
Lemon	12 fl oz	144	0	26	36	—
Orange	12 fl oz	144	0	26	36	—
Wild Berry	12 fl oz	144	0	34	36	—
Shasta						
Ice Tea	12 oz	124	0	—	—	—
Sipps						
Ice Tea	8.45 oz	100	0	—	—	—
Snapple						
Cranberry	8 fl oz	110	0	10	27	—
Diet	8 fl oz	0	0	10	1	—
Diet Peach	8 fl oz	0	0	10	1	—
Diet Raspberry	8 fl oz	0	0	10	1	—
Lemon	8 fl oz	110	0	10	27	—
Mango	8 fl oz	110	0	5	27	—
Mint	8 fl oz	120	0	10	29	—
Old Fashioned	8 fl oz	80	0	10	20	—
Orange	8 fl oz	110	0	10	27	—
Peach	8 fl oz	110	0	10	27	—
Raspberry	8 fl oz	120	0	10	29	—
Strawberry	8 fl oz	100	0	10	26	—
Tropicana						
Diet Lemon Fruit	8 fl oz	15	0	25	4	—
Lemon Fruit	8 fl oz	100	0	25	25	—
Peach Fruit	8 fl oz	120	0	15	28	—
Peach Fruit	1 bottle (10 fl oz)	140	0	20	35	—
Peach Fruit	1 can (11.5 oz)	160	0	20	41	—
Raspberry Fruit	1 bottle (10 fl oz)	140	0	20	34	—
Raspberry Fruit	8 fl oz	120	0	15	28	—
Raspberry Fruit	1 can (11.5 oz)	160	0	15	41	—
Tangerine Fruit	1 can (11.5 oz)	170	0	30	42	—
Tangerine Fruit	1 bottle (10 fl oz)	140	0	30	34	—

FOOD	PORTION	CAL.	FAT	SOD.	CARB.	FIB.
Tropicana (CONT.)						
Tangerine Fruit	8 fl oz	110	0	20	27	—
Twister Apple Berry	8 fl oz	100	0	15	28	—
Twister Lemon Citrus	8 fl oz	110	0	5	28	—
Turkey Hill						
Diet Decaffeinated	1 cup (8 oz)	0	0	0	0	—
Raspberry Cooler	1 cup (8 oz)	110	0	0	28	—
Regular	1 cup (8 oz)	90	0	0	22	—
Veryfine						
With Lemon	8 oz	80	0	<10	16	—

ICES AND ICE POPS

(*see also* ICE CREAM AND FROZEN DESSERTS, PUDDING POPS, SHERBET, SORBET, YOGURT FROZEN)

FOOD	PORTION	CAL.	FAT	SOD.	CARB.	FIB.
Ben & Jerry's						
Cherry Pop	1	330	24	—	28	—
Bresler's						
All Flavors Ice	3.5 oz	120	0	—	30	—
Chiquita						
Fruit & Cream Banana	1 bar	80	2	—	—	—
Fruit & Cream Blueberry	1 bar	80	1	—	—	—
Fruit & Cream Peach	1 bar	80	1	—	—	—
Fruit & Cream Raspberry	1 bar	80	1	—	—	—
Fruit & Cream Strawberry	1 bar	80	1	—	—	—
Fruit & Cream Strawberry Banana	1 bar	80	2	—	—	—
Fruit & Juice Bar Cherry	1 bar (2 oz)	50	0	—	—	—
Fruit & Juice Bar Raspberry	1 bar (2 oz)	50	0	—	—	—
Fruit & Juice Bar Raspberry Banana	1 bar (2 oz)	50	0	—	—	—
Fruit & Juice Bar Strawberry	1 bar (2 oz)	50	0	—	—	—
Fruit & Juice Bar Strawberry Banana	1 bar (2 oz)	50	0	—	—	—
Cool Creations						
10 Pack	1 pop (2 oz)	60	0	5	14	0
Lion King Cone	1 (4 oz)	280	14	90	36	1
Mickey Mouse Bar	1 (4 oz)	170	11	40	17	0
Mickey Mouse Bar	1 (2.5 oz)	110	7	25	12	0
Surprise Pops	1 (2 oz)	60	0	5	14	0
Crystal Light						
Berry Blend	1 bar	13	0	2	2	—

FOOD	PORTION	CAL.	FAT	SOD.	CARB.	FIB.
Crystal Light (CONT.)						
Cherry	1 bar	13	0	4	2	—
Fruit Punch	1 bar	14	0	2	2	—
Orange	1 bar	13	0	3	2	—
Pina Colada	1 bar	14	0	2	2	—
Pineapple	1 bar	14	0	2	2	—
Pink Lemonade	1 bar	14	0	2	2	—
Raspberry	1 bar	13	0	4	2	—
Strawberry	1 bar	13	0	2	2	—
Strawberry Daiquiri	1 bar	14	0	2	2	—
Cyrk						
Ice Chocolate	4 oz	85	1	19	21	—
Ice Vanilla	4 oz	75	tr	14	17	—
Sorbet Apricot	4 oz	104	tr	2	27	1
Sorbet Blueberry	4 oz	77	tr	1	20	2
Sorbet Cherry	4 oz	98	tr	1	25	1
Sorbet Lemon	4 oz	66	0	2	18	0
Sorbet Mango	4 oz	83	tr	2	22	tr
Sorbet Pina Colada	4 oz	107	3	3	23	tr
Sorbet Plum	4 oz	90	tr	1	23	1
Sorbet Raspberry	4 oz	88	tr	1	23	2
Sorbet Strawberry	4 oz	79	tr	2	21	1
Sorbet Sugar Free Apricot	4 oz	36	tr	1	9	1
Sorbet Sugar Free Mango	4 oz	48	tr	2	13	2
Sorbet Sugar Free Pina Colada	4 oz	66	3	3	11	1
Sorbet Sugar Free Raspberry	4 oz	35	tr	1	9	3
Sorbet White Peach	4 oz	96	tr	1	26	1
Dole						
Fruit Juice Grape	1 bar (1.75 oz)	45	0	5	11	0
Fruit Juice No Sugar Added Grape	1 bar (1.75 oz)	25	0	5	6	0
Fruit Juice No Sugar Added Strawberry	1 bar (1.75 oz)	25	0	5	6	0
Fruit Juice Raspberry	1 bar (1.75 oz)	45	0	5	11	0
Fruit Juice Strawberry	1 bar (1.75 oz)	45	0	5	11	0
Fruit 'n Juice Coconut	1 bar (4 oz)	210	7	50	33	0
Fruit 'n Juice Lemonade	1 bar (4 oz)	120	0	55	28	0
Fruit 'n Juice Lime	1 bar (4 oz)	110	0	55	28	0
Fruit 'n Juice Peach Passion	1 bar (2.5 oz)	70	0	5	17	0

FOOD	PORTION	CAL.	FAT	SOD.	CARB.	FIB.
Dole (CONT.)						
Fruit 'n Juice Pineapple Coconut	1 bar (4 oz)	140	4	5	27	0
Fruit 'n Juice Pineapple Orange Banana	1 bar (2.5 oz)	70	0	5	16	0
Fruit 'n Juice Pineapple Orange Banana	1 bar (4 oz)	110	0	5	26	0
Fruit 'n Juice Raspberry	1 bar (2.5 oz)	70	0	5	16	0
Fruit 'n Juice Strawberry	1 bar (2.5 oz)	70	0	5	17	0
Fruit 'n Juice Strawberry	1 bar (4 oz)	110	0	5	26	0
Fi-Bar						
Juice Bar Lemoney-Lime	1 bar	63	tr	—	15	—
Juice Bar Strawberry Nectar	1 bar	63	tr	—	15	—
Juice Bar Tropical Delight	1 bar	63	tr	—	15	—
Flintstones						
Rock Pops	1 (3.5 oz)	80	0	5	20	0
Frozfruit						
Strawberry	1 (4 oz)	80	0	20	20	1
Good Humor						
Big Stick Cherry Pineapple	1 (3.6 fl oz)	50	0	—	12	0
Big Stick Popsicle	1 (3.6 fl oz)	50	0	5	12	—
Calippo Cherry	1 (3.8 fl oz)	100	0	5	23	—
Calippo Grape Lemon	1 (3.9 fl oz)	90	0	0	22	—
Calippo Orange	1 (3.9 fl oz)	90	0	0	23	—
Citrus Bites	1 (1.8 fl oz)	35	0	0	9	—
Creamsicle Orange	1 (1.8 fl oz)	70	2	15	13	0
Creamsicle Orange	1 (2.8 fl oz)	110	3	30	20	0
Creamsicle Orange Raspberry	1 (2.6 fl oz)	100	3	25	19	0
Creamsicle Sugar Free	1 (1.8 fl oz)	25	0	10	5	—
Flintstones Push-Up Yabba Dabba Doo Orange	1 (2.75 fl oz)	90	1	20	20	—
Fudgsicle Bar	1 (2.8 fl oz)	90	1	55	17	1
Fudgsicle Pop	1 (1.8 fl oz)	60	1	40	12	0
Fudgsicle Sugar Free	1 (1.8 fl oz)	40	1	35	8	1
Fun Box Fudge Bar	1 (2.3 fl oz)	80	1	65	16	0
Fun Box Pops	1 (2 fl oz)	35	0	5	10	—
Fun Box Twin Box Cherry	1 (2.6 fl oz)	50	0	10	14	—
Fun Box Twin Pop Banana	1 (2.6 fl oz)	50	0	10	14	—

FOOD	PORTION	CAL.	FAT	SOD.	CARB.	FIB.
Good Humor (CONT.)						
Fun Box Twin Pop Blue Raspberry	1 (2.6 fl oz)	50	0	10	14	—
Fun Box Twin Pop Cherry Lemon	1 (2.6 fl oz)	50	0	10	14	—
Fun Box Twin Pop Orange Cherry Grape	1 (2.6 fl oz)	50	0	10	14	—
Fun Box Twin Pop Root Beer	1 (2.6 fl oz)	50	0	10	14	—
Garfield Bar	1 (3.9 fl oz)	90	0	0	22	—
Great White	1 (3.1 fl oz)	70	1	0	18	—
Hyperstripe	1 (2.8 fl oz)	80	0	0	21	—
Ice Stripe Cherry Orange	1 (1.5 fl oz)	35	0	0	9	0
Ice Stripe Grape Lemon	1 (1.5 fl oz)	35	0	0	9	0
Jumbo Jet Star	1 (4.7 fl oz)	80	0	0	20	—
Laser Blazer	1 (2.6 oz)	70	0	5	16	—
Popsicle All Natural	1 (1.8 fl oz)	45	0	5	10	—
Popsicle Orange Cherry Grape	1 (1.8 fl oz)	45	0	0	11	—
Popsicle Rainbow Pops	1 (1.8 fl oz)	45	0	0	11	—
Popsicle Rootbeer Banana Lime	1 (1.8 fl oz)	45	0	0	11	—
Popsicle Strawberry Raspberry Wildberry	1 (1.8 fl oz)	45	0	0	11	—
Popsicle Supersicle Traffic Signal	1	80	0	0	20	—
Popsicle Twin Pop Cherry	1 (2.6 fl oz)	70	0	0	16	—
Popsicle Twin Pop Orange Cherry Grape Lime	1 (2.6 fl oz)	70	0	5	16	—
Snow Cone	1	60	0	5	14	—
Snowfruit Coconut Bar	1 (3.75 fl oz)	150	4	35	27	1
Snowfruit Orange Bar	1	140	0	10	34	tr
Snowfruit Strawberry Bar	1	120	0	15	31	tr
Snowfruit Tropical Fruit Bar	1	110	0	10	28	—
Sugar Free Pop Orange Cherry Grape	1 (1.8 fl oz)	15	0	0	3	—
Super Mario Bar	1	120	1	10	27	—
Supersicle Cherry Banana	1 (4.7 fl oz)	80	0	0	20	—
Supersicle Cherry Cola	1 (4.7 fl oz)	80	0	0	20	—

FOOD	PORTION	CAL.	FAT	SOD.	CARB.	FIB.
Good Humor (CONT.)						
Supersicle Double Fudge	1 (4.7 fl oz)	150	2	95	29	1
Supersicle Firecracker	1 (4.7 fl oz)	90	0	0	20	—
Supersicle Firecracker Jr.	1	72	0	0	10	—
Supersicle Sour Tower	1	80	0	0	20	—
Swirl Bubble Gum	1 (2.7 fl oz)	55	0	0	13	—
Swirl Cherry Banana	1 (2.7 fl oz)	55	0	0	13	—
Torpedo Cherry	1 (1.8 fl oz)	35	0	5	10	0
Twister Blue Raspberry Cherry Cherry Cola Cherry	1 (1.8 fl oz)	45	0	0	10	—
Twister Cherry Lemon Orange Lemon	1 (1.8 fl oz)	45	0	0	10	—
Vampire's Deadly Secret	1 (2.8 fl oz)	100	0	10	24	—
Watermelon Bar	1 (3.6 fl oz)	80	0	0	20	—
Haagen-Dazs						
Sorbet & Cream Blueberry	4 oz	190	8	35	25	—
Sorbet & Cream Keylime	4 oz	190	7	30	29	—
Sorbet & Cream Orange	4 oz	190	8	35	27	—
Sorbet & Cream Orange	½ cup (3.7 oz)	200	9	45	27	0
Sorbet & Cream Raspberry	½ cup (3.7 oz)	190	9	45	23	tr
Sorbet Bar Chocolate	1 (2.7 oz)	80	0	50	20	1
Sorbet Bar Wild Berry	1 (2.7 oz)	90	0	5	22	tr
Sorbet Chocolate	½ cup (4 oz)	130	0	80	30	2
Sorbet Mango	½ cup (4 oz)	120	0	0	30	tr
Sorbet Raspberry	½ cup (4 oz)	120	0	5	29	1
Sorbet Strawberry	½ cup (4 oz)	130	0	0	33	1
Sorbet Zesty Lemon	½ cup (4 oz)	130	0	5	32	tr
Hood						
Hendrie's Sizzle'N Sour Stix	1 bar (2 oz)	80	tr	15	15	0
Hoodsie Pop	1 (3.3 oz)	60	0	0	16	—
Natural Blenders Pineapple	1 bar (1 oz)	60	0	0	16	—
Natural Blenders Raspberry	1 bar (1 oz)	60	0	0	16	—
Natural Blenders Strawberry	1 bar (1 oz)	60	0	0	16	—
Pop Banana	1 (3.3 oz)	60	0	0	16	—
Pop Blue Raspberry	1 (3.3 oz)	60	0	0	16	—
Pop Cherry	1 (3.3 oz)	60	0	0	16	—

FOOD	PORTION	CAL.	FAT	SOD.	CARB.	FIB.
Hood (CONT.)						
Pop Grape	1 (3.3 oz)	60	0	0	16	—
Pop Orange	1 (3.3 oz)	60	0	0	16	—
Pop Root Beer	1 (3.3 oz)	60	0	0	16	—
Super Sortment Juice Bars	1 bar (1.9 oz)	40	0	0	10	—
Jell-O						
Lemon Lime	1 bar	33	tr	23	8	—
Mixed Berry	1 bar	31	tr	23	7	—
Orange	1 bar	31	tr	23	7	—
Orange Pineapple	1 bar	31	tr	23	7	—
Raspberry	1 bar	29	tr	24	7	—
Raspberry Peach	1 bar	29	tr	24	7	—
Side By Side Apple Cherry	1 bar	36	tr	7	8	—
Side By Side Grape Lemon	1 bar	36	tr	7	8	—
Strawberry	1 bar	31	tr	23	7	—
Strawberry Banana	1 bar	31	tr	23	7	—
Kool-Aid						
Berry Punch	1 bar	31	tr	23	7	—
Cherry	1 bar	42	0	2	11	—
Grape	1 bar	42	0	2	11	—
Mountain Berry Punch	1 bar	42	0	2	11	—
Lifesavers						
Ice Pops	1 (1.75 oz)	35	0	0	9	0
Sunkist						
Orange Juice Bar	1 (3.4 fl oz)	80	1	5	19	—
Wildberry	1 (3.4 fl oz)	120	1	10	27	—
Tofutti						
Frutti Apricot Mango	4 fl oz	100	0	90	20	—
Frutti Three Berry	4 fl oz	100	0	90	20	—
Vitari						
Passion-Fruit	4 oz	80	0	—	—	—
Peach	4 oz	80	0	—	—	—
fruit & juice bar	1 (3 fl oz)	75	tr	3	19	—
gelatin pop	1 (1.5 oz)	31	0	20	7	—
ice coconut pineapple	½ cup (4 fl oz)	109	3	34	23	—
ice fruit w/ Equal	1 bar (1.7 oz)	12	0	3	3	—
ice lime	½ cup (4 fl oz)	75	0	—	31	—
ice pop	1 (2 fl oz)	42	0	7	11	—

ICING

(*see* CAKE)

FOOD	PORTION	CAL.	FAT	SOD.	CARB.	FIB.

INSTANT BREAKFAST
(see BREAKFAST DRINKS)

JACKFRUIT
| fresh | 3½ oz | 70 | tr | 2 | 4 | — |

JALAPENO
(see PEPPERS)

JAM/JELLY/PRESERVES
BAMA

Apple Butter	2 tsp	25	0	5	6	—
Apple Jelly	2 tsp	30	0	5	8	—
Grape Jelly	2 tsp	30	0	5	8	—
Peach Preserves	2 tsp	30	0	5	8	—
Red Plum Jam	2 tsp	30	0	5	8	—
Strawberry Preserves	2 tsp	30	0	5	8	—

Eden

| Apple Butter | 1 tbsp (0.5 fl oz) | 25 | 0 | 0 | 3 | 0 |

Estee

Apple Reduced Calorie	1 pkg (0.5 oz)	10	0	25	2	—
Apple Slice	1 tbsp (0.5 oz)	10	0	20	2	—
Apricot	1 tbsp (0.5 oz)	5	0	20	1	—
Blackberry	1 tbsp (0.5 oz)	5	0	25	1	—
Cherry	1 tbsp (0.5 oz)	5	0	20	1	—
Grape	1 tbsp (0.5 oz)	10	0	20	2	—
Orange	1 tbsp (0.5 oz)	10	0	20	2	—
Peach	1 tbsp (0.5 oz)	5	0	20	1	—
Red Raspberry	1 tbsp (0.5 oz)	5	0	25	1	—
Strawberry	1 tbsp (0.5 oz)	10	0	20	2	—

Harvest Moon

Apricot Fruit Spread	1 tbsp (0.6 oz)	35	0	0	9	—
Blueberry Fruit Spread	1 tbsp (0.6 oz)	35	0	0	9	—
Cherry Fruit Spread	1 tbsp (0.6 oz)	35	0	0	9	—
Grape Fruit Spread	1 tbsp (0.6 oz)	35	0	0	9	—
Peach Fruit Spread	1 tbsp (0.6 oz)	35	0	0	9	—
Raspberry Fruit Spread	1 tbsp (0.6 oz)	35	0	0	9	—
Strawberry Fruit Spread	1 tbsp (0.6 oz)	35	0	0	9	—

Home Brands

| All Flavors Jelly | 2 tsp | 35 | 0 | — | — | — |
| All Flavors Preserves | 2 tsp | 35 | 0 | — | — | — |

Kraft

Apple Jelly	1 tbsp (0.7 oz)	60	0	10	14	0
Apple Strawberry Jelly	1 tbsp (0.7 oz)	50	0	10	13	0
Apricot Preserves	1 tbsp (0.7 oz)	50	0	10	13	0

FOOD	PORTION	CAL.	FAT	SOD.	CARB.	FIB.
Kraft (CONT.)						
Blackberry Jelly	1 tbsp (0.7 oz)	50	0	10	13	0
Blackberry Preserves	1 tbsp (0.7 oz)	50	0	10	13	tr
Grape Jam	1 tbsp (0.7 oz)	60	0	10	14	0
Grape Jelly	1 tbsp (0.7 oz)	50	0	10	14	0
Grape Reduced Calorie	1 tbsp (0.6 oz)	20	0	20	5	0
Guava Jelly	1 tbsp (0.7 oz)	50	0	10	13	0
Orange Marmalade	1 tbsp (0.7 oz)	50	0	10	14	0
Peach Preserves	1 tbsp (0.7 oz)	50	0	10	14	0
Pineapple Preserves	1 tbsp (0.7 oz)	50	0	10	14	0
Red Currant Jelly	1 tbsp (0.7 oz)	50	0	10	13	0
Red Plum Jam	1 tbsp (0.7 oz)	60	0	10	13	0
Red Raspberry Preserves	1 tbsp (0.7 oz)	50	0	10	13	0
Strawberry Jam	1 tbsp (0.7 oz)	50	0	10	13	0
Strawberry Jelly	1 tbsp (0.7 oz)	60	0	10	14	0
Strawberry Preserves	1 tbsp (0.7 oz)	50	0	10	13	0
Strawberry Reduced Calorie	1 tbsp	20	0	20	5	0
Red Wing						
Apple Blackberry Jelly	1 tbsp (0.7 oz)	50	0	5	13	0
Apple Cherry Jelly	1 tbsp (0.7 oz)	50	0	10	13	0
Apple Currant Jelly	1 tbsp (0.7 oz)	50	0	15	13	0
Apple Grape Jelly	1 tbsp (0.7 oz)	50	0	10	13	0
Apple Jelly	1 tbsp (0.7 oz)	50	0	5	13	0
Apple Raspberry Jelly	1 tbsp (0.7 oz)	50	0	5	13	0
Apple Strawberry Jelly	1 tbsp (0.7 oz)	50	0	5	13	0
Black Raspberry Jelly	1 tbsp (0.7 oz)	50	0	5	13	0
Blackberry Jelly	1 tbsp (0.7 oz)	50	0	5	13	0
Cherry Jelly	1 tbsp (0.7 oz)	50	0	5	13	0
Concord Grape Jelly	1 tbsp (0.7 oz)	50	0	5	13	0
Crabapple Jelly	1 tbsp (0.7 oz)	50	0	10	13	0
Cranberry Jelly	1 tbsp (0.7 oz)	50	0	10	13	0
Cranberry Grape Jelly	1 tbsp (0.7 oz)	50	0	10	13	0
Currant Jelly	1 tbsp (0.7 oz)	50	0	10	13	0
Damson Plum Jelly	1 tbsp (0.7 oz)	50	0	5	13	0
Elderberry Jelly	1 tbsp (0.7 oz)	50	0	5	13	0
Grape Jelly	1 tbsp (0.7 oz)	50	0	5	13	0
Mint Apple Jelly	1 tbsp (0.7 oz)	50	0	5	13	0
Mint Jelly	1 tbsp (0.7 oz)	50	0	5	13	0
Mixed Fruit Jelly	1 tbsp (0.7 oz)	50	0	5	13	0
Red Plum Jelly	1 tbsp (0.7 oz)	50	0	10	13	0
Red Raspberry Jelly	1 tbsp (0.7 oz)	50	0	5	13	0
Strawberry Apple Jelly	1 tbsp (0.7 oz)	50	0	10	13	0

FOOD	PORTION	CAL.	FAT	SOD.	CARB.	FIB.
Red Wing (CONT.)						
Strawberry Jelly	1 tbsp (0.7 oz)	50	0	5	13	0
S&W						
Apricot Pineapple Reduced Calorie Preserves	1 tsp	4	0	0	1	—
Blueberry Reduced Calorie Jam	1 tsp	4	0	0	1	—
Concord Grape Reduced Calorie Jelly	1 tsp	4	0	0	1	—
Orange Marmalade Reduced Calorie	1 tsp	4	0	0	1	—
Red Raspberry Reduced Calorie Jam	1 tsp	4	0	0	1	—
Red Tart Cherry Reduced Calorie Preserves	1 tsp	4	0	0	1	—
Strawberry Reduced Calorie Jam	1 tsp	4	0	0	1	—
Smucker's						
All Flavors Jam	1 tsp	18	0	0	4	—
All Flavors Jelly	1 tsp	18	0	0	4	—
All Flavors Low Sugar Spread	1 tsp	8	0	<10	2	—
All Flavors Preserves	1 tsp	18	0	0	4	—
All Flavors Simply Fruit	1 tsp	16	0	0	4	—
All Flavors Single Serving Jelly	½ oz	38	0	<10	9	—
All Flavors Single Serving Preserves	½ oz	38	0	<10	9	—
All Flavors Slenderella	1 tsp	7	0	0	2	—
Apple Butter Autumn Harvest	1 tsp	12	0	0	3	—
Apple Butter Natural	1 tsp	12	0	0	3	—
Apple Butter Simply Fruit	1 tsp	12	0	0	3	—
Apple Cider Butter	1 tsp	12	0	0	3	—
Blackberry Single Serving Imitation Jelly	1 pkg (0.4 oz)	4	0	<10	1	—
Cherry Single Serving Imitation Jelly	1 pkg (0.4 oz)	4	0	<10	1	—
Grape Single Serving Imitation Jelly	1 pkg (0.4 oz)	4	0	<10	1	—
Orange Marmalade	1 tsp	18	0	0	4	—
Peach Butter	1 tsp	15	0	0	4	—
Pumpkin Butter Autumn Harvest	1 tsp	12	0	14	3	—

FOOD	PORTION	CAL.	FAT	SOD.	CARB.	FIB.
Tree Of Life						
Apricot Fruit Spread	1 tbsp (0.6 oz)	45	0	0	12	—
Blueberry Fruit Spread	1 tbsp (0.6 oz)	35	0	0	9	—
Cherry Fruit Spread	1 tbsp (0.6 oz)	40	0	0	10	—
Grape Fruit Spread	1 tbsp (0.6 oz)	35	0	0	8	—
Peach Fruit Spread	1 tbsp (0.6 oz)	45	0	0	12	—
Raspberry Fruit Spread	1 tbsp (0.6 oz)	30	0	0	7	—
Strawberry Fruit Spread	1 tbsp (0.6 oz)	35	0	0	9	—
Weight Watchers						
Grape Spread	1 tsp	8	0	0	2	—
Raspberry Spread	1 tsp	8	0	0	2	—
Strawberry Spread	1 tsp	8	0	0	2	—
Whistling Wings						
Blueberry Jam	1 oz	50	tr	2	12	tr
Raspberry Jam	1 oz	60	tr	1	14	1
White House						
Apple Butter	1 oz	50	0	5	12	1
all flavors jam	1 pkg (0.5 oz)	34	0	—	9	tr
all flavors jam	1 tbsp (0.7 oz)	48	0	—	13	tr
all flavors jelly	1 tbsp (0.7 oz)	52	0	—	14	tr
all flavors jelly	1 pkg (0.5 oz)	38	0	—	10	tr
all flavors preserve	1 tbsp (0.7 oz)	48	0	—	13	tr
all flavors preserve	1 pkg (0.5 oz)	34	0	—	9	tr
apple butter	1 cup (9.9 oz)	519	1	1	135	—
apple butter	1 tbsp (0.6 oz)	33	0	0	9	—
apple jelly	3½ oz	259	0	15	65	—
apple jelly	1 tbsp (0.7 oz)	52	0	7	14	—
apple jelly	1 pkg (0.5 oz)	38	0	5	10	tr
apricot jam	3½ oz	250	0	—	62	—
blackberry jam	3½ oz	237	0	—	59	—
cherry jam	3½ oz	250	0	—	62	—
lingonberry jam	0.5 oz	23	tr	—	6	tr
orange jam	3½ oz	243	0	11	60	—
orange marmalade	1 tbsp (0.7 oz)	49	0	11	13	—
orange marmalade	1 pkg (0.5 oz)	34	0	8	9	—
plum jam	3½ oz	241	0	—	60	—
quince jam	3½ oz	236	0	—	59	—
raspberry jam	3½ oz	248	0	—	61	—
raspberry jelly	3½ oz	259	0	—	65	—
red currant jam	3½ oz	237	0	—	59	—
red currant jelly	3½ oz	265	0	4	66	—
rose hip jam	3½ oz	250	0	5	62	—
strawberry jam	1 tbsp (0.7 oz)	48	0	8	13	tr
strawberry jam	1 pkg (0.5 oz)	34	0	6	9	tr

FOOD	PORTION	CAL.	FAT	SOD.	CARB.	FIB.
strawberry preserve	1 pkg (0.5 oz)	34	0	6	9	tr
strawberry preserve	1 tbsp (0.7 oz)	48	0	8	13	tr

JAPANESE FOOD
(see ORIENTAL FOOD)

JAVA PLUM
fresh	1 cup	82	tr	18	21	—
fresh	3	5	tr	1	1	—

JELLY
(see JAM/JELLY/PRESERVES)

JERUSALEM ARTICHOKE
(see ARTICHOKE)

JEW'S EAR
pepeao dried	½ cup	36	tr	8	10	—
pepeao raw sliced	1 cup	25	tr	9	7	—

JUJUBE
fresh	3½ oz	105	tr	3	24	—

KALE
FRESH
Dole
Chopped	½ cup	17	1	15	3	—
chopped cooked	½ cup	21	tr	15	4	—
raw chopped	½ cup	21	tr	15	3	—
scotch chopped cooked	½ cup	18	tr	29	4	—
FROZEN						
chopped cooked	½ cup	20	tr	10	4	—

KEFIR
kefir	3½ oz	66	4	46	5	—

KETCHUP
Del Monte
	1 tbsp (0.5 oz)	15	0	190	4	0
Hain						
Natural	1 tbsp	16	0	155	4	—
Natural No Salt Added	1 tbsp	16	0	5	4	—
Heinz						
Hot	1 tbsp	14	0	185	3	—
Lite	1 tbsp	8	0	115	2	—
Hunt's						
No Salt Added	1 tbsp	20	tr	0	5	tr
McIlhenny						
Spicy	1 tbsp (0.6 oz)	23	tr	128	5	tr

FOOD	PORTION	CAL.	FAT	SOD.	CARB.	FIB.
Muir Glen						
Organic	1 tbsp (0.6 oz)	15	0	190	3	0
Red Wing						
Extra Fancy	1 tbsp (0.6 oz)	20	0	190	5	0
Smucker's						
Ketchup	1 tsp	8	0	0	2	—
Tree Of Life						
Salsa Ketchup	1 tbsp (0.5 oz)	10	0	50	3	—
catsup	1 pkg (0.2 oz)	6	tr	71	2	tr
catsup	1 tbsp	16	tr	178	4	tr
low sodium	1 tbsp	16	tr	3	4	tr

KIDNEY

FOOD	PORTION	CAL.	FAT	SOD.	CARB.	FIB.
beef simmered	3 oz	122	3	114	0	—
lamb braised	3 oz	117	3	128	1	—
pork braised	3 oz	128	4	—	0	—
veal braised	3 oz	139	5	93	0	—

KIDNEY BEANS
CANNED

FOOD	PORTION	CAL.	FAT	SOD.	CARB.	FIB.
B&M						
Red Baked Beans	8 oz	250	7	640	42	11
Eden						
Organic	½ cup (4.4 oz)	100	0	15	18	10
Friends						
Red Beans	8 oz	340	4	1060	57	—
Goya						
Spanish Style	7.5 oz	140	1	760	29	10
Green Giant						
Dark Red	½ cup	90	0	250	20	5
Light Red	½ cup	90	0	250	20	5
Hanover						
Dark Red	½ cup	110	0	—	—	—
Light Red In Sauce	½ cup	120	0	—	—	—
Hunt's						
Red	4 oz	100	tr	400	20	5
Luck's						
Seasoned w/ Pork	7.5 oz	220	6	—	—	—
Special Cook Red	7.5 oz	190	4	—	—	—
Progresso						
Red	½ cup	100	tr	210	21	7
S&W						
Dark Red Lite 50% Less Salt	½ cup	120	0	355	22	—
Dark Red Premium	½ cup	120	1	—	22	—

FOOD	PORTION	CAL.	FAT	SOD.	CARB.	FIB.
S&W (CONT.)						
Water Pack	½ cup	90	0	0	16	—
Trappey						
Dark Red	½ cup (4.5 oz)	130	1	310	22	8
Light Red	½ cup (4.5 oz)	120	1	340	22	8
Light Red New Orleans Style With Bacon	½ cup (4.5 oz)	110	1	410	20	6
Light Red With Jalapeno	½ cup (4.5 oz)	110	1	420	19	6
With Chili Gravy	½ cup (4.5 oz)	110	1	510	20	7
Van Camp's						
Dark Red	½ cup (4.6 oz)	90	0	760	20	6
Light Red	½ cup (4.6 oz)	90	0	390	20	6
kidney beans	1 cup	208	1	889	38	—
red	1 cup	216	1	873	40	—
DRIED						
Arrowhead						
Red	¼ cup (1.6 oz)	160	1	0	29	10
Hurst						
Kidney Beans	1.2 oz	120	1	10	21	10
california red cooked	1 cup	219	tr	7	40	—
cooked	1 cup	225	1	4	40	—
red cooked	1 cup	225	1	4	40	—
royal red cooked	1 cup	218	tr	8	39	—
SPROUTS						
cooked	1 lb	152	3	—	21	—
raw	½ cup	27	tr	—	4	—
KIWI JUICE						
After The Fall						
Kiwi Bear	1 cup (8 oz)	100	0	15	24	0
KIWIS						
Dole	2	90	1	0	18	4
California Kiwifruit	2 (4.9 oz)	90	1	0	18	4
fresh	1 med	46	tr	4	11	3
DRIED						
Sonoma	7-8 pieces (1 oz)	90	1	0	19	2
KNISH						
Brand's						
Cheese 'N Blueberry	1 (7 oz)	378	13	—	40	—
Cheese 'N Cherry	1 (7 oz)	378	13	—	40	—
Everything	1 (7 oz)	221	8	—	34	—
Kashe	1 (7 oz)	270	8	—	45	—
Potato	1 (7 oz)	290	9	—	47	—

FOOD	PORTION	CAL.	FAT	SOD.	CARB.	FIB.
Brand's (CONT.)						
Potato w/ Broccoli & Cheese	1 (7 oz)	312	15	—	33	—
Potato w/ Spinach & Mushroom	1 (7 oz)	214	8	—	32	—
Joshua's						
Coney Island Potato	1 (4.6 oz)	280	8	610	52	1
TAKE-OUT						
cheese & blueberry	1 (7 oz)	378	13	—	40	—
cheese & cherry	1 (7 oz)	378	13	—	40	—
everything	1 (7 oz)	221	8	—	34	—
kashe	1 (7 oz)	270	8	—	45	—
potato	1 lg (7 oz)	332	12	470	49	1
potato	1 med (3.5 oz)	166	6	235	25	tr
potato w/ broccoli & cheese	1 (7 oz)	312	15	—	33	—
potato w/ spinach & mushroom	1 (7 oz)	214	8	—	32	—
KOHLRABI						
raw sliced	½ cup	19	tr	14	4	—
sliced cooked	½ cup	24	tr	17	5	—
KUMQUATS						
fresh	1	12	tr	1	3	—
LAMB						
(*see also* LAMB DISHES)						
FRESH						
cubed lean only braised	3 oz	190	7	60	0	—
cubed lean only broiled	3 oz	158	6	65	0	—
ground broiled	3 oz	240	17	69	0	—
leg lean & fat Choice roasted	3 oz	219	14	56	14	—
loin chop w/ bone lean & fat Choice broiled	1 chop (2.3 oz)	201	15	49	0	—
loin chop w/ bone lean only Choice broiled	1 chop (1.6 oz)	100	5	39	0	—
rib chop lean & fat Choice broiled	3 oz	307	25	64	0	—
rib chop lean only Choice broiled	3 oz	200	11	73	0	—
shank lean & fat Choice braised	3 oz	206	11	61	0	—
shank lean & fat Choice roasted	3 oz	191	11	55	0	—

FOOD	PORTION	CAL.	FAT	SOD.	CARB.	FIB.
shoulder chop w/ bone lean & fat Choice braised	1 chop (2.5 oz)	244	17	51	0	—
shoulder chop w/ bone lean only Choice braised	1 chop (1.9 oz)	152	8	41	0	—
sirloin lean & fat Choice roasted	3 oz	248	21	58	0	—
FROZEN						
New Zealand lean & fat cooked	3 oz	259	19	39	0	—
New Zealand lean only cooked	3 oz	175	8	43	0	—

LAMB DISHES
TAKE-OUT

FOOD	PORTION	CAL.	FAT	SOD.	CARB.	FIB.
curry	¾ cup	345	17	258	22	—
moussaka	5.6 oz	312	21	—	16	1
stew	¾ cup	124	5	140	11	2

LAMB'S QUARTERS

FOOD	PORTION	CAL.	FAT	SOD.	CARB.	FIB.
chopped cooked	½ cup	29	1	—	5	—

LECITHIN
(see SOY)

LEEKS

FOOD	PORTION	CAL.	FAT	SOD.	CARB.	FIB.
chopped cooked	¼ cup	8	tr	3	2	—
cooked	1 (4.4 oz)	38	tr	13	9	—
freeze dried	1 tbsp	1	0	0	tr	—
raw	1 (4.4 oz)	76	tr	25	18	—
raw chopped	¼ cup	16	tr	5	4	—

LEMON
FRESH

FOOD	PORTION	CAL.	FAT	SOD.	CARB.	FIB.
Dole	1	18	0	0	4	0
lemon	1 med	22	tr	3	12	—
peel	1 tbsp	0	tr	0	1	—
wedge	1	5	tr	1	3	—

LEMON CURD

FOOD	PORTION	CAL.	FAT	SOD.	CARB.	FIB.
lemon curd made w/ egg	2 tsp	29	1	—	4	0
lemon curd made w/ starch	2 tsp	28	—	—	6	0

LEMON EXTRACT

FOOD	PORTION	CAL.	FAT	SOD.	CARB.	FIB.
Virginia Dare	1 tsp	22	0	—	—	—

LEMON JUICE

FOOD	PORTION	CAL.	FAT	SOD.	CARB.	FIB.
Realemon	1 fl oz	6	0	5	2	—
bottled	1 tbsp	3	tr	3	1	—

FOOD	PORTION	CAL.	FAT	SOD.	CARB.	FIB.
fresh	1 tbsp	4	0	0	1	—
frzn	1 tbsp	3	tr	0	1	—

LEMONADE

FROZEN

FOOD	PORTION	CAL.	FAT	SOD.	CARB.	FIB.
Bright & Early	8 fl oz	120	0	5	30	—
Minute Maid	8 fl oz	110	0	0	29	—
Country Style	8 fl oz	120	0	0	30	—
Cranberry Lemonade	8 fl oz	80	0	0	30	—
Pink	8 fl oz	120	0	0	30	—
Raspberry	8 fl oz	120	0	0	30	—
Seneca						
as prep	8 fl oz	110	0	0	27	1
as prep w/ water	1 cup	100	tr	8	26	—
not prep	1 can (6 oz)	397	tr	8	103	—

MIX

FOOD	PORTION	CAL.	FAT	SOD.	CARB.	FIB.
4C						
Instant as prep	8 fl oz	80	0	0	20	—
Country Time						
Mix	8 fl oz	82	0	21	21	—
Pink	8 fl oz	82	0	21	21	—
Pink Sugar Free	8 fl oz	4	0	—	0	—
Sugar Free	8 fl oz	4	0	—	0	—
Crystal Light						
Mix	8 fl oz	5	0		0	—
Kool-Aid						
Mix	8 fl oz	99	0	8	25	—
Pink	8 fl oz	99	0	8	25	—
Sugar Free	8 fl oz	4	0	—	0	—
Sugar Sweetened Pink	8 fl oz	82	0	—	21	—
Wylers						
Drink Mix Unsweetened	8 oz	3	0	19	1	—
powder as prep w/ water	9 fl oz	113	tr	19	29	—
powder w/ Nutrasweet	1 pitcher (67 oz)	40	0	58	10	—

READY-TO-DRINK

FOOD	PORTION	CAL.	FAT	SOD.	CARB.	FIB.
After The Fall						
Apple Raspberry	1 bottle (10 oz)	120	0	15	29	—
Crystal Geyser						
Juice Squeeze Pink	1 bottle (12 fl oz)	140	0	20	34	—
Diet Rite						
Salt/Sodium Free	8 fl oz	2	0	0	1	—
Kool-Aid						
Koolers	1 pkg (8.45 fl oz)	120	0	3	32	—
Minute Maid						
Chilled	8 fl oz	110	0	25	28	—

FOOD	PORTION	CAL.	FAT	SOD.	CARB.	FIB.
Minute Maid (CONT.)						
Cranberry Chilled	8 fl oz	120	0	25	31	—
Juices To Go	1 bottle (16 fl oz)	110	0	25	28	—
Juices To Go	1 can (11.5 fl oz)	160	0	40	40	—
Juices To Go Cranberry Lemonade	1 bottle (16 fl oz)	110	0	25	29	—
Juices To Go Raspberry Lemonade	1 bottle (16 fl oz)	120	0	25	29	—
Pink Chilled	8 fl oz	110	0	25	28	—
Raspberry Chilled	8 fl oz	120	0	0	30	—
Mott's						
Lemonade	10 fl oz	160	0	20	41	0
Newman's Own						
Roadside Virginia	8 fl oz	100	tr	0	22	—
Ocean Spray						
With Cranberry Juice	8 fl oz	110	0	35	26	0
With Raspberry Juice	8 fl oz	110	0	35	27	0
Odwalla						
Honey	8 fl oz	70	0	10	26	0
Strawberry	8 fl oz	150	0	35	40	2
Royal Mistic						
Lemonade Limeade	16 fl oz	230	0	19	57	—
Tropical Pink	16 fl oz	230	0	11	57	—
Shasta						
Lemonade	12 fl oz	146	0	—	—	—
Sipps	8.45 fl oz	85	0	—	—	—
Snapple						
Diet Pink	8 fl oz	13	0	10	3	—
Pink	8 fl oz	110	0	15	26	—
Strawberry	8 fl oz	110	0	5	26	—
Tropicana						
Twister Orange Cranberry	8 fl oz	130	0	5	32	—
Twister Wild Berry	8 fl oz	120	0	5	30	—

LENTILS
CANNED
Health Valley

FOOD	PORTION	CAL.	FAT	SOD.	CARB.	FIB.
Fast Menu Hearty Lentils Garden Vegetables	7½ oz	150	4	200	16	16
Fast Menu Organic Lentils With Tofu Wiener	7½ oz	170	5	260	15	15

FOOD	PORTION	CAL.	FAT	SOD.	CARB.	FIB.
DRIED						
Hurst						
Lentils	1.2 oz	120	1	5	20	11
cooked	1 cup	231	1	4	40	—
FROZEN						
Natural Touch						
Lentil Rice Loaf	2.5 in slice (113 g)	200	11	420	18	—
MIX						
Casbah						
Pilaf as prep	1 cup	200	tr	400	38	2
SPROUTS						
raw	½ cup	40	tr	4	8	—
LETTUCE						
(see also SALAD)						
Dole						
Butter	1 head	21	tr	8	4	2
Iceberg	⅙ med head	20	0	10	4	1
Leaf shredded	1½ cup	12	0	40	1	1
Romaine shredded	1½ cups	18	1	40	2	1
Western Express						
Heart's Of Romaine	6 leaves (3 oz)	20	1	0	3	1
bibb	1 head (6 oz)	21	tr	8	4	2
boston	2 leaves	2	tr	1	tr	tr
boston	1 head (6 oz)	21	tr	8	4	2
iceberg	1 leaf	3	tr	2	tr	tr
iceberg	1 head (19 oz)	70	1	48	11	5
looseleaf shredded	½ cup	5	tr	3	1	—
romaine shredded	½ cup	4	tr	2	1	—
LIMA BEANS						
CANNED						
Allen						
Green	½ cup (4.5 oz)	120	1	370	23	8
Green & White	½ cup (4.5 oz)	110	1	280	20	9
Del Monte						
Green	½ cup (4.4 oz)	80	0	360	15	4
Dennison's						
With Ham	7.5 oz	250	7	—	—	—
East Texas Fair						
Green	½ cup (4.5 oz)	120	1	370	23	8
Luck's						
Small Seasoned w/ Pork	7.5 oz	220	7	—	—	—
S&W						
Small Fancy	½ cup	80	0	390	16	—

FOOD	PORTION	CAL.	FAT	SOD.	CARB.	FIB.
Seneca						
Limas	½ cup	80	0	240	15	5
Trappey						
Baby Green With Bacon	½ cup (4.5 oz)	120	1	330	22	6
large	1 cup	191	tr	809	36	—
lima beans	½ cup	93	tr	309	17	—
DRIED						
baby cooked	1 cup	229	1	5	42	17
cooked	½ cup	104	tr	14	20	—
large cooked	1 cup	217	1	4	39	14
FROZEN						
Birds Eye						
Baby	½ cup	130	0	115	24	—
Fordhook	½ cup	100	0	10	19	—
Fresh Like						
Baby	3.5 oz	138	1	106	25	2
Green Giant						
Harvest Fresh	½ cup	80	0	170	18	4
In Butter Sauce	½ cup	100	3	390	17	5
Hanover						
Baby	½ cup	110	0	—	—	—
Fordhook	½ cup	100	0	—	—	—
cooked	½ cup	94	tr	26	18	—
fordhook cooked	½ cup	85	tr	45	16	—
LIME						
fresh	1	20	tr	1	7	—
LIME JUICE						
After The Fall						
Caribbean Lime	1 can (12 oz)	170	0	25	42	0
Key West	1 cup (8 oz)	100	0	10	25	0
Lifesavers						
Lime Punch	8 fl oz	140	0	25	34	—
Odwalla						
Summertime Lime	8 fl oz	90	0	10	23	0
bottled	1 tbsp	3	tr	2	1	—
fresh	1 tbsp	4	tr	0	1	—
LING						
blue raw	3½ oz	83	1	—	0	—
fresh baked	3 oz	95	1	147	0	—
fresh fillet baked	5.3 oz	168	1	261	0	—
LINGCOD						
baked	3 oz	93	1	64	0	—
fillet baked	5.3 oz	164	2	114	0	—

FOOD	PORTION	CAL.	FAT	SOD.	CARB.	FIB.

LIQUOR/LIQUEUR

(see also BEER AND ALE, CHAMPAGNE, DRINK MIXERS, MALT, WINE, WINE
COOLERS)

FOOD	PORTION	CAL.	FAT	SOD.	CARB.	FIB.
anisette	⅔ oz	74	0	—	7	0
apricot brandy	⅔ oz	64	0	—	6	0
aquavit	3.5 oz	229	0	—	0	0
benedictine	⅔ oz	69	0	—	7	0
bloody mary	5 oz	116	tr	332	5	—
bourbon & soda	4 oz	105	0	16	0	—
coffee liqueur	1½ oz	174	tr	4	24	—
coffee w/ cream liqueur	1½ oz	154	7	43	10	—
cognac	3.5 oz	233	0	—	1	0
creme de menthe	1½ oz	186	tr	3	21	—
curacao liqueur	⅔ oz	54	0	—	6	0
daiquiri	2 oz	111	0	1	4	—
gin	1½ oz	110	0	1	0	—
gin & tonic	7.5 oz	171	0	10	16	—
gin ricky	4 oz	150	0	—	—	—
manhattan	2 oz	128	0	2	2	—
martini	2½ oz	156	0	2	tr	—
mint julep	10 oz	210	0	—	3	0
old-fashioned	2½ oz	127	0	—	3	0
pina colada	4½ oz	262	3	9	40	—
planter's punch	3½ oz	175	0	—	—	—
rum	1½ oz	97	0	0	0	—
screwdriver	7 oz	174	tr	2	18	—
sloe gin fizz	2½ oz	132	0	1	4	0
tequila sunrise	5½ oz	189	tr	7	15	—
tom collins	7½ oz	121	0	39	3	—
vodka	1½ oz	97	0	0	0	—
whiskey	1½ oz	105	0	0	tr	—
whiskey sour	3 oz	123	tr	10	5	—
whiskey sour mix not prep	1 pkg (0.6 oz)	64	0	46	16	—

LIVER

(see also PATE)

Dakota Lean

FOOD	PORTION	CAL.	FAT	SOD.	CARB.	FIB.
Beef raw	3 oz	100	1	—	8	—
beef braised	3 oz	137	4	59	3	—
beef pan-fried	3 oz	184	7	90	7	—
chicken stewed	1 cup (5 oz)	219	8	71	1	—
duck raw	1 (1.5 oz)	60	2	—	2	—
goose raw	1 (3.3 oz)	125	4	132	6	—
lamb braised	3 oz	187	7	48	2	—

FOOD	PORTION	CAL.	FAT	SOD.	CARB.	FIB.
lamb fried	3 oz	202	11	105	3	—
pork braised	3 oz	141	4	42	3	—
sheep raw	3½ oz	131	4	95	0	—
turkey simmered	1 cup (5 oz)	237	8	89	5	—
veal braised	3 oz	140	6	45	2	—
veal fried	3 oz	208	10	112	3	—

LOBSTER
(see also CRAYFISH)

CANNED

Progresso

Rock Lobster Sauce	½ cup	120	8	430	11	2

FRESH

northern cooked	1 cup	142	1	551	2	—
northern cooked	3 oz	83	1	323	1	—
northern raw	1 lobster (5.3 oz)	136	1	—	1	—
northern raw	3 oz	77	1	—	tr	—
spiny steamed	3 oz	122	2	193	3	—
spiny steamed	1 (5.7 oz)	233	3	370	5	—

FROZEN

Cajun Cookin'

Crawfish Etouffee	12 oz	390	10	1110	51	—

TAKE-OUT

newburg	1 cup	485	27	127	13	—

LOGANBERRIES

frzn	1 cup	80	tr	1	19	—

LONGANS

fresh	1	2	tr	0	tr	—

LOQUATS

fresh	1	5	tr	0	1	—

LOTUS

root raw sliced	10 slices	45	tr	33	14	—
root sliced cooked	10 slices	59	tr	40	14	—
seeds dried	1 oz	94	1	1	18	—

LOX
(see SALMON)

LUNCHEON MEATS/COLD CUTS

Armour

Beef Bologna Lower Salt	1 oz	90	8	—	—	—
Bologna Lower Salt	1 oz	90	8	—	—	—
Salami Lower Salt	1 oz	80	7	—	—	—

FOOD	PORTION	CAL.	FAT	SOD.	CARB.	FIB.
Carl Buddig						
Beef	1 oz	40	2	430	1	0
Corned Beef	1 oz	40	2	380	1	0
Pastrami	1 oz	40	2	320	1	0
DiLusso						
Genoa	1 oz	100	8	500	0	0
Hansel n' Gretel						
Healthy Deli Bologna Beef & Pork	1 oz	41	2	200	1	—
Healthy Deli Cooked Corn Beef	1 oz	35	1	210	1	—
Healthy Deli Italian Roast Beef	1 oz	31	1	140	tr	—
Healthy Deli Pastrami Round	1 oz	34	1	195	1	—
Healthy Deli Regular Roast Beef	1 oz	30	tr	130	tr	—
Healthy Deli St Paddy's Corned Beef	1 oz	24	tr	290	1	—
Healthy Choice						
Bologna	1 slice (1 oz)	30	1	290	1	0
Bologna Beef	1 slice (1 oz)	35	1	280	3	0
Hebrew National						
Bologna Beef	2 oz	180	16	440	—	—
Bologna Beef Reduced Fat	2 oz	130	12	320	—	—
Bologna Lean Chub	2 oz	90	6	430	—	—
Bologna Midget	2 oz	180	16	440	—	—
Deli Express Corned Beef	2 oz	80	3	450	—	—
Deli Express Tongue Sliced	2 oz	120	9	330	—	—
Deli Pastrami	2 oz	80	3	510	—	—
Salami Beef	2 oz	170	14	420	—	—
Salami Beef Reduced Fat	2 oz	110	8	380	—	—
Salami Lean Chub	2 oz	90	6	340	—	—
Salami Midget	2 oz	170	14	420	—	—
Hillshire						
Bologna Large	1 oz	90	8	260	tr	—
Bologna Ring	1 oz	90	8	230	tr	—
Braunschweiger	1 oz	95	8	270	2	—
Deli Select Corned Beef	1 slice	10	tr	100	tr	—
Deli Select Light Bologna	1 slice	12	1	85	tr	—
Deli Select Oven Roasted Cured Beef	1 slice	10	tr	95	tr	—

FOOD	PORTION	CAL.	FAT	SOD.	CARB.	FIB.
Hillshire (CONT.)						
Deli Select Pastrami	1 slice	10	tr	100	tr	—
Deli Select Roast Beef	1 slice	10	tr	135	tr	—
Deli Select Smoked Beef	1 slice	10	tr	100	tr	—
Flavor Pack 90-99% Fat Free Light Bologna	1 slice (0.73 oz)	30	2	190	1	—
Flavor Pack 90-99% Fat Free Pastrami	1 slice (0.6 oz)	18	tr	180	tr	—
Lunch 'N Munch Bologna/ American	1 pkg (4.5 oz)	480	37	1390	20	—
Lunch 'N Munch Bologna/ American/ Snickers	1 pkg (4.25 oz)	490	34	1110	31	—
Lunch 'N Munch Bologna/ American/ Snickers/ Hi-C	1 pkg (4.25 oz + 6 fl oz)	590	34	1130	55	—
Lunch 'N Munch Cotto Salami/ Monterey Jack	1 pkg (4.5 oz)	440	32	1270	21	—
Lunch 'N Munch Pepperoni/ American	1 pkg (4.5 oz)	570	46	1670	20	—
Pepperoni	1 oz	110	10	450	0	—
Salami Hard	1 oz	90	7	470	1	—
Summer Sausage	2 oz	180	16	670	1	—
Summer Sausage Beef	2 oz	190	17	612	1	—
Summer Sausage Light	2 oz	150	12	630	1	—
Summer Sausage w/ Cheddar Cheese	2 oz	200	18	605	1	—
Homeland						
Hard Salami	1 oz	110	10	450	0	0
Hormel						
Liverwurst Spread	4 tbsp (2 oz)	130	10	650	2	0
Pepperoni Chunk	1 oz	140	13	470	0	0
Pepperoni Sliced	15 slices (1 oz)	140	13	470	0	0
Pepperoni Twin	1 oz	140	13	470	0	0
Pillow Pack Genoa Salami	4 slices (1.1 oz)	120	10	540	0	0
Pillow Pack Pepperoni	1 oz	140	13	470	0	0
Pillow Pack Pepperoni	16 slices (1 oz)	140	13	470	0	0
Jones						
Liver Sausage	1 slice	80	7	180	tr	—
Liver Sausage Chub	1 slice	80	7	230	tr	—
Oscar Mayer						
Bologna Beef	1 slice (1 oz)	90	8	300	1	0

FOOD	PORTION	CAL.	FAT	SOD.	CARB.	FIB.
Oscar Mayer (CONT.)						
Bologna Garlic	1 slice (1.4 oz)	110	12	400	1	0
Bologna Light	1 slice (1 oz)	60	4	310	2	0
Bologna Light Beef	1 slice (1 oz)	60	4	310	2	0
Bologna Pork & Chicken & Beef	1 slice (1 oz)	90	8	270	0	0
Bologna Wisconsin Made Ring	2 oz	140	16	470	1	0
Braunschweiger	1 slice (1 oz)	100	9	320	1	0
Braunschweiger	2 oz	190	17	610	2	0
Braunschweiger German Brand	2 oz	200	18	650	1	0
Cotto Salami	2 slices (1.6 oz)	100	8	520	1	0
Cotto Salami Beef	2 slices (1.6 oz)	90	7	590	0	0
Free Bologna	2 slices (1.6 oz)	35	0	480	2	—
Genoa Salami	3 slices (1 oz)	100	9	490	0	0
Hard Salami	3 slices (1 oz)	100	9	510	0	0
Head Cheese	1 slice (1 oz)	50	4	360	0	0
Healthy Favorites Bologna	2 slices (1.6 oz)	45	1	510	2	0
Honey Loaf	1 slice (1 oz)	35	1	380	1	0
Liver Cheese	1 slice (1.3 oz)	120	10	420	1	0
Lunchables Bologna/ American	1 pkg (4.5 oz)	450	34	1620	19	0
Lunchables Deluxe Turkey/Ham	1 pkg (5.1 oz)	360	19	1930	23	1
Lunchables Dessert Jello/Honey Turkey/ Cheddar	1 pkg (5.7 oz)	320	16	1360	27	tr
Lunchables Fun Pack Bologna/Wild Cherry	1 pkg (11.2 oz)	530	29	1120	58	tr
Lunchables Fun Pack Ham/Fruit Punch	1 pkg (11.2 oz)	450	20	1260	53	tr
Lunchables Ham/Swiss	1 pkg (4.5 oz)	320	17	1770	19	0
Lunchables Pepperoni/ American	1 pkg (4.5 oz)	480	36	1840	19	0
Lunchables Salami/ American	1 pkg (4.5 oz)	430	32	1740	18	0
Luncheon Loaf Spiced	1 slice (1 oz)	70	5	340	2	0
New England Brand Sausage	2 slices (1.6 oz)	60	3	570	1	0
Old Fashioned Loaf	1 slice (1 oz)	60	5	340	2	0
Olive Loaf	1 slice (1 oz)	70	5	370	2	0
Peppered Loaf	1 slice (1 oz)	39	2	367	1	—

FOOD	PORTION	CAL.	FAT	SOD.	CARB.	FIB.
Oscar Mayer (CONT.)						
Pickle And Pimiento Loaf	1 slice (1 oz)	70	6	360	2	0
Salami For Beer	1 slices (1.6 oz)	110	9	580	1	0
Salami Machaich Brand Beef	2 slices (1.6 oz)	120	10	510	1	0
Sandwich Spread	2 oz	140	10	530	9	0
Summer Sausage	2 slices (1.6 oz)	140	13	650	0	0
Summer Sausage Beef	2 slices (1.6 oz)	140	12	640	1	0
Russer						
Bologna	2 oz	180	15	540	3	—
Bologna Jalapeno Pepper	2 oz	170	14	600	3	—
Bologna Wunderbar German Brand	2 oz	190	16	600	5	—
Bologna Beef	2 oz	180	15	600	3	—
Bologna Garlic	2 oz	180	16	520	3	—
Bologna Italian Brand Sweet Red Pepper	2 oz	180	15	540	3	—
Braunschweiger	2 oz	170	14	600	3	—
Cooked Salami	2 oz	120	8	600	3	—
Dutch Brand	2 oz	130	8	600	6	—
Hot Cooked Salami	2 oz	110	7	600	3	—
Italian Brand Loaf	2 oz	130	8	600	5	—
Jalapeno Loaf With Monterey Jack Cheese	2 oz	160	13	650	4	—
Kielbasa Loaf	2 oz	120	8	600	5	—
Light Bologna	2 oz	120	8	400	3	—
Light Bologna Beef	2 oz	120	8	400	3	—
Light Braunschweiger	2 oz	120	8	400	3	—
Light Old Fashioned Loaf	2 oz	90	4	430	4	—
Light P&P Loaf	2 oz	100	6	430	4	—
Light Salami Cooked	2 oz	90	5	400	4	—
Olive Loaf	2 oz	160	13	600	4	—
P&P Loaf	2 oz	160	13	600	4	—
Pepper Loaf	2 oz	90	3	600	6	—
Polish Loaf	2 oz	140	10	600	7	—
Sara Lee						
Pastrami Beef	2 oz	100	6	540	1	1
Peppered Beef	2 oz	70	2	200	1	—
Shofar						
Salami Beef	2 oz	160	15	410	0	0
Spam						
Less Salt	2 oz	170	16	560	0	0
Lite	2 oz	110	8	560	0	0

FOOD	PORTION	CAL.	FAT	SOD.	CARB.	FIB.
Underwood						
Liverwurst	2.08 oz	180	15	470	4	—
Weight Watchers						
Bologna	2 slices (¾ oz)	35	2	220	1	—
barbecue loaf pork & beef	1 oz	49	3	378	2	—
beerwurst beef	1 slice	20	2	62	tr	—
	(2¾ in x ¹⁄₁₆ in)					
beerwurst beef	1 slice (4 in x ⅛ in)	75	7	214	tr	—
beerwurst pork	1 slice	14	1	74	tr	—
	(2¾ in x ¹⁄₁₆ in)					
beerwurst pork	1 slice (4 in x ⅛ in)	55	4	285	tr	—
berliner pork & beef	1 oz	65	4	368	1	—
blood sausage	1 oz	95	9	—	tr	—
bologna beef	1 oz	88	8	278	tr	—
bologna beef & pork	1 oz	89	8	289	1	—
bologna pork	1 oz	70	6	336	tr	—
braunschweiger pork	1 oz	102	9	324	1	—
braunschweiger pork	1 slice	65	6	206	1	—
	(2½ in x ¼ in)					
corned beef loaf	1 oz	43	2	270	0	—
dried beef	5 slices (21 g)	35	tr	—	tr	—
dried beef	1 oz	47	1	—	tr	—
dutch brand loaf pork & beef	1 oz	68	5	354	2	—
headcheese pork	1 oz	60	5	356	tr	—
honey loaf pork & beef	1 oz	36	1	374	2	—
honey roll sausage beef	1 oz	42	2	304	1	—
lebanon bologna beef	1 oz	60	4	379	1	—
liver cheese pork	1 oz	86	7	347	1	—
liverwurst pork	1 oz	92	8	—	1	—
luncheon meat beef	1 oz	87	7	377	1	—
luncheon meat pork & beef	1 oz	100	9	367	1	—
luncheon meat pork canned	1 oz	95	9	365	1	—
luncheon sausage pork & beef	1 oz	74	6	335	tr	—
luxury loaf pork	1 oz	40	1	347	1	—
mortadella beef & pork	1 oz	88	7	353	1	—
mother's loaf pork	1 oz	80	6	320	2	—
new england sausage pork & beef	1 oz	46	2	346	1	—
olive loaf pork	1 oz	67	5	421	3	—
peppered loaf pork & beef	1 oz	42	2	432	1	—
pepperoni pork & beef	1 slice (0.2 oz)	27	2	112	tr	—

FOOD	PORTION	CAL.	FAT	SOD.	CARB.	FIB.
pepperoni pork & beef	1 (9 oz)	1248	110	5120	7	—
pickle & pimiento loaf pork	1 oz	74	6	394	2	—
picnic loaf pork & beef	1 oz	66	5	330	1	—
salami cooked beef & pork	1 oz	71	6	302	1	—
salami hard pork	1 slice (⅓ oz)	41	4	226	3	—
salami hard pork	1 pkg (4 oz)	460	38	2554	2	—
salami hard pork & beef	1 slice (⅓ oz)	42	3	186	tr	—
salami hard pork & beef	1 pkg (4 oz)	472	39	2101	3	—
sandwich spread pork & beef	1 tbsp	35	3	152	2	—
sandwich spread pork & beef	1 oz	67	5	287	3	—
summer sausage thuringer cervelat	1 oz	98	8	412	1	—
TAKE-OUT						
corned beef	2 oz	70	2	390	0	—
corned beef brisket	2 oz	90	5	370	0	—
submarine w/ salami ham cheese lettuce tomato onion & oil	1	456	19	1650	51	—
LUPINES						
dried cooked	1 cup	197	5	7	16	—
LYCHEES						
Ka-Me						
Whole Pitted In Syrup	15 pieces (5 oz)	130	0	26	32	0
fresh	1	6	tr	0	2	—
MACADAMIA NUTS						
Mauna Loa						
Candy Glazed	1 oz	170	14	80	11	—
Chocolate Covered	1 oz	170	13	21	12	—
Honey Roasted	1 oz	200	17	80	8	—
Macadamia Nut Brittle	1 oz	150	8	140	19	—
Roasted & Salted	1 oz	210	21	75	4	—
dried	1 oz	199	21	1	4	—
oil roasted	1 oz	204	22	3	4	—
MACARONI						
(see PASTA)						
MACE						
ground	1 tsp	8	1	1	1	—
MACKEREL						
CANNED						
Empress						
Jack	4 oz	140	8	480	0	—

FOOD	PORTION	CAL.	FAT	SOD.	CARB.	FIB.
jack	1 cup	296	12	720	0	—
jack	1 can (12.7 oz)	563	23	1368	0	—
FRESH						
atlantic cooked	3 oz	223	15	71	0	—
atlantic raw	3 oz	174	12	76	0	—
jack baked	3 oz	171	9	94	0	—
jack fillet baked	6.2 oz	354	18	194	0	—
king baked	3 oz	114	2	172	0	—
king fillet baked	5.4 oz	207	4	312	0	—
pacific baked	3 oz	171	9	94	0	—
pacific fillet baked	6.2 oz	354	18	194	0	—
spanish cooked	3 oz	134	5	56	0	—
spanish cooked	1 fillet (5.1 oz)	230	9	96	0	—
spanish raw	3 oz	118	5	50	0	—

MALT

Bartles & Jaymes

FOOD	PORTION	CAL.	FAT	SOD.	CARB.	FIB.
Malt Cooler Berry	12 fl oz	210	0	5	32	—
Malt Cooler Black Cherry	12 fl oz	190	0	5	30	—
Malt Cooler Light Berry	12 fl oz	140	0	0	29	—
Malt Cooler Mandarin Lemon	12 fl oz	210	0	5	34	—
Malt Cooler Margarita	12 fl oz	250	0	40	44	—
Malt Cooler Original	12 fl oz	180	0	0	27	—
Malt Cooler Peach	12 fl oz	200	0	5	31	—
Malt Cooler Pina Colada	12 fl oz	270	0	5	48	—
Malt Cooler Planter's Punch	12 fl oz	220	0	5	35	—
Malt Cooler Red Sangria	12 fl oz	190	0	5	29	—
Malt Cooler Strawberry	12 fl oz	200	0	5	31	—
Malt Cooler Strawberry Daiquiri	12 fl oz	220	0	5	35	—
Malt Cooler Tropical	12 fl oz	220	0	5	36	—
nonalcoholic	12 fl oz	32	0	—	5	—

MALTED MILK

Carnation

FOOD	PORTION	CAL.	FAT	SOD.	CARB.	FIB.
Chocolate	3 heaping tsp (21 g)	79	tr	—	—	—
Original	3 heaping tsp (21 g)	90	2	—	—	—
Kraft						
Instant Chocolate	3 tsp (0.7 oz)	80	1	40	17	tr
Instant Chocolate as prep w/ 2% milk	1 serv (9.5 oz)	200	6	160	29	tr

FOOD	PORTION	CAL.	FAT	SOD.	CARB.	FIB.
Kraft (CONT.)						
Instant Natural	3 tsp (0.7 oz)	90	2	85	15	0
Instant Natural as prep w/ 2% milk	1 serv (9.5 oz)	210	7	205	27	0
chocolate as prep w/ milk	1 cup	229	9	172	30	—
chocolate flavor powder	3 heaping tsp (¾ oz)	79	1	53	18	—
natural flavor as prep w/ milk	1 cup	237	10	223	27	—
natural flavor powder	3 heaping tsp (¾ oz)	87	2	103	19	—

MAMMY-APPLE
fresh	1	431	4	127	106	—

MANGO
fresh	1	135	1	4	35	—
Ka-Me canned	4 pieces (5 oz)	102	0	10	25	0
Sonoma						
Pieces dried	8 pieces (2 oz)	180	1	50	44	0

MANGO JUICE
After The Fall						
Hawaiian Mango	1 can (12 oz)	180	0	20	45	0
Mango Ginger	1 can (12 oz)	150	0	25	35	0
Kern's						
Nectar	6 fl oz	100	0	0	28	—
Libby						
Nectar	1 can (11.5 fl oz)	210	0	10	52	—
Snapple						
Diet Mango Madness	8 fl oz	13	0	10	3	—
Mango Madness Cocktail	8 fl oz	110	0	10	29	—

MARGARINE
(*see also* BUTTER BLENDS, BUTTER SUBSTITUTES)

Blue Bonnet						
Stick	1 tbsp	100	11	95	0	—
Tub	1 tbsp	100	11	95	0	—
Whipped	1 tbsp	80	9	100	0	—
Chiffon						
Stick	1 tbsp	100	11	105	0	—
Tub	1 tbsp (0.5 oz)	100	11	105	0	0
Whipped	1 tbsp (0.3 oz)	70	7	70	0	0
Fleischmann's						
Stick	1 tbsp	100	11	95	0	—

FOOD	PORTION	CAL.	FAT	SOD.	CARB.	FIB.
Fleischmann's (CONT.)						
Stick Light Corn Oil	1 tbsp	80	8	70	0	—
Stick Sweet Unsalted	1 tbsp	100	11	0	0	—
Hain						
Stick Safflower	1 tbsp	100	11	170	0	—
Stick Safflower Unsalted	1 tbsp	100	11	<5	0	—
Tub Safflower	1 tbsp	100	11	170	0	—
Hollywood						
Safflower	1 tbsp	100	11	130	0	—
Safflower Unsalted Sweet	1 tbsp	100	11	2	0	—
Soft Spread	1 tbsp	90	10	135	1	0
I Can't Believe It's Not Butter						
Tub	1 tbsp	90	10	—	—	—
Krona						
Stick	1 tbsp	100	11	—	—	—
Land O'Lakes						
Stick	1 tbsp (0.5 oz)	90	10	95	0	—
Stick With Sweet Cream	1 tbsp (0.5 oz)	90	10	95	0	—
Tub	1 tbsp (0.5 oz)	80	8	90	0	—
Tub With Sweet Cream	1 tbsp (0.5 oz)	80	8	70	0	—
Mazola						
Stick	1 tbsp (14 g)	100	11	100	0	—
Stick	1 cup (229 g)	1650	184	1650	3	—
Stick Unsalted	1 tbsp (14 g)	100	11	1	0	—
Stick Unsalted	1 cup (229 g)	1635	184	8	0	—
Tub Diet	1 tbsp (14 g)	50	6	130	0	—
Tub Diet	1 cup (235 g)	815	93	2160	1	—
Tub Light Corn Oil Spread	1 tbsp (14 g)	50	6	100	0	—
Mother's						
Stick Unsalted	1 tbsp	100	11	—	—	—
Sticks	1 tbsp	100	11	—	—	—
Tub Salted	1 tbsp	100	11	—	—	—
Tub Unsalted	1 tbsp	100	11	—	—	—
Nucanola						
Stick	1 tbsp (14 g)	90	10	90	0	—
Stick	1 tbsp	90	10	90	0	—
Parkay						
Squeeze	1 tbsp (0.5 oz)	80	9	120	0	0
Stick	1 tbsp (0.5 oz)	90	10	110	0	0
Stick ⅓ Less Fat	1 tbsp (0.5 oz)	70	7	120	0	0
Tub	1 tbsp (0.5 oz)	60	7	110	0	0
Tub Light	1 tbsp (0.5 oz)	50	6	120	0	0

FOOD	PORTION	CAL.	FAT	SOD.	CARB.	FIB.
Parkay (CONT.)						
Tub Soft	1 tbsp (0.5 oz)	100	11	105	0	0
Tub Soft Diet	1 tbsp (0.5 oz)	50	6	110	0	0
Whipped	1 tbsp (0.3 oz)	70	7	70	0	0
Promise						
Stick	1 tbsp	90	10	—	—	—
Smart Beat						
Tub	1 tbsp	25	3	110	0	—
Tub Unsalted	1 tbsp	25	3	0	0	—
Touch Of Butter						
Squeeze	1 tbsp (0.5 oz)	80	9	115	0	0
Stick	1 tbsp (0.5 oz)	90	10	110	0	0
Tree Of Life						
Canola Soft	1 tbsp (0.5 oz)	100	11	110	0	—
Stick 100% Soy	1 tbsp (0.5 oz)	100	11	110	0	—
Stick 100% Soy Salt Free	1 tbsp (0.5 oz)	100	11	0	0	—
Stick Canola Soy	1 tbsp (0.5 oz)	100	11	110	0	—
Stick Canola Soy Salt Free	1 tbsp (0.5 oz)	100	11	0	0	—
Weight Watchers						
Stick Light	1 tbsp	60	7	130	0	—
Tub Extra Light	1 tbsp	50	6	130	0	—
Tub Extra Light Sweet Unsalted	1 tbsp	50	6	0	0	—
squeeze soybean & cottonseed	1 tsp	34	4	37	0	—
stick corn	1 tsp	34	4	44	0	—
stick corn	1 stick (4 oz)	815	91	1070	1	—
stick salted	1 tsp	39	4	44	0	—
stick salted	1 stick (4 oz)	815	91	1069	1	—
stick unsalted	1 stick (4 oz)	809	91	2	1	—
stick unsalted	1 tsp	34	4	tr	0	—
tub corn	1 cup	1626	183	2449	1	—
tub corn	1 tsp	34	4	51	0	—
tub diet	1 tsp	17	2	46	0	—
tub diet	1 cup	800	90	2226	1	—
tub safflower	1 cup	1626	183	2449	1	—
tub safflower	1 tsp	34	4	51	0	—
tub salted	1 cup	1626	183	2449	1	—
tub salted	1 tsp	34	4	51	0	—
tub soybean salted	1 tsp	34	4	51	0	—
tub soybean salted	1 cup	1626	183	2449	1	—
tub soybean unsalted	1 cup	1626	182	63	2	—

FOOD	PORTION	CAL.	FAT	SOD.	CARB.	FIB.
tub soybean unsalted	1 tsp	34	4	1	0	—
tub unsalted	1 cup	1626	182	63	0	—
tub unsalted	1 tsp	34	4	1	0	—

MARINADE
(see SAUCE)

MARJORAM
dried	1 tsp	2	tr	tr	tr	—

MARSHMALLOW
Campfire						
Campfire	2 lg	40	0	10	10	—
Campfire						
Miniature	24	40	0	10	10	—
Joyva						
Twists Chocolate Covered	2 (1.5 oz)	190	4	20	21	0
Kraft						
Funmallows	4 (1.1 oz)	110	0	20	26	0
Funmallows Miniature	½ cup (1.1 oz)	100	0	20	25	0
Jet-Puffed	5 (1.2 oz)	110	0	40	27	0
Marshmallow Creme	2 tbsp (0.4 oz)	40	0	10	10	0
Miniature	½ cup (1.1 oz)	100	0	30	25	0
Teddy Bear Cocoa-Flavored	½ cup (1.1 oz)	100	0	25	23	0
Marshmallow Fluff	1 heaping tsp (18 g)	59	tr	12	14	—
marshmallow	1 cup (1.6 oz)	146	tr	22	37	—
marshmallow	1 reg (0.3 oz)	23	0	3	6	—

MATZO
Goodman's						
Matzo Ball Mix 50% Less Salt	2 tbsp (0.5 oz)	50	0	150	11	0
Matzo Ball Mix as prep	2 tbsp (0.5 oz)	60	0	190	12	1
Horowitz Margareten						
Egg Milk Chocolate Coated	1 oz	97	4	7	16	1
Manischewitz						
American Matzo	1	115	2	—	22	—
Daily Thin Tea	1	103	tr	1	22	tr
Dietetic Thins	1	91	tr	tr	19	tr
Egg Dark Chocolate Coated	½ matzo (1 oz)	97	3	7	17	1
Egg n' Onion	1	112	tr	180	23	—
Matzo Cracker Miniatures	10	90	tr	—	20	—

FOOD	PORTION	CAL.	FAT	SOD.	CARB.	FIB.
Manischewitz (CONT.)						
Matzo Farfel	1 cup	180	1	2	60	—
Matzo Meal	1 cup	514	1	3	109	tr
Passover	1	129	tr	—	27	—
Passover Egg	1	132	2	—	27	—
Passover Egg Matzo Crackers	10	108	2	—	20	—
Salted Thin	1	100	tr	—	21	tr
Unsalted	1	110	tr	1	24	tr
Wheat Matzo Crackers	10	90	1	—	18	—
Whole Wheat w/ Bran	1	110	1	1	21	1
Streit's						
Dietetic	1 (1 oz)	100	0	0	23	1
Lightly Salted	1 (1 oz)	110	1	65	23	1
Matzoh Meal	¼ cup (1 oz)	110	1	0	24	1
Passover	1 (1 oz)	110	1	0	25	1
Unsalted	1 (0.9 oz)	100	1	0	22	1
Whole Wheat	1 (1 oz)	110	1	0	24	4
egg	1 (1 oz)	111	1	6	22	1
egg & onion	1 (1 oz)	111	1	81	22	1
plain	1 (1 oz)	112	tr	0	24	1
whole wheat	1 (1 oz)	99	tr	1	22	3

MAYONNAISE

(*see also* MAYONNAISE TYPE SALAD DRESSING, RELISH)

FOOD	PORTION	CAL.	FAT	SOD.	CARB.	FIB.
BAMA	1 tbsp	100	11	65	0	—
Bennett's	1 tbsp	110	12	65	1	—
Best Foods						
Cholesterol Free Reduced Calorie	1 tbsp (15 g)	50	5	80	1	—
Cholesterol Free Reduced Calorie	1 cup (233 g)	760	75	1210	17	—
Light	1 tbsp (15 g)	50	5	115	1	—
Light	1 cup (233 g)	760	78	1815	16	—
Real	1 cup	1570	175	1255	tr	—
Real	1 tbsp	100	11	80	tr	—
Hain						
Canola	1 tbsp	60	5	160	2	—
Canola	1 tbsp	100	11	100	tr	—
Cold Processed	1 tbsp	110	12	70	0	—
Eggless No Salt Added	1 tbsp	110	12	<5	0	—
Light Low Sodium	1 tbsp	60	6	95	2	—
Real No Salt Added	1 tbsp	110	12	0	0	—
Safflower	1 tbsp	110	12	70	0	—

FOOD	PORTION	CAL.	FAT	SOD.	CARB.	FIB.
Hellman's						
Cholesterol Free Reduced Calorie	1 tbsp (15 g)	50	5	80	1	—
Cholesterol Free Reduced Calorie	1 cup (233 g)	760	75	1210	17	—
Light Reduced Calorie	1 tbsp (15 g)	50	5	115	1	—
Light Reduced Calorie	1 cup (233 g)	760	78	1815	16	—
Mayonnaise	1 tbsp	100	11	80	tr	—
Mayonnaise	1 cup (220 g)	1570	173	1255	1	—
Hollywood						
Canola	1 tbsp	100	11	100	tr	—
Safflower	1 tbsp	100	12	75	0	—
Kraft						
Free	1 tbsp (0.6 oz)	10	0	105	2	0
Light	1 tbsp (0.5 oz)	50	5	110	1	0
Real	1 tbsp (0.5 oz)	100	11	75	0	0
McIlhenny						
Spicy	1 tbsp (0.5 oz)	108	12	94	1	tr
Mother's						
Mayonnaise	1 tbsp	100	11	—	—	—
Red Wing						
"H" Style	1 tbsp (0.5 oz)	110	11	80	1	0
Smart Beat						
Canola Oil	1 tbsp	40	4	110	1	—
Corn Beat	1 tbsp	40	4	110	1	—
Weight Watchers						
Fat Free	1 tbsp	12	0	125	4	—
Light	1 tbsp	50	5	100	1	—
Low Sodium	1 tbsp	50	1	45	1	—
mayonnaise	1 cup	1577	175	1250	6	—
mayonnaise	1 tbsp	99	11	78	tr	—
reduced calorie	1 cup	556	46	1193	38	—
reduced calorie	1 tbsp	34	3	75	2	—
sandwich spread	1 tbsp	60	5	—	3	—

MAYONNAISE TYPE SALAD DRESSING

(*see also* MAYONNAISE, RELISH)

FOOD	PORTION	CAL.	FAT	SOD.	CARB.	FIB.
BAMA	1 tbsp	50	4	105	3	—
Bright Day						
Salad Dressing	1 tbsp	60	6	—	—	—
Miracle Whip						
Free	1 tbsp (0.6 oz)	15	0	120	3	0
Light	1 tbsp (0.5 oz)	40	3	120	3	0
Salad Dressing	1 tbsp (0.5 oz)	70	7	85	2	0

FOOD	PORTION	CAL.	FAT	SOD.	CARB.	FIB.
Spin Blend						
Cholesterol Free	1 tbsp	40	4	110	2	—
Weight Watchers						
Fat Free Whipped Dressing	1 tbsp	16	0	115	4	—
home recipe	1 cup	400	24	1872	38	—
home recipe	1 tbsp	25	2	117	2	—
mayonnaise type salad dressing	1 tbsp	57	5	—	4	—
mayonnaise type salad dressing	1 cup	916	78	1670	56	—
reduced calorie w/o cholesterol	1 cup	1084	107	794	36	—
reduced calorie w/o cholesterol	1 tbsp	68	7	49	2	—

MEAT STICKS

Tombstone						
Beef Jerky	1 stick (0.5 oz)	35	0	310	tr	0
Beef Sticks	1 (0.8 oz)	110	10	270	0	0
Snappy Sticks	1 (0.8 oz)	110	10	260	tr	0
jerky beef	1 oz	96	4	815	4	—
jerky beef	1 lg piece (0.7 oz)	67	3	569	3	—
smoked	1 oz	156	14	420	2	—
smoked	1 (0.7 oz)	109	10	293	1	—

MEAT SUBSTITUTES

(*see also* BACON SUBSTITUTES, CHICKEN SUBSTITUTES, SAUSAGE SUBSTITUTES, TURKEY SUBSTITUTES)

Green Giant						
Harvest Burgers Original	1 (3 oz)	140	4	380	8	5
Harvest Direct						
TVP Beef Chunks	3.5 oz	280	1	15	32	18
TVP Beef Chunks Flavored	3.5 oz	250	1	2000	30	17
TVP Beef Strips	3.5 oz	280	1	15	32	18
TVP Ground Beef	3.5 oz	280	1	15	32	18
TVP Ground Beef Flavored	3.5 oz	250	1	2000	30	17
Jaclyn's						
Salisbury Steak Style Dinner	11 oz	260	8	320	37	—
Sirloin Strips Style Dinner	12 oz	290	6	320	37	—

FOOD	PORTION	CAL.	FAT	SOD.	CARB.	FIB.
Ken & Robert's						
Veggie Burger	1 (62 g)	110	2	390	19	—
Knox Mountain Farm						
Wheat Balls Mix	1 serv (1/10 pkg)	110	1	360	9	2
LaLoma						
Big Franks	1 (51 g)	110	6	190	2	—
Corn Dogs	1 (71 g)	190	8	400	15	—
Dinner Cuts	2 pieces (99 g)	110	1	340	2	—
Griddle Steaks	1 piece (54 g)	140	7	390	4	—
Nuteena	½ in slice (65 g)	160	12	110	6	—
Patty Mix	¼ cup (16 g)	50	0	200	4	—
Redi-Burger	½ in slice (68 g)	130	6	340	5	—
Sandwich Spread	3 tbsp (48 g)	70	4	300	4	—
Savory Dinner Loaf Mix not prep	¼ cup (16 g)	50	0	380	4	—
Savory Meatballs	7 (70 g)	190	8	420	7	—
Sizzle Burger	1 patty (71 g)	220	12	420	10	—
Sizzle Franks	2 (68 g)	170	13	340	3	—
Swiss Steak	1 piece (92 g)	170	10	360	7	—
Tender Bits	4 pieces (57 g)	80	3	260	5	—
Tender Rounds	6 pieces (73 g)	120	4	310	7	—
Vege-Burger	½ cup (108 g)	110	2	190	3	—
Vita-Burger Chunk	¼ cup (21 g)	70	0	150	6	—
Vita-Burger Granules	3 tbsp (21 g)	70	0	150	6	—
Lightlife						
American Grill	2.75 oz	110	3	325	8	—
Barbecue Grill	2.75 oz	130	6	336	10	—
Smart Deli Slices	2 slices (1.5 oz)	44	0	290	1	—
Smart Dogs	1 (1.5 oz)	40	0	290	1	—
Smart Dogs To Go	1 (5 oz)	115	0	300	19	—
Tofu Pups	1 (1.5 oz)	92	5	—	—	—
Vegetarian Sloppy Joe	4.3 oz	130	6	310	11	—
Midland Harvest						
Burger n' Loaf Chili w/o Beans	0.8 oz	90	3	225	7	2
Burger n' Loaf Herbs & Spice	3.2 oz	140	5	250	7	4
Burger n' Loaf Italian	3.2 oz	140	5	375	7	4
Burger n' Loaf Original	3.2 oz	140	5	350	7	4
Burger n' Loaf Sloppy Joe w/o Sauce	0.8 oz	80	2	165	9	—
Burger n' Loaf Taco	2.7 oz	90	2	250	7	1
Morningstar Farms						
Breaded Cutlet	1 patty (71 g)	230	14	390	12	—

FOOD	PORTION	CAL.	FAT	SOD.	CARB.	FIB.
Morningstar Farms (CONT.)						
Deli Franks	1 (35 g)	90	6	420	2	—
Sandwich Burger Pattie w/ Cheese	1 (4.75 oz)	370	17	700	32	—
Sandwich Pattie Biscuit	1 (3.5 oz)	280	11	570	31	—
Natural Touch						
Dinner Entree	1 patty (85 g)	230	14	300	6	—
Garden Pattie	1 (67 g)	120	4	300	8	—
Loaf Mix as prep	4 oz	180	7	670	12	—
Okra Pattie	1 (64 g)	160	10	420	7	—
Stroganoff Mix as prep	4 oz	90	3	700	10	—
Taco Mix as prep	2 tbsp	90	2	210	6	—
Sovex						
Better Than Burger?	½ cup (1.9 oz)	165	2	52	25	9
Spring Creek						
Soysage	1 patty (1.6 oz)	63	tr	237	11	—
White Wave						
Meatless Healthy Franks	1 (1.5 oz)	90	2	350	6	0
Meatless Jumbo Franks	1 (3 oz)	170	3	690	11	0
Meatless Sandwich Slices Beef	2 slices (1.6 oz)	90	0	270	8	1
Meatless Sandwich Slices Bologna	2 slices (1.6 oz)	120	8	370	5	1
Meatless Sandwich Slices Pastrami	2 slices (1.6 oz)	90	0	270	8	1
Meatless Healthy Franks	1 (1.5 oz)	90	2	350	6	—
Veggie Burger	1 patty (2.5 oz)	110	3	210	16	2
Worthington						
Beef Style Meatless	4 slices (70 g)	130	6	750	7	—
Bolono	2 slices (38 g)	60	2	390	2	—
Choplets	2 slices (92 g)	100	2	440	4	—
Corn Beef Sliced	4 slices (57 g)	120	6	740	8	—
Country Stew	9.5 oz (270 g)	220	10	760	23	—
Dinner Roast	2 oz	120	8	440	5	—
FriPats	1 (64 g)	180	12	360	5	—
Granburger not prep	6 tbsp (33 g)	110	1	730	7	—
Multigrain Cutlet	2 slices (92 g)	90	2	550	5	—
Non-Meat Balls	3 (54 g)	100	6	210	5	—
Numete	½ in slice (68 g)	150	11	410	7	—
Prime Stakes	1 piece (92 g)	160	10	410	7	—
Prosage Patties	2 (76 g)	210	14	780	4	—
Prosage Roll	2⅜ in slice (70 g)	180	12	570	4	—
Protose	½ in slice (76 g)	180	8	470	9	—
Salami Meatless	2 slices (38 g)	70	4	460	2	—

FOOD	PORTION	CAL.	FAT	SOD.	CARB.	FIB.
Worthington (cont.)						
Savory Slices	2 slices (56 g)	100	6	340	4	—
Smoked Beef Slices	6 slices (56 g)	120	6	790	7	—
Stakelets	1 piece (71 g)	150	8	460	7	—
Veelets	1 patty (71 g)	230	14	390	12	—
Vegetable Skallops	½ cup (85 g)	90	2	430	4	—
Vegetable Skallops No Added Salt	½ cup (85 g)	80	1	80	4	—
Vegetable Steaks	2.5 pieces (90 g)	110	2	400	5	—
Vegetarian Beef Pie	1 (227 g)	360	16	1940	44	—
Vegetarian Burger	½ cup (113 g)	150	4	780	9	—
Vegetarian Burger No Added Salt	½ cup (113 g)	150	4	170	7	—
Wham	3 slices (68 g)	120	7	940	3	—
Zoglo's						
Crispy Vegetarian Cutlets	1 (3.5 oz)	200	10	300	10	2
Savory Vegetarian Kebabs	1 serv (2.8 oz)	135	5	240	5	2
Tender Vegetarian Burgers	1 (2.6 oz)	150	7	230	5	2
Vegetable Patties	1 (2.6 oz)	130	5	270	10	2
Vegetarian Franks	1 (2.6 oz)	125	5	240	5	2
simulated sausage	1 link (25 g)	64	5	222	2	—
simulated sausage	1 patty (38 g)	97	7	137	4	—
simulated meat product	1 oz	88	1	3	11	—

MELON
(see also individual names)

FRESH

Chiquita

Cantalene	1 cup	60	0	—	—	—
Honey Mist	1 cup	80	0	—	—	—

FROZEN

Big Valley

Mixed	¾ cup (4.9 oz)	40	0	16	10	1
melon balls	1 cup	55	tr	53	14	—

MEXICAN FOOD
(see SALSA, SAUCE, TORTILLA)

MILK
(see also CHOCOLATE, COCOA, MILK DRINKS)

CANNED

Carnation

Evaporated	2 tbsp	40	3	35	3	—

FOOD	PORTION	CAL.	FAT	SOD.	CARB.	FIB.
Carnation (CONT.)						
Evaporated Lowfat	2 tbsp	25	1	35	3	—
Lite Evaporated Skimmed	½ cup (4 fl oz)	100	tr	150	14	—
Sweetened Condensed	2 tbsp	130	3	45	22	—
Eagle						
Sweetened Condensed	⅓ cup	320	9	120	52	—
Pet						
Evaporated	½ cup	170	10	140	12	—
Evaporated Filled	½ cup	150	8	140	12	—
Evaporated Light Skimmed	½ cup	100	tr	150	14	—
condensed sweetened	1 cup	982	27	389	166	—
condensed sweetened	1 oz	123	3	49	21	—
evaporated	½ cup	169	10	122	13	—
evaporated skim	½ cup	99	tr	147	14	—
DRIED						
Carnation						
Nonfat	⅓ cup dry	80	0	125	12	—
Nutra/Balance						
Lactose Reduced as prep	8 oz	80	tr	125	12	—
buttermilk	1 tbsp	25	tr	34	3	—
nonfat instantized	1 pkg (3.2 oz)	244	tr	499	47	—
REFRIGERATED						
BodyWise						
Nonfat	8 fl oz	100	0	150	14	0
Borden						
Acidophilus 1%	8 fl oz	100	2	130	11	—
Buttermilk Lowfat Golden Churn	8 fl oz	120	4	250	11	—
Hi-Calcium	8 fl oz	150	8	130	11	—
Hi-Protein 2%	8 fl oz	140	5	150	13	—
Skim	8 fl oz	90	1	130	12	—
Skim-line	8 fl oz	100	1	150	13	—
CalciMilk	8 fl oz	102	3	123	12	0
Farmland						
1%	8 fl oz	100	3	130	12	0
2%	8 fl oz	130	5	130	12	0
Cholesterol Reduced	8 fl oz	150	8	125	11	—
Easylac 1%	8 fl oz	100	2	125	11	—
Easylac Nonfat	8 fl oz	90	0	125	12	—
Skim	8 fl oz	80	0	130	12	0
Skim Plus	8 fl oz	100	tr	150	13	—

FOOD	PORTION	CAL.	FAT	SOD.	CARB.	FIB.
Friendship						
Buttermilk	8 fl oz	120	4	125	12	0
Hood						
1%	1 cup (8 oz)	110	3	125	13	0
Better Taste 2%	1 cup (8 oz)	130	5	125	13	0
Buttermilk	1 cup (8 oz)	90	0	220	13	0
Whole	1 cup (8 oz)	150	8	125	12	0
Lactaid						
1%	8 fl oz	102	3	123	12	0
Nonfat	8 fl oz	86	tr	126	12	0
Nuform						
1%	1 cup (8 oz)	120	3	150	15	0
Skim	1 cup (8 oz)	100	0	150	15	0
Silovet						
Skim	1 cup (8 oz)	90	0	125	13	0
Viva						
2%	8 fl oz	120	5	125	11	—
Skim	8 fl oz	100	1	150	13	—
1%	1 qt	409	10	493	47	—
1%	1 cup	102	3	123	12	—
1% protein fortified	1 qt	477	12	574	54	—
1% protein fortified	1 cup	119	3	143	14	—
2%	1 qt	485	19	487	47	—
2%	1 cup	121	5	122	12	—
buffalo	3½ oz	112	8	40	5	—
buttermilk	1 qt	396	9	1028	47	—
buttermilk	1 cup	99	2	257	12	—
camel	3½ oz	80	4	30	5	—
donkey	3½ oz	43	1	—	6	—
goat	1 cup	168	10	122	11	—
goat	1 qt	672	40	486	43	—
human	1 cup	171	11	42	17	—
indian buffalo	1 cup	236	17	127	13	—
low sodium	1 cup	149	8	6	11	—
mare	3½ oz	49	2	—	6	—
sheep	1 cup	264	17	108	13	—
skim	1 cup	86	tr	125	12	—
skim	1 qt	342	2	505	48	—
skim protein fortified	1 qt	400	2	578	55	—
skim protein fortified	1 cup	100	1	144	14	—
whole	1 cup	150	8	120	11	—
SHELF-STABLE						
Parmalat						
1%	1 cup (8 oz)	110	3	135	13	0

FOOD	PORTION	CAL.	FAT	SOD.	CARB.	FIB.
Parmalat (CONT.)						
2%	1 cup (8 oz)	130	5	130	13	0
Skim	1 cup (8 oz)	90	1	130	13	0
Whole	1 cup (8 oz)	160	8	130	13	0

MILK DRINKS
(*see also* BREAKFAST DRINKS, CHOCOLATE, COCOA)

FOOD	PORTION	CAL.	FAT	SOD.	CARB.	FIB.
Body Wise						
Chocolate Nonfat Milk	1 cup (8 fl oz)	180	0	170	35	1
Borden						
Chocolate Lowfat Dutch Brand	8 fl oz	180	5	180	25	—
Bosco						
Chocolate Milk	1 cup (8 fl oz)	230	8	110	33	—
Hershey						
Chocolate Milk 2%	1 cup	190	5	130	29	—
Whole Chocolate Milk	8 oz	210	9	120	28	—
Hood						
Chocolate Lowfat	1 cup (8 oz)	150	2	240	27	0
Lactaid						
Chocolate Milk 1%	8 fl oz	158	3	152	26	tr
Meadow Gold						
Chocolate Milk	8 fl oz	210	8	240	25	—
Parmalat						
Chocolate 2%	1 box (8 oz)	180	5	115	28	1
Quik						
Banana Lowfat Milk	8 oz	190	4	115	30	—
Chocolate	2½ tsp (0.75 oz)	90	1	25	20	—
Chocolate as prep w/ 2% milk	8 oz	210	5	150	31	—
Chocolate as prep w/ skim milk	8 oz	170	1	150	31	—
Chocolate as prep w/ whole milk	8 oz	230	9	140	31	—
Chocolate Lowfat Milk	8 oz	200	5	150	29	—
Ready To Drink Chocolate	8 oz	230	9	120	30	—
Ready To Drink Lite Chocolate Lowfat	8 oz	130	5	150	13	—
Ready To Drink Strawberry	8 oz	230	8	140	32	—
Strawberry	2½ tsp (0.75 oz)	80	0	0	21	—
Strawberry as prep w/ 2% milk	8 oz	200	5	120	32	—
Strawberry as prep w/ skim milk	8 oz	160	0	125	32	—

FOOD	PORTION	CAL.	FAT	SOD.	CARB.	FIB.
Quik (CONT.)						
Strawberry as prep w/ whole milk	8 oz	220	8	120	32	—
Strawberry Lowfat Milk	8 oz	200	4	120	33	—
Sugar Free Chocolate	1 heaping tsp (5.8 g)	18	tr	35	3	—
Sugar Free Chocolate as prep w/ 2% milk	8 oz	140	5	150	15	—
Syrup Chocolate as prep w/ 2% milk	8 oz	220	5	160	34	—
Syrup Chocolate as prep w/ skim milk	8 oz	220	9	160	34	—
Syrup Chocolate as prep w/ whole milk	8 oz	240	9	160	33	—
Syrup Strawberry as prep w/ 2% milk	8 oz	220	5	120	36	—
Syrup Strawberry as prep w/ skim milk	8 oz	180	0	130	36	—
Syrup Strawberry as prep w/ whole milk	8 oz	240	8	120	36	—
Vanilla Lowfat Milk	8 oz	200	4	115	31	—
chocolate milk	1 cup	208	8	149	26	—
chocolate milk	1 qt	833	34	596	103	—
chocolate milk 1%	1 qt	630	10	607	104	—
chocolate milk 1%	1 cup	158	3	152	26	—
chocolate milk 2%	1 cup	179	5	150	26	—
strawberry flavor mix as prep w/ whole milk	9 oz	234	8	128	33	—

MILK SUBSTITUTES

(*see also* COFFEE WHITENERS)

FOOD	PORTION	CAL.	FAT	SOD.	CARB.	FIB.
Better Than Milk						
Carob	8 fl oz	130	5	175	20	—
Chocolate	8 fl oz	125	5	175	17	—
Light	8 fl oz	80	tr	120	15	—
Natural	8 fl oz	90	5	120	10	—
Eden						
Original	1 pkg (8.8 oz)	135	4	110	14	0
Original	8 fl oz	130	4	105	13	0
EdenBlend						
Original	8 fl oz	120	3	85	16	0
Edensoy						
Carob	8 fl oz	150	4	105	23	0
Extra Original	1 pkg (8.8 oz)	140	5	105	13	0

FOOD	PORTION	CAL.	FAT	SOD.	CARB.	FIB.
Edensoy (CONT.)						
Extra Original	8 fl oz	130	5	100	12	0
Extra Vanilla	1 pkg (8.8 fl oz)	150	3	95	24	0
Extra Vanilla	8 fl oz	140	3	90	23	0
Vanilla	8 fl oz	150	3	90	23	0
Vanilla	1 pkg (8.8 fl oz)	150	3	95	24	0
Health Valley						
Soo Moo	1 cup	120	6	55	12	0
Rice Dream						
Carob Lite	8 fl oz	150	3	80	32	—
Chocolate	8 fl oz	190	3	80	44	—
Lite Organic Original	8 fl oz	130	2	80	28	—
Lite Vanilla	8 fl oz	130	2	80	30	—
Spring Creek						
IHoney Vanilla	1 oz	23	5	7	3	—
Original	1 oz	21	5	6	3	—
Plain	1 oz	15	5	4	1	—
Vitasoy						
Carob Supreme	8 fl oz	150	4	110	22	—
Cocoa Light	8 fl oz	140	2	80	25	—
Cocoa Rich	8 fl oz	160	4	130	24	—
Original Creamy	8 fl oz	100	5	130	10	—
Original Light	8 fl oz	90	2	90	15	—
Vanilla Delite	8 fl oz	150	4	100	23	—
Vanilla Light	8 fl oz	110	2	100	20	—
Westsoy						
Cocoa Lite	8 fl oz	140	2	95	25	—
Plain Lite	8 fl oz	100	2	100	16	—
Vanilla Lite	8 fl oz	110	2	80	20	—
imitation milk	1 qt	600	33	764	60	—
imitation milk	1 cup	150	8	191	15	—
MILKFISH						
baked	3 oz	162	7	—	0	—
MILKSHAKE						
Frostee						
Chocolate	8 fl oz	200	8	160	30	—
Strawberry	8 fl oz	180	7	150	27	—
Hood						
Shake Up Chocolate	1 cup (8 oz)	240	6	290	38	0
Shake Up Strawberry	1 cup (8 oz)	220	5	270	36	0
Shake Up Vanilla	1 cup (8 oz)	220	5	270	36	0
MicroMagic						
Chocolate	1 (10.5 oz)	290	8	90	46	—

FOOD	PORTION	CAL.	FAT	SOD.	CARB.	FIB.
Milky Way						
Shake	1 (10 fl oz)	390	16	235	54	0
Parmalat						
Shake A Shake Chocolate	1 box (6 oz)	180	4	140	29	1
Shake A Shake Orange Vanilla	1 box (6 oz)	110	3	55	14	0
Shake A Shake Vanilla	1 box (6 oz)	170	3	140	28	0
Weight Watchers						
Chocolate Fudge	1 pkg	70	tr	150	11	—
Orange Sherbet	1 pkg	70	tr	210	12	—
chocolate	10 oz	360	11	273	58	—
strawberry	10 oz	319	8	234	53	—
thick shake chocolate	10.6 oz	356	8	333	63	—
thick shake vanilla	11 oz	350	10	299	56	—
vanilla	10 oz	314	8	232	51	—

MILLET

FOOD	PORTION	CAL.	FAT	SOD.	CARB.	FIB.
cooked	½ cup	143	1	2	28	—

MINERAL/BOTTLED WATER

FOOD	PORTION	CAL.	FAT	SOD.	CARB.	FIB.
Artesia						
Almund	7 oz	0	0	—	—	—
Cranberi	7 oz	0	0	—	—	—
Lemin	7 oz	0	0	—	—	—
Orange	7 oz	0	0	—	—	—
Plain	7 oz	0	0	—	—	—
Canada Dry						
Sparkling Water	8 fl oz	0	0	10	0	0
Crystal Geyser						
Sparkling Lemon	1 bottle (12 fl oz)	0	0	70	0	—
Sparkling Mineral	1 bottle (12 fl oz)	0	0	70	0	—
Sparkling Natural Cola Berry	1 bottle (12 fl oz)	0	0	70	0	—
Sparkling Natural Wild Cherry	1 bottle 12 fl oz	0	0	70	0	—
Sparkling Orange	1 bottle (12 fl oz)	0	0	70	0	—
Glennpatrick						
Irish Spring Pure	8 oz	0	0	—	—	—
LaCroix						
Sparking Berry	12 fl oz	0	0	—	—	—
Sparkling Lemon	12 fl oz	0	0	—	—	—
Sparkling Lime	12 fl oz	0	0	—	—	—
Sparkling Orange	12 fl oz	0	0	—	—	—
Sparkling Regular	12 fl oz	0	0	—	—	—

FOOD	PORTION	CAL.	FAT	SOD.	CARB.	FIB.
Saratoga						
Sparkling	1 liter	0	0	19	0	—
MISO						
Eden						
Genmai Miso Organic	1 tbsp (0.5 oz)	25	1	810	3	tr
Hacho Miso Organic	1 tbsp (0.5 oz)	35	2	600	2	1
Kome Miso Organic	1 tbsp (0.6 oz)	25	1	850	3	tr
Mugi Miso Organic	1 tbsp (0.6 oz)	25	1	760	3	1
Shiro Miso Organic	1 tbsp (0.6 oz)	35	1	410	5	1
miso	½ cup	284	8	5036	39	7
MOLASSES						
Brer Rabbit						
Dark	2 tbsp	110	0	20	28	—
Light	2 tbsp	110	0	15	29	—
Tree Of Life						
Blackstrap	1 tbsp (0.5 oz)	45	0	15	11	—
blackstrap	1 tbsp (0.7 oz)	47	0	11	12	—
blackstrap	1 cup (11.5 oz)	771	tr	180	199	—
molasses	1 cup (11.5 oz)	873	1	120	226	—
molasses	1 tbsp (0.7 oz)	53	0	7	14	—
MONKFISH						
baked	3 oz	82	2	20	0	—
MOOSE						
roasted	3 oz	114	1	58	0	—
MOTH BEANS						
dried cooked	1 cup	207	1	17	37	—
MOUSSE						
FROZEN						
Pepperidge Farm						
San Francisco Chocolate Mousse	1	490	34	75	41	—
Sara Lee						
Chocolate	1 slice (2.7 oz)	260	17	100	23	—
Chocolate Light	1 (3 oz)	170	8	60	20	—
Light Classics Strawberry	1 slice (53.8 g)	180	11	—	—	—
Weight Watchers						
Chocolate	1 (2.5 oz)	160	3	160	27	—
Praline Pecan	1 (2.71 oz)	180	4	180	30	—
HOME RECIPE						
chocolate	½ cup (7.1 oz)	447	33	87	33	—

FOOD	PORTION	CAL.	FAT	SOD.	CARB.	FIB.
crab	¼ cup	364	20	—	—	—
orange	½ cup	87	5	24	19	—
MIX						
Jell-O						
Rich & Luscious Chocolate	½ cup	145	6	73	21	—
Rich & Luscious Chocolate Fudge	½ cup	143	6	74	20	—
Knorr						
Dark Chocolate as prep	½ cup	90	5	50	10	—
Milk Chocolate as prep	½ cup	90	5	50	11	—
Unflavored as prep	½ cup	80	5	45	8	—
White Chocolate as prep	½ cup	80	4	50	10	—
Royal						
Chocolate Mousse No-Bake	⅛ pie	130	4	190	21	—
Weight Watchers						
Chocolate	½ cup	70	3	—	7	—
White Chocolate Almond Mousse	½ cup	70	3	105	7	—
TAKE-OUT						
chocolate	½ cup (7.1 oz)	447	33	87	33	—

MUFFIN

FOOD	PORTION	CAL.	FAT	SOD.	CARB.	FIB.
FROZEN						
Health Valley						
Almond & Date Oat Bran Fancy Fruit	1	180	4	80	31	8
Fat Free Apple Spice	1	140	tr	110	30	5
Fat Free Banana	1	130	tr	110	29	5
Fat Free Raisin Spice	1	140	tr	100	32	5
Oat Bran Fancy Fruit Blueberry	1	140	4	100	32	8
Oat Bran Fancy Fruit Raisin	1	180	5	90	5	8
Rice Bran Fancy Fruit Raisin	1	210	7	125	7	6
Pepperidge Farm						
Banana Nut	1	170	6	220	28	—
Blueberry	1	170	7	250	27	1
Cholesterol Free Multi Grain Muesli	1	200	8	230	30	—
Cholesterol Free Oatbran With Apple	1	190	7	200	29	—

FOOD	PORTION	CAL.	FAT	SOD.	CARB.	FIB.
Pepperidge Farm (CONT.)						
Cholesterol Free Raisin Bran	1	170	6	280	30	—
Cinnamon Swirl	1	190	6	170	30	1
Corn	1	180	7	260	27	—
Sara Lee						
Apple Oat Bran	1	190	6	300	36	—
Apple Spice	1	220	8	280	36	—
Blueberry	1	200	8	290	34	—
Blueberry Free & Light	1	120	0	140	28	—
Cheese Streusel	1	220	11	170	27	—
Chocolate Chunk	1	220	8	210	33	—
Golden Corn	1	240	13	310	31	—
Oat Bran	1	210	8	320	35	—
Raisin Bran	1	220	7	400	37	—
Weight Watchers						
Banana Nut	1 (2.5 oz)	170	5	—	32	—
Blueberry	1 (2.5 oz)	170	5	—	32	—
HOME RECIPE						
blueberry as prep w/ 2% milk	1 (2 oz)	163	6	251	23	—
blueberry as prep w/ whole milk	1 (2 oz)	165	6	251	23	—
corn as prep w/ 2% milk	1 (2 oz)	180	7	334	25	—
corn as prep w/ whole milk	1 (2 oz)	183	7	333	25	—
plain as prep w/ 2% milk	1 (2 oz)	169	7	266	24	—
plain as prep w/ whole milk	1 (2 oz)	172	7	266	24	—
wheat bran as prep w/ 2% milk	1 (2 oz)	161	7	335	24	—
wheat bran as prep w/ whole milk	1 (2 oz)	164	7	335	24	—
MIX						
Arrowhead						
Bran	⅓ cup (1.4 oz)	150	2	160	26	7
Oat Bran Wheat Free	⅓ cup (1.5 oz)	160	4	310	23	7
Betty Crocker						
Apple Cinnamon	1	120	4	140	18	—
Apple Cinnamon No Cholesterol Recipe	1	110	2	140	18	—
Banana Nut	1	120	5	140	17	—
Banana Nut No Cholesterol Recipe	1	110	4	140	17	—
Blueberry Streusel Bake Shop	1	210	8	230	31	—

FOOD	PORTION	CAL.	FAT	SOD.	CARB.	FIB.
Betty Crocker (CONT.)						
Cinnamon Streusel	1	200	9	240	17	—
Oat Bran	1	190	8	240	25	—
Oat Bran No Cholesterol Recipe	1	180	7	240	25	—
Twice The Blueberries	1	120	4	140	18	—
Twice The Blueberries No Cholesterol Recipe	1	110	3	140	18	—
Wild Blueberry	1	120	4	150	18	—
Wild Blueberry Light	1	70	tr	140	16	—
Wild Blueberry Light No Cholesterol Recipe	1	70	tr	140	16	—
Wild Blueberry No Cholesterol Recipe	1	110	3	150	18	—
Dromedary						
Corn Muffin	1	120	4	270	20	—
Flako						
Corn	⅓ cup (1.4 oz)	160	4	380	29	1
Hain						
Oat Bran Apple Cinnamon	1	140	3	200	28	5
Oat Bran Banana Nut	1	140	4	190	26	4
Oat Bran Raspberry Spice	1	140	3	190	27	4
Jiffy						
Apple Cinnamon as prep	1	190	7	360	28	1
Banana Nut as prep	1	180	7	420	25	1
Blueberry as prep	1	190	7	288	28	1
Bran Date	1	110	—	—	—	—
Bran With Dates as prep	1	170	6	240	26	3
Corn as prep	1	180	4	320	28	1
Honey Date as prep	1	170	5	240	27	1
Oatmeal as prep	1	180	7	270	26	2
Wanda's						
Blue Corn	¼ cup mix per serv (1.2 oz)	130	1	350	25	1
blueberry	1 (1¾ oz)	149	4	219	24	—
corn	1 (1.75 oz)	160	5	397	25	—
wheat bran as prep	1 (1¾ oz)	138	5	233	23	—
READY-TO-EAT						
Arnold						
Bran'nola	1 (2.3 oz)	160	1	220	30	2
Raisin	1 (2.3 oz)	160	1	220	33	2

FOOD	PORTION	CAL.	FAT	SOD.	CARB.	FIB.
Dutch Mill						
Apple Oat Bran	1 (2 oz)	180	5	210	31	1
Banana Walnut	1 (2 oz)	220	6	210	33	1
Carrot	1 (2 oz)	190	7	230	31	1
Corn	1 (2 oz)	190	6	280	31	1
Cranberry Orange	1 (2 oz)	170	6	290	26	1
Raisin Bran	1 (2 oz)	230	5	330	37	3
Entenmann's						
Blueberry	1 (2 oz)	200	8	250	29	—
Freihofer's						
Corn Toasters	1 (1.3 oz)	130	6	210	18	0
Hostess						
Mini Apple Cinnamon	5 (2 oz)	260	16	180	28	3
Mini Banana Nut	5 (2 oz)	260	16	160	28	tr
Mini Blueberry	5 (2 oz)	240	13	180	30	tr
Mini Chocolate Chip	5 (2 oz)	260	15	170	29	1
Muffin Loaf Blueberry	1 (3.8 oz)	440	19	460	62	2
Oat Bran	1 (1.5 oz)	160	8	150	22	tr
Oat Bran Banana Nut	1 (1.5 oz)	150	6	160	22	1
Weight Watchers						
Apple Cinnamon	1 (2.5 oz)	200	5	250	36	1
Lemon Poppy Seed	1 (2.5 oz)	200	5	250	37	1
blueberry	1 (2 oz)	158	4	255	27	2
corn	1 (2 oz)	174	5	297	29	—
oat bran wheat free	1 (2 oz)	154	4	224	28	4
toaster type blueberry	1	103	3	158	18	—
toaster type corn	1	114	4	142	19	—
toaster type wheat bran w/ raisins	1 (36 g)	106	3	178	19	—

MULBERRIES

fresh	1 cup	61	1	14	14	—

MULLET

striped cooked	3 oz	127	4	61	0	—
striped raw	3 oz	99	3	55	0	—

MUNG BEANS
DRIED

cooked	1 cup	213	1	4	39	—
SPROUTS						
canned	½ cup	8	tr	—	1	—
cooked	½ cup	13	tr	6	3	—
raw	½ cup	16	tr	3	3	—
stir fried	½ cup	31	tr	—	7	—

FOOD	PORTION	CAL.	FAT	SOD.	CARB.	FIB.
MUNGO BEANS						
dried cooked	1 cup	190	1	13	33	—
MUSHROOMS						
CANNED						
B In B	¼ cup	12	0	240	2	1
With Garlic	¼ cup	12	0	200	2	1
Empress						
Button	2 oz	14	0	260	2	—
Button Sliced	2 oz	14	0	260	2	—
Pieces & Stems	2 oz	14	0	260	2	—
Straw Broken	2 oz	10	0	180	2	—
Green Giant						
Oriental Straw	¼ cup	12	0	290	2	1
Pieces And Stems	¼ cup	12	0	220	2	1
Sliced	¼ cup	12	0	220	2	1
Whole	¼ cup	12	0	220	2	1
Ka-Me						
Stir Fry	½ cup (4.5 oz)	20	0	380	3	2
Straw Whole Peeled	½ cup (4.5 oz)	20	0	380	3	2
Seneca						
Mushrooms	½ cup	25	0	552	3	2
chanterelle	3½ oz	12	1	165	tr	6
pieces	½ cup	19	tr	—	4	—
whole	1 (0.4 oz)	3	tr	—	1	—
DRIED						
chanterelle	3½ oz	89	2	32	2	60
shitake	4 (½ oz)	44	tr	2	11	—
FRESH						
chanterelle	3½ oz	11	tr	3	tr	6
enoki raw	1 (4 in)	2	tr	0	tr	—
morel	3½ oz	9	tr	2	0	7
oyster	3.5 oz	11	tr	6	0	6
raw	1 (½ oz)	5	tr	1	1	tr
raw sliced	½ cup	9	tr	1	2	tr
shitake cooked	4 (2.5 oz)	40	tr	3	10	—
sliced cooked	½ cup	21	tr	2	4	1
whole cooked	1 (0.4 oz)	3	tr	0	1	—
FROZEN						
Fresh Like	3.5 oz	28	tr	15	4	—
Empire						
Breaded	7 (2.8 oz)	90	1	390	16	1
MUSKRAT						
roasted	3 oz	199	10	81	0	—

FOOD	PORTION	CAL.	FAT	SOD.	CARB.	FIB.
MUSSELS						
blue raw	1 cup	129	3	429	6	—
blue raw	3 oz	73	2	243	3	—
fresh blue cooked	3 oz	147	4	313	6	—
MUSTARD						
Blanchard & Blanchard						
Mustard	1 tsp (5 g)	0	0	45	0	0
Eden						
Hot Organic	1 tsp (5 g)	0	0	65	tr	0
Estee						
Sodium Free	1 pkg (0.5 oz)	5	1	0	tr	—
Grey Poupon						
Country Dijon	1 tsp	6	0	120	0	0
Dijon	1 tsp	6	0	120	0	0
Parisian	1 tsp	6	0	55	0	0
Gulden's						
Diablo	1 tsp	8	0	—	—	—
Mild	1 tsp	6	0	—	—	—
Spicy Brown	1 tsp	8	0	—	—	—
Hain						
Stone Ground	1 tbsp	14	1	185	1	—
Stone Ground No Salt Added	1 tbsp	14	1	10	1	—
Heinz						
Mild Yellow	1 tbsp	8	tr	175	1	—
Spicy Brown	1 tbsp	14	1	115	1	—
Ka-Me						
Hot Mustard Powder Chinese Style	¼ tsp (1 g)	5	0	0	1	1
Kosciuszko						
Spicy Brown	1 tsp	5	tr	60	tr	—
McIlhenny						
Coarse Ground	1 tsp (0.2 oz)	4	tr	39	tr	tr
Spicy	1 tsp (0.2 oz)	6	tr	28	tr	1
Plochman						
Dijon	1 tsp (5 g)	7	tr	82	tr	—
Spoonable Salad	1 tsp (5 g)	4	tr	53	tr	—
Squeeze Salad	1 tsp (5 g)	4	tr	53	tr	—
Stone Ground	1 tsp (5 g)	6	tr	60	tr	—
Russer						
Deli	1 tsp (5 g)	4	0	65	0	—
Tree Of Life						
Dijon	1 tsp (5 g)	0	0	66	0	—

FOOD	PORTION	CAL.	FAT	SOD.	CARB.	FIB.
Tree Of Life (CONT.)						
Dijon Imported	1 tsp (5 g)	5	0	120	tr	—
Low Sodium	1 tsp (5 g)	3	0	50	tr	—
Stone Ground	1 tsp (5 g)	0	0	55	0	—
Yellow	1 tsp (5 g)	0	0	55	0	—
Watkins						
Country Mill	1 tsp (7 oz)	15	1	110	2	0
Dusseldorf	1 tsp (7 oz)	10	0	110	1	0
Horseradish	1 tsp (7 oz)	10	0	120	1	0
Jalapeno	1 tsp (7 oz)	10	0	150	1	0
Onion	1 tsp (7 oz)	10	0	110	1	0
Parisienne	1 tsp (7 oz)	10	0	110	1	0
dry mustard seed yellow	1 tsp	15	1	tr	1	—
yellow ready-to-use	1 tsp	5	tr	63	tr	—

MUSTARD GREENS
CANNED

FOOD	PORTION	CAL.	FAT	SOD.	CARB.	FIB.
Allen	½ cup (4.1 oz)	30	1	10	5	3
Sunshine	½ cup (4.1 oz)	30	1	10	5	3
FRESH						
chopped cooked	½ cup	11	tr	11	1	—
raw chopped	½ cup	7	tr	7	1	—
FROZEN						
chopped cooked	½ cup	14	tr	19	2	—

NATTO

FOOD	PORTION	CAL.	FAT	SOD.	CARB.	FIB.
natto	½ cup	187	10	6	13	—

NAVY BEANS
CANNED

FOOD	PORTION	CAL.	FAT	SOD.	CARB.	FIB.
Allen	½ cup (4.5 oz)	110	1	380	19	6
Eden						
Organic	½ cup (4.3 oz)	100	1	15	18	7
Hanover						
Navy	½ cup	100	0	—	—	—
Luck's						
Seasoned w/ Pork	7.5 oz	230	7	—	—	—
Trappey						
With Bacon	½ cup (4.5 oz)	110	2	420	17	7
With Bacon & Jalapeno	½ cup (4.5 oz)	110	2	420	17	7
navy	1 cup	296	1	1173	54	—
DRIED						
cooked	1 cup	259	1	2	48	—
SPROUTS						
cooked	3½ oz	78	1	—	—	—
raw	½ cup	35	tr	—	—	—

FOOD	PORTION	CAL.	FAT	SOD.	CARB.	FIB.
NECTARINE						
Dole	1	70	1	0	16	3
fresh	1	67	1	0	16	2
NEUFCHATEL						
Philadelphia	1 oz	70	6	120	tr	0
Spreadery						
Classic Ranch	2 tbsp (1 oz)	60	7	210	1	0
Garden Vegetable	2 tbsp (1 oz)	70	6	230	2	0
Garlic & Herb	2 tbsp (1 oz)	80	7	180	1	0
With Strawberry	1 oz	70	5	270	tr	—
WisPride						
Garden Vegetable Cup	2 tbsp (1.1 oz)	60	5	180	2	0
Garlic & Herb Cup	2 tbsp (1.1 oz)	60	5	180	2	0
neufchatel	1 pkg (3 oz)	221	20	339	3	—
neufchatel	1 oz	74	7	113	1	—
NON-DAIRY CREAMERS						
(see COFFEE WHITENERS)						
NON-DAIRY WHIPPED TOPPINGS						
(see WHIPPED TOPPINGS)						
NOODLES						
(see also PASTA DINNERS)						
CANNED						
Dinty Moore						
Noodles & Chicken	1 can (7.5 oz)	180	8	1010	19	1
Micro Cup Meals						
Noodles & Chicken	1 cup (10.4 oz)	250	11	1410	27	2
Noodles & Chicken	1 cup (7.5 oz)	180	8	1010	19	1
Van Camp's						
Noodlee Weenee	1 can (8 oz)	230	8	680	34	1
DRY						
Azumaya						
Chinese	4 oz	293	1	530	60	—
Japanese	4 oz	289	1	542	59	—
Creamette						
Egg	2 oz	221	3	—	—	—
Egg not prep	2 oz	220	3	20	40	—
Golden Grain						
Egg	2 oz	210	2	10	39	2
Hodgson Mill						
Veggie Egg not prep	2 oz	200	2	25	37	2
Whole Wheat Egg not prep	2 oz	190	2	20	34	4

FOOD	PORTION	CAL.	FAT	SOD.	CARB.	FIB.
Hodgson Mill (CONT.)						
Whole Wheat Spinach Egg not prep	2 oz	190	2	45	32	5
Ka-Me						
Chinese Egg	½ cup (2 oz)	210	2	3	40	2
Chinese Plain	½ cup (2 oz)	200	0	1	45	1
Chuka Soba Curly Noodles	2 oz	200	1	310	42	1
Lo Mein Wide Chinese	½ cup (2 oz)	200	0	1	45	1
Py Mai Fun Rice Sticks	2 oz	193	0	100	48	0
Sai Fun Bean Thread	1 cup (2 oz)	190	0	0	50	1
Soba Shin Shu Japanese Buckwheat	2 oz	200	1	80	40	2
Tomoshiraga Somen Noodles	2 oz	190	1	670	41	1
Udon Japanese Thick	2 oz	190	1	670	41	1
La Choy						
Chow Mein Narrow	½ cup	150	8	320	16	tr
Chow Mein Wide	½ cup	150	8	300	16	tr
Rice	½ cup	130	5	420	21	tr
Mueller's						
Egg	2 oz (57 g)	220	3	8	40	—
Noodle Trio	2 oz (57 g)	220	2	18	40	—
Noodles By Leonardo						
Egg Fine not prep	1 cup (2 oz)	210	2	10	39	2
Egg Medium not prep	1 cup (2 oz)	210	2	30	39	2
Egg Wide not prep	1 cup (2 oz)	210	2	30	39	2
San Giorgio						
Egg	2 oz	210	3	15	38	—
Shofar						
No Yolks	2 oz	210	0	30	41	3
cellophane	1 cup	492	tr	14	121	—
chow mein	1 cup	237	14	197	26	—
egg	1 cup (38 g)	145	2	8	27	—
egg cooked	1 cup	212	2	11	40	—
japanese soba	2 oz	192	tr	451	43	—
japanese soba cooked	½ cup	56	tr	34	12	—
japanese somen	2 oz	203	tr	1049	42	—
japanese somen cooked	½ cup	115	tr	142	24	—
spinach/egg	1 cup	145	2	27	27	—
spinach/egg cooked	1 cup	211	3	20	39	—
FRESH						
Herb's						
Egg Fine	2 oz	220	2	5	42	2

FOOD	PORTION	CAL.	FAT	SOD.	CARB.	FIB.
Herb's (CONT.)						
Egg Medium	2 oz	220	2	5	42	2
Kluski Medium	2 oz	220	2	5	42	2
Kluski Wide	2 oz	220	2	5	42	2
FROZEN						
Luigino's						
Stroganoff	1 cup (7.5 oz)	290	16	870	23	2
Stroganoff	1 pkg (8 oz)	310	17	920	25	2
MIX						
Kraft						
Chicken Egg Noodle	1 cup	330	12	1430	45	1
La Choy						
Ramen Noodles Beef as prep	1 cup	200	8	865	33	4
Ramen Noodles Chicken as prep	1 cup	200	7	740	29	4
Lipton						
Noodles & Sauce Alfredo	½ cup	131	3	530	20	tr
Noodles & Sauce Beef	½ cup	120	2	513	22	0
Noodles & Sauce Butter	½ cup	142	4	461	22	0
Noodles & Sauce Butter & Herb	½ cup	136	3	458	22	0
Noodles & Sauce Carbonara Alfredo	½ cup	126	3	465	20	0
Noodles & Sauce Cheese	½ cup	136	2	470	24	0
Noodles & Sauce Chicken	½ cup	125	2	391	22	tr
Noodles & Sauce Chicken Broccoli	½ cup	124	2	425	22	—
Noodles & Sauce Creamy Chicken	½ cup	125	2	390	22	—
Noodles & Sauce Parmesan	½ cup	138	4	409	20	0
Noodles & Sauce Romanoff	½ cup	136	3	504	23	—
Noodles & Sauce Sour Cream & Chive	½ cup	142	3	442	23	0
Noodles & Sauce Stroganoff	½ cup	110	2	406	19	0
Noodles & Sauce Tomato Alfredo	½ cup	126	3	562	20	—
Minute						
Microwave Chicken Flavored	½ cup	157	5	471	23	—

FOOD	PORTION	CAL.	FAT	SOD.	CARB.	FIB.
Minute (CONT.)						
Microwave Parmesan	½ cup	178	6	491	24	—
Noodle Roni						
Chicken & Mushroom	½ cup	160	4	550	25	—
Fettuccini	½ cup	300	18	560	29	—
Herb & Butter	½ cup	160	7	290	19	—
Parmesano	½ cup	240	13	140	23	—
Romanoff	½ cup	240	11	730	28	—
Stroganoff	½ cup	350	17	1190	37	—
Noodles By Leonardo						
Macaroni & Cheese as prep	1 cup (2.5 oz)	250	1	530	49	2
Ultra Slim-Fast						
Noodles & Alfredo Sauce	2.3 oz	240	4	1110	47	4
Noodles & Beef	2.3 oz	230	3	1070	45	4
Noodles & Cheese	2.3 oz	230	4	770	44	4
Noodles & Chicken Sauce	2.3 oz	220	3	980	45	4
Noodles & Tomato Herb Sauce	2.3 oz	220	3	1090	46	5
TAKE-OUT						
noodle pudding	½ cup	132	7	222	11	—

NOPALES

FOOD	PORTION	CAL.	FAT	SOD.	CARB.	FIB.
cooked	1 cup (5.2 oz)	23	tr	30	5	—
raw sliced	½ cup (1.5 oz)	7	tr	9	1	—
raw sliced	1 cup (3 oz)	14	tr	19	3	—

NUTMEG

FOOD	PORTION	CAL.	FAT	SOD.	CARB.	FIB.
Watkins	¼ tsp (0.5 g)	0	0	0	0	0
ground	1 tsp	12	1	tr	1	—

NUTRITIONAL SUPPLEMENTS

(*see also* BREAKFAST BAR, BREAKFAST DRINKS)

FOOD	PORTION	CAL.	FAT	SOD.	CARB.	FIB.
DIET						
Dynatrim						
Dutch Chocolate as prep w/ 1% milk	8 oz	220	4	300	33	6
Strawberry Royale as prep w/ 1% milk	8 oz	220	4	300	33	6
Vanilla as prep w/ 1% milk	8 oz	220	4	300	33	6
Figurines						
Chocolate	1 bar	100	5	45	11	—
Chocolate Caramel	1 bar	100	6	55	10	—

FOOD	PORTION	CAL.	FAT	SOD.	CARB.	FIB.
Figurines (CONT.)						
Chocolate Peanut Butter	1 bar	100	6	45	10	—
S'Mores	1 bar	100	5	54	11	—
Vanilla	1 bar	100	5	45	11	—
Sego						
Lite Chocolate	10 fl oz	150	3	480	20	—
Lite Dutch Chocolate	10 fl oz	150	3	480	20	—
Lite French Vanilla	10 fl oz	150	4	390	17	—
Lite Strawberry	10 fl oz	150	4	390	17	—
Lite Vanilla	10 fl oz	150	4	390	17	—
Very Chocolate	10 fl oz	225	1	450	43	—
Very Chocolate Malt	10 fl oz	225	1	450	43	—
Very Strawberry	10 fl oz	225	5	360	34	—
Very Vanilla	10 fl oz	225	5	360	34	—
Slim-Fast						
Powder Chocolate as prep w/ skim milk	8 oz	190	1	210	32	2
Powder Chocolate Malt as prep w/ skim milk	8 oz	190	tr	230	32	2
Powder Strawberry as prep w/ skim milk	8 oz	190	1	220	32	2
Powder Vanilla as prep w/ skim milk	8 oz	190	1	220	32	2
Sweet Success						
Chewy Bar Chocolate Brownie	1 (1.6 oz)	120	4	35	28	3
Chewy Bar Chocolate Chip	1 (1.6 oz)	120	4	35	23	3
Chewy Bar Chocolate Peanut Butter	1 (1.6 oz)	120	4	35	23	3
Chewy Bar Chocolate Raspberry	1 (1.6 oz)	120	4	35	23	3
Chewy Bar Oatmeal Raisin	1 (1.6 oz)	120	4	30	23	3
Chocolate Raspberry Truffle	1 can (10 fl oz)	200	3	220	38	6
Chocolate Raspberry as prep w/ skim milk	9 fl oz	180	1	360	30	6
Chocolate Mocha Supreme	1 can (10 fl oz)	200	3	220	38	6
Chocolate Mocha Supreme as prep w/ skim milk	9 fl oz	180	tr	356	30	6
Classic Chocolate Chip as prep w/ skim milk	9 fl oz	180	1	288	30	6

FOOD	PORTION	CAL.	FAT	SOD.	CARB.	FIB.
Sweet Success (CONT.)						
Creamy Milk Chocolate	1 can (10 fl oz)	200	3	240	38	6
Creamy Milk Chocolate	1 carton (12 fl oz)	220	2	300	45	6
Creamy Milk Chocolate as prep w/ skim milk	9 fl oz	180	1	336	30	6
Creamy Vanilla Delight as prep w/ skim milk	9 fl oz	180	tr	312	33	6
Dark Chocolate Fudge	1 can (10 fl oz)	200	3	220	38	6
Dark Chocolate Fudge	1 carton (12 fl oz)	220	2	310	45	6
Dark Chocolate Fudge as prep w/ skim milk	9 fl oz	180	1	356	30	6
Rich Chocolate Almond	1 can (10 fl oz)	200	3	240	38	6
Rich Chocolate Almond	1 carton (12 fl oz)	220	2	300	45	6
Rich Chocolate Almond as prep w/ skim milk	9 fl oz	180	tr	356	30	6
Smooth Vanilla Creme	1 can (10 fl oz)	200	3	220	38	6
Ultra Slim-Fast						
Cafe Mocha as prep w/ skim milk	8 oz	200	tr	280	38	6
Chocolate Royale as prep w/ skim milk	8 oz	200	1	230	36	5
Crunch Bar Cocoa Almond	1	110	3	30	19	3
Crunch Bar Cocoa Raspberry	1	100	3	30	21	3
Crunch Bar Vanilla Almond	1	110	4	30	18	3
Dutch Chocolate as prep w/ water	8 oz	220	tr	260	40	5
French Vanilla as prep w/ skim milk	8 oz	190	tr	250	36	4
French Vanilla as prep w/ water	8 oz	220	tr	260	40	4
Fruit Juice Mix as prep w/ fruit juice	8 oz	200	tr	80	43	6
Nutrition Bar Dutch Chocolate	1	130	4	90	17	6
Nutrition Bar Peanut Butter	1	140	6	100	15	7
Pina Colada as prep w/ skim milk	8 oz	180	tr	250	36	6
Ready-To-Drink Chocolate Royale	11 oz	230	3	220	42	5
Ready-To-Drink Chocolate Royale	12 oz	250	1	240	45	5

FOOD	PORTION	CAL.	FAT	SOD.	CARB.	FIB.
Ultra Slim-Fast (CONT.)						
Ready-To-Drink French Vanilla	11 oz	230	5	190	38	5
Ready-To-Drink French Vanilla	12 oz	220	tr	240	38	5
Ready-To-Drink Strawberry Supreme	12 oz	220	1	240	38	5
Strawberry as prep w/ skim milk	8 oz	190	1	250	36	4
Strawberry Supreme as prep w/ water	8 oz	220	tr	260	40	4
REGULAR						
BeneFit						
Chocolate	1 serv	120	2	200	15	1
Nutrition Bar	1 (2 oz)	240	8	190	33	tr
Vanilla	1 serv	120	2	220	15	tr
Boost						
Vanilla	8 oz	240	4	130	40	0
EggPro	4 oz	200	4	105	33	—
Fi-Bar						
Apple	1 (1 oz)	90	3	12	15	5
Cocoa Almond	1	130	4	20	21	4
Cocoa Peanut	1	130	4	20	20	4
Cranberry & Wild Berries	1 (1 oz)	100	3	20	13	4
Lemon	1 (1 oz)	90	3	12	15	5
Mandarin Orange	1 (1 oz)	99	4	12	15	5
Nuggets Almond Butter Crunch	1 pkg	163	11	—	12	—
Nuggets Almond Cappuccino Crunch	1 pkg	136	6	—	18	—
Nuggets Coconut Almond Crunch	1 pkg	136	6	—	18	—
Nuggets Peanut Butter Crunch	1 pkg	160	10	—	12	—
Raspberry	1 (1 oz)	100	3	20	13	4
Strawberry	1 (1 oz)	100	3	20	13	4
Treat Yourself Right Almond	1	152	6	38	22	5
Treat Yourself Right Peanutty Butter	1	152	5	56	18	5
Vanilla Almond	1	130	4	20	21	4
Vanilla Peanut	1	130	4	20	20	4
Gatorade						
GatorBar	1 (1.17 oz)	110	1	10	13	1

FOOD	PORTION	CAL.	FAT	SOD.	CARB.	FIB.
Gatorade (CONT.)						
GatorLode	1 can (11.6 fl oz)	280	0	90	71	—
GatorPro	1 can (11 fl oz)	360	6	270	59	0
ReLode	1 pkt (0.75 oz)	80	0	25	17	—
Gookinaid						
Lemonade	1 cup (8 fl oz)	45	0	70	12	—
Malsovit						
Mealwafers	2	152	8	—	—	—
Meal On The Go						
Apple	1 bar (3 oz)	294	5	114	50	5
Banana w/ Pecans	1 bar (3 oz)	289	10	109	50	8
Original	1 bar (3 oz)	286	9	119	52	7
Nutra/Balance						
Frozen Pudding Butterscotch	4 oz	225	8	220	31	—
Frozen Pudding Chocolate	4 oz	225	8	220	31	—
Frozen Pudding Tapioca	4 oz	225	8	220	31	—
Frozen Pudding Vanilla	4 oz	225	8	220	31	—
NutraShake						
Chocolate	4 oz	200	6	55	31	—
Strawberry	4 oz	200	6	55	31	—
Vanilla	4 oz	200	6	55	31	—
With Fiber Strawberry	6 oz	300	2	110	60	—
With Fiber Vanilla	6 oz	300	2	110	60	—
Resource						
Fructose Sweetened	1 pkg (8 oz)	250	11	230	23	3
Fruit Beverage	1 pkg (8 oz)	180	0	55	36	—
Liquid Food	1 pkg (8 oz)	250	9	210	34	—
Plus Liquid Food	1 pkg (8 oz)	355	13	300	47	—
Sustacal						
Vanilla Sustacal	8 oz	240	6	220	33	tr
Vita-J						
Apple Juice	11.5 fl oz	8	0	25	2	—
Fruit Punch	11.5 fl oz	8	0	25	2	—
Grapefruit Cocktail w/ Raspberry	11.5 fl oz	8	0	25	2	—
Orange Juice	11.5 fl oz	8	0	25	2	—

NUTS MIXED
(see also individual names)

FOOD	PORTION	CAL.	FAT	SOD.	CARB.	FIB.
Eagle						
Cashews & Peanuts Honey Roasted	1 oz	170	8	130	8	—

FOOD	PORTION	CAL.	FAT	SOD.	CARB.	FIB.
Eagle (CONT.)						
Mixed	1 oz	180	16	130	6	—
Mixed Deluxe	1 oz	180	17	130	6	—
Fisher						
Mixed Deluxe Lightly Salted	1 oz	180	16	—	5	—
Mixed Deluxe Salted	1 oz	180	16	95	5	—
Mixed Oil Roasted 25% More Cashews Lightly Salted	1 oz	180	16	50	5	—
Mixed Oil Roasted 25% More Cashews Salted	1 oz	180	16	110	5	—
Nut & Fruit Pina Colada	1 oz	150	10	50	13	—
Nut & Fruit Raisin Cranberry	1 oz	150	10	70	12	—
Nut & Fruit Tropical Fruit	1 oz	140	8	90	15	—
Nut Toppings Oil Roasted With Peanuts	1 oz	190	17	150	6	—
Peanuts Cashews	1 oz	170	13	110	8	—
Guy's						
Mixed With Peanuts	1 oz	180	16	140	3	—
Tasty Mix	1 oz	130	7	510	14	—
Planters						
Cashews & Peanuts Honey Roasted	1 oz	150	12	125	10	2
Deluxe Oil Roasted	1 oz	170	16	110	6	2
Dry Roasted	1 oz	170	14	250	7	2
Honey Roasted	1 oz	140	13	85	9	2
Lightly Salted Oil Roasted	1 oz	170	15	55	6	2
No Brazils Lightly Salted Oil Roasted	1 oz	170	15	55	6	2
No Brazils Oil Roasted	1 oz	170	15	110	6	2
Oil Roasted	1 oz	170	15	115	5	2
Select Mix Cashews Almonds & Macadamias Oil Roasted	1 oz	170	16	90	6	2
Select Mix Cashews Almonds & Pecans Oil Roasted	1 oz	170	15	95	7	2
Unsalted Oil Roasted	1 oz	170	15	0	6	3
dry roasted w/ peanuts	1 oz	169	15	3	7	—
dry roasted w/ peanuts salted	1 oz	169	15	223	7	—

FOOD	PORTION	CAL.	FAT	SOD.	CARB.	FIB.
oil roasted w/ peanuts	1 oz	175	16	3	6	—
oil roasted w/ peanuts salted	1 oz	175	16	217	6	—
oil roasted w/o peanuts	1 oz	175	16	3	6	—
oil roasted w/o peanuts salted	1 oz	175	16	233	6	—

OCTOBER BEANS
Luck's
Seasoned w/ Pork	7.25 oz	230	6	—	—	—

OCTOPUS
fresh steamed	3 oz	140	2	—	4	—

OHELOBERRIES
fresh	1 cup	39	tr	2	10	—

OIL
(*see also* FAT)
Arrowhead
Flax Seed	1 tbsp (0.5 fl oz)	120	14	0	0	0
Hazelnut	1 tbsp (0.5 fl oz)	120	14	0	0	0

Bertolli
Classico	1 tbsp	120	14	—	—	—
Extra Light	1 tbsp	120	14	—	—	—
Extra Virgin	1 tbsp	120	14	—	—	—

Crisco
Corn Canola	1 tbsp (0.5 fl oz)	120	14	0	0	0
Puritan Canola	1 tbsp (0.5 fl oz)	120	14	0	0	0

Eden
Hot Pepper Sesame	1 tbsp (0.5 oz)	130	14	0	0	0
Toasted Sesame	1 tbsp (0.5 oz)	130	14	0	0	0

Hain
All Blend	1 tbsp	120	14	0	0	—
Almond	1 tbsp	120	14	0	0	—
Apricot Kernel	1 tbsp	120	14	0	0	—
Avocado	1 tbsp	120	14	0	0	—
Canola	1 tbsp	120	14	0	0	—
Canola Organic	1 tbsp	120	14	0	0	—
Coconut	1 tbsp	120	14	0	0	—
Corn	1 tbsp	120	14	0	0	—
Garlic & Oil	1 tbsp	120	14	0	0	—
Olive	1 tbsp	120	14	0	0	—
Peanut	1 tbsp	120	14	0	0	—
Rice Bran	1 tbsp	120	14	0	0	—
Safflower	1 tbsp	120	14	0	0	—

FOOD	PORTION	CAL.	FAT	SOD.	CARB.	FIB.
Hain (CONT.)						
Safflower Hi-Oleic	1 tbsp	120	14	0	0	—
Safflower Organic	1 tbsp	120	14	0	0	—
Sesame	1 tbsp	120	14	0	0	—
Soy	1 tbsp	120	14	0	0	—
Sunflower	1 tbsp	120	14	0	0	—
Sunflower Organic	1 tbsp	120	14	0	0	—
Walnut	1 tbsp	120	14	0	0	—
Hollywood						
Canola	1 tbsp	120	14	0	0	—
Peanut	1 tbsp	120	14	0	0	—
Safflower	1 tbsp	120	14	0	0	—
Soy	1 tbsp	120	14	0	0	—
Sunflower	1 tbsp	120	14	0	0	—
House Of Tsang						
Hot Chili Sesame	1 tsp (5 g)	45	5	0	0	0
Mongolian Fire	1 tsp (5 g)	45	5	0	0	0
Pure Sesame	1 tsp (5 g)	45	5	0	0	0
Singapore Curry	1 tsp (5 g)	45	5	0	0	0
Wok Oil	1 tbsp (0.5 oz)	130	14	0	0	0
Italica						
Olive Oil	1 tbsp	120	9	—	0	—
Ka-Me						
Chili Hot	1 tbsp (0.5 fl oz)	130	14	0	0	0
Sesame	1 tbsp (0.5 fl oz)	130	14	0	0	0
Sesame Tempura	1 tbsp (0.5 fl oz)	130	14	0	0	0
Mazola						
No Stick	2.5 second spray (0.2 g)	2	tr	0	0	—
Oil	1 tbsp (14 g)	120	14	0	0	—
Oil	1 cup (221 g)	1955	221	0	0	—
Orville Redenbacher's	1 tbsp	120	14	0	0	0
Pam						
Butter	1 sec spray (0.266 g)	2	tr	0	0	—
Cooking Spray	1 sec spray (0.266 g)	2	tr	0	0	—
Olive Oil	1 sec spray (0.266 g)	2	tr	0	0	—
Pump	1 spray (0.43 g)	4	tr	0	0	—
Planters						
Peanut	1 tbsp (0.5 oz)	120	14	0	0	—
Popcorn	1 tbsp (0.5 oz)	120	14	0	0	—

FOOD	PORTION	CAL.	FAT	SOD.	CARB.	FIB.
Pompeian						
Olive	1 tbsp	130	14	—	—	—
Progresso						
Olive	1 tbsp	119	14	0	0	0
Olive Extra Light	1 tbsp	119	14	0	0	0
Olive Extra Virgin	1 tbsp	119	14	0	0	0
Smart Beat						
Canola	1 tbsp (14 g)	120	14	0	0	—
Tree Of Life						
Almond	1 tbsp (0.5 g)	130	14	0	0	—
Apricot Kernel	1 tbsp (0.5 g)	130	14	0	0	—
Avocado	1 tbsp (0.5 g)	130	14	0	0	—
Macadamia Nut	1 tbsp (0.5 g)	130	14	0	0	—
Olive Extra Virgin Organic	1 tbsp (0.5 g)	130	14	0	0	—
Sesame	1 tbsp (0.5 g)	130	14	0	0	—
Toasted Sesame	1 tbsp (0.5 oz)	130	14	0	0	0
Weight Watchers						
Butter Spray	1 second spray	2	tr	0	0	—
Cooking Spray	1 second spray	2	tr	0	0	—
Wesson						
Canola	1 tbsp	120	14	0	0	0
Cooking Spray Lite	0.5 sec spray	0	0	0	0	0
Corn	1 tbsp	120	14	0	0	0
Olive	1 tbsp	120	14	0	0	0
Sunflower	1 tbsp	120	14	0	0	0
Vegetable	1 tbsp	120	14	0	0	0
almond	1 cup	1927	218	—	0	—
almond	1 tbsp	120	14	—	0	—
apricot kernel	1 cup	1927	218	—	0	—
apricot kernel	1 tbsp	120	14	—	0	—
avocado	1 tbsp	124	14	—	0	—
avocado	1 cup	1927	218	—	0	—
babassu palm	1 tbsp	120	14	—	0	—
butter oil	1 tbsp	112	13	—	0	—
butter oil	1 cup	1795	204	—	0	—
canola	1 cup	1927	218	—	0	—
canola	1 tbsp	124	14	—	0	—
coconut	1 tbsp	117	14	—	0	—
corn	1 tbsp	120	14	—	0	—
corn	1 cup	1927	218	—	0	—
cottonseed	1 cup	1927	218	—	0	—
cottonseed	1 tbsp	120	14	—	0	—
cupu assu	1 tbsp	120	14	—	0	—

FOOD	PORTION	CAL.	FAT	SOD.	CARB.	FIB.
grapeseed	1 tbsp	120	14	—	0	—
hazelnut	1 cup	1927	218	—	0	—
hazelnut	1 tbsp	120	14	—	0	—
mustard	1 tbsp	124	14	—	0	—
mustard	1 cup	1927	218	—	0	—
oat	1 tbsp	120	14	—	0	—
olive	1 cup	1909	216	tr	0	—
olive	1 tbsp	119	14	0	0	—
palm	1 cup	1927	218	—	0	—
palm	1 tbsp	120	14	—	0	—
palm kernel	1 cup	1879	218	—	0	—
palm kernel	1 tbsp	117	14	—	0	—
peanut	1 tbsp	119	14	tr	0	—
peanut	1 cup	1909	216	tr	0	—
poppyseed	1 tbsp	120	14	—	0	—
poppyseed	3.5 fl oz	900	100	—	0	—
pumpkin seed	3.5 oz	925	100	—	0	—
rice bran	1 tbsp	120	14	—	0	—
safflower	1 cup	1927	218	—	0	—
safflower	1 tbsp	120	14	—	0	—
sesame	1 tbsp	120	14	—	0	—
sheanut	1 tbsp	120	14	—	0	—
soybean	1 tbsp	120	14	0	0	—
soybean	1 cup	1927	218	tr	0	—
sunflower	1 cup	1927	218	—	0	—
sunflower	1 tbsp	120	14	—	0	—
teaseed	1 tbsp	120	14	—	0	—
tomatoseed	1 tbsp	120	14	—	0	—
vegetable soybean & cottonseed	1 tbsp	120	14	—	0	—
vegetable soybean & cottonseed	1 cup	1927	218	—	0	—
walnut	1 tbsp	120	14	—	0	—
walnut	1 cup	1927	218	—	0	1
wheat germ	1 tbsp	120	14	—	0	—
FISH OIL						
Hain						
Cod Liver	1 tbsp	120	14	0	0	—
Cod Liver Cherry	1 tbsp	120	14	0	0	—
Cod Liver Mint	1 tbsp	120	14	0	0	—
cod liver	1 tbsp	123	14	—	0	—
herring	1 tbsp	123	14	—	0	—
menhaden	1 tbsp	123	14	—	0	—
salmon	1 tbsp	123	14	—	0	—

FOOD	PORTION	CAL.	FAT	SOD.	CARB.	FIB.
sardine	1 tbsp	123	14	—	0	—
shark	3½ oz	945	100	—	0	—
whale	3½ oz	945	100	—	0	—

OKRA
CANNED
Allen
Cut	½ cup (4.4 oz)	25	0	400	6	3
McIlhenny						
Pickled	2 pieces (1 oz)	7	tr	18	1	1
Trappey						
Cocktail Hot	2 pieces (1 oz)	8	tr	139	2	1
Cocktail Mild	1 piece (1 oz)	9	tr	207	1	1
Creole Gumbo	½ cup (4.2 oz)	35	0	290	6	3
Cut	½ cup (4.4 oz)	25	0	400	6	3

FRESH
raw	8 pods	36	tr	8	7	—
raw sliced	½ cup	19	tr	4	4	—
sliced cooked	½ cup	25	tr	4	6	—
sliced cooked	8 pods	27	tr	5	6	—

FROZEN
Fresh Like
Cut	3.5 oz	26	tr	3	6	1
Whole	3.5 oz	32	tr	2	7	1
Hanover						
Cut	½ cup	25	0	—	—	—
Whole	½ cup	35	0	—	—	—
sliced cooked	½ cup	34	tr	3	8	—
sliced cooked	1 pkg (10 oz)	94	1	8	21	—

OLIVES
California
Ripe	3 sm	4	tr	29	tr	3
Ripe	2 jumbo	188	9	—	—	—
Progresso						
Olive Appetizer	½ cup	180	21	1600	6	—
Olive Condite	½ cup	130	14	870	5	—
Salad Olives	½ cup	120	15	2400	1	—
S&W						
Ripe Extra Large	3.5 oz	163	18	760	1	—
Ripe Pitted Large	3.5 oz	163	18	760	1	—
Tee Pee						
Spanish Green	2 oz	98	10	—	1	—
green	4 med	15	2	312	tr	tr
green	3 extra lg	15	2	312	tr	tr

FOOD	PORTION	CAL.	FAT	SOD.	CARB.	FIB.
ripe	1 colossal	12	1	136	1	—
ripe	1 jumbo	7	1	75	tr	—
ripe	1 lg	5	tr	38	tr	tr
ripe	1 sm	4	tr	28	tr	tr
ONION						
CANNED						
S&W						
Whole Small	½ cup	35	0	345	9	—
Vlasic						
Lightly Spiced Cocktail Onions	1 oz	4	0	365	1	—
Watkins						
Liquid Spice	1 tbsp (0.5 oz)	120	14	0	0	0
chopped	½ cup	21	tr	416	5	—
whole	1 (2.2 oz)	12	tr	234	3	—
DRIED						
Watkins						
Flakes	¼ tsp (1 g)	0	0	0	0	0
flakes	1 tbsp	16	tr	1	4	—
powder	1 tsp	7	tr	1	2	—
FRESH						
Antioch Farms						
Vidalia	1 med	60	0	10	14	3
Dole						
Green chopped	1 tbsp	2	tr	0	tr	tr
chopped cooked	½ cup	47	tr	3	11	—
raw chopped	1 tbsp	4	tr	0	1	tr
raw chopped	½ cup	30	tr	2	7	—
scallions raw chopped	1 tbsp	2	tr	1	tr	tr
scallions raw sliced	½ cup	16	tr	8	4	1
welsh raw	3½ oz	34	tr	—	7	—
FROZEN						
Birds Eye						
Polybag Whole Small	½ cup	30	0	10	8	2
Small With Cream Sauce	½ cup	100	3	340	12	1
Fresh Like						
Diced	3.5 oz	29	0	7	7	0
Whole	3.5 oz	37	tr	10	8	1
Kineret						
Rings	6 (3 oz)	200	10	310	25	—
Mrs. Paul's						
Crispy Onion Rings	2½ oz	190	12	230	19	—
Ore Ida						
Chopped	¾ cup (3 oz)	25	0	20	6	1

FOOD	PORTION	CAL.	FAT	SOD.	CARB.	FIB.
Ore Ida (CONT.)						
Onion Ringers	6 pieces (3 oz)	240	14	250	26	2
Southland						
Chopped	2 oz	15	0	—	—	—
chopped cooked	½ cup	30	tr	12	7	—
chopped cooked	1 tbsp	4	tr	2	1	—
rings	7 (2.5 oz)	285	19	263	27	—
rings cooked	2 (0.7 oz)	81	5	75	8	—
whole cooked	3½ oz	28	tr	8	7	—
TAKE-OUT						
fried	½ cup (7.5 oz)	176	11	—	17	—
rings breaded & fried	8 to 9	275	16	430	31	—
OPOSSUM						
roasted	3 oz	188	9	—	0	—
ORANGE						
CANNED						
Del Monte						
Mandarin in Heavy Syrup	½ cup (4.4 oz)	80	0	10	19	tr
Dole						
Mandarin Segments	½ cup	70	tr	10	19	—
Pineapple Mandarin Segments	½ cup	80	tr	5	19	—
Empress						
Mandarin	5.5 oz	100	0	10	25	—
Mandarin From Japan	5.5 oz	35	0	—	8	—
S&W						
Mandarin Natural Style	½ cup	60	0	10	15	—
Mandarin Selected Sections in Heavy Syrup	½ cup	76	0	10	20	—
Mandarin Unsweetened	½ cup	28	0	10	7	—
FRESH						
Dole	1	50	0	0	13	6
california navel	1	65	tr	1	16	3
california valencia	1	59	tr	0	14	3
florida	1	69	tr	1	17	4
peel	1 tbsp	6	tr	0	2	—
sections	1 cup	85	tr	0	21	4
ORANGE EXTRACT						
Virginia Dare	1 tsp	22	0	—	—	—
ORANGE JUICE						
After The Fall	1 bottle (10 oz)	110	0	10	26	—

FOOD	PORTION	CAL.	FAT	SOD.	CARB.	FIB.
Bright & Early						
Chilled	8 fl oz	120	0	30	30	—
Frozen	8 fl oz	120	0	10	30	—
Hi-C						
Box	8.45 fl oz	130	0	30	33	—
Hood						
From Concentrate	1 cup (8 oz)	120	0	20	30	—
Select	1 cup (8 oz)	120	0	2	30	—
With Calcium	1 cup (8 oz)	120	0	20	30	—
Kool-Aid						
Drink	8 oz	98	0	—	25	—
Koolers	1 (8.45 oz)	115	0	2	30	—
Sugar Sweetened	8 oz	79	0	—	20	—
Minute Maid						
Box	8.45 fl oz	120	0	25	28	—
Calcium Rich Chilled	8 fl oz	120	0	25	27	—
Calcium Rich frzn	8 fl oz	120	0	0	27	—
Chilled	8 fl oz	110	0	25	27	—
Country Style Chilled	8 fl oz	110	0	25	27	—
Country Style frzn	8 fl oz	110	0	0	27	—
Juices To Go	1 bottle (16 fl oz)	110	0	25	27	—
Juices To Go	1 bottle (10 fl oz)	140	0	30	34	—
Juices To Go	1 can (11.5 fl oz)	160	0	35	39	—
Orange Punch Box	8.45 fl oz	130	0	25	33	—
Premium Choice Chilled	8 fl oz	110	0	0	27	—
Pulp Free Chilled	8 fl oz	110	0	25	27	—
Pulp Free frzn	8 fl oz	110	0	0	27	—
Reduced Acid frzn	8 fl oz	110	0	0	27	—
Mott's						
From Concentrate	10 fl oz	130	1	20	29	0
Ocean Spray						
Juice	8 fl oz	120	0	35	31	0
S&W						
100% Unsweetened	6 oz	83	0	2	18	—
Sippin' Pak						
100% Pure	8.45 fl oz	110	0	25	26	—
Snapple						
Juice	10 fl oz	130	0	55	29	—
Orangeade	8 fl oz	120	0	10	31	—
Tang						
Breakfast Crystals Sugar Free as prep	6 oz	5	0	2	0	—
Breakfast Crystals as prep	6 oz	86	0	1	22	—

FOOD	PORTION	CAL.	FAT	SOD.	CARB.	FIB.
Tang (CONT.)						
Fruit Box	8.45 oz	127	0	1	31	—
Tropical Orange	8.45 fl oz	146	0	3	37	—
Tree Top						
Juice	6 oz	90	0	5	22	—
Tropicana						
Frozen as prep	6 fl oz	110	0	5	27	—
Season's Best	8 fl oz	110	0	5	27	—
Season's Best	1 bottle (10 fl oz)	130	0	5	33	—
Season's Best	1 bottle (7 fl oz)	90	0	0	23	—
Season's Best	1 can (11.5 fl oz)	140	0	5	36	—
Season's Best Calcium	8 fl oz	110	0	5	27	—
Season's Best Homestyle	8 fl oz	110	0	5	27	—
Season's Best Vitamin	8 fl oz	110	0	5	27	—
Veryfine						
100%	8 oz	121	0	<10	24	—
Orange Drink	8 oz	140	0	<70	33	—
canned	1 cup	104	tr	6	25	—
chilled	1 cup	110	1	2	25	—
fresh	1 cup	111	tr	2	26	—
frzn as prep	1 cup	112	tr	2	27	1
frzn not prep	6 oz	339	tr	7	81	2
mandarin orange	3½ oz	47	tr	—	10	—
orange drink	6 oz	94	0	31	24	—

OREGANO

Watkins

Liquid Spice	1 tbsp (0.5 oz)	120	14	0	0	0
ground	1 tsp	5	tr	tr	1	—

ORGAN MEATS

(*see* BRAINS, GIBLETS, GIZZARD, HEART, KIDNEY, LIVER, SWEETBREADS)

ORIENTAL FOOD

(*see also* DINNER, NOODLES, RICE)

CANNED

La Choy

Bi-Pack Beef Pepper	¾ cup	80	2	950	10	2
Bi-Pack Chow Mein Chicken	¾ cup	80	3	970	8	1
Bi-Pack Chow Mein Pork	¾ cup	80	4	950	7	2
Bi-Pack Chow Mein Shrimp	¾ cup	70	1	860	6	1
Bi-Pack Sweet & Sour Chicken	¾ cup	120	2	440	18	2

FOOD	PORTION	CAL.	FAT	SOD.	CARB.	FIB.
La Choy (CONT.)						
Bi-Pack Teriyaki Chicken	¾ cup	85	2	850	8	1
Dinner Chow Mein Chicken	¾ pkg	300	17	1800	29	2
Entree Beef Pepper Oriental	¾ cup	100	4	1340	12	2
Entree Chow Mein Beef	¾ cup	40	2	960	5	2
Entree Chow Mein Chicken	¾ cup	70	4	850	2	4
Entree Chow Mein Meatless	¾ cup	25	tr	860	5	2
Entree Chow Mein Shrimp	¾ cup	35	1	940	4	2
Entree Sweet & Sour Chicken	¾ cup	240	2	1420	47	1
Entree Sweet & Sour Pork	¾ cup	250	4	1540	48	1
chow mein chicken	1 cup	95	tr	725	18	—
FRESH						
Azumaya						
Won Ton Wraps	1 (8 g)	23	tr	50	5	—
egg roll wrapper	1	83	tr	162	16	—
wonton wrappers	1	23	tr	46	5	—
FROZEN						
Banquet						
Chow Mein Chicken	1 pkg (9 oz)	400	7	850	28	3
Birds Eye						
Easy Recipe Chicken Teriyaki not prep	½ pkg	160	4	600	28	4
Easy Recipe Oriental Beef not prep	½ pkg	100	7	620	11	8
Internationals Chinese Stir Fry not prep	3.3 oz	35	0	125	6	2
Japanese Stir Fry International not prep	3.3 oz	30	0	310	5	2
Chun King						
Beef Pepper Steak	1 pkg (13 oz)	300	4	1670	50	5
Chow Mein Chicken	1 pkg (13 oz)	370	14	2010	45	4
Egg Rolls Chicken	8 (4.4 oz)	270	9	350	40	4
Egg Rolls Pork & Shrimp	8 (4.4 oz)	290	11	350	39	4
Egg Rolls Shrimp	8 (4.4 oz)	260	8	480	39	4
Imperial Chicken	1 pkg (13 oz)	460	10	1670	59	5
Sweet & Sour Pork	1 pkg (13 oz)	450	6	1180	66	4
Walnut Chicken	1 pkg (13 oz)	460	19	1820	56	5

FOOD	PORTION	CAL.	FAT	SOD.	CARB.	FIB.
Empire						
Large Egg Rolls	1 (3 oz)	190	6	350	28	2
Miniature Egg Rolls	6 (4.8 oz)	280	8	740	43	4
La Choy						
Egg Roll Restaurant Style Almond Chicken	1 (3 oz)	170	6	390	23	3
Egg Roll Restaurant Style Chicken	1 (3 oz)	170	5	450	25	4
Egg Roll Restaurant Style Mu Sho Pork	1 (3 oz)	190	7	330	25	2
Egg Roll Restaurant Style Shrimp	1 (3 oz)	150	4	420	24	3
Egg Roll Restaurant Style Sweet & Sour	1 (3 oz)	180	4	300	29	3
Egg Roll Mini Chicken	14 (7.25 oz)	430	11	900	67	6
Egg Roll Mini Lobster	14 (7.25 oz)	410	11	690	65	9
Egg Roll Mini Meat & Shrimp	15 (3.75 oz)	240	9	350	31	3
Egg Roll Mini Pork & Shrimp	14 (7.25 oz)	430	12	890	65	7
Egg Roll Mini Shrimp	14 (7.25 oz)	410	9	990	68	7
Restaurant Style Egg Roll Pork	1 (3 oz)	150	5	480	20	—
Lean Cuisine						
Chicken Chow Mein With Rice	1 meal (9 oz)	210	5	510	28	2
Luigino's						
Chicken & Almonds With Rice	1 pkg (8 oz)	250	8	770	33	3
Chop Suey Pork With Rice	1 pkg (8.5 oz)	210	4	980	34	2
Egg Rolls Chicken	1 pkg (6 oz)	360	13	590	48	2
Egg Rolls Pork & Shrimp	1 pkg (6 oz)	340	9	760	51	3
Egg Rolls Shrimp	1 pkg (6 oz)	350	11	460	39	4
Egg Rolls Sweet & Sour Chicken	1 pkg (6 oz)	400	12	460	59	4
Egg Rolls Sweet & Sour Pork	1 pkg (6 oz)	360	10	270	56	4
Egg Rolls Szechwan Vegetable	1 pkg (6 oz)	350	12	920	38	3
Lo Mein Chicken	1 pkg (8 oz)	320	5	950	35	3
Lo Mein Shrimp	1 pkg (8 oz)	190	3	980	31	4
Oriental Beef & Peppers With Rice	1 pkg (8 oz)	230	5	820	38	2

FOOD	PORTION	CAL.	FAT	SOD.	CARB.	FIB.
Pasta Favorites						
Chicken Lo Mein	1 pkg (10.5 oz)	270	6	1060	43	5
Stouffer's						
Chicken Chow Mein With Rice	1 pkg (10.6 oz)	260	4	940	43	3
Chicken Oriental	1 pkg (9.75 oz)	320	9	930	45	2
Stir-Fry Teriyaki	1 pkg (9 oz)	260	5	550	39	4
Tyson						
Stir Fry Kit With Yoshida Oriental Sauce	10.6 oz	330	10	1740	37	—
Sweet & Sour Kit With Sweet & Sour Sauce	14.85 oz	440	9	1300	71	—
Worthington						
Vegetarian Egg Rolls	1 (85 g)	160	6	530	20	—
MIX						
Kikkoman						
Chow Mein Seasoning	1⅛ oz pkg	98	tr	—	—	—
Teriyaki Baste & Glaze	1 tbsp	24	tr	310	5	—
La Choy						
Dinner Classics Pepper Steak	¾ cup	180	9	760	9	1
Dinner Classics Egg Foo Young	2 patties + 3 oz sauce	170	7	1390	20	1
Dinner Classics Sweet & Sour	¾ cup	310	6	860	30	tr
TAKE-OUT						
chicken teriyaki	¾ cup	399	27	2190	7	—
chop suey w/ beef & pork	1 cup	300	17	1053	13	—
chop suey w/ pork	1 cup	375	29	1378	29	2
chow mein chicken	1 cup	255	10	718	10	—
chow mein pork	1 cup	425	24	1673	21	3
chow mein shrimp	1 cup	221	10	1658	21	3
chow mein vegetable	1 serv (8 oz)	90	3	1010	15	4
egg roll lobster	1 (4.8 oz)	270	7	460	43	6
egg roll meat & shrimp	1 (4.8 oz)	320	12	470	41	4
egg roll pork & shrimp	1 (5 oz)	300	10	890	41	7
egg roll shrimp	1 (3 oz)	170	5	420	24	4
egg roll vegetable	1 (3 oz)	170	4	520	28	4
fried rice	6.6 oz	249	6	—	48	2
fried rice w/ egg	6.7 oz	395	20	—	49	2
oriental pepper & beef	1 serv (8 oz)	90	0	780	12	2
spring roll deep fried	3.5 oz	202	9	—	24	—
sweet & sour pork	1 serv (8 oz)	250	8	1500	37	2
wonton fried	½ cup (1 oz)	111	8	147	8	1
wonton soup	1 cup	205	3	322	26	1

FOOD	PORTION	CAL.	FAT	SOD.	CARB.	FIB.

OYSTERS
CANNED
Bumble Bee

Whole	½ cup (3.5 oz)	100	4	490	6	0
Empress						
Whole	4 oz	100	4	390	8	—
S&W						
Fancy Whole	2 oz	95	3	—	4	—
eastern	1 cup	170	6	277	10	—
eastern	3 oz	58	2	95	3	—
FRESH						
eastern cooked	3 oz	117	4	190	7	—
eastern cooked	6 med	58	2	94	3	—
eastern raw	6 med	58	2	94	3	—
eastern raw	1 cup	170	6	277	10	—
pacific raw	1 med	41	1	53	2	—
pacific raw	3 oz	69	2	90	4	—
steamed	1 med	41	1	53	2	—
steamed	3 oz	138	4	180	8	—
TAKE-OUT						
battered & fried	6 (4.9 oz)	368	18	677	40	—
breaded & fried	6 (4.9 oz)	368	18	677	40	—
eastern breaded & fried	3 oz	167	11	355	10	—
eastern breaded & fried	6 med (88 g)	173	11	367	10	—
oysters rockefeller	3 oysters	66	2	80	5	—
stew	1 cup	278	18	928	15	tr

PANCAKE/WAFFLE SYRUP
(see also SYRUP)
Alaga

Breakfast	2 tbsp	108	0	—	—	—
Butter Lite	2 tbsp	54	0	—	—	—
Honey Flavored	2 tbsp	124	0	—	—	—
Lite	2 tbsp	54	0	—	—	—
Aunt Jemima						
Butter Rich	¼ cup (2.8 oz)	210	0	170	52	—
Butterlite	¼ cup (2.5 oz)	100	0	150	26	—
Lite	¼ cup (2.5 oz)	100	0	160	27	—
Brer Rabbit						
Dark	2 tbsp	120	0	0	31	—
Light	2 tbsp	120	0	0	31	—
Estee						
Lite Maple	¼ cup (2.4 oz)	80	0	125	20	—
Golden Griddle						
Syrup	1 cup (321 g)	885	0	225	229	—

FOOD	PORTION	CAL.	FAT	SOD.	CARB.	FIB.
Golden Griddle (CONT.)						
Syrup	1 tbsp (20 g)	50	0	55	14	—
Karo						
Syrup	1 tbsp (21 g)	60	0	35	15	—
Log Cabin						
Country Kitchen	1 oz	103	0	22	27	—
Lite	1 oz	49	0	92	13	—
Mrs. Richardson's						
Lite	¼ cup (2.5 oz)	100	0	160	26	—
Original Recipe	¼ cup (2.8 oz)	210	0	115	52	—
Red Wing						
Lite	¼ cup (2 oz)	100	0	115	26	0
Tastee						
Maple	2 tbsp	113	0	—	—	—
Syrup	2 tbsp	121	0	—	—	—
Tree Of Life						
Maple	¼ cup (2.1 oz)	200	0	7	53	—
Whitfield						
White Label	2 tbsp	121	0	—	—	—
Yellow Label	2 tbsp	125	0	—	—	—
Yellow Label Butter Flavor	2 tbsp	117	0	—	—	—
Yellow Label Maple Flavor	2 tbsp	117	0	—	—	—
low calorie	1 tbsp	12	0	—	3	0
maple	1 tbsp (0.8 oz)	52	0	2	13	—
maple	1 cup (11.1 oz)	824	1	27	212	—
maple	2 tbsp	122	0	19	32	—
pancake syrup	1 cup (11 oz)	903	0	290	238	—
pancake syrup	1 tbsp (0.7 oz)	57	0	17	15	—
pancake syrup light	1 oz	46	0	57	13	—
pancake syrup w/ butter	1 tbsp (0.7 oz)	59	tr	20	15	—
pancake syrup w/ butter	1 cup (11 oz)	933	5	307	234	—
PANCAKES						
FROZEN						
Aunt Jemima						
Blueberry	3 (3.4 oz)	210	4	670	40	2
Buttermilk	3 (3 oz)	180	3	590	34	2
Lowfat	3 (3.4 oz)	130	2	580	33	8
Original	3 (3.4 oz)	200	3	700	40	2
Downyflake						
Blueberry	3	290	9	920	48	—
Buttermilk	3	280	9	920	45	—

FOOD	PORTION	CAL.	FAT	SOD.	CARB.	FIB.
Downyflake (CONT.)						
Pancakes And Sausages	1 pkg (5.5 oz)	430	23	1170	47	—
Regular	3	280	9	920	45	—
Great Starts						
Pancakes And Sausages	6 oz	460	22	920	52	—
Pancakes With Bacon	4½ oz	400	20	1000	43	—
Silver Dollar Pancakes And Sausage	3¾ oz	310	14	680	37	—
Whole Wheat Pancakes With Lite Links	5½ oz	350	16	600	39	—
Healthy Starts						
Pancakes w/ LeanLinks	6 oz	360	8	490	48	—
Jimmy Dean						
Flapstick	1 (2.5 oz)	240	14	320	22	1
Flapstick Blueberry	1 (2.5 oz)	260	15	320	23	1
Morningstar Farms						
Pancakes/Links	1 pkg (4 oz)	240	8	700	31	—
Pillsbury						
Buttermilk Microwave	3	260	4	590	51	—
Harvest Wheat Microwave	3	240	4	420	48	—
Microwave	3	250	4	540	49	—
Original Microwave	3	240	4	550	47	—
Quaker						
Lite Pancakes & Lite Links	1 pkg (6 oz)	310	10	970	43	—
Lite Pancakes & Lite Syrup	1 pkg (6 oz)	260	3	860	53	—
Pancakes & Sausages	1 pkg (6 oz)	420	16	1140	57	—
Weight Watchers						
Buttermilk	2 (2.5 oz)	140	3	270	22	—
Pancakes With Links	4 oz	220	10	—	21	—
buttermilk	1, 4 in diam (1.3 oz)	83	1	183	16	—
plain	1, 4 in diam (1.3 oz)	83	1	183	16	—
HOME RECIPE						
blueberry	1 (4 in diam)	84	4	157	11	—
plain	1 (4 in diam)	86	4	157	11	—
MIX						
Arrowhead						
Multigrain Pancake & Waffle Mix	¼ cup (1.2 oz)	120	1	260	24	3
Aunt Jemima						
Buckwheat Pancake & Waffle Mix	¼ cup (1.4 oz)	120	1	560	28	4

FOOD	PORTION	CAL.	FAT	SOD.	CARB.	FIB.
Aunt Jemima (cont.)						
Buttermilk Pancake & Waffle Mix	⅓ cup (1.9 oz)	190	2	480	38	2
Original Pancake & Waffle Mix	⅓ cup (1.6 oz)	150	1	620	34	1
Pancake & Waffle Mix Regular	⅓ cup (1.9 oz)	190	2	470	39	1
Pancake & Waffle Mix Whole Wheat	¼ cup (1.4 oz)	130	1	560	28	3
Betty Crocker						
Buttermilk	3 (4 in diam)	280	10	810	39	—
Bisquick						
Apple Cinnamon Shake 'N Pour	3 (4 in diam)	240	3	880	47	—
Blueberry Shake 'N Pour	3 (4 in diam)	270	3	840	54	—
Buttermilk Shake 'N Pour	3 (4 in diam)	250	3	880	49	—
Original Shake 'N Pour	3 (4 in diam)	250	3	880	49	—
Estee						
Pancake Mix Fat Free as prep	4 (4 in diam)	180	0	255	40	1
Fast Shake						
Blueberry	1 serv (2.5 oz)	251	3	685	50	—
Buttermilk	1 serv (2.5 oz)	258	3	770	50	—
Original	1 serv (2.5 oz)	266	4	736	50	—
Health Valley						
Pancake Mix not prep	1 oz	100	1	170	20	3
Hodgson Mill						
Buckwheat	⅓ cup (1.8 oz)	160	1	550	35	1
Hungry Jack						
Blueberry	3 (4 in diam)	320	15	820	41	—
Buttermilk	3 (4 in diam)	240	11	820	29	—
Buttermilk Complete	3 (4 in diam)	180	1	710	39	—
Buttermilk Complete Packets	3 (4 in diam)	180	3	680	35	—
Extra Lights	3 (4 in diam)	210	7	490	30	—
Extra Lights Complete	3 (4 in diam)	190	2	700	37	—
Panshakes	3 (4 in diam)	250	6	880	43	—
Stone-Buhr						
Buckwheat	¼ cup (1.4 oz)	130	1	410	29	3
Oat Bran	¼ cup (1.4 oz)	130	0	330	30	2
Whole Wheat	¼ cup (1.4 oz)	120	1	330	25	3
Wanda's						
Blue Corn	⅓ cup mix per serv (1.7 oz)	170	2	480	32	2

FOOD	PORTION	CAL.	FAT	SOD.	CARB.	FIB.
buckwheat	1 (4 in diam)	62	2	160	9	—
buttermilk	1, 4 in diam (1.3 oz)	74	1	239	14	tr
plain	1, 4 in diam (1.3 oz)	74	1	239	14	tr
sugar free low sodium	1 (3 in diam)	44	tr	58	9	—
whole wheat	1 (4 in diam)	92	3	252	13	—
TAKE-OUT						
buckwheat	1 (4 in diam)	55	2	125	6	—
potato	1 (4 in diam)	78	6	238	4	tr
w/ butter & syrup	3	519	14	1103	91	—

PANCREAS
(see SWEETBREADS)

PAPAYA
CANNED
Ka-Me

Ka-Me	¾ cup	120	0	15	29	1

DRIED
Sonoma

Pieces	2 pieces (2 oz)	200	4	60	41	6

FRESH
Produce Marketing Assoc

Papaya	½	80	0	—	—	—
cubed	1 cup	54	tr	4	14	—
papaya	1	117	tr	8	30	—

PAPAYA JUICE
Goya

Nectar	6 oz	110	0	10	27	—

Kern's

Nectar	6 fl oz	110	0	5	27	—

Libby

Nectar	1 can (11.5 fl oz)	210	0	10	51	—
nectar	1 cup	142	tr	14	36	—

PAPRIKA
Watkins

Watkins	¼ tsp (0.5 oz)	0	0	0	0	0
paprika	1 tsp	6	tr	1	1	—

PARSLEY
Dole

Chopped	1 tbsp	10	tr	4	1	tr
dry	1 tbsp	1	tr	2	tr	—
dry	1 tsp	1	tr	1	tr	—
fresh chopped	½ cup	11	tr	17	2	—

PARSNIPS

fresh cooked	1 (5.6 oz)	130	tr	17	31	—

FOOD	PORTION	CAL.	FAT	SOD.	CARB.	FIB.
fresh sliced cooked	½ cup	63	tr	8	15	—
raw sliced	½ cup	50	tr	7	12	—
PASSION FRUIT						
purple fresh	1	18	tr	5	4	—
PASSION FRUIT JUICE						
Snapple						
Passion Supreme	10 fl oz	160	0	20	39	—
purple	1 cup	126	tr	—	34	—
yellow	1 cup	149	tr	15	36	—
PASTA						
(see also NOODLES, PASTA DINNERS, PASTA SALAD)						
DRY						
Anthony						
Pasta	2 oz	210	1	0	42	tr
Bella Via						
Angel Hair	2 oz	200	0	0	40	—
Artichoke Angel Hair as prep	⅝ cup	200	0	0	40	—
Artichoke Spaghetti as prep	⅝ cup	200	0	0	40	—
Elbows	2 oz	200	0	0	40	—
Fettucini as prep	⅝ cup	200	0	0	40	—
Linguini	2 oz	200	0	0	40	—
Penne as prep	⅝ cup	200	0	0	40	—
Rotelli	2 oz	200	0	0	40	—
Shells	2 oz	200	0	0	40	—
Spaghetti	2 oz	200	0	0	40	—
Ziti	2 oz	200	0	0	40	—
Classico						
Gnocchi Di Toscana	1 cup (2 oz)	210	1	0	42	2
Creamette						
Elbow Macaroni not prep	2 oz	210	1	5	42	—
Linguini Egg	2 oz	221	3	—	—	—
Rotelle	2 oz	210	1	—	—	—
Rotini Rainbow	2 oz	210	1	—	—	—
Spaghetti not prep	2 oz	210	1	5	42	—
Spaghetti Egg	2 oz	221	3	—	—	—
Spaghetti Thin	2 oz	210	1	—	—	—
Spinach Ribbons not prep	2 oz	210	1	70	42	—
Ziti	2 oz	210	1	—	—	—
DeFino						
Lasagna No Boil	1 oz	102	tr	2	20	—

FOOD	PORTION	CAL.	FAT	SOD.	CARB.	FIB.
DeFino (CONT.)						
Ribbons No Boil	2 oz	204	2	3	40	—
Delverde						
Spaghetti Whole Wheat	2 oz	206	1	1	42	5
Eden						
Elbows Whole Wheat Organic	2 oz	210	2	0	39	6
Elbows Whole Wheat Vegetable Organic	2 oz	210	2	0	39	6
Kudzu And Sweet Potato Pasta	2 oz	190	0	0	47	0
Kudzu Kiri Pasta	2 oz	190	0	0	47	0
Mung Bean Pasta Harusame	2 oz	190	0	5	47	0
Ribbons Durum Wheat Curry Organic	2 oz	220	1	0	44	3
Ribbons Durum Wheat Organic	2 oz	220	1	0	44	3
Ribbons Durum Wheat Paella Organic	2 oz	220	1	0	44	3
Ribbons Durum Wheat Parsley Garlic Organic	2 oz	220	1	0	44	3
Ribbons Durum Wheat Pesto Organic	2 oz	220	1	0	44	3
Ribbons Whole Wheat Spinach Organic	2 oz	200	2	10	40	7
Rice Pasta Bifun	2 oz	200	1	5	44	0
Shells Durum Wheat Vegetable Organic	2 oz	210	1	10	42	2
Soba 100% Buckwheat	2 oz	200	0	30	41	3
Soba 40% Buckwheat	2 oz	190	1	490	37	3
Soba Lotus Root	2 oz	190	1	470	37	4
Soba Mugwort	2 oz	190	1	550	37	2
Soba Wild Yam Jinenjo	2 oz	190	1	510	37	2
Spaghetti Durum Wheat Organic	2 oz	210	1	10	42	2
Spaghetti Kamut Organic	2 oz	210	2	0	38	6
Spaghetti Parsley Garlic Organic	2 oz	210	1	10	42	2
Spaghetti Whole Wheat Organic	2 oz	210	2	0	39	6
Spirals Durum Wheat Vegetable Organic	2 oz	210	1	10	42	2
Spirals Kamut Organic	2 oz	210	2	0	38	6

FOOD	PORTION	CAL.	FAT	SOD.	CARB.	FIB.
Eden (CONT.)						
Spirals Sesame Rice Organic	2 oz	200	2	0	37	6
Spirals Whole Wheat Vegetable Organic	2 oz	210	2	0	39	6
Udon	2 oz	190	1	660	37	3
Udon Brown Rice	2 oz	190	1	510	38	2
Gioia						
Pasta	2 oz	210	1	0	42	tr
Golden Grain						
Pasta	2 oz	203	1	26	41	0
Hanover						
Spaghetti Wheels	½ cup	90	0	—	—	—
Health Valley						
Lasagna Spinach Whole Wheat	2 oz	170	1	15	40	7
Lasagna Whole Wheat	2 oz	170	1	10	40	7
Spaghetti Amaranth	2 oz	170	1	10	40	9
Spaghetti Oat Bran	2 oz	120	1	2	23	4
Spaghetti Spinach Whole Wheat	2 oz	170	1	15	40	7
Spaghetti Whole Wheat	2 oz	170	1	10	40	7
Hodgson Mill						
Spaghetti Whole Wheat Spinach not prep	2 oz	190	2	25	35	5
Veggie Bows not prep	2 oz	200	1	15	41	1
Veggie Rotini not prep	2 oz	200	1	15	41	1
Veggie Wagon Wheels not prep	2 oz	200	1	15	41	1
Whole Wheat Spirals not prep	2 oz	190	1	10	34	6
La Molisana						
Radiatori	2 oz	230	1	30	48	—
Lupini						
Elbow uncooked	½ cup (2 oz)	190	2	0	37	5
Spaghetti Light uncooked	½ cup (2 oz)	190	2	0	37	5
Spaghetti With Triticale	⅓ pkg (2 oz)	190	3	5	38	6
Luxury						
Pasta	2 oz	210	1	0	42	tr
Merlino's						
Pasta	2 oz	210	1	0	42	tr
Mueller's						
Dinosaurs	2 oz (57 g)	210	1	3	42	—

FOOD	PORTION	CAL.	FAT	SOD.	CARB.	FIB.
Mueller's (CONT.)						
Jungle Animals	2 oz (57 g)	210	1	3	42	—
Lasagne	2 oz (57 g)	210	1	4	42	—
Monsters	2 oz (57 g)	210	1	3	42	—
Outer Space	2 oz	210	1	3	42	—
Spaghetti	2 oz (57 g)	210	1	3	42	—
Teddy Bears	2 oz (57 g)	210	1	3	42	—
Twists Tri Color	2 oz (57 g)	210	1	10	41	—
Noodles By Leonardo						
Capellini not prep	½ cup (2 oz)	200	1	10	40	2
Elbows not prep	½ cup (2 oz)	200	1	10	40	2
Fettucini not prep	½ cup (2 oz)	200	1	10	40	2
Linguine not prep	½ cup (2 oz)	200	1	10	40	2
Rigatoni not prep	½ cup (2 oz)	200	1	10	40	2
Rotini not prep	½ cup (2 oz)	200	1	10	40	2
Shells not prep	½ cup (2 oz)	200	1	10	40	2
Spaghetti not prep	½ cup (2 oz)	200	1	10	40	2
Spaghettini not prep	½ cup (2 oz)	200	1	10	40	2
Vermicelli not prep	½ cup (2 oz)	200	1	10	40	2
Penn Dutch						
Pasta	2 oz	210	1	0	42	tr
Pomi						
Capellini	2 oz	210	1	<5	41	—
Prince						
Egg	2 oz	221	3	3	40	1
Pasta	2 oz	210	1	0	42	tr
Rainbow	2 oz	210	1	5	42	1
Spinach Egg	2 oz	220	3	65	40	1
Pritikin						
Spaghetti Whole Wheat	⅛ box (2 oz)	190	1	0	40	—
Spiral	⅔ cup (2 oz)	190	1	10	40	—
Red Cross						
Pasta	2 oz	210	1	0	42	tr
Ronco						
Pasta	2 oz	210	1	0	42	tr
Ronzoni						
Elbows	¾ cup (2 oz)	210	1	0	40	—
Fettucini	¾ cup (2 oz)	210	1	0	40	—
Fusilli	¾ cup (2 oz)	210	1	0	40	—
Lasagne	¾ cup (2 oz)	210	1	0	40	—
Manicotti	¾ cup (2 oz)	210	1	0	40	—
Mostaccioli	¾ cup (2 oz)	210	1	0	40	—
Rigatoni	¾ cup (2 oz)	210	1	0	40	—
Rotelle uncooked	¾ cup (2 oz)	210	1	0	40	—

FOOD	PORTION	CAL.	FAT	SOD.	CARB.	FIB.
Ronzoni (CONT.)						
Rotini uncooked	¾ cup (2 oz)	210	1	0	40	—
Shells uncooked	¾ cup (2 oz)	210	1	0	40	—
Shells Jumbo	¾ cup (2 oz)	210	1	0	40	—
Spaghetti not prep	¾ cup (2 oz)	210	1	0	40	—
Tubettini	¾ cup (2 oz)	210	1	0	40	—
San Giorgio						
Bowties Egg	2 oz	210	3	15	38	—
Capellini	2 oz	210	1	0	40	2
Elbow Macaroni	2 oz	210	1	0	40	2
Fettuccine Egg	2 oz	210	3	15	38	—
Fettuccini Florentine	2 oz	210	3	15	38	—
Lasagne	2 oz	210	1	0	40	2
Linguini	2 oz	210	1	0	40	2
Manicotti	2 oz	210	1	0	40	2
Mostaccioli Rigati	2 oz	210	1	—	—	2
Rigatoni	2 oz	210	1	0	40	2
Rotini	2 oz	210	1	0	40	2
Shells	2 oz	210	1	0	40	2
Spaghetti	2 oz	210	1	0	40	2
Spaghetti Thin	2 oz	210	1	0	40	2
Vermicelli	2 oz	210	1	0	40	2
Ziti Cut	2 oz	210	1	0	40	2
Tree Of Life						
Cajun as prep	⅝ cup (4.9 oz)	200	1	50	40	1
Confetti as prep	⅝ cup (4.9 oz)	200	1	50	40	1
Garlic & Parsley as prep	⅝ cup (4.9 oz)	200	1	50	40	1
Jamaican Spice as prep	⅝ cup (4.9 oz)	200	1	50	40	1
Lemon Pepper as prep	⅝ cup (4.9 oz)	200	1	50	40	1
Spinach as prep	⅝ cup (4.9 oz)	200	1	50	40	1
Tex Mex as prep	⅝ cup (4.9 oz)	200	1	50	40	1
Thai as prep	⅝ cup (4.9 oz)	200	1	50	40	1
Tomato Basil as prep	⅝ cup (4.9 oz)	200	1	50	40	1
Vimco						
Pasta	2 oz	210	1	0	42	tr
Weight Watchers						
Elbow Style	2 oz	160	1	35	30	—
Spaghettini	2 oz	160	1	35	30	—
corn cooked	1 cup	176	1	1	39	—
elbows	1 cup	389	2	8	78	—
elbows cooked	1 cup	197	tr	1	40	—
protein-fortified cooked	1 cup	188	tr	6	36	—
shells	1 cup	389	2	4	78	—
shells cooked	1 cup	197	tr	1	40	—

FOOD	PORTION	CAL.	FAT	SOD.	CARB.	FIB.
spaghetti	2 oz	211	tr	4	43	—
spaghetti cooked	1 cup	197	tr	1	40	—
spaghetti protein-fortified cooked	1 cup	229	tr	7	44	—
spinach spaghetti	2 oz	212	tr	20	43	—
spinach spaghetti cooked	1 cup	183	tr	20	37	—
spirals	1 cup	389	2	8	78	—
spirals cooked	1 cup	197	tr	1	40	—
vegetable	1 cup	308	tr	36	63	—
vegetable cooked	1 cup	171	tr	9	36	—
whole wheat	1 cup	365	1	8	79	—
whole wheat cooked	1 cup (4.9 oz)	174	tr	4	37	—
whole wheat spaghetti	2 oz	198	tr	5	43	—
whole wheat spaghetti cooked	1 cup	174	tr	4	37	—
FRESH						
Contadina						
Angel's Hair	1¼ cup (2.8 oz)	240	3	30	43	2
Fettuccine	1¼ cup (2.9 oz)	250	4	30	45	2
Fettuccine Cholesterol Free	1 cup (2.9 oz)	240	3	16	46	2
Light Ravioli Cheese	1 cup (3.1 oz)	240	5	340	35	2
Light Ravioli Garden Vegetable	1¼ cup (3.8 oz)	290	6	370	43	3
Light Tortellini Garlic & Cheese	1 cup (3.6 oz)	280	5	390	50	3
Linguine	1¼ cup (3 oz)	260	4	30	47	2
Linguine Cholesterol Free	1¼ cup (3.1 oz)	250	3	20	49	2
Ravioli Beef And Garlic	1¼ cup (4 oz)	350	14	350	39	3
Ravioli Cheese	1 cup (3.1 oz)	280	12	350	31	2
Ravioli Chicken And Rosemary	1¼ cup (4 oz)	330	12	420	43	3
Tagliatelli Spinach	1¼ cup (3.1 oz)	270	4	110	46	4
Tortellini Cheese	¾ cup (3 oz)	260	6	330	39	3
Tortellini Cheese And Basil	1 cup (4 oz)	360	11	380	49	3
Tortellini Chicken And Prosciutto	1 cup (3.8 oz)	360	13	440	46	3
Tortellini Chicken And Vegetable	¾ cup (2.9 oz)	260	7	220	39	2
Tortellini Spicy Italian Sausage And Bell Pepper	1 cup (3.6 oz)	330	10	280	47	3

FOOD	PORTION	CAL.	FAT	SOD.	CARB.	FIB.
Contadina (cont.)						
Tortellini Spinach Three Cheese	¾ cup (3.1 oz)	280	5	380	38	3
Di Giorno						
Angel's Hair	2 oz	160	1	190	31	1
Fettuccine	2.5 oz	190	2	125	39	2
Fettuccine Spinach	2.5 oz	190	2	140	38	2
Linguine	2.5 oz	190	2	125	39	2
Linguine Herb	2.5 oz	190	2	125	39	2
Ravioli Italian Herb Cheese	1 cup (3.8 oz)	350	13	610	44	2
Ravioli Light Cheese & Garlic	1 cup (3.7 oz)	270	2	580	45	1
Ravioli Light Tomato & Cheese	1 cup (3.7 oz)	280	3	490	49	2
Ravioli With Italian Sausage	¾ cup (3.6 oz)	340	12	630	41	2
Tortellini Cheese	¾ cup (2.8 oz)	260	6	230	37	1
Tortellini Mozzarella Garlic	1 cup (3.5 oz)	300	9	440	40	1
Tortellini Mushroom	1 cup (3.4 oz)	290	7	510	42	2
Tortellini Red Hot Pepper Cheese	1 cup (3.4 oz)	310	9	310	41	3
Tortellini With Chicken And Herbs	1 cup (3.2 oz)	260	5	290	40	1
Tortellini With Meat	¾ cup (3.1 oz)	290	9	380	40	1
Herb's						
Fettucine Bell Pepper Basil	2 oz	220	2	5	42	2
Fettucine Parsley Garlic	2 oz	220	2	5	42	2
Fettucine Spinach	2 oz	220	2	5	42	2
Ribbons Vegetable	2 oz	220	2	5	42	2
Ribbons Whole Wheat	2 oz	200	2	10	40	7
Rotini Mixed Vegetable	2 oz	210	1	10	42	2
Shells Mixed Vegetable	2 oz	210	1	10	42	2
Trios						
Ravioli Cracked Pepper Garlic Cheese	1 cup (4.3 oz)	340	9	380	48	0
plain made w/ egg cooked	2 oz	75	tr	3	14	—
spinach made w/ egg cooked	2 oz	74	tr	3	14	—
HOME RECIPE						
made w/ egg cooked	2 oz	74	tr	47	13	—
made w/o egg cooked	2 oz	71	tr	42	14	—

FOOD	PORTION	CAL.	FAT	SOD.	CARB.	FIB.

PASTA DINNERS
(see also DINNER, PASTA SALAD)

CANNED

Chef Boyardee

FOOD	PORTION	CAL.	FAT	SOD.	CARB.	FIB.
ABC's & 1,2,3's In Cheese Flavor Sauce	7.5 oz	180	1	940	37	—
ABC's & 1,2, 3's w/ Mini Meatballs	7.5 oz	260	11	1005	32	2
Beef Ravioli	7.5 oz	190	4	1160	31	2
Beefaroni	7.5 oz	220	7	1145	31	2
Cheese Ravioli In Meat Sauce	7.5 oz	200	3	1010	37	—
Dinosaurs In Cheese Flavor Sauce	7.5 oz	180	1	880	36	—
Dinosaurs w/ Meatballs	7.5 oz	240	9	900	32	4
Elbows In Beef Sauce	7.5 oz	210	7	1000	29	—
Lasagna	7.5 oz	230	9	1080	31	—
Lasagna In Garden Vegetable Sauce	7.5 oz	170	1	940	34	—
Macaroni & Cheese	7.5 oz	180	5	970	27	1
Microwave Main Meal Beans & Pasta	10.5 oz	200	1	1030	44	10
Microwave Main Meal Beef Ravioli Suprema	10.5 oz	290	4	1390	52	5
Microwave Main Meal Cheese Ravioli Suprema	10.5 oz	290	4	1360	52	5
Microwave Main Meal Fettuccine	10.5 oz	290	9	1010	46	6
Microwave Main Meal Lasagna	10.5 oz	290	8	1000	41	5
Microwave Main Meal Meat Tortellini	10.5 oz	220	4	980	53	6
Microwave Main Meal Noodles w/ Chicken	10.5 oz	170	1	1120	27	3
Microwave Main Meal Peas & Pasta	10.5 oz	190	2	1020	39	6
Microwave Main Meal Spaghetti Suprema	10.5 oz	200	7	1000	37	7
Microwave Main Meal Zesty Macaroni	10.5 oz	290	8	1300	40	5
Microwave Main Meal Ziti In Sauce	10.5 oz	210	tr	1030	52	7
Pasta Rings & Meatballs	7.5 oz	220	8	990	33	4

FOOD	PORTION	CAL.	FAT	SOD.	CARB.	FIB.
Chef Boyardee (CONT.)						
Rigatoni	7.5 oz	210	6	1080	31	—
Rings & Franks	7.5 oz	190	5	980	31	3
Shells In Meat Sauce	7.5 oz	210	6	1090	32	—
Shells In Mushroom Sauce	7.5 oz	170	1	1080	35	—
Spaghetti & Meat Balls	7.5 oz	230	7	1060	29	—
Tic Tac Toes In Cheese Flavor Sauce	7.5 oz	170	1	930	36	3
Tic Tac Toes w/ Mini Meatballs	7.5 oz	250	10	1035	32	3
Turtles In Sauce	7.5 oz	160	1	870	33	2
Turtles w/ Meatballs	7.5 oz	210	8	990	30	2
Dinty Moore						
American Classics Lasagna With Meat & Sauce	1 bowl (10 oz)	260	4	990	33	3
Franco-American						
Beef RavioliO's In Meat Sauce	½ can (7½ oz)	250	8	920	35	—
CircusO's Pasta In Tomato & Cheese Sauce	½ can (7⅜ oz)	170	2	860	33	—
Macaroni & Cheese	½ can (7⅜ oz)	170	6	870	24	—
Spaghetti In Tomato Sauce w/ Cheese	½ can (7⅜ oz)	180	2	840	36	—
Spaghetti w/ Meatballs In Tomato Sauce	½ can (7⅜ oz)	220	8	870	28	—
SpaghettiO's In Tomato & Cheese Sauce	½ can (7⅜ oz)	170	2	860	33	—
SpaghettiO's With Meatballs	½ can (7⅜ oz)	220	9	950	25	—
SpaghettiO's With Sliced Franks	½ can (7⅜ oz)	220	9	1000	26	—
SportyO's In Tomato & Cheese Sauce	½ can (7½ oz)	170	2	860	33	—
SportyO's Pasta With Meatballs In Tomato Sauce	½ can (7⅜ oz)	210	8	950	25	—
TeddyO's In Tomato & Cheese Sauce	½ can (7½ oz)	170	2	900	33	—
TeddyO's Pasta With Meatballs	½ can (7⅜ oz)	210	8	950	25	—

FOOD	PORTION	CAL.	FAT	SOD.	CARB.	FIB.
Hormel						
Lasagna	1 can (7.5 oz)	250	14	940	24	1
Spaghetti & Meatballs	1 can (7.5 oz)	210	7	940	28	2
Kid's Kitchen						
Cheezy Mac & Beef	1 cup (7.5 oz)	250	7	1180	34	0
Microwave Meals Beefy Macaroni	1 cup (7.5 oz)	190	6	790	23	2
Microwave Meals Macaroni & Cheese	1 cup (7.5 oz)	260	11	690	30	1
Microwave Meals Mini Ravioli	1 cup (7.5 oz)	240	7	920	35	3
Microwave Meals Spaghetti Ring & Meatballs	1 cup (7.5 oz)	250	7	1200	35	3
Noodle Rings & Chicken	1 cup (7.5 oz)	150	5	860	16	1
Spaghetti Rings & Franks	1 cup (7.5 oz)	230	6	880	36	3
Micro Cup Meals						
Lasagna	1 cup (7.5 oz)	230	7	650	34	2
Lasagna & Beef Tomato Sauce	1 cup	359	19	1384	34	3
Macaroni & Beef With Vegetables	1 cup	285	8	918	37	6
Macaroni & Cheese	1 cup (7.5 oz)	260	11	690	30	1
Ravioli Tomato Sauce	1 cup (7.5 oz)	260	10	990	34	3
Spaghetti & Meat Sauce	1 cup (7.5 oz)	220	5	670	33	4
Top Shelf						
Italian Lasagna	1 bowl (10 oz)	350	15	860	29	3
Spaghetti With Meat Sauce	1 bowl (10 oz)	240	5	940	36	3
Van Camp's						
Spaghetti Weenee	1 can (8 oz)	230	8	670	34	1
FROZEN						
Armour						
Classics Chicken Fettucini	1 meal (10 oz)	230	8	520	25	6
Banquet						
Family Entree Lasagna w/ Meat Sauce	1 serv (8 oz)	240	7	650	32	5
Family Entree Macaroni & Beef	1 serv (8 oz)	230	7	810	31	3
Family Entree Macaroni & Cheese	1 serv (8 oz)	300	10	1190	39	2
Family Entree Noodles & Beef	1 serv (7.47 oz)	140	4	1120	16	2

FOOD	PORTION	CAL.	FAT	SOD.	CARB.	FIB.
Banquet (CONT.)						
Family Entree Noodles & Chicken	1 serv (8 oz)	210	9	810	24	2
Birds Eye						
Easy Recipe Chicken Alfredo not prep	½ pkg	160	7	430	22	3
Easy Recipe Chicken Primavera not prep	½ pkg	80	3	540	14	7
Budget Gourmet						
Cheese Ravioli	1 meal (9.5 oz)	290	13	750	34	—
Lasagna Italian Sausage	1 meal (10 oz)	430	23	830	34	—
Lasagna Three Cheese	1 meal (10 oz)	390	17	640	26	—
Lasagna Vegetable	1 meal (10.5 oz)	390	10	770	36	—
Lasagna With Meat Sauce	1 meal (9.4 oz)	290	11	720	30	—
Linguini With Shrimp & Clams	1 meal (9.5 oz)	280	10	710	34	—
Macaroni & Cheese	1 meal (5.75 oz)	230	12	570	22	—
Macaroni & Cheese With Cheddar & Parmesan	1 meal (10.5 oz)	330	8	760	49	—
Manicotti Cheese	1 meal (10 oz)	440	24	740	36	—
Pasta Alfredo With Broccoli	1 meal (5.5 oz)	210	10	630	22	—
Penne Pasta With Chunky Tomato Sauce & Italian Sausage	1 meal (10 oz)	320	9	590	34	—
Rigatoni In Cream Sauce With Broccoli & Chicken	1 meal (10.8 oz)	290	7	710	44	—
Spaghetti With Chunky Tomato & Meat Sauce	1 meal (10 oz)	300	8	470	44	—
Tortellini Cheese	1 meal (5.5 oz)	200	8	530	25	—
Ziti In Marinara Sauce	1 meal (6.25 oz)	200	9	600	23	—
Dining Light						
Cheese Cannelloni	9 oz	310	9	650	38	—
Formagg						
Penne Pasta Alfredo	⅔ cup (5 oz)	190	2	470	35	0
Penne Pasta Primavera	⅔ cup (5 oz)	190	2	470	35	0
Vegetable Pasta & Caesar Italian Garden	⅔ cup (5 oz)	190	2	470	35	0
Green Giant						
Garden Gourmet Creamy Mushroom	1 pkg	220	11	860	29	3

FOOD	PORTION	CAL.	FAT	SOD.	CARB.	FIB.
Green Giant (CONT.)						
Garden Gourmet Pasta Dijon	1 pkg	260	17	630	21	4
Garden Gourmet Pasta Florentine	1 pkg	230	9	840	27	4
Garden Gourmet Rotini Cheddar	1 pkg	230	10	570	32	5
One Serve Cheese Tortellini	1 pkg	260	9	660	37	—
One Serve Macaroni & Cheese	1 pkg	230	9	590	28	—
One Serve Pasta Marinara	1 pkg	180	5	440	29	—
One Serve Pasta Parmesan With Green Peas	1 pkg	170	5	510	23	—
Pasta Accents Creamy Cheddar	½ cup	100	5	310	12	—
Pasta Accents Garden Herb	½ cup	80	3	220	11	—
Pasta Accents Garlic Seasoning	½ cup	110	5	280	13	—
Pasta Accents Pasta Primavera	½ cup	110	5	180	13	—
Healthy Choice						
Beef Macaroni Casserole	1 meal (8.5 oz)	200	1	450	34	5
Cheese Ravioli Parmigiana	1 meal (9 oz)	250	4	290	44	6
Chicken Broccoli Alfredo	1 meal (12.1 oz)	370	8	470	53	6
Chicken Fettucini Alfredo	1 meal (8.5 oz)	250	3	370	34	3
Classics Pasta Shells Marinara	1 meal (12 oz)	360	3	390	59	5
Classics Turkey Fettucini Alla Crema	1 meal (12.5 oz)	350	4	370	50	5
Fettucini Alfredo	1 meal (8 oz)	240	5	430	39	3
Lasagna Roma	1 meal (13.5 oz)	390	5	580	60	9
Macaroni & Cheese	1 meal (9 oz)	290	5	580	45	4
Spaghetti Bolognese	1 meal (10 oz)	260	3	470	43	5
Three Cheese Manicotti	1 meal (11 oz)	310	9	450	41	7
Vegetable Pasta Italiano	1 meal (10 oz)	220	1	340	44	6
Zucchini Lasagna	1 meal (14 oz)	330	2	310	58	11
Kid Cuisine						
Macaroni & Cheese	1 pkg (10.6 oz)	420	12	920	68	3
Mini Cheese Ravioli	1 pkg (9.82 oz)	320	5	780	63	6

FOOD	PORTION	CAL.	FAT	SOD.	CARB.	FIB.
Le Menu						
Entree LightStyle Garden Vegetables Lasagna	10½ oz	260	8	500	35	—
Entree LightStyle Lasagna With Meat Sauce	10 oz	290	8	510	36	—
Entree LightStyle Meat Sauce & Cheese Tortellini	8 oz	250	8	480	34	—
Entree LightStyle Spaghetti With Beef Sauce And Mushrooms	9 oz	280	6	450	45	—
LightStyle 3-Cheese Stuffed Shells	10 oz	280	8	690	34	—
LightStyle Cheese Tortellini	10 oz	230	6	460	35	—
Manicotti With Three Cheeses	11¾ oz	390	15	870	44	—
Lean Cuisine						
Angel Hair Pasta	1 meal (10 oz)	210	4	420	35	4
Cannelioni Cheese	1 meal (9.1 oz)	270	8	500	28	3
Cheddar Bake With Pasta	1 meal (9 oz)	220	6	560	29	3
Chicken Fettucini	1 pkg (9 oz)	270	6	580	33	2
Fettucini Alfredo	1 meal (9 oz)	270	7	590	38	2
Fettucini Primavera	1 meal (10 oz)	260	8	580	33	4
Lasagna Classic Cheese	1 meal (11.5 oz)	290	6	560	38	5
Lasagna Tuna	1 meal (9.75 oz)	230	6	540	29	3
Lasagne With Meat Sauce	1 pkg (10.25 oz)	270	6	560	34	5
Lasagna Zucchini	1 meal (11 oz)	240	4	470	33	4
Macaroni & Beef	1 pkg (10 oz)	280	8	550	40	3
Macaroni & Cheese	1 pkg (9 oz)	270	7	550	39	2
Marinara Twist	1 pkg (10 oz)	240	3	440	42	4
Ravioli Cheese	1 meal (8.5 oz)	250	8	500	32	4
Rigatoni	1 pkg (9 oz)	180	4	560	25	4
Spaghetti & Meatballs	1 pkg (9.5 oz)	290	7	520	40	4
Spaghetti With Meat Sauce	1 meal (11.5 oz)	290	6	550	45	4
Life Choice						
Linguini Roma	1 meal (13.2 oz)	230	1	580	48	6
Sun Dried Tomato Manicotti	1 meal (11.65 oz)	220	3	540	39	7

FOOD	PORTION	CAL.	FAT	SOD.	CARB.	FIB.
Life Choice (CONT.)						
Vegetable Lasagna Primavera	1 meal (11.2 oz)	170	1	600	30	8
Luigino's						
& Pomodoro Sauce With Meatballs	1 pkg (9 oz)	320	11	890	43	2
& Pomodoro Sauce With Meatballs	1 cup (6.3 oz)	270	9	740	36	2
Cheese Ravioli & Alfredo With Broccoli Sauce	1 pkg (8.5 oz)	420	25	890	30	2
Cheese Tortellini & Alfredo Sauce With Broccoli	1 pkg (8 oz)	390	24	840	28	2
Fettuccine Alfredo	1 cup (7.5 oz)	330	11	510	36	3
Fettuccine Alfredo	1 pkg (9.4 oz)	390	14	630	45	4
Fettuccine Alfredo With Broccoli	1 pkg (9.2 oz)	360	16	500	39	4
Fettuccine Carbonara	1 pkg (9 oz)	360	13	760	47	3
Lasagna Alfredo	1 pkg (9 oz)	360	20	660	30	2
Lasagna Alfredo	1 cup (6.3 oz)	300	17	550	25	2
Lasagna Pollo	1 pkg (9 oz)	320	14	610	33	3
Lasagna With Meat Sauce	1 cup (7.2 oz)	240	8	680	30	2
Lasagna With Meat Sauce	1 pkg (9 oz)	290	10	820	36	2
Lasagna With Vegetables	1 pkg (9 oz)	290	10	630	35	2
Linguini With Clams & Sauce	1 pkg (9 oz)	270	6	650	42	2
Linguini With Red Sauce & Clams	1 pkg (9 oz)	260	6	540	41	3
Linguini With Seafood	1 pkg (9 oz)	290	8	740	45	4
Macaroni & Cheese	1 cup (7.2 oz)	310	12	620	37	2
Macaroni & Cheese	1 pkg (9 oz)	370	15	750	45	3
Marinara Sauce Penne Pasta Italian Sausage & Peppers	1 cup (7.4 oz)	290	14	730	27	2
Marinara Sauce Penne Pasta Italian Sausage & Peppers	1 pkg (9 oz)	350	17	880	32	2
Meat Ravioli & Pomodoro Sauce	1 pkg (8.5 oz)	320	13	1060	37	2
Minestrone With Penne Pasta	1 cup (6.3 oz)	180	6	640	21	1
Penne Pollo	1 pkg (9 oz)	330	14	530	36	3

FOOD	PORTION	CAL.	FAT	SOD.	CARB.	FIB.
Luigino's (CONT.)						
Penne Primavera	1 pkg (9 oz)	350	10	330	50	3
Rigatoni Pomodoro Italiano	1 pkg (9 oz)	290	8	710	40	4
Shells & Cheese With Jalapenos	1 pkg (8.5 oz)	360	15	700	41	2
Spaghetti Bolognese	1 pkg (9 oz)	270	8	820	38	4
Spaghetti Marinara	1 pkg (10 oz)	250	2	680	49	3
Spinach Ravioli & Primavera Sauce	1 pkg (8.5 oz)	360	17	800	36	2
Morton						
Macaroni & Cheese	1 serv (8 oz)	220	6	960	34	2
Mrs. Paul's						
Entrees Light Seafood Lasagne	9½ oz	290	8	750	39	—
Entrees Light Seafood Rotini	9 oz	240	6	570	34	—
Seafood Rotini	9 oz	240	6	570	34	—
Palmazone						
Macaroni 'n Cheese	½ pkg (6 oz)	260	7	320	36	—
Pasta Favorites						
Chicken Pasta Primavera	1 pkg (10.5 oz)	330	13	930	40	6
Fettuccini Alfredo	1 pkg (10.5 oz)	370	18	940	39	4
Italian Sausage & Peppers	1 pkg (10.5 oz)	340	13	840	43	7
Lasagna	1 pkg (10.5 oz)	290	9	900	39	6
Macaroni & Cheese	1 pkg (10.5 oz)	350	12	1070	47	5
Pasta Primavera	1 pkg (10.5 oz)	320	14	920	40	7
Spaghetti w/ Meatballs	1 pkg (10.5 oz)	370	16	1040	40	6
Vegetable Lasagna	1 pkg (10.5 oz)	260	6	850	41	7
White Cheddar & Rotini	1 pkg (10.5 oz)	350	12	900	48	6
Senor Felix's						
Lasagna Southwestern	1 serv (6 oz)	160	7	380	15	2
Stouffer's						
Beef Ravioli	1 pkg (9.5 oz)	370	14	680	43	5
Cheese Manicotti	1 pkg (9 oz)	340	16	810	32	7
Cheese Ravioli With Tomato Sauce	1 pkg (9.5 oz)	360	16	720	42	4
Cheese Shells With Tomato Sauce	1 pkg (9.25 oz)	340	16	920	29	5
Cheese Tortellini With Alfredo Sauce	1 pkg (8.9 oz)	550	33	720	38	5
Cheese Tortellini With Tomato Sauce	1 pkg (9.25 oz)	290	6	740	40	4

FOOD	PORTION	CAL.	FAT	SOD.	CARB.	FIB.
Stouffer's (CONT.)						
Fettucini Alfredo	1 pkg (10 oz)	480	29	850	40	3
Four Cheese Lasagna	1 pkg (10.75 oz)	410	19	840	37	3
Homestyle Chicken Fettucini	1 pkg (10.5 oz)	380	15	1250	32	3
Lasagna With Meat Sauce	1 cup (7 oz)	260	10	560	24	4
Lasagna With Meat Sauce	1 pkg (10.5 oz)	360	13	780	34	5
Lunch Express Cheese Lasagna Casserole	1 pkg (9.5 oz)	270	7	590	38	5
Lunch Express Cheese Ravioli	1 pkg (8.5 oz)	310	12	620	38	2
Lunch Express Chicken Alfredo	1 pkg (9.6 oz)	360	17	620	34	3
Lunch Express Chicken Fettucini	1 pkg (10.25 oz)	250	6	540	32	4
Lunch Express Fettucini Primavera	1 pkg (10.25 oz)	420	25	690	33	4
Lunch Express Lasagna With Meat Sauce	1 pkg (10 oz)	350	12	940	42	4
Lunch Express Macaroni & Cheese With Broccoli	1 pkg (10.4 oz)	360	19	900	32	3
Lunch Express Pasta & Chicken Marinara	1 pkg (9.1 oz)	270	6	540	38	4
Lunch Express Pasta & Tuna Casserole	1 pkg (9.6 oz)	280	6	590	39	4
Lunch Express Pasta & Turkey Dijon	1 pkg (9.9 oz)	270	6	570	37	6
Lunch Express Rigatoni With Meat Sauce	1 pkg (10.75 oz)	340	12	710	44	3
Lunch Express Spaghetti With Meat Sauce	1 pkg (9.6 oz)	320	10	580	43	5
Lunch Express Swedish Meatballs With Pasta	1 pkg (10.25 oz)	530	32	1010	41	3
Macaroni & Beef	1 pkg (11.5 oz)	340	12	1530	40	4
Macaroni & Cheese	1 cup (6 oz)	330	17	940	31	2
Noodles Romanoff	1 pkg (12 oz)	460	23	1400	48	4
Spaghetti With Meat Sauce	1 pkg (12.9 oz)	430	13	760	57	6
Spaghetti With Meatballs	1 pkg (12.6 oz)	420	15	680	51	5
Tuna Noodle Casserole	1 pkg (10 oz)	330	14	1130	31	3
Turkey Tettrazini	1 pkg (10 oz)	360	19	1140	28	2

FOOD	PORTION	CAL.	FAT	SOD.	CARB.	FIB.
Stouffer's (CONT.)						
Vegetable Lasagna	1 cup (8 oz)	280	12	280	29	2
Vegetable Lasagna	1 pkg (10.5 oz)	370	19	820	31	3
Swanson						
Homestyle Lasagne With Meat Sauce	10½ oz	400	15	1070	39	—
Homestyle Macaroni & Cheese	10 oz	390	19	1150	37	—
Homestyle Spaghetti With Italian Style Meatballs	13 oz	490	18	940	60	—
Macaroni & Cheese	12¼ oz	370	15	1070	48	—
Macaroni & Cheese	7 oz	200	8	740	24	—
Spaghetti & Meatballs	12½ oz	390	17	1100	46	—
Tabatchnick						
Macaroni & Cheese	7.5 oz	280	12	840	30	2
Tyson						
Parmigiana	1 pkg (11.25 oz)	380	17	1100	37	—
Ultra Slim-Fast						
Pasta Primavera	12 oz	340	9	730	52	5
Spaghetti With Beef & Mushroom Sauce	12 oz	370	10	990	49	0
Weight Watchers						
Angel Hair Pasta	10 oz	200	4	330	28	—
Baked Cheese Ravioli	9 oz	240	6	370	27	—
Cheese Tortellini	9 oz	310	6	570	50	—
Cheese Manicotti	9.25 oz	260	8	510	31	—
Chicken Fettucini	8.25 oz	280	9	590	25	—
Fettucini Alfredo	8 oz	230	7	550	28	—
Garden Lasagne	11 oz	260	7	430	30	—
Italian Cheese Lasagna	11 oz	290	6	510	29	—
Lasagne	10.25 oz	240	6	510	29	—
Spaghetti With Meat Sauce	10 oz	240	7	490	28	—
HOME RECIPE						
macaroni & cheese	1 cup	430	22	1086	40	—
spaghetti w/ meatballs & tomato sauce	1 cup	330	12	1009	39	—
MIX						
Casbah						
Pasta Fasul	1 pkg (1.6 oz)	150	1	490	10	2
Golden Grain						
Macaroni & Cheese	½ cup	310	15	620	36	—

FOOD	PORTION	CAL.	FAT	SOD.	CARB.	FIB.
Hain						
Pasta & Sauce Creamy Parmesan	¼ pkg	150	3	400	22	—
Pasta & Sauce Creamy Swiss	¼ pkg	170	4	360	26	—
Pasta & Sauce Fettuccine Alfredo	¼ pkg	180	4	420	27	—
Pasta & Sauce Italian Herb	¼ pkg	110	2	160	17	—
Pasta & Sauce Primavera	¼ pkg	140	4	430	20	—
Pasta & Sauce Tangy Cheddar	¼ pkg	180	6	350	24	—
Kraft						
Cheddar Cheese Egg Noodle	1 cup (8 oz)	430	21	780	46	1
Macaroni & Cheese Deluxe Original	1 cup (6.1 oz)	320	10	730	44	1
Macaroni & Cheese Dinosaurs	1 cup (6.8 oz)	390	17	770	48	1
Macaroni & Cheese Flintstones	1 cup (6.8 oz)	390	17	770	48	1
Macaroni & Cheese Milk White Cheddar	1 cup (6.8 oz)	390	17	730	48	1
Macaroni & Cheese Original	1 cup (6.9 oz)	390	17	730	48	1
Macaroni & Cheese Santa Mac	1 cup	390	17	770	48	1
Macaroni & Cheese Spirals	1 cup (6.8 oz)	390	17	770	48	1
Macaroni & Cheese Super Mario Bros	1 cup (6.8 oz)	390	17	770	48	1
Macaroni & Cheese Teddy Bears	1 cup (6.8 oz)	390	17	770	48	1
Macaroni & Cheese Thick 'N Creamy	1 cup (6.1 oz)	320	10	730	50	2
Spaghetti Mild American	1 cup (8.1 oz)	270	5	690	48	3
Spaghetti Tangy Italian	1 cup (7.9 oz)	270	5	780	46	3
Spaghetti With Meat Sauce	1 cup (8.2 oz)	330	11	830	46	3
Lipton						
Pasta & Sauce Cheddar Broccoli	½ cup	132	2	458	24	—
Pasta & Sauce Creamy Garlic	½ cup	146	2	447	26	—

FOOD	PORTION	CAL.	FAT	SOD.	CARB.	FIB.
Lipton (CONT.)						
Pasta & Sauce Creamy Mushroom	½ cup	143	3	424	25	0
Pasta & Sauce Herb Tomato	½ cup	130	1	356	26	—
Minute						
Microwave Cheddar Cheese Broccoli And Pasta as prep	½ cup	160	5	538	23	—
Nile Spice						
Pasta'n Sauce Mediterranean	1 pkg	210	5	640	33	2
Pasta'n Sauce Parmesan	1 pkg	200	3	470	36	1
Pasta'n Sauce Primavera	1 pkg	200	4	610	34	2
Terrazza						
Pasta E Fagioli as prep	½ cup	150	3	135	23	—
Ultra Slim-Fast						
Macaroni & Cheese	2.3 oz	230	3	770	46	4
Uncle Ben						
Country Inn Pasta & Sauce Angel Hair Parmesan	1 serv (2.2 oz)	245	5	926	39	3
Country Inn Pasta & Sauce Broccoli & White Cheddar	1 serv (2.2 oz)	240	5	799	40	2
Country Inn Pasta & Sauce Butter & Herb	1 serv (2 oz)	230	6	885	36	1
Country Inn Pasta & Sauce Creamy Garlic	1 serv (2.4 oz)	261	5	599	45	2
Country Inn Pasta & Sauce Fettuccine Alfredo	1 serv (2.2 oz)	310	6	656	41	2
Country Inn Pasta & Sauce Herb Linguine	1 serv (2.2 oz)	240	3	654	43	2
Country Inn Pasta & Sauce Mushroom Fettuccine	1 serv (2.2 oz)	250	6	638	41	2
Country Inn Pasta & Sauce Vegetable Alfredo	1 serv (2.2 oz)	240	5	548	42	2
Velveeta						
Rotini & Cheese Broccoli	1 cup (7.2 oz)	400	16	1240	46	2
Shells & Cheese Bacon	1 cup (6.8 oz)	360	14	1140	43	1
Shells & Cheese Original	1 cup (6.6 oz)	360	13	1030	44	1

FOOD	PORTION	CAL.	FAT	SOD.	CARB.	FIB.
Velveeta (CONT.)						
Shells & Cheese Salsa	1 cup (7.5 oz)	380	14	1180	47	2
SHELF-STABLE						
Lunch Bucket						
Elbows In Tomato Sauce	1 pkg (7.5 oz)	190	2	860	38	—
Lasagna With Meatsauce	1 pkg (7.5 oz)	220	4	870	38	—
Light'n Healthy Italian Style Pasta	1 pkg (7.5 oz)	130	1	630	23	—
Light'n Healthy Pasta In Wine Sauce	1 pkg (7.5 oz)	130	3	600	21	—
Light'n Healthy Pasta'n Garden Vegetables	1 pkg (7.5 oz)	150	1	630	30	—
Macaroni'n Cheese	1 pkg (7.5 oz)	210	9	990	24	—
Pasta'n Chicken	1 pkg (7.5 oz)	180	6	860	22	—
Spaghetti'n Meatsauce	1 pkg (7.5 oz)	240	5	870	39	—
My Own Meal						
Cheese Tortellini	1 pkg (10 oz)	340	10	1000	49	6
TAKE-OUT						
lasagna	1 piece (2.5 in x 2.5 in)	374	21	668	25	2
macaroni & cheese	1 cup	230	10	730	26	—
manicotti	¾ cup (6.4 oz)	273	12	414	28	2
rigatoni w/ sausage sauce	¾ cup	260	12	106	28	3
spaghetti w/ meatballs & cheese	1 cup	407	19	696	38	—

PASTA MACHINE MIX

Wanda's

FOOD	PORTION	CAL.	FAT	SOD.	CARB.	FIB.
Dried Tomato	⅓ cup mix per serv (1.9 oz)	202	1	0	42	1
Durum & Semolina	⅓ cup mix per serv (1.9 oz)	199	1	0	42	1
Semolina Blend	⅓ cup mix per serv (1.9 oz)	202	1	0	42	1
Spinach	⅓ cup mix per serv (1.9 oz)	202	1	0	42	1
Whole Wheat & Semolina	⅓ cup mix per serv (1.9 oz)	196	1	2	41	4

PASTA SALAD

MIX

Kraft

FOOD	PORTION	CAL.	FAT	SOD.	CARB.	FIB.
Pasta Salad Classic Ranch With Bacon	¾ cup (4.7 oz)	360	23	500	30	2
Pasta Salad Creamy Caesar	¾ cup (4.8 oz)	350	22	650	30	2

FOOD	PORTION	CAL.	FAT	SOD.	CARB.	FIB.
Kraft (CONT.)						
Pasta Salad Garden Primavera	¾ cup (5 oz)	280	12	730	34	2
Pasta Salad Light Italian	¾ cup (5 oz)	190	2	660	34	2
Pasta Salad Parmesan Peppercorn	¾ cup (4.9 oz)	360	25	610	28	2
Lipton						
Robust Italian	½ cup	126	1	118	25	tr
Suddenly Salad						
Classic Pasta as prep	½ cup	160	6	530	23	—
Creamy Macaroni as prep	½ cup	200	10	280	21	—
Creamy Macaroni as prep low fat recipe	½ cup	140	4	310	21	—
Italian Pasta as prep	½ cup	160	6	480	22	—
Pasta Primavera as prep	½ cup	190	10	340	20	—
Pasta Primavera as prep low fat recipe	½ cup	150	5	370	21	—
Tortellini Italiano as prep	½ cup	160	7	450	21	—
TAKE-OUT						
elbow macaroni salad	3.5 oz	160	5	590	26	—
italian style pasta salad	3.5 oz	140	7	480	15	—
mustard macaroni salad	3.5 oz	190	10	560	23	—
pasta salad w/ vegetables	3.5 oz	140	4	210	21	—

PASTRY

(*see* BROWNIE, CAKE, DANISH PASTRY)

PATE

CANNED

Sells

FOOD	PORTION	CAL.	FAT	SOD.	CARB.	FIB.
Liver	2.08 oz	190	16	470	4	—
chicken liver	1 oz	238	4	—	2	—
chicken liver	1 tbsp (13 g)	109	2	—	1	—
goose liver smoked	1 tbsp (13 g)	60	6	—	1	—
goose liver smoked	1 oz	131	12	—	1	—
liver	1 tbsp (13 g)	41	4	91	tr	—
liver	1 oz	90	8	198	tr	—

PEACH

CANNED

Del Monte

FOOD	PORTION	CAL.	FAT	SOD.	CARB.	FIB.
Halves Cling In Heavy Syrup	½ cup (4.5 oz)	100	0	10	24	1
Halves Cling Lite	½ cup (4.4 oz)	60	0	10	15	1

FOOD	PORTION	CAL.	FAT	SOD.	CARB.	FIB.
Del Monte (CONT.)						
Halves Cling Melba In Heavy Syrup	½ cup (4.5 oz)	100	0	10	24	1
Halves Freestone In Heavy Syrup	½ cup (4.5 oz)	100	0	10	24	1
Sliced Cling Fruit Naturals	½ cup (4.4 oz)	60	0	10	15	1
Sliced Cling In Heavy Syrup	½ cup (4.5 oz)	100	0	10	24	1
Sliced Cling Lite	½ cup (4.4 oz)	60	0	10	15	1
Sliced Freestone In Heavy Syrup	½ cup (4.5 oz)	100	0	10	24	1
Sliced Freestone Lite	½ cup (4.4 oz)	60	0	10	14	1
Snack Cups Diced Fruit Naturals	1 serv (4.5 oz)	60	0	10	16	1
Snack Cups Diced Fruit Naturals EZ-Open Lid	1 serv (4.2 oz)	60	0	10	15	1
Snack Cups Diced In Heavy Syrup	1 serv (4.5 oz)	100	0	10	24	1
Snack Cups Diced In Heavy Syrup EZ-Open Lid	1 serv (4.2 oz)	90	0	10	23	1
Snack Cups Diced Lite	1 serv (4.5 oz)	60	0	10	16	1
Snack Cups Diced Lite EZ-Open Lid	1 serv (4.2 oz)	60	0	10	15	1
Whole Cling In Heavy Syrup	½ cup (4.2 oz)	100	0	10	24	tr
Hunt's						
Halves	4 oz	90	tr	7	23	tr
Slices	4 oz	90	tr	7	23	tr
Libby						
Halves Yellow Cling Lite	½ cup (4.4 oz)	60	0	10	13	1
Sliced Yellow Cling Lite	½ cup (4.4 oz)	60	0	10	13	1
S&W						
Halves Clingstone	½ cup	100	0	10	25	—
Halves Clingstone Diet	½ cup	30	0	5	8	—
Halves Clingstone Unsweetened	½ cup	30	0	5	8	—
Halves Freesstone Diet	½ cup	30	0	10	7	—
Halves Freestone In Heavy Syrup	½ cup	100	0	10	26	—
Sliced Clingstone Diet	½ cup	30	0	5	8	—
Sliced Clingstone Unsweetened	½ cup	30	0	5	8	—

FOOD	PORTION	CAL.	FAT	SOD.	CARB.	FIB.
S&W (CONT.)						
Sliced Freestone Diet	½ cup	30	0	10	7	—
Sliced Freestone In Heavy Syrup	½ cup	100	0	10	26	—
Sliced Yellow Cling Natural Style	½ cup	90	0	10	20	—
Sliced Yellow Cling Premium In Heavy Syrup	½ cup	100	0	10	25	—
Whole Yellow Cling Spiced In Heavy Syrup	½ cup	90	0	10	23	—
Yellow Cling Natural Lite	½ cup	50	0	10	13	—
halves in heavy syrup	1 half	60	tr	5	16	—
halves in light syrup	1 half	44	tr	4	12	—
halves juice pack	1 half	34	tr	3	9	—
halves water pack	1 half	18	tr	3	5	—
spiced in heavy syrup	1 cup	180	tr	9	49	—
spiced in heavy syrup	1 fruit	66	tr	3	18	—
DRIED						
Del Monte						
Sun Dried	⅓ cup (1.4 oz)	90	0	0	28	5
Mariani						
Peaches	¼ cup	140	0	—	—	—
Sonoma						
Pieces	3-5 pieces (1.4 oz)	120	0	0	31	1
halves	1 cup	383	1	12	98	13
halves	10	311	1	9	80	11
halves cooked w/ sugar	½ cup	139	tr	3	36	—
halves cooked w/o sugar	½ cup	99	tr	3	25	—
FRESH						
Dole	2	70	0	0	19	1
peach	1	37	tr	0	10	1
sliced	1 cup	73	tr	1	19	—
FROZEN						
Big Valley						
Freestone	⅔ cup (4.9 oz)	50	0	0	13	1
slices sweetened	1 cup	235	tr	16	60	—
PEACH JUICE						
Goya						
Nectar	6 oz	110	0	30	27	—
Kern's						
Nectar	6 fl oz	110	0	0	26	—

FOOD	PORTION	CAL.	FAT	SOD.	CARB.	FIB.
Libby						
Nectar	1 can (11.5 fl oz)	210	0	5	52	—
Mott's						
Fruit Basket Orchard Peach Juice Cocktail as prep	8 fl oz	130	0	0	32	0
Smucker's						
Juice	8 oz	120	0	10	30	—
Snapple						
Dixie Peach	10 fl oz	140	0	20	39	—
nectar	1 cup	134	tr	17	35	—

PEANUT BUTTER

FOOD	PORTION	CAL.	FAT	SOD.	CARB.	FIB.
Arrowhead						
Creamy	2 tbsp (1.1 oz)	200	15	0	6	1
Crunchy	2 tbsp (1.1 oz)	200	15	0	6	1
BAMA						
Creamy	2 tbsp	200	17	140	6	—
Crunchy	2 tbsp	200	17	115	6	—
Jelly & Peanut Butter	2 tbsp	150	7	75	20	—
Crazy Richard's						
Natural Creamy	2 tbsp (1.1 oz)	190	16	0	6	2
Erewhon						
Chunky	2 tbsp (32 g)	190	14	75	7	—
Chunky Unsalted	2 tbsp (32 g)	190	14	10	7	—
Creamy	2 tbsp (32 g)	190	14	75	7	—
Creamy Unsalted	2 tbsp (32 g)	190	14	10	7	—
Estee						
Chunky Sodium Free	2 tbsp (1 oz)	190	15	0	7	2
Chunky Sodium Free Sorbitol Sweetened	2 tbsp (1 oz)	190	15	0	7	2
Creamy Sodium Free	2 tbsp (1 oz)	190	15	0	7	2
Creamy Sodium Free Sorbitol Sweetened	2 tbsp (1 oz)	190	15	0	7	2
Health Valley						
Chunky No Salt	2 tbsp	170	14	2	6	2
Creamy No Salt	2 tbsp	170	14	2	6	3
Hollywood						
Creamy	1 tbsp	35	3	25	1	1
Crunchy	1 tbsp	35	3	25	1	1
Unsalted	1 tbsp	35	3	0	1	1
Home Brand						
Natural Lightly Salted	2 tbsp	210	17	—	—	—
Natural Unsalted	2 tbsp	210	17	—	—	—

FOOD	PORTION	CAL.	FAT	SOD.	CARB.	FIB.
Home Brand (CONT.)						
No Sugar Added	2 tbsp	180	16	—	—	—
Peanut Butter	2 tbsp	210	17	—	—	—
Jif						
Creamy	2 tbsp (1.1 oz)	190	16	150	7	2
Extra Crunchy	2 tbsp (1.1 oz)	190	16	130	7	2
Reduced Fat	2 tbsp (1.3 oz)	190	12	250	15	2
Simply Creamy	2 tbsp (1.1 oz)	190	16	65	6	2
Simply Extra Crunchy	2 tbsp (1.1 oz)	190	16	50	6	2
Peter Pan						
Creamy	2 tbsp	190	16	150	6	2
Creamy Salt Free	2 tbsp	190	17	0	5	2
Crunchy	2 tbsp	190	16	150	6	2
Crunchy Salt Free	2 tbsp	190	17	0	5	2
Red Wing						
Creamy	2 tbsp (1.1 oz)	200	16	140	6	2
Crunchy	2 tbsp (1.1 oz)	200	16	120	6	2
Reese's						
Peanut Butter Chips	¼ cup (1.5 oz)	230	13	90	19	—
Skippy						
Creamy	1 cup (263 g)	1540	135	1240	38	—
Creamy w/ 2 slices white bread	1 sandwich	340	19	430	33	—
Reduced Fat Creamy	2 tbsp	190	12	200	13	1
Super Chunk	2 tbsp (32 g)	190	17	130	4	—
Super Chunk	1 cup (260 g)	1540	138	1120	36	—
Super Chunk w/ 2 slices white bread	1 sandwich	340	19	410	32	—
Smucker's						
Goober Grape	2 tbsp	180	10	120	18	—
Honey Sweetened	2 tbsp	200	16	155	7	—
Natural	2 tbsp	200	16	125	6	—
Natural No Salt Added	2 tbsp	200	16	<10	6	—
Tree Of Life						
Creamy	2 tbsp (1 oz)	190	15	150	7	1
Creamy No Salt	2 tbsp (1 oz)	190	15	0	7	1
Creamy Organic	2 tbsp (1 oz)	190	16	45	7	1
Creamy Organic No Salt	2 tbsp (1 oz)	190	16	0	7	1
Crunchy	2 tbsp (1 oz)	190	15	150	7	1
Crunchy No Salt	2 tbsp (1 oz)	190	15	0	7	1
Crunchy Organic	2 tbsp (1 oz)	190	16	45	7	1
Crunchy Organic No Salt	2 tbsp (1 oz)	190	16	0	7	1
Peanut Wonder 78% Less Fat	2 tbsp (1 oz)	100	4	250	11	1

FOOD	PORTION	CAL.	FAT	SOD.	CARB.	FIB.
chunky	1 cup	1520	129	1255	56	17
chunky	2 tbsp	188	16	156	7	2
chunky w/o salt	1 cup	1520	129	44	56	17
chunky w/o salt	2 tbsp	188	16	5	7	2
smooth	2 tbsp	188	16	153	7	2
smooth	1 cup	1517	128	1234	53	15
smooth w/o salt	1 cup	1517	129	44	53	15
smooth w/o salt	2 tbsp	188	16	5	7	2

PEANUTS

Beer Nuts
Peanuts	1 pkg (1 oz)	180	14	60	7	—

Eagle
Honey Roasted	1 oz	170	13	130	7	—
Honey Roasted Cinnamon	1 oz	170	13	90	7	—
Honey Roasted Maple	1 oz	170	13	90	7	—
Low Salt	1 oz	170	15	90	5	—
Virginia Fancy	1 oz	90	8	65	3	—

Fisher
Party Peanuts	1 oz	160	14	—	—	—
Salted-In-Shell shelled	1 oz	170	14	170	6	—
Spanish Roasted	1 oz	180	16	130	6	—

Frito Lay
Dry Roasted	1.2 oz	190	16	300	7	—
Salted	1 oz	170	15	170	6	—

Guy's
Dry Roasted	1 oz	170	14	310	3	—
Spanish Salted	1 oz	170	14	170	3	—

Lance
Honey Toasted	1 pkg (39 g)	230	17	240	11	—
Roasted w/ Shell	1 pkg (50 g)	190	15	0	8	—
Salted	1 pkg (32 g)	190	15	105	7	—
Salted Tube	1 pkg (42 g)	240	20	120	9	—

Little Debbie
Salted	1 pkg (1.2 oz)	230	21	45	3	2

Pennant
Oil Roasted	1 oz	170	14	115	6	3

Planters
Cocktail Lightly Salted Oil Roasted	1 oz	170	15	55	5	2
Cocktail Oil Roasted	1 oz	170	14	115	6	3
Cocktail Unsalted Oil Roasted	1 oz	170	14	0	6	2

FOOD	PORTION	CAL.	FAT	SOD.	CARB.	FIB.
Planters (CONT.)						
Dry Roasted	1 oz	160	13	250	6	3
Fun Size! Oil Roasted	2 pkg (1 oz)	170	15	140	6	2
Heat Hot Spicy Oil Roasted	1 pkg (2 oz)	330	29	390	10	5
Heat Hot Spicy Oil Roasted	1 oz	160	14	190	5	2
Heat Hot Spicy Oil Roasted	1 pkg (1.7 oz)	290	25	370	9	4
Heat Mild Spicy Oil Roasted	1 oz	160	14	130	5	2
Honey Roasted	1 oz	160	13	90	8	2
Honey Roasted Dry Roasted	1 pkg (1.7 oz)	260	19	260	17	3
Lightly Salted Dry Roasted	1 pkg (1.75 oz)	290	25	190	9	4
Lightly Salted Dry Roasted	1 oz	160	14	110	5	3
Lightly Salted Oil Roasted	1 pkg (1.8 oz)	300	27	95	8	4
Munch'N Go Singles Heat Hot Spicy Oil Roasted	1 pkg (2.5 oz)	410	36	480	13	6
Salted Oil Roasted	1 pkg (1 oz)	170	15	110	5	2
Spanish Oil Roasted	1 oz	170	14	105	5	2
Spanish Raw	1 oz	150	13	5	6	3
Sweet N Crunchy	1 oz	140	7	20	16	2
Unsalted Dry Roasted	1 oz	160	14	0	6	3
Weight Watchers						
Honey Roasted	0.7 oz	100	6	100	7	—
chocolate coated	1 cup (5.2 oz)	773	50	61	74	—
chocolate coated	10 (1.4 oz)	208	13	16	20	—
cooked	½ cup	102	7	240	7	—
dry roasted	1 cup	855	73	1187	31	12
dry roasted	1 oz	164	14	228	6	2
oil roasted	1 oz	163	14	121	5	2
oil roasted	1 cup	837	71	624	27	13
oil roasted w/o salt	1 cup	837	71	9	27	13
oil roasted w/o salt	1 oz	163	14	2	5	2
spanish oil roasted	1 oz	162	14	121	5	2
spanish oil roasted w/o salt	1 oz	162	14	2	5	2
unroasted	1 oz	159	14	5	5	—
valencia oil roasted	1 cup	848	74	1111	23	9
valencia oil roasted	1 oz	165	14	216	5	2

FOOD	PORTION	CAL.	FAT	SOD.	CARB.	FIB.
valencia oil roasted w/o salt	1 cup	848	74	9	23	9
valencia oil roasted w/o salt	1 oz	165	14	2	5	2
virginia oil roasted	1 oz	161	14	121	5	—
virginia oil roasted	1 cup	826	70	619	28	—

PEAR
CANNED
Del Monte

FOOD	PORTION	CAL.	FAT	SOD.	CARB.	FIB.
Halves Fruit Naturals	½ cup (4.4 oz)	60	0	10	15	1
Halves In Heavy Syrup	½ cup (4.5 oz)	100	0	10	24	1
Halves Lite	½ cup (4.4 oz)	60	0	10	15	1
Sliced In Heavy Syrup	½ cup (4.5 oz)	100	0	10	24	1
Sliced Lite	½ cup (4.4 oz)	60	0	10	15	1
Snack Cups Diced In Heavy Syrup	1 serv (4.5 oz)	100	0	10	24	1
Snack Cups Diced In Heavy Syrup EZ-Open Lid	1 serv (4.2 oz)	90	0	10	23	1
Snack Cups Diced Lite	1 serv (4.5 oz)	60	0	10	15	1
Snack Cups Diced Lite EZ-Open Lid	1 serv (4.2 oz)	60	0	10	15	1

Hunt's

FOOD	PORTION	CAL.	FAT	SOD.	CARB.	FIB.
Halves	4 oz	90	tr	6	22	tr

Libby

FOOD	PORTION	CAL.	FAT	SOD.	CARB.	FIB.
Halves Lite	½ cup (4.3 oz)	60	0	10	13	1
Sliced Lite	½ cup (4.3 oz)	60	0	10	13	1

S&W

FOOD	PORTION	CAL.	FAT	SOD.	CARB.	FIB.
Halves Bartlett In Heavy Syrup	½ cup	100	0	—	25	—
Halves Bartlett Peeled Unsweetened	½ cup	35	0	10	10	—
Halves Peeled Diet	½ cup	35	0	10	10	—
Quartered Peeled Diet	½ cup	35	0	10	10	—
Sliced Natural Light Bartlett	½ cup	60	0	10	15	—
Sliced Natural Style	½ cup	80	0	10	20	—
halves in heavy syrup	1 cup	188	tr	13	49	—
halves in heavy syrup	1 half	68	tr	4	15	—
halves in light syrup	1 half	45	tr	4	12	—
halves juice pack	1 cup	123	tr	10	32	—
halves water pack	1 half	22	tr	41	6	—

DRIED
Mariani

FOOD	PORTION	CAL.	FAT	SOD.	CARB.	FIB.
Pears	¼ cup	150	0	—	—	—

FOOD	PORTION	CAL.	FAT	SOD.	CARB.	FIB.
Sonoma						
Pieces	3-4 pieces (1.4 oz)	120	0	0	33	3
halves	1 cup	472	1	10	125	—
halves	10	459	1	10	122	—
halves cooked w/ sugar	½ cup	196	tr	4	52	—
halves cooked w/o sugar	½ cup	163	tr	4	43	—
FRESH						
Dole	1	100	1	1	25	4
asian	1 (4.3 oz)	51	tr	0	13	—
pear	1	98	1	1	25	4
sliced w/ skin	1 cup	97	1	1	25	4
PEAR JUICE						
Goya						
Nectar	6 oz	120	0	15	29	—
Kern's						
Nectar	6 fl oz	120	0	0	28	—
Libby						
Nectar	1 can (11.5 fl oz)	220	0	5	54	3
nectar	1 cup	149	tr	9	39	—
PEAS						
CANNED						
Allen						
Crowder	½ cup (4.5 oz)	110	1	460	19	8
Purple Hull	½ cup (4.4 oz)	120	1	350	21	6
Crest Top						
Early June	½ cup (4.5 oz)	100	1	300	20	6
Del Monte						
Sweet	½ cup (4.4 oz)	60	0	360	11	4
Sweet 50% Less Salt	½ cup (4.4 oz)	60	0	180	11	4
Sweet No Salt Added	½ cup (4.4 oz)	60	0	10	11	4
Sweet Very Young	½ cup (4.4 oz)	60	0	360	10	4
East Texas Fair						
Cream Peas	½ cup (4.4 oz)	120	1	420	20	5
Crowder	½ cup (4.5 oz)	110	1	460	19	8
Lady Peas With Snaps	½ cup (4.3 oz)	100	1	420	17	4
Peas 'n Pork	½ cup (4.5 oz)	110	2	540	19	5
Pepper Peas	½ cup (4.5 oz)	120	1	580	22	6
Purple Hull	½ cup (4.4 oz)	120	1	350	21	6
White Acre	½ cup (4.3 oz)	100	1	460	17	5
Friends						
Small Pea Beans	8 oz	360	4	1040	62	—
Green Giant						
Sweet	½ cup	50	0	320	11	4

FOOD	PORTION	CAL.	FAT	SOD.	CARB.	FIB.
Homefolks						
Crowder	½ cup (4.5 oz)	110	1	460	19	8
Purple Hull	½ cup (4.4 oz)	120	1	350	21	6
Luck's						
Crowder Peas Seasoned w/ Pork	7.5 oz	200	7	—		
Owatonna						
Early June or Sweet	½ cup	70	0	—		
S&W						
Petit Pois	½ cup	70	0	330	12	—
Sweet	½ cup	70	0	330	12	—
Sweet Water Pack	½ cup	40	0	5	8	—
Veri-Green Sweet	½ cup	70	0	320	14	—
Seneca						
Natural Pack	½ cup	60	0	0	9	4
Peas	½ cup	50	0	360	9	5
Sunshine						
Field Peas	½ cup (4.4 oz)	120	1	350	21	6
Lady Peas	½ cup (4.3 oz)	100	1	460	17	5
Trappey						
Field Peas With Bacon	½ cup (4.5 oz)	90	1	380	15	5
Field Peas With Snaps And Bacon	½ cup (4.5 oz)	110	1	380	19	4
Van De Kamp's						
Baked Pea Beans	8 oz	270	6	750	50	11
green	½ cup	59	tr	186	11	—
green low sodium	½ cup	59	tr	2	11	—
DRIED						
split cooked	1 cup	231	1	4	41	—
FRESH						
Dole						
Sugar Peas	½ cup	30	tr	3	5	2
edible-pod cooked	½ cup	34	tr	3	6	2
edible-pod raw	½ cup	30	tr	3	5	2
green cooked	½ cup	67	tr	2	13	—
green raw	½ cup	58	tr	3	11	—
FROZEN						
Birds Eye						
Green	½ cup	80	0	130	13	4
In Butter Sauce	½ cup	80	2	170	12	3
Polybag Deluxe Tender Tiny	½ cup	60	0	120	11	4
Polybag Green	½ cup	70	0	125	12	2
Sugar Snap Deluxe	½ cup	45	0	5	9	4

FOOD	PORTION	CAL.	FAT	SOD.	CARB.	FIB.
Birds Eye (CONT.)						
Tender Tiny Deluxe	½ cup	60	0	120	11	4
Chun King						
Snow Pea Pods	½ pkg (3 oz)	35	2	0	4	2
Fresh Like						
Green	3.5 oz	85	1	79	14	2
Tiny Green	3.5 oz	63	tr	79	12	1
Green Giant						
Harvest Fresh Early June	½ cup	60	1	140	12	3
Harvest Fresh Sugar Snap	½ cup	30	0	100	8	2
Harvest Fresh Sweet	½ cup	50	0	95	12	3
In Butter Sauce	½ cup	80	2	410	14	4
One Serve In Butter Sauce	1 pkg	90	2	500	16	5
Sugar Snap Sweet Select	½ cup	30	0	0	8	2
Sweet	½ cup	50	0	95	11	4
Hanover						
Petite	½ cup	70	0	—	—	—
Snow Peas	½ cup	35	0	—	—	—
Sweet	½ cup	70	0	—	—	—
Le Seur						
Early In Butter Sauce	½ cup	80	2	440	14	3
Early Select	½ cup	60	0	115	13	4
edible-pod cooked	1 pkg (10 oz)	132	1	12	23	—
edible-pod cooked	½ cup	42	tr	4	7	—
green cooked	½ cup	63	tr	70	11	—
SHELF-STABLE						
Green Giant						
Mini Sweet	½ cup	60	tr	240	12	4
SPROUTS						
raw	½ cup	77	tr	12	17	—
TAKE-OUT						
pea & potato curry	1 serving (7 oz)	264	22	—	19	6
pea curry	1 serving (4.4 oz)	438	42	—	11	4

PECANS

FOOD	PORTION	CAL.	FAT	SOD.	CARB.	FIB.
Eagle						
Honey Roasted	1 oz	200	19	130	5	—
Planters						
Chips	1 pkg (2 oz)	390	40	5	9	7
Gold Measure Halves	1 pkg (2 oz)	390	40	5	9	3
Halves	1 oz	190	20	0	4	2
Honey Roasted	1 oz	180	16	75	9	2

FOOD	PORTION	CAL.	FAT	SOD.	CARB.	FIB.
Planters (CONT.)						
Pieces	1 pkg (2 oz)	390	40	5	9	3
Pieces	1 oz	190	20	0	4	2
dried	1 oz	190	19	0	5	2
dry roasted	1 oz	187	18	0	6	—
dry roasted salted	1 oz	187	18	260	6	—
halves dried	1 cup	721	73	1	20	7
oil roasted	1 oz	195	20	0	5	—
oil roasted salted	1 oz	195	20	252	5	—
PECTIN						
Certo	1 tbsp	2	0	—	—	—
Slim Set	1 pkg	208	0	42	44	14
Slim Set	1 tbsp	3	0	1	1	tr
Sure-Jell	¼ pkg	38	0	—	—	—
Light	¼ pkg	33	0	—	—	—
powder	1 pkg (1.75 oz)	163	tr	100	45	—
powder	¼ pkg (0.4 oz)	39	0	24	11	—
PEPPER						
Ac'cent						
Lemon	½ tsp	0	0	0	0	0
Seasoned	½ tsp	0	0	0	0	0
Lawry's						
Lemon	1 tsp	6	tr	340	1	tr
Watkins						
Black	¼ tbsp (0.5 g)	0	0	0	0	0
Cajun	¼ tbsp (0.5 g)	0	0	25	0	0
Cracked Black	¼ tbsp (0.5 g)	0	0	0	0	0
Dijon	¼ tbsp (0.5 g)	0	0	15	0	0
Garlic Peppercorn Blend	¼ tbsp (1 g)	0	0	0	0	0
Herb	¼ tbsp (0.5 g)	0	0	0	0	0
Italian	¼ tbsp (0.5 g)	0	0	0	0	0
Lemon	¼ tbsp (1 g)	0	0	55	0	0
Mexican	¼ tbsp (0.5 g)	0	0	0	0	0
Red Pepper Flakes	¼ tsp (0.5 oz)	0	0	0	0	0
Royal Pepper Blend	¼ tbsp (0.5 g)	0	0	0	0	0
black	1 tsp	5	tr	1	1	—
cayenne	1 tsp	6	tr	1	1	—
red	1 tsp	6	tr	1	1	—
white	1 tsp	7	tr	tr	2	—
PEPPERS						
CANNED						
Chi-Chi's						
Chilies Diced Green	2 tbsp (1.2 oz)	10	0	5	1	0

FOOD	PORTION	CAL.	FAT	SOD.	CARB.	FIB.
Chi-Chi's (CONT.)						
Chilies Green Whole	¾ pepper (1 oz)	10	0	5	1	0
Jalapenos Green Wheels	1 oz	10	0	110	1	0
Jalapenos Green Whole	1 oz	10	0	110	2	0
Jalapenos Red Wheels	1 oz	10	0	110	1	0
Jalapenos Red Whole	1 oz	15	0	110	3	0
Del Monte						
Chilpotle In Spice Sauce	2 tbsp (1.1 oz)	20	1	430	4	1
Hot Chili	4 (1 oz)	10	0	610	3	tr
Jalapeno Nacho Pickled Sliced	2 tbsp (1 oz)	5	0	340	1	tr
Jalapeno Pickled Sliced	2 tbsp (1.1 oz)	5	0	530	1	tr
Jalapeno Pickled Whole	2 tbsp (1.1 oz)	5	0	560	1	tr
Jalapeno Whole	1 (0.7 oz)	3	0	230	tr	tr
Hebrew National						
Filet	¼ pepper (1 oz)	9	0	310	2	—
Hot Cherry	⅓ pepper (1 oz)	11	0	270	2	—
Red Filet	¼ pepper (1 oz)	9	0	310	2	—
McIlhenny						
Jalapeno Nacho Slices	12 slices (1.1 oz)	7	tr	70	1	1
Old El Paso						
Green Chilies Chopped	2 tbsp	5	0	110	1	1
Green Chilies Whole	1	10	0	230	1	1
Jalapenos Peeled	3	10	0	200	1	1
Jalapenos Slices	2 tbsp	15	0	400	1	1
Progresso						
Hot Cherry	½ cup	190	20	130	3	—
Hot Cherry Pickled	½ cup	130	12	110	3	—
Piccalilli	½ cup	190	20	220	4	—
Roasted	½ cup	20	tr	2	5	2
Sweet Fried	½ jar	37	tr	17	4	1
Tuscan	½ cup	20	0	5	7	—
Rosoff's						
Sweet	¼ pepper (1 oz)	9	0	310	2	—
Schorr's						
Filet Peppers	1 oz	9	0	310	2	—
Trappey						
Banana Mild	3 peppers (1 oz)	6	tr	100	1	1
Banana Sliced Rings	21 slices (1 oz)	6	tr	529	1	1
Cherry Hot	2 peppers (1 oz)	7	tr	373	1	1
Cherry Mild	2 peppers (1 oz)	10	tr	225	2	1
Dulcito Italian Pepperoncini	4 peppers (1 oz)	8	tr	178	2	1
In Vinegar Hot	15 peppers (1 oz)	9	tr	573	2	tr

FOOD	PORTION	CAL.	FAT	SOD.	CARB.	FIB.
Trappey (CONT.)						
Jalapeno Hot Sliced	21 slices (1 oz)	4	tr	296	1	1
Jalapeno Whole	2 peppers (1 oz)	11	0	658	2	1
Serano	7 peppers (1 oz)	7	tr	37	1	tr
Tempero Golden Greek Pepperoncini	4 peppers (1 oz)	7	tr	470	1	1
Torrido Santa Fe Grande	3 peppers (1 oz)	10	tr	492	2	tr
Vlasic						
Hot Banana Pepper Rings	1 oz	4	0	465	1	—
Hot Cherry	1 oz	10	0	425	2	—
Jalapeno Mexican Hot	1 oz	8	0	380	2	—
Mexican Tiny Hot	1 oz	6	0	430	2	—
Mild Cherry	1 oz	8	0	410	2	—
Mild Greek Pepperoncini Salad Peppers	1 oz	4	0	450	1	—
chili green hot	1 (2.6 oz)	18	tr	—	4	—
chili green hot chopped	½ cup	17	tr	—	4	—
chili red hot	1 (2.6 oz)	18	tr	—	4	—
chili red hot chopped	½ cup	17	tr	—	4	—
green halves	½ cup	13	tr	958	3	—
jalapeno chopped	½ cup	17	tr	995	3	—
red halves	½ cup	13	tr	958	3	—
DRIED						
green	1 tbsp	1	tr	1	tr	—
red	1 tbsp	1	tr	1	tr	—
FRESH						
Dole						
Bell	1 med	25	1	0	5	2
chili green hot raw	1	18	tr	3	4	—
chili green hot raw chopped	½ cup	30	tr	5	7	—
chili red hot raw	1 (1.6 oz)	18	tr	3	4	—
chili red raw chopped	½ cup	30	tr	5	7	—
green chopped cooked	½ cup	19	tr	1	5	—
green cooked	1 (2.6 oz)	20	tr	1	5	—
green raw	1 (2.6 oz)	20	tr	1	5	1
green raw chopped	½ cup	13	tr	1	3	1
red chopped cooked	½ cup	19	tr	1	5	—
red cooked	1 (2.6 oz)	20	tr	1	5	—
red raw	1 (2.6 oz)	20	tr	1	5	1
red raw chopped	½ cup	13	tr	1	3	1
yellow raw	1 (6.5 oz)	50	tr	3	12	—
yellow raw	10 strips	14	tr	1	3	—

FOOD	PORTION	CAL.	FAT	SOD.	CARB.	FIB.
FROZEN						
Old El Paso						
Jalapenos Pickled	2	5	0	380	1	—
Southland						
Green Diced	2 oz	10	0	—	—	—
Sweet Red & Green Cut	2 oz	15	0	—	—	—
green chopped not prep	1 oz	6	tr	1	1	—
red chopped	1 oz	6	tr	1	1	—
PERCH						
FRESH						
cooked	1 fillet (1.6 oz)	54	1	36	0	—
cooked	3 oz	99	1	67	0	—
ocean perch atlantic cooked	1 fillet (1.8 oz)	60	1	48	0	—
ocean perch atlantic cooked	3 oz	103	2	82	0	—
ocean perch atlantic raw	3 oz	80	1	64	0	—
raw	3 oz	77	1	52	0	—
red raw	3½ oz	114	4	80	0	—
FROZEN						
Gorton's						
Fishmarket Fresh Ocean Perch	5 oz	140	3	100	2	—
Van De Kamp's						
Battered	2 pieces	310	21	500	18	—
Ocean Perch Light Fillets	1 piece	280	14	450	21	—
Ocean Perch Natural Fillets	4 oz	130	5	65	0	—
PERSIMMONS						
Sonoma						
Dried	6-8 pieces (1.4 oz)	140	0	10	35	3
dried japanese	1	93	tr	1	25	—
fresh	1	32	tr	0	8	—
fresh japanese	1	118	tr	3	31	—
PHEASANT						
breast w/o skin raw	½ breast (6.4 oz)	243	6	60	0	—
leg w/o skin raw	1 (3.6 oz)	143	5	48	0	—
w/ skin raw	½ pheasant (14 oz)	723	37	161	0	—
w/o skin raw	½ pheasant (12.4 oz)	470	13	131	0	—
PHYLLO DOUGH						
Ekizian						
	½ lb	865	17	573	151	—

FOOD	PORTION	CAL.	FAT	SOD.	CARB.	FIB.
phyllo dough	1 oz	85	2	137	15	—
sheet	1	57	1	92	10	—

PICKLES

Claussen
Bread 'N Butter Slices	1 slice	7	tr	—	—	—
Dill Spears	1 spear	4	tr	—	—	—
Kosher Halves	1 half	9	tr	—	—	—
Kosher Slices	1 slice	1	tr	—	—	—
Kosher Whole	1	9	tr	—	—	—
No Garlic Dills	1	17	tr	—	—	—

Del Monte
Dill Halves	¼ pickle (1 oz)	5	0	370	tr	tr
Dill Hamburger Chips	5 pieces (1 oz)	5	0	310	1	0
Dill Sweet Chips	5 pieces (1 oz)	40	0	210	10	tr
Dill Sweet Gherkin	2 pickles (1 oz)	40	0	210	10	tr
Dill Sweet Midgets	3 pickles (1 oz)	40	0	210	10	tr
Dill Sweet Whole	2 pickles (1 oz)	40	0	210	10	tr
Dill Tiny Kosher	1½ pickles (1 oz)	5	0	240	1	tr
Dill Whole Pickles	1½ pickles (1 oz)	5	0	370	tr	tr

Hebrew National
Half Sour	½ pickle (1 oz)	4	0	210	1	—
Kosher	⅓ pickle (1 oz)	4	0	260	1	—
Kosher Barrel Cured Dill	1 pkg	23	0	1570	4	—
Kosher Barrel Cured Hot Dill	1 pkg	23	0	1570	4	—
Kosher Chips	3 slices (1 oz)	4	0	300	1	—
Kosher Halves	⅓ pickle (1 oz)	4	0	290	1	—
Kosher Large	⅕ pickle (1 oz)	4	0	300	1	—
Kosher Spears	½ spear (1 oz)	4	0	260	1	—
Sour Garlic	⅓ pickle (1 oz)	3	0	250	1	—

Mcilhenny
Hot N' Sweet	4 (1 oz)	42	tr	28	10	tr

Rosoff's
Half Sour	⅓ pickle (1 oz)	4	0	210	1	—
Half Sour Spears	½ spear (1 oz)	4	0	200	1	—
Kosher	⅓ pickle (1 oz)	4	0	260	1	—
Kosher Halves	⅓ pickle (1 oz)	4	0	290	1	—

Schorr's
Garlic	⅓ pickle (1 oz)	3	0	250	1	—
Half Sour	½ spear (1 oz)	4	0	200	1	—
Half Sour	⅓ pickle (1 oz)	4	0	210	1	—
Kosher Deli	½ pickle (1 oz)	4	0	160	1	—
Kosher Halves	⅓ pickle (1 oz)	4	0	290	1	—

FOOD	PORTION	CAL.	FAT	SOD.	CARB.	FIB.
Schorr's (CONT.)						
Kosher Spears	½ spear (1 oz)	4	0	260	1	—
Kosher Whole	⅓ pickle (1 oz)	4	0	260	1	—
Vlasic						
Bread & Butter Chips	1 oz	30	0	160	7	—
Bread & Butter Chunks	1 oz	25	0	120	6	—
Bread & Butter Stixs	1 oz	18	0	110	5	—
Deli Bread & Butter	1 oz	25	0	120	6	—
Deli Dill Halves	1 oz	4	0	290	1	—
Half-The-Salt Hamburger Dill Chips	1 oz	2	0	175	1	—
Half-The-Salt Kosher Crunchy Dills	1 oz	4	0	125	1	—
Half-The-Salt Kosher Dill Spears	1 oz	4	0	120	1	—
Half-The-Salt Sweet Butter Chips	1 oz	30	0	80	7	—
Hot & Spicy Garden Mix	1 oz	4	0	380	1	—
Kosher Baby Dills	1 oz	4	0	210	1	—
Kosher Crunchy Dills	1 oz	4	0	210	1	—
Kosher Dill Gherkins	1 oz	4	0	210	1	—
Kosher Dill Spears	1 oz	4	0	175	1	—
Kosher Snack Chunks	1 oz	4	0	220	1	—
No Garlic Dill Spears	1 oz	4	0	210	1	—
Original Dills	1 oz	2	0	375	1	—
Polish Snack Chunk Dills	1 oz	4	0	300	1	—
Zesty Crunchy Dills	1 oz	4	0	250	1	—
Zesty Dill Snack Chunks	1 oz	4	0	290	1	—
Zesty Dill Spears	1 oz	4	0	230	1	—
dill	1 (2.3 oz)	12	tr	833	3	—
dill low sodium	1 (2.3 oz)	12	tr	12	3	1
dill low sodium sliced	1 slice	1	tr	1	tr	tr
dill sliced	1 slice	1	tr	77	tr	tr
gerkins	3½ oz	21	tr	960	4	—
kosher dill	1 (2.3 oz)	12	tr	833	3	1
polish dill	1 (2.3 oz)	12	tr	833	3	1
quick sour	1 (1.2 oz)	4	tr	423	1	—
quick sour low sodium	1 (1.2 oz)	4	tr	6	1	—
quick sour sliced	1 slice	1	tr	85	tr	—
sweet	1 (1.2 oz)	41	tr	328	11	tr
sweet gherkin	1 sm (½ oz)	20	tr	107	5	—
sweet low sodium	1 (1.2 oz)	41	tr	6	11	tr
sweet sliced	1 slice	7	tr	56	2	tr

FOOD	PORTION	CAL.	FAT	SOD.	CARB.	FIB.
PIE						
(*see also* PIE CRUST)						
CANNED FILLING						
Libby						
Pumpkin Pie Mix	½ cup	100	0	150	25	2
None Such						
Mincemeat Condensed	¼ pkg	220	2	310	50	—
Mincemeat Ready-to-Use	⅓ cup	200	1	360	48	—
Mincemeat Ready-to-Use With Brandy & Rum	⅓ cup	220	2	260	48	—
S&W						
Mincemeat Old Fashioned	½ cup	206	2	206	49	—
apple	⅛ can (2.6 oz)	74	tr	32	19	1
apple	1 can (21 oz)	599	1	259	156	6
cherry	1 can (21 oz)	683	1	54	175	—
cherry	⅛ can (2.6 oz)	85	tr	7	22	—
pumpkin pie mix	1 cup	282	tr	561	71	—
FROZEN						
Banquet						
Apple	⅕ pie (4 oz)	300	13	370	41	2
Banana Cream	⅓ pie (4.7 oz)	350	21	290	39	1
Cherry	⅕ pie (4 oz)	290	14	310	39	2
Chocolate Cream	⅓ pie (4.7 oz)	360	20	240	43	3
Coconut Cream	⅓ pie (4.7 oz)	350	20	250	39	2
Lemon Cream	⅓ pie (4.7 oz)	360	20	240	43	2
Mincemeat	⅕ pie (4 oz)	310	13	430	46	2
Peach	⅕ pie (4 oz)	260	12	340	36	2
Pumpkin	⅙ pie (4 oz)	250	8	340	40	3
Kineret						
Apple Homestyle	⅙ pie (4 oz)	313	16	175	41	1
McMillin's						
Apple	4 oz	430	23	340	51	—
Berry	4 oz	430	23	410	52	—
Cherry	4 oz	430	24	350	51	—
Chocolate Pudding	4 oz	420	21	350	54	—
Coconut Pudding	4 oz	450	26	420	50	—
Lemon	4 oz	450	25	330	52	—
Peach	4 oz	430	24	370	52	—
Strawberry	4 oz	400	20	370	50	—
Mrs. Smith's						
Apple	⅒ of 10 in pie (4.6 oz)	280	12	310	43	1

FOOD	PORTION	CAL.	FAT	SOD.	CARB.	FIB.
Mrs. Smith's (CONT.)						
Apple	1/8 of 9 in pie (4.6 oz)	370	18	430	50	2
Apple	1/6 of 8 in pie (4.3 oz)	270	11	300	41	1
Apple Cranberry	1/6 of 8 in pie (4.3 oz)	280	11	290	43	1
Apple Lattice Ready To Serve	1/5 of 8 in pie (4.6 oz)	310	13	350	45	2
Banana Cream	1/4 of 8 in pie (3.4 oz)	250	9	170	40	1
Berry	1/6 of 8 in pie (4.3 oz)	280	11	340	44	0
Blackberry	1/6 of 8 in pie (4.3 oz)	280	11	320	43	1
Blueberry	1/6 of 8 in pie	260	11	320	39	1
Boston Cream	1/8 of 8 in pie (2.4 oz)	170	5	140	29	0
Cherry	1/10 of 10 in pie (4.6 oz)	410	18	—	—	—
Cherry	1/8 of 9 in pie (4.6 oz)	320	13	350	48	1
Cherry	1/6 of 8 in pie	270	11	320	41	1
Cherry Lattice Ready To Serve	1/5 of 8 in pie (4.6 oz)	320	13	340	47	1
Chocolate Cream	1/4 of 8 in pie (3.4 oz)	290	14	180	37	1
Coconut Cream	1/4 of 8 in pie (3.4 oz)	280	14	160	36	0
Coconut Custard	1/5 of 8 in pie (5 oz)	280	12	350	35	0
Dutch Apple	1/10 of 10 in pie (4.6 oz)	320	12	270	50	1
Dutch Apple	1/6 of 8 in pie	310	13	270	48	1
Dutch Apple	1/9 of 9 in pie (4.5 oz)	300	12	240	48	2
French Silk Cream	1/5 of 8 in pie (4.8 oz)	410	21	250	55	1
Hearty Pumpkin	1/5 of 8 in pie (5.2 oz)	280	10	350	46	2
Lemon Cream	1/4 of 8 in pie (3.4 oz)	270	13	150	36	0
Lemon Meringue	1/5 of 8 in pie (4.8 oz)	300	8	220	54	0

FOOD	PORTION	CAL.	FAT	SOD.	CARB.	FIB.
Mrs. Smith's (CONT.)						
Mince	⅙ of 8 in pie (4.3 oz)	300	11	400	48	2
Peach	⅙ of 8 in pie	260	11	310	38	1
Peach	⅛ of 9 in pie (4.6 oz)	310	13	350	46	1
Pecan	⅛ of 10 in pie (4.5 oz)	500	23	460	68	1
Pumpkin	⅕ of 8 in pie (5.2 oz)	270	8	350	44	1
Pumpkin	⅛ of 10 in pie (5.1 oz)	250	8	330	42	1
Red Raspberry	⅙ of 8 in pie (4.3 oz)	280	11	310	43	0
Strawberry Rhubarb	⅕ of 8 in pie (4.8 oz)	520	23	450	73	1
Strawberry Rhubarb	⅙ of 8 in pie (4.3 oz)	280	11	380	44	0
Pepperidge Farm						
Hyannis Boston Cream Pie	1	230	10	125	34	2
Mississippi Mud	1	310	23	45	23	—
Pet-Ritz						
Apple	⅙ pie (4.33 oz)	330	12	385	53	—
Banana Cream	⅙ pie (2.33 oz)	170	9	155	22	—
Blueberry	⅙ pie (4.33 oz)	370	12	330	50	—
Cherry	⅙ pie (4.33 oz)	300	12	330	48	—
Chocolate Cream	⅙ pie (2.33 oz)	190	8	145	27	—
Coconut Cream	⅙ pie (2.33 oz)	190	8	145	27	—
Egg Custard	⅙ pie (4.0 oz)	200	8	—	28	—
Lemon Cream	⅙ pie (2.33 oz)	190	9	150	26	—
Mince	⅙ pie (4.33 oz)	280	9	—	48	—
Neapolitan Cream	⅙ pie (2.33 oz)	180	10	185	17	—
Peach	⅙ pie (4.33 oz)	320	12	320	51	—
Pumpkin Custard	⅙ pie (4.33 oz)	250	9	—	39	—
Strawberry Cream	⅙ pie (2.33 oz)	170	9	145	20	—
Sweet Potato	⅙ pie (3.33 oz)	150	7	110	21	—
Sara Lee						
Apple Homestyle	1 slice (4 oz)	280	12	220	42	—
Apple Homestyle High	1 slice (4.9 oz)	400	23	450	46	—
Apple Streusel Free & Light	1 slice (2.9 oz)	170	2	140	36	—
Blueberry Homestyle	1 slice (4 oz)	300	12	210	45	—
Cherry Homestyle	1 slice (4 oz)	270	13	270	37	—

FOOD	PORTION	CAL.	FAT	SOD.	CARB.	FIB.
Sara Lee (CONT.)						
Cherry Streusel Free & Light	1 slice (3.6 oz)	160	2	140	34	—
Dutch Apple Homestyle	1 slice (4 oz)	300	12	310	45	—
Mince Homestyle	1 slice (4 oz)	300	13	340	43	—
Peach Homestyle	1 slice (3.4 oz)	280	12	170	41	—
Pecan Homestyle	1 slice (3.4 oz)	400	18	290	56	—
Pumpkin Homestyle	1 slice (4 oz)	240	10	250	34	—
Raspberry Homestyle	1 slice (4 oz)	280	13	150	39	—
Weight Watchers						
Apple	1 slice (3.5 oz)	165	4	90	30	—
Chocolate Mocha	1 (2.75 oz)	180	4	150	30	—
apple	⅛ of 9 in pie (4.4 oz)	297	14	333	43	2
blueberry	⅛ of 9 in pie (4.4 oz)	289	13	406	44	—
cherry	⅛ of 9 in pie (4.4 oz)	325	14	308	50	1
chocolate creme	⅙ of 8 in pie (4 oz)	344	22	153	38	—
coconut creme	⅙ of 7 in pie (2.2 oz)	191	11	163	24	1
lemon meringue	⅙ of 8 in pie (4.5 oz)	303	10	165	53	1
peach	⅙ of 8 in pie (4.1 oz)	261	12	316	39	—
HOME RECIPE						
apple	⅛ of 9 in pie (5.4 oz)	411	19	327	58	3
banana cream	⅛ of 9 in pie (5.2 oz)	398	20	355	49	—
blueberry	⅛ of 9 in pie (5.2 oz)	360	18	272	49	—
butterscotch	⅛ of 9 in pie (4.5 oz)	355	18	335	42	—
cherry	⅛ of 9 in pie (6.3 oz)	486	22	343	69	—
coconut creme	⅛ of 9 in pie (4.7 oz)	396	21	356	46	—
custard	⅛ of 9 in pie (4.5 oz)	262	11	256	34	2
lemon meringue	⅛ of 9 in pie (4.5 oz)	362	16	307	50	2
mince	⅛ of 9 in pie (5.8 oz)	477	18	419	79	—

FOOD	PORTION	CAL.	FAT	SOD.	CARB.	FIB.
pecan	⅛ of 9 in pie (4.3 oz)	502	27	320	64	4
pumpkin	⅛ of 9 in pie (5.4 oz)	316	14	349	41	4
vanilla cream	⅛ of 9 in pie (4.4 oz)	350	18	327	41	—
MIX						
Betty Crocker						
Boston Cream Classic Dessert	⅛ pie	270	6	390	50	—
Jell-O						
Banana Cream as prep w/ whole milk	⅛ of 8 in pie	103	3	161	18	—
Chocolate Cream Pie No Bake Dessert	⅛ pie	260	17	—	—	—
Chocolate Mousse	⅛ pie	259	17	426	25	—
Coconut Cream	⅛ pie	258	16	304	27	—
Coconut Cream as prep w/ whole milk	⅛ of 8 in pie	111	4	140	16	—
Lemon	⅛ of 8 in pie	175	2	95	38	—
Pumpkin	⅛ pie	253	13	448	31	—
Royal						
Key Lime Pie Filling	mix for 1 serving	50	0	120	13	—
Lemon Pie Filling	mix for 1 serving	50	0	120	13	0
Lemon Meringue No-Bake	⅛ pie	210	5	170	38	—
banana cream no-bake	⅛ of 9 in pie (3.2 oz)	231	12	267	29	—
chocolate mousse no-bake	⅛ of 9 in pie (3.3 oz)	247	15	437	28	—
coconut creme no-bake	⅛ of 9 in pie (3.3 oz)	259	17	309	27	—
READY-TO-EAT						
Entenmann's						
Apple Homestyle	1 serving (2.1 oz)	140	7	150	21	—
Coconut Custard	1 serving (1.8 oz)	140	8	160	16	—
SNACK						
Drake's						
Apple	1 (2 oz)	210	10	135	29	—
Blueberry	1 (2 oz)	210	10	135	30	—
Cherry	1 (2 oz)	220	10	135	30	—
Lemon	1 (2 oz)	210	11	115	27	—
Lance						
Pecan	1 (38 g)	350	15	70	51	—

FOOD	PORTION	CAL.	FAT	SOD.	CARB.	FIB.
Little Debbie						
Marshmallow Banana	1 pkg (1.4 oz)	160	5	95	27	0
Marshmallow Banana	1 pkg (2 oz)	240	8	140	40	0
Marshmallow Banana	1 pkg (2.7 oz)	320	11	190	54	0
Marshmallow Chocolate	1 pkg (2.7 oz)	320	11	190	53	1
Marshmallow Chocolate	1 pkg (1.4 oz)	160	5	95	27	1
Marshmallow Chocolate	1 pkg (2 oz)	240	9	135	40	1
Oatmeal Creme	1 pkg (1.3 oz)	170	8	200	25	1
Oatmeal Creme	1 pkg (2.5 oz)	300	11	330	48	1
Oatmeal Creme	1 pkg (3 oz)	360	14	400	58	2
Raisin Creme	1 pkg (1.2 oz)	140	5	120	23	1
Raisin Creme	1 pkg (2.5 oz)	290	12	240	47	0
Tastykake						
Apple	1 pkg (113 g)	300	12	340	46	2
Banana Creme	1 pkg (120 g)	380	16	430	54	2
Blueberry	1 pkg (113 g)	310	9	410	55	2
Cherry	1 pkg (113 g)	300	10	310	49	2
Coconut Creme	1 pkg (113 g)	380	20	420	46	2
French Apple	1 pkg (120 g)	350	11	220	63	2
Lemon	1 pkg (113 g)	320	13	380	48	2
Lemon Lime	1 pkg (113 g)	320	13	310	49	1
Peach	1 pkg (113 g)	300	12	360	47	—
Pineapple Cheese	1 pkg (120 g)	340	13	410	54	2
Pumpkin	1 pkg (4 oz)	320	14	520	46	2
Strawberry	1 pkg (113 g)	340	11	300	57	1
Tasty Klair	1 pkg (113 g)	400	20	320	51	2
apple	1 (3 oz)	266	14	325	33	—
apple fried	1 (6.4 oz)	404	21	479	55	3
blueberry fried	1 (6.4 oz)	404	21	479	55	3
cherry	1 (3 oz)	266	14	325	33	—
cherry fried	1 (6.4 oz)	404	21	479	55	3
lemon	1 (3 oz)	266	14	325	33	—
lemon fried	1 (6.4 oz)	404	21	479	55	3
peach fried	1 (6.4 oz)	404	21	479	55	3
strawberry fried	1 (6.4 oz)	404	21	479	55	3
TAKE-OUT						
coconut custard	⅛ of 8 in pie (3.6 oz)	271	14	348	32	—
custard	⅙ pie 9 in	330	17	436	36	—
pecan	⅛ of 8 in pie (4 oz)	452	21	480	65	4
pumpkin	⅛ of 8 in pie (3.8 oz)	229	10	308	30	3

FOOD	PORTION	CAL.	FAT	SOD.	CARB.	FIB.
PIE CRUST						
(see also PIE*)*						
FROZEN						
Oronoque	⅙ pie (1.23 oz)	170	12	170	14	—
Deep Dish	⅙ pie (1.41 oz)	200	13	200	16	—
Pepperidge Farm						
Patty Shells	1	210	15	180	16	—
Puff Pastry Sheets	¼ sheet	260	17	290	22	—
Pet-Ritz						
Deep Dish	⅙ pie (1 oz)	130	8	120	12	—
Graham Cracker	⅙ pie (0.83 oz)	110	6	80	8	—
Regular	⅙ pie (0.83 oz)	110	7	110	11	—
Tart Shells	1	150	10	150	12	—
baked	⅛ of 9 in pie (0.6 oz)	82	5	104	8	—
baked	9 in shell (4.4 oz)	647	41	815	63	—
puff pastry baked	1 shell (1.4 oz)	223	15	101	18	—
HOME RECIPE						
9-inch crust	1	900	60	1100	79	—
baked	9 in shell (6.3 oz)	949	62	975	86	—
baked	⅛ 9 in crust (0.8 oz)	119	8	122	11	—
MIX						
Betty Crocker	¹⁄₁₆ pkg	120	8	140	10	—
Sticks	¹⁄₁₆ pkg	120	8	140	10	—
Jiffy						
As prep	⅐ crust	180	10	250	19	tr
Pillsbury						
Mix	⅙ of 2 crust pie	270	17	420	25	—
Stick	⅙ of a 2 crust pie	270	17	420	25	—
as prep	9 in crust (5.6 oz)	801	49	1167	81	—
as prep	⅛ of 9 in pie (0.7 oz)	100	6	146	10	—
READY-TO-EAT						
Generic Label						
Graham	⅛ pie (0.7 oz)	110	5	110	14	1
Honey Maid						
Graham	⅙ crust (1 oz)	140	7	125	18	tr
Nabisco						
Nilla	⅙ crust (1 oz)	140	8	65	18	0
Oreo						
Crumb Crust	⅙ crust (1 oz)	140	11	180	18	tr
Ready Crust						
Chocolate	1 (3 in diam)	110	5	135	15	—

FOOD	PORTION	CAL.	FAT	SOD.	CARB.	FIB.
Ready Crust (CONT.)						
Chocolate	⅛ pie 9 in	100	5	120	14	—
Graham	⅛ pie 9 in	100	5	130	13	—
Graham	1 (3 in diam)	110	5	145	15	—
chocolate cookie crumb baked	9 in crust (7.7 oz)	1130	69	1502	122	—
chocolate cookie crumb baked	⅛ of 9 in pie (1 oz)	139	9	185	15	—
chocolate cookie crumb chilled	⅛ of 9 in pie (1 oz)	142	9	188	15	—
chocolate cookie crumb chilled	9 in crust (7.8 oz)	1127	69	1499	121	—
graham cracker baked	⅛ of 9 in pie (1 oz)	148	8	171	20	—
graham cracker baked	9 in crust (8.4 oz)	1181	60	1365	156	—
graham cracker chilled	⅛ of 9 in pie (1 oz)	150	8	173	20	—
graham cracker chilled	9 in crust (8.6 oz)	1182	60	1365	155	—
vanilla wafer cracker crumbs baked	9 in crust (6.1 oz)	937	64	909	89	—
vanilla wafer cracker crumbs baked	⅛ of 9 in pie (0.8 oz)	119	8	116	11	—
vanilla wafer cracker crumbs chilled	⅛ of 9 in pie (0.8 oz)	117	8	113	11	—
vanilla wafer cracker crumbs chilled	9 in crust (6.2 oz)	934	64	906	88	—
REFRIGERATED						
Pillsbury						
All Ready	⅛ of 2 crust pie	240	15	200	24	—
PIEROGI						
FROZEN						
Empire						
Potato Cheese	3 (4.6 oz)	260	6	200	40	5
Potato Onion	3 (4.6 oz)	250	5	210	43	4
Golden						
Potato Cheese	3 (4 oz)	250	8	260	38	—
Potato Onion	3 (4 oz)	210	6	220	36	—
Mrs. T's						
Potato And Cheddar Cheese	1 (1.3 oz)	60	tr	170	11	—
Potato And Onion	1 (1.3 oz)	50	tr	140	10	—
Sauerkraut	1	60	0	—	—	—
TAKE-OUT						
pierogi	¾ cup (4.4 oz)	307	19	369	24	—
PIGEON						
w/ skin & bone	3.5 oz	169	10	90	0	—

FOOD	PORTION	CAL.	FAT	SOD.	CARB.	FIB.
PIGEON PEAS						
dried cooked	½ cup	102	tr	5	20	—
dried cooked	1 cup	204	1	9	39	—
PIGNOLIA						
(see PINE NUTS)						
PIG'S EARS AND FEET						
Hormel						
Pickled Feet	2 oz	80	6	530	0	0
Pickled Hocks	2 oz	110	8	530	0	0
ears frzn simmered	1 ear (3.7 oz)	183	12	183	0	—
feet pickled	1 oz	58	5	—	tr	—
feet pickled	1 lb	923	73	—	tr	—
feet simmered	2.5 oz	138	9	—	0	—
PIKE						
northern cooked	½ fillet (5.4 oz)	176	1	76	0	—
northern cooked	3 oz	96	1	42	0	—
northern raw	3 oz	75	1	33	0	—
roe raw	3½ oz	130	2	—	2	—
walleye baked	3 oz	101	1	56	0	—
walleye fillet baked	4.4 oz	147	2	81	0	—
PILLNUTS						
canarytree dried	1 oz	204	23	1	1	—
PIMIENTOS						
Dromedary						
canned	1 oz	10	0	5	2	—
canned	1 slice	0	0	0	tr	—
canned	1 tbsp	3	tr	2	1	—
PINE NUTS						
pignolia dried	1 oz	146	14	1	4	—
pignolia dried	1 tbsp	51	5	0	1	—
pinyon dried	1 oz	161	17	20	5	—
PINEAPPLE						
CANNED						
Del Monte						
Chunks In Heavy Syrup	½ cup (4.3 oz)	90	0	10	24	1
Chunks In Its Own Juice	½ cup (4.4 oz)	70	0	5	17	1
Crushed In Heavy Syrup	½ cup (4.4 oz)	90	0	10	24	1
Crushed In Its Own Juice	½ cup (4.3 oz)	70	0	10	17	1
Sliced In Heavy Syrup	½ cup (4.1 oz)	90	0	10	23	1
Sliced In Its Own Juice	½ cup (4 oz)	60	0	10	16	1
Snack Cups Tidbits In Juice	1 serv (4.5 oz)	70	0	10	18	1

FOOD	PORTION	CAL.	FAT	SOD.	CARB.	FIB.
Del Monte (CONT.)						
Snack Cups Tidbits In Juice EZ-Open Lid	1 serv (4.2 oz)	60	0	10	17	1
Spears In Its Own Juice	½ cup (4.3 oz)	70	0	5	17	1
Tidbits In Its Own Juice	½ cup (4.3 oz)	70	0	5	17	1
Wedges In Its Own Juice	½ cup (4.3 oz)	70	0	5	17	1
Dole						
All Cuts Juice Pack	½ cup	70	tr	10	18	—
All Cuts Syrup Pack	½ cup	90	0	10	23	—
Empress						
Chunk	4 oz	70	0	—	18	—
Crushed	4 oz	70	0	—	18	—
Sliced	4 oz	70	0	—	18	—
Libby						
Crushed	1 cup with juice	140	0	10	35	—
Sliced In Unsweetened Juice	1 cup with juice	140	0	<10	35	—
S&W						
Hawaiian Slice In Heavy Syrup	½ cup	90	0	0	23	—
Hawaiian Slice Juice Pack	½ cup	70	0	10	17	—
Sliced Unsweetened	½ cup	60	0	10	15	—
chunks in heavy syrup	1 cup	199	tr	3	52	—
chunks juice pack	1 cup	150	tr	4	39	—
crushed in heavy syrup	1 cup	199	tr	3	52	—
slices in heavy syrup	1 slice	45	tr	1	12	—
slices in light syrup	1 slice	30	tr	1	8	—
slices juice pack	1 slice	35	tr	1	9	—
slices water pack	1 slice	19	tr	1	5	—
tidbits in heavy syrup	1 cup	199	tr	3	52	—
tidbits in juice	1 cup	150	tr	4	19	—
tidbits in water	1 cup	79	tr	3	20	—
DRIED						
Sonoma						
Pieces	2 pieces (1.4 oz)	140	2	30	30	2
FRESH						
Chiquita						
Fresh	1 cup	90	1	—	—	—
diced	1 cup	77	tr	1	19	2
slice	1 slice	42	tr	1	10	1
FROZEN						
chunks sweetened	½ cup	104	tr	2	27	—

FOOD	PORTION	CAL.	FAT	SOD.	CARB.	FIB.
PINEAPPLE JUICE						
After The Fall						
Mandarin Pineapple	1 can (12 oz)	150	0	25	37	0
Bright & Early						
Frozen	8 fl oz	120	0	10	30	—
Dole						
100% frzn as prep	8 fl oz	130	0	20	30	0
Chilled	6 fl oz	90	0	5	22	—
Minute Maid						
Box	8.45 fl oz	130	0	25	33	—
Frozen	8 fl oz	110	0	5	28	—
S&W						
Unsweetened	6 oz	100	0	0	25	—
Tree Top						
Juice	6 oz	100	0	0	24	—
Veryfine						
100%	8 oz	125	0	<10	31	—
canned	1 cup	139	tr	2	34	—
frzn as prep	1 cup	129	tr	3	32	—
frzn not prep	6 oz	387	tr	6	96	—
PINK BEANS						
CANNED						
Goya						
Spanish Style	7.5 oz	140	tr	800	32	10
DRIED						
cooked	1 cup	252	1	3	47	—
PINTO BEANS						
CANNED						
Allen	½ cup (4.5 oz)	110	1	290	20	7
Brown Beauty	½ cup (4.5 oz)	110	1	290	20	7
East Texas Fair	½ cup (4.5 oz)	110	1	290	20	7
Eden						
Organic	½ cup (4.4 oz)	90	1	15	17	6
Goya						
Spanish Style	7.5 oz	140	1	860	31	10
Green Giant						
Picante	½ cup	100	1	580	21	6
Luck's						
Seasoned w/ Pork w/ Onions	7.5 oz	220	6	—	—	—
Trappey						
Jalapinto With Bacon	½ cup (4.5 oz)	120	1	540	22	8
With Bacon	½ cup (4.5 oz)	120	1	270	20	7
pinto	1 cup	186	1	998	35	—

FOOD	PORTION	CAL.	FAT	SOD.	CARB.	FIB.
DRIED						
Arrowhead	¼ cup (1.5 oz)	150	1	0	27	8
Bean Cuisine	½ cup	115	1	5	—	5
Hurst						
Pinto Beans	1.2 oz	120	1	5	22	10
With Spanish Seasoning	1.3 oz	120	1	350	22	6
cooked	1 cup	235	1	3	44	—
FROZEN						
cooked	3 oz	152	tr	—	29	—
SPROUTS						
cooked	3½ oz	22	tr	—	4	—
raw	3½ oz	62	1	—	12	—
PINYON						
(*see* PINE NUTS)						
PISTACHIOS						
Dole						
Shelled	1 oz	163	14	—	7	—
Shells On	1 oz	90	7	250	3	—
Fisher						
Red Tint	1 oz	170	15	220	6	—
Lance						
Pistachios	1 pkg (32 g)	100	8	100	4	—
Planters						
Munch'N Go Singles	1 pkg (2 oz)	330	29	450	14	6
Shelled Dry Roasted						
Red Salted Dry Roasted	1 pkg	160	14	250	7	3
Uncolored Dry Roasted	½ cup	160	14	180	7	3
Sonoma						
Salted Shelled	¼ cup (1 oz)	190	14	220	9	3
dried	1 oz	164	14	2	7	3
dried	1 cup	739	62	7	32	14
dry roasted	1 oz	172	15	2	8	—
dry roasted salted	1 oz	172	15	260	8	—
dry roasted salted	1 cup	776	68	1040	35	—
PITANGA						
fresh	1 cup	57	1	5	13	—
fresh	1	2	tr	0	1	—
PIZZA						
DOUGH						
Boboli						
Shell + Sauce	⅛ lg shell (2.6 oz)	170	3	460	28	1
Shell + Sauce	⅙ sm shell (2.6 oz)	170	3	540	29	1

FOOD	PORTION	CAL.	FAT	SOD.	CARB.	FIB.
House of Pasta						
Frozen	⅛ of 14 in pie (1.9 oz)	140	1	140	27	1
Jiffy						
As prep	¼ crust	180	3	264	33	2
Sassafras						
Cornmeal Pizza Crust	1 slice (1.4 oz)	140	0	240	30	1
Italian Pizza Crust Mix	1 slice (1.4 oz)	140	0	135	30	1
Wanda's						
Crust Mix Oregano & Basil	⅒ pie (1.4 oz)	149	0	227	32	1
Crust Mix Oregano & Basil Whole Wheat	⅒ pie (1.4 oz)	141	1	227	30	5
Watkins						
Crust Mix	⅛ pkg (1.8 oz)	180	1	60	36	2
FROZEN						
Celeste						
Italian Bread Deluxe	1 (5.1 oz)	290	11	1000	36	3
Italian Bread Garlic & Herb Zesty Chicken	1 (5 oz)	260	8	960	34	3
Italian Bread Pepperoni	1 (5 oz)	320	13	1140	37	3
Italian Bread Zesty Four Cheese	1 (4.6 oz)	300	12	820	32	3
Large Cheese	¼ pie (4.4 oz)	320	16	590	32	3
Large Deluxe	¼ pie (5.5 oz)	350	18	880	35	4
Large Pepperoni	¼ pie (4.7 oz)	350	20	990	33	3
Large Suprema With Meat	⅕ pie (4.6 oz)	290	16	770	27	3
Large Zesty Four Cheese	¼ pie (4.4 oz)	330	16	610	34	3
Small Cheese	1 (7.5 oz)	540	25	1090	60	4
Small Deluxe	1 (8.2 oz)	540	29	1320	53	6
Small Hot & Zesty Four Cheese	1 (7 oz)	530	27	1090	50	4
Small Original Four Cheese	1 (7 oz)	540	30	1040	47	4
Small Pepperoni	1 (6.7 oz)	520	27	1280	53	4
Small Sausage	1 (7.5 oz)	530	27	1400	52	5
Small Suprema Vegetable	1 (7.5 oz)	480	23	1270	52	5
Small Suprema With Meat	1 (9 oz)	580	31	1480	56	7
Small Zesty Four Cheese	1 (7 oz)	530	27	1090	50	4
Croissant Pocket						
Stuffed Sandwich Pepperoni Pizza	1 piece (4.5 oz)	350	15	870	39	3

FOOD	PORTION	CAL.	FAT	SOD.	CARB.	FIB.
Empire						
3 Pack	1 (3 oz)	210	9	630	23	7
Bagel	1 (2 oz)	150	5	390	15	0
English Muffin	1 (2 oz)	130	5	390	15	1
Fox						
Deluxe Golden Topping	½ pizza	240	11	600	25	—
Deluxe Hamburger	½ pizza	260	12	700	26	—
Deluxe Pepperoni	½ pizza	250	13	640	26	—
Deluxe Sausage	½ pizza	260	13	630	26	—
Deluxe Sausage & Pepperoni	½ pizza	260	13	640	26	—
Healthy Choice						
French Bread Cheese	1 (5.6 oz)	310	4	470	49	6
French Bread Pepperoni	1 (6 oz)	360	9	580	48	5
French Bread Sausage	1 (6 oz)	330	4	470	52	6
French Bread Supreme	1 (6.35 oz)	340	6	510	49	5
Hot Pocket						
Stuffed Sandwich Pepperoni & Sausage Pizza	1 (4.5 oz)	340	16	630	38	3
Stuffed Sandwich Pepperoni Pizza	1 (4.5 oz)	350	17	780	38	2
Jeno's						
4-Pack Cheese	1 pizza	160	8	460	17	—
4-Pack Combination	1 pizza	180	9	470	17	—
4-Pack Hamburger	1 pizza	180	9	500	17	—
4-Pack Pepperoni	1 pizza	170	9	460	17	—
4-Pack Sausage	1 pizza	180	9	460	17	—
Crisp 'n Tasty Canandian Bacon	½ pizza	250	11	880	27	—
Crisp 'n Tasty Cheese	½ pizza	270	14	770	28	—
Crisp 'n Tasty Hamburger	½ pizza	290	15	810	28	—
Crisp 'n Tasty Pepperoni	½ pizza	280	15	760	27	—
Crisp 'n Tasty Sausage	½ pizza	300	16	850	28	—
Crisp 'n Tasty Sausage & Pepperoni	½ pizza	300	16	840	27	—
Microwave Pizza Rolls Pepperoni & Cheese	6	240	13	440	23	—
Microwave Pizza Rolls Sausage & Cheese	6	250	13	440	24	—
Pizza Rolls Cheese	6	240	12	350	23	—
Pizza Rolls Hamburger	6	240	13	280	21	—
Pizza Rolls Pepperoni & Cheese	6	230	13	390	22	—

FOOD	PORTION	CAL.	FAT	SOD.	CARB.	FIB.
Jeno's (CONT.)						
Pizza Rolls Sausage & Pepperoni	6	230	13	380	22	—
Kid Cuisine						
Cheese	1 (8 oz)	430	11	440	71	5
Hamburger	1 (8.30 oz)	400	11	530	61	6
Kineret						
Bagel Pizza	2 (4 oz)	300	10	700	39	1
Lean Cuisine						
French Bread Cheese	1 pkg (6 oz)	350	8	400	48	4
French Bread Deluxe	1 pkg (6.1 oz)	350	6	560	45	5
French Bread Pepperoni	1 pkg (5.25 oz)	330	7	590	46	4
Lean Pockets						
Stuffed Sandwich Pizza Deluxe	1 (4.5 oz)	270	8	680	37	2
MicroMagic						
Deep Dish Combination	1 (6.5 oz)	605	34	1280	60	—
Deep Dish Pepperoni	1 (6.5 oz)	615	32	1300	65	—
Deep Dish Sausage	1 (6.5 oz)	590	31	1250	62	—
Mrs. P's						
Combination	½ pizza	260	13	640	26	—
Golden Topping	½ pizza	240	11	600	25	—
Hamburger	½ pizza	260	12	700	26	—
Pepperoni	½ pizza	250	13	640	26	—
Sausage	½ pizza	260	13	630	26	—
Old El Paso						
Pizza Burrito Cheese	1	320	9	430	27	0
Pizza Burrito Pepperoni	1	260	10	510	31	0
Pizza Burrito Sausage	1	260	9	420	32	0
Pappalo's						
French Bread Cheese	1 pizza	360	15	830	40	—
French Bread Combination	1 pizza	430	21	1120	41	—
French Bread Pepperoni	1 pizza	410	20	1130	41	—
French Bread Sausage	1 pizza	410	18	1000	41	—
Pan Combination	⅙ pizza	340	15	700	34	—
Pan Hamburger	⅙ pizza	310	12	580	34	—
Pan Pepperoni	⅙ pizza	330	14	710	34	—
Pan Sausage	⅙ pizza	360	18	550	34	—
Thin Crust Combination	⅙ pizza	260	10	590	29	—
Thin Crust Hamburger	⅙ pizza	240	8	470	28	—
Thin Crust Pepperoni	⅙ pizza	270	11	600	28	—
Thin Crust Sausage	⅙ pizza	250	9	490	28	—

FOOD	PORTION	CAL.	FAT	SOD.	CARB.	FIB.
Pepperidge Farm						
Croissant Pastry Cheese	1	430	23	640	41	—
Croissant Pastry Deluxe	1	440	23	790	43	—
Croissant Pastry Pepperoni	1	420	22	690	43	—
Pillsbury						
Microwave Cheese	½ pizza	240	10	540	28	—
Microwave Combination	½ pizza	310	15	780	29	—
Microwave French Bread	1 pizza	370	15	680	41	—
Microwave French Bread Pepperoni	1 pizza	430	19	940	46	—
Microwave French Bread Sausage	1 pizza	410	16	860	48	—
Microwave French Bread Sausage & Pepperoni	1 pizza	450	21	950	47	—
Microwave Pepperoni	½ pizza	300	15	790	29	—
Microwave Sausage	½ pizza	280	13	680	29	—
Small World						
Four Cheese	1 (4 oz)	240	6	350	38	1
Special Delivery						
Organic	⅓ pizza (5.3 oz)	320	9	500	46	1
Organic Soy Kaas	⅓ pizza (5.3 oz)	320	7	600	47	1
Stouffer's						
French Bread Bacon Cheddar	1 piece (5.8 oz)	440	22	940	44	4
French Bread Cheese	1 piece (5.2 oz)	350	14	660	42	3
French Bread Cheeseburger	1 piece (6 oz)	440	26	1110	31	5
French Bread Deluxe	1 piece (6.2 oz)	440	22	980	42	5
French Bread Double Cheese	1 piece (5.9 oz)	420	19	790	44	5
French Bread Garden Vegetable	1 piece (5.8 oz)	340	12	540	45	4
French Bread Pepperoni	1 piece (5.6 oz)	420	20	930	42	3
French Bread Pepperoni & Mushroom	1 piece (6.1 oz)	430	21	1000	43	3
French Bread Sausage	1 piece (6 oz)	420	20	900	41	4
French Bread Sausage & Pepperoni	1 piece (6.25 oz)	460	25	1130	45	4
French Bread Vegetable Deluxe	1 piece (6.4 oz)	380	17	830	43	5
French Bread White Pizza	1 piece (5.1 oz)	460	28	760	43	5

FOOD	PORTION	CAL.	FAT	SOD.	CARB.	FIB.
Stouffer's (CONT.)						
Lunch Express Deluxe	1 pkg (6.6 oz)	460	25	1000	40	4
Lunch Express Double Cheese	1 pkg (5.9 oz)	420	19	710	41	3
Lunch Express Pepperoni	1 pkg (5.75 oz)	440	23	960	39	4
Lunch Express Sausage	1 pkg (6.5 oz)	460	25	1090	40	3
Lunch Express Sausage & Pepperoni	1 pkg (6.4 oz)	500	27	1140	41	4
Tombstone						
12 in Canadian Bacon	⅕ pie (5.5 oz)	360	15	920	36	2
12 in Cheese & Hamburger	⅕ pie (4.4 oz)	320	16	660	29	2
12 in Cheese & Pepperoni	⅕ pie (4.4 oz)	340	18	750	29	2
12 in Cheese & Sausage	⅕ pie (4.4 oz)	320	16	650	29	2
12 in Cheese Sausage & Mushroom	⅕ pie (4.5 oz)	320	16	630	29	2
12 in Deluxe	⅕ pie (4.7 oz)	320	16	640	29	2
12 in Extra Cheese	⅕ pie (5.1 oz)	370	17	680	36	2
12 in Sausage & Pepperoni	⅕ pie (4.4 oz)	340	18	740	29	2
12 in Special Order Four Cheese	⅕ pie (5.2 oz)	400	19	760	37	2
12 in Special Order Four Meat	⅙ pie (4.7 oz)	350	18	810	31	2
12 in Special Order Pepperoni	⅙ pie (4.5 oz)	360	19	790	31	2
12 in Special Order Super Supreme	⅙ pie (4.8 oz)	350	18	800	31	2
12 in Special Order Three Sausage	⅙ pie (4.6 oz)	340	17	740	31	2
12 in Supreme	⅕ pie (4.6 oz)	330	17	720	29	2
12 in ThinCrust Italian Style Three Cheese	¼ pie (4.8 oz)	380	22	730	25	2
9 in Cheese & Hamburger	⅓ pie (4.1 oz)	310	16	620	28	2
9 in Cheese & Pepperoni	⅓ pie (4.1 oz)	340	19	740	28	2
9 in Cheese & Sausage	⅓ pie (4.1 oz)	310	16	610	28	2
9 in Deluxe	⅓ pie (4.5 oz)	320	16	620	28	2
9 in Extra Cheese	⅓ pie (5.6 oz)	420	19	730	42	3
9 in Pepperoni & Sausage	⅓ pie (4.4 oz)	360	21	820	28	2
9 in Special Order Four Meat	⅓ pie (5.3 oz)	400	20	910	35	2

FOOD	PORTION	CAL.	FAT	SOD.	CARB.	FIB.
Tombstone (CONT.)						
9 in Special Order Pepperoni	⅓ pie (5.1 oz)	400	21	880	35	2
9 in Special Order Super Supreme	⅓ pie (5.5 oz)	400	21	900	36	2
9 in Special Order Three Sausage	⅓ pie (5.2 oz)	390	19	830	35	2
Double Top Pepperoni With Double Cheese	⅙ pie (4.5 oz)	350	20	850	25	2
Double Top Sausage & Pepperoni With Double Cheese	⅙ pie (4.7 oz)	360	20	800	25	2
Double Top Sausage With Double Cheese	⅙ pie (4.7 oz)	350	19	740	25	2
For One ½ Less Fat Cheese	1 pie (6.5 oz)	360	10	920	45	3
For One ½ Less Fat Pepperoni	1 pie (6.7 oz)	400	13	1040	45	4
For One ½ Less Fat Supreme	1 pie (7.7 oz)	400	13	1090	45	4
For One ½ Less Fat Vegetable	1 pie (7.2 oz)	360	10	730	46	5
For One Cheese & Pepperoni	1 pie (7 oz)	580	35	1170	41	3
For One Extra Cheese	1 pie (7 oz)	540	30	910	41	3
For One Italian Sausage	1 pie (7 oz)	560	33	1130	40	2
For One Sausage & Pepperoni	1 pie (7 oz)	590	37	1200	40	3
For One Supreme	1 pie (7.5 oz)	570	34	1130	41	3
Light Supreme	⅕ pie (4.8 oz)	270	9	710	30	3
Light Vegetable	⅕ pie (4.6 oz)	240	7	500	31	3
ThinCrust Italian Style Four Meat Combo	¼ pie (5.1 oz)	410	25	940	25	2
ThinCrust Italian Style Pepperoni	¼ pie (5 oz)	420	27	950	25	2
ThinCrust Italian Style Sausage	¼ pie (5.1 oz)	400	24	880	25	2
ThinCrust Italian Style Supreme	¼ pie (5.3 oz)	400	24	880	26	2
ThinCrust Mexican Style Supreme Taco	¼ pie (5.1 oz)	380	23	850	26	2
Totino's						
Microwave Cheese	1 pizza	250	8	760	34	—
Microwave Pepperoni	1 pizza	280	12	880	34	—

FOOD	PORTION	CAL.	FAT	SOD.	CARB.	FIB.
Totino's (CONT.)						
Microwave Sausage	1 pizza	320	16	870	33	—
Microwave Sausage Pepperoni Combination	1 pizza	310	15	970	31	—
My Classic Deluxe Cheese	⅙ pizza	210	9	420	23	—
My Classic Deluxe Combination	⅙ pizza	270	14	630	23	—
My Classic Deluxe Pepperoni	⅙ pizza	260	13	630	23	—
Pan Pepperoni	⅙ pizza	330	14	730	34	—
Pan Sausage	⅙ pizza	320	13	630	34	—
Pan Sausage & Pepperoni Combination	⅙ pizza	340	15	720	34	—
Pan Three Cheese	⅙ pizza	290	10	510	33	—
Party Bacon	½ pizza	370	20	1030	35	—
Party Canadian Bacon	½ pizza	310	14	1150	35	—
Party Cheese	½ pizza	340	17	1000	34	—
Party Combination	½ pizza	380	21	1230	35	—
Party Hamburger	½ pizza	370	19	1060	35	—
Party Mexican Style	½ pizza	380	21	970	35	—
Party Pepperoni	½ pizza	370	20	1310	35	—
Party Sausage	½ pizza	390	21	1180	35	—
Party Vegetable	½ pizza	300	13	910	36	—
Slices Cheese	1	170	7	350	20	—
Slices Combination	1	200	10	630	20	—
Slices Pepperoni	1	190	9	530	20	—
Slices Sausage	1	200	10	540	20	—
Weight Watchers						
Cheese	1 (6.03 oz)	300	7	310	36	—
Deluxe Combination	1 (7.32 oz)	320	9	370	36	—
Deluxe French Bread	1 (5.94 oz)	260	7	480	29	—
Pepperoni	1 (6.08 oz)	320	8	550	36	—
Sausage	1 (6.43 oz)	340	10	380	37	—
SAUCE						
Boboli	1 pkg (1.2 oz)	20	0	200	4	1
Boboli	¼ cup (2.5 oz)	40	0	410	9	1
Contadina						
Flavored With Pepperoni	¼ cup	40	2	420	6	1
Pizza Sauce	¼ cup	35	2	350	6	1
Squeeze	¼ cup	35	2	350	6	1
With Italian Cheeses	¼ cup	40	2	420	6	1

FOOD	PORTION	CAL.	FAT	SOD.	CARB.	FIB.
Eden						
Pizza Pasta Sauce	½ cup (4.4 oz)	80	3	320	12	3
Muir Glen						
Organic	¼ cup (2.2 oz)	40	1	230	6	2
Ragu						
Quick Traditional	3 tbsp (1.7 oz)	35	2	330	3	—
TAKE-OUT						
cheese	12 in pie	1121	26	2680	164	—
cheese	⅛ of 12 in pie	140	3	336	21	—
cheese deep dish individual	1 (5.5 oz)	460	24	750	47	2
cheese meat & vegetables	12 in pie	1472	43	3054	170	—
cheese meat & vegetables	⅛ of 12 in pie	184	5	382	21	—
pepperoni	12 in pie	1445	56	2133	157	—
pepperoni	⅛ of 12 in pie	181	7	267	20	—

PLANTAINS
Top Banana

FOOD	PORTION	CAL.	FAT	SOD.	CARB.	FIB.
All Natural Plantain Chips	1 oz	150	8	85	17	—
fresh uncooked	1 (6.3 oz)	218	1	7	57	—
sliced cooked	½ cup	89	tr	4	24	—
TAKE-OUT						
ripe fried	2.8 oz	214	7	—	38	4

PLUMS
CANNED
S&W

FOOD	PORTION	CAL.	FAT	SOD.	CARB.	FIB.
Halves Purple Fancy Unpeeled In Extra Heavy Syrup	½ cup	135	0	25	35	—
Whole Purple Fancy Unpeeled In Extra Heavy Syrup	½ cup	135	0	25	35	—
Whole Unpeeled Diet	½ cup	52	0	0	13	—
purple in heavy syrup	3	119	tr	26	31	—
purple in heavy syrup	1 cup	320	tr	50	60	—
purple in light syrup	3	83	tr	26	22	—
purple in light syrup	1 cup	158	tr	50	41	—
purple juice pack	1 cup	146	tr	3	38	—
purple juice pack	3	55	tr	1	14	—
purple water pack	3	39	tr	1	10	—
purple water pack	1 cup	102	tr	2	27	—
FRESH						
Dole						
	2	70	1	0	17	1
plum	1	36	tr	0	9	—
sliced	1 cup	91	1	1	21	—

FOOD	PORTION	CAL.	FAT	SOD.	CARB.	FIB.
POI						
poi	½ cup	134	tr	14	33	—
POKEBERRY SHOOTS						
Allen	½ cup (4.1 oz)	35	1	5	5	3
cooked	½ cup	16	tr	—	3	—
raw	½ cup	18	tr	—	3	—
POLENTA						
(*see* CORNMEAL)						
POLLACK						
atlantic baked	3 oz	100	1	94	0	—
atlantic fillet baked	5.3 oz	178	2	166	0	—
FROZEN						
Mrs. Paul's						
Fillets Light	1 fillet (4.5 oz)	240	11	530	18	—
POMEGRANATES						
pomegranate	1	104	tr	5	26	—
POMPANO						
florida cooked	3 oz	179	10	65	0	—
florida raw	3 oz	140	8	55	0	—
POPCORN						
(*see also* CHIPS, POPCORN CAKES, PRETZELS, SNACKS)						
Barrel O' Fun	1 oz	160	12	240	13	1
Baked Curl	1 oz	150	9	260	17	0
Caramel Corn	1 oz	115	1	170	25	1
Corn Pop	1 oz	190	16	230	10	0
White Cheddar Pops	1 oz	170	13	370	11	0
Cape Cod						
Light	½ oz	60	3	95	8	—
Cheetos						
Cheddar Cheese	0.5 oz	80	6	160	6	—
Chesters						
Cheddar Cheese	0.5 oz	80	5	200	7	—
Microwave	3 cups	110	7	170	13	—
Microwave Butter	3 cups	120	7	180	13	—
Microwave Cheese	3 cups	110	8	230	11	—
Estee						
No Sugar Added Caramel	1 cup (1 oz)	120	2	90	26	1
Greenfield						
Caramel	1 cup (1 oz)	120	2	100	22	—

FOOD	PORTION	CAL.	FAT	SOD.	CARB.	FIB.
Jiffy Pop						
Bag Butter	3 cups	90	5	140	11	2
Bag Lite	3 cups	70	3	110	11	2
Bag Regular	3 cups	100	6	140	11	2
Glazed Popcorn Clusters	1 oz	120	2	120	25	1
Microwave Butter	4 cup	140	7	270	17	3
Microwave Regular	4 cup	140	7	270	17	3
Pan Butter	4 cup	130	6	270	16	2
Pan Regular	4 cup	130	6	270	16	2
Lance						
Cheese	1 pkg (25 g)	130	8	280	13	—
Plain	1 pkg (25 g)	140	9	210	13	—
White Cheddar Cheese	1 pkg (25 g)	140	9	170	12	—
Louise's						
Fat-Free Apple Cinnamon	1 oz	100	0	80	24	1
Fat-Free Buttery Toffee	1 oz	100	0	80	24	1
Fat-Free Caramel	1 oz	100	0	80	24	1
Newman's Own						
Oldstyle Picture Show	3 ⅓ cups	80	1	0	16	—
Oldstyle Picture Show Microwave Light Butter	3 cups	90	3	100	18	4
Oldstyle Picture Show Microwave Light Natural	3 cups	90	3	100	18	4
Oldstyle Picture Show Microwave Natural Butter	3 cups	150	8	200	18	4
Oldstyle Picture Show Microwave No Salt	3 cups	150	8	0	18	4
Orville Redenbacher's						
Gourmet Hot Air	3 cups	40	tr	0	10	3
Gourmet Original	3 cups	80	4	0	10	3
Gourmet White	3 cups	80	4	0	10	3
Microwave Gourmet	3 cups	100	6	200	11	3
Microwave Gourmet Butter	3 cups	100	6	240	11	3
Microwave Gourmet Butter Toffee	2½ cups	210	12	85	26	2
Microwave Gourmet Caramel	2½ cups	240	14	90	29	2
Microwave Gourmet Cheddar Cheese	3 cups	130	8	280	14	3

FOOD	PORTION	CAL.	FAT	SOD.	CARB.	FIB.
Orville Redenbacher's (CONT.)						
Microwave Gourmet Frozen	3 cups	100	6	200	11	3
Microwave Gourmet Frozen Butter	3 cups	100	6	240	11	3
Microwave Gourmet Light	3 cups	70	3	115	8	3
Microwave Gourmet Light Butter	3 cups	70	3	110	8	3
Microwave Gourmet Salt Free	3 cups	100	6	0	11	3
Microwave Gourmet Salt Free Butter	3 cups	100	6	0	11	3
Microwave Gourmet Sour Cream 'n Onion	3 cups	160	12	270	12	3
Pillsbury						
Microwave Butter	3 cups	210	13	410	20	—
Microwave Original	3 cups	210	13	410	20	—
Microwave Salt Free	3 cups	170	7	0	23	—
Pop Secret						
Butter Flavor	3 cups	100	6	170	11	2
Butter Flavor Singles	6 cups	250	16	310	23	4
Light Butter Flavor	3 cups	70	3	115	12	2
Light Butter Flavor Singles	6 cups	140	6	190	23	4
Light Natural Flavor	3 cups	70	3	160	12	2
Light Natural Flavor Singles	6 cups	150	6	320	23	4
Natural Flavor	3 cups	100	6	170	11	2
Natural Flavor Salt Free	3 cups	100	6	<5	11	2
Pop Chips	1½ cups (1 oz)	130	4	400	23	1
Pop Qwiz Butter Flavor	3 cups	100	6	170	11	2
Pop Qwiz Natural Flavor	3 cups	100	6	170	11	2
Smartfood						
Cheddar Cheese	0.5 oz	80	5	130	7	—
Light Butter	0.5 oz	70	3	105	9	—
Snyder's						
Butter	1 oz	140	9	140	13	3
Ultra Slim-Fast						
Lite N' Tasty	½ oz	60	2	150	10	2
Weight Watchers						
Microwave	1 oz	100	1	5	22	—

FOOD	PORTION	CAL.	FAT	SOD.	CARB.	FIB.
Weight Watchers (CONT.)						
Ready-To-Eat Butter	0.7 oz	90	3	100	13	—
Ready-To-Eat White Cheddar Cheese	0.7 oz	90	4	120	11	—
Wise						
Tender Eating	0.5 oz	70	6	120	4	—
With Real Premium White Cheddar Cheese	0.5 oz	70	5	170	4	—
air-popped	1 oz	108	1	1	22	4
air-popped	1 cup (0.3 oz)	31	tr	0	6	2
caramel coated	1 oz	122	4	58	22	1
caramel coated	1 cup (1.2 oz)	152	5	72	28	2
caramel coated w/ peanuts	⅔ cup (1 oz)	114	2	84	23	1
cheese	1 oz	149	9	252	15	3
cheese	1 cup (0.4 oz)	58	4	98	6	1
oil popped	1 oz	142	8	251	16	3
oil popped	1 cup (0.4 oz)	55	3	97	6	1

POPCORN CAKES

FOOD	PORTION	CAL.	FAT	SOD.	CARB.	FIB.
Lundberg						
Organic Lightly Salted	1	60	1	140	12	—
Organic Unsalted	1	60	1	3	12	—
Rye With Caraway Lightly Salted	1	59	0	5	14	—
Mother's						
Butter Flavor	1 (0.3 oz)	35	0	0	7	0
Unsalted	1 (0.3 oz)	35	0	0	7	0
Quaker						
Blueberry Crunch	1 (0.5 oz)	50	0	0	11	—
Butter Popped	1 (0.3 oz)	35	0	45	7	—
Caramel	1 (0.5 oz)	50	0	30	12	—
Monterey Jack	1 (0.4 oz)	40	0	80	8	—
Strawberry Crunch	1 (0.5 oz)	50	0	0	11	—
White Cheddar	1 (0.4 oz)	40	0	90	8	—
popcorn cake	1 (0.3 oz)	38	tr	29	8	—

POPOVER

FOOD	PORTION	CAL.	FAT	SOD.	CARB.	FIB.
home recipe as prep w/ 2% milk	1 (1.4 oz)	87	3	82	11	—
home recipe as prep w/ whole milk	1 (1.4 oz)	90	3	82	11	—
mix as prep	1 (1.2 oz)	67	2	143	10	—

FOOD	PORTION	CAL.	FAT	SOD.	CARB.	FIB.

POPPY SEEDS

| poppy seeds | 1 tsp | 15 | 1 | 1 | 1 | — |

PORK

(see also BACON, BACON SUBSTITUTES, CANADIAN BACON, HAM, LUNCHEON MEAT/COLD CUTS, SAUSAGE)

The values for cooked pork may differ slightly from values for raw pork. When meat is cooked some moisture and fat are lost, changing the nutritive value slightly. As a rule of thumb, it can be assumed that a 4 oz raw portion will equal a 3 oz cooked portion of meat.

CANNED

Hormel

| Pickled Tidbits | 2 oz | 100 | 8 | 530 | 0 | 0 |

FRESH

Oscar Mayer

Sweet Morsel Smoked Boneless Pork Shoulder	3 oz	180	15	990	0	0
blade chop roasted	1 (3.1 oz)	321	27	54	0	—
center loin chop broiled	1 (3.1 oz)	275	24	61	0	—
center loin chop lean & fat braised	1 chop (2.6 oz)	266	19	—	—	—
center loin chop lean & fat broiled	1 chop (3.1 oz)	275	19	—	—	—
center loin chop lean & fat panfried	1 chop (3.1 oz)	333	27	—	—	—
center loin chop lean & fat roasted	1 chop (3.1 oz)	268	19	—	—	—
center loin chop lean only braised	1 chop (2.1 oz)	166	8	—	—	—
center loin chop lean only broiled	1 chop (2.5 oz)	166	8	—	—	—
center loin chop lean only panfried	1 chop (2.4 oz)	178	11	—	—	—
center loin chop lean only roasted	1 chop (2.4 oz)	180	10	—	—	—
center loin lean & fat braised	3 oz	301	22	—	—	—
center loin lean & fat panfried	3 oz	318	26	—	—	—
center loin lean only broiled	3 oz	196	9	—	—	—
center loin lean only panfried	3 oz	226	14	—	—	—

FOOD	PORTION	CAL.	FAT	SOD.	CARB.	FIB.
center loin lean only roasted	3 oz	204	11	—	—	—
center loin roasted	3 oz	259	18	54	0	—
ham fresh rump half lean & fat roasted	3 oz	233	23	—	—	—
ham fresh rump half lean only roasted	3 oz	187	9	—	—	—
ham fresh shank half lean & fat roasted	3 oz	258	19	—	—	—
ham fresh shank half lean only roasted	3 oz	183	9	—	—	—
ham fresh whole lean & fat roasted	3 oz	250	18	—	—	—
ham fresh whole lean only roasted	3 oz	187	9	—	—	—
leg loin & shoulder lean only roasted	3 oz	198	11	—	—	—
loin blade chop lean & fat braised	1 chop (3.1 oz)	321	27	—	—	—
loin blade chop lean & fat braised	1 chop (2.4 oz)	275	23	—	—	—
loin blade chop lean & fat panfried	1 chop (3.1 oz)	368	33	—	—	—
loin blade chop lean only braised	1 chop (1.8 oz)	156	10	—	—	—
loin blade chop lean only broiled	1 chop (2.1 oz)	177	13	—	—	—
loin blade chop lean only panfried	1 chop (2.2 oz)	175	12	—	—	—
loin blade chop lean only roasted	1 chop (2.5 oz)	198	14	—	—	—
loin blade lean & fat braised	3 oz	348	29	—	—	—
loin blade lean & fat broiled	3 oz	334	29	—	—	—
loin blade lean & fat panfried	3 oz	352	31	—	—	—
loin blade lean & fat roasted	3 oz	310	26	—	—	—
loin blade lean only broiled	3 oz	255	18	—	—	—
loin blade lean only panfried	3 oz	240	17	—	—	—
loin blade lean only roasted	3 oz	238	16	—	—	—
loin chop lean & fat braised	1 chop (2.5 oz)	261	20	—	—	—
loin chop lean & fat braised	1 chop (2.3 oz)	267	20	—	—	—

FOOD	PORTION	CAL.	FAT	SOD.	CARB.	FIB.
loin chop lean & fat broiled	1 chop (2.7 oz)	295	23	—	—	—
loin chop lean & fat panfried	1 chop (2.9 oz)	337	29	—	—	—
loin chop lean & fat roasted	1 chop (2.8 oz)	274	21	—	—	—
loin chop lean & fat roasted	1 chop (2.9 oz)	262	20	—	—	—
loin chop lean only braised	1 chop (1.8 oz)	147	8	—	—	—
loin chop lean only broiled	1 chop (2.1 oz)	165	10	—	—	—
loin chop lean only panfried	1 chop (2oz)	157	9	—	—	—
loin chop lean only roasted	1 chop (2.3 oz)	167	9	—	—	—
loin lean & fat braised	3 oz	312	24	—	—	—
loin lean & fat broiled	3 oz	294	23	—	—	—
loin lean only braised	3 oz	232	12	—	—	—
loin lean only broiled	3 oz	218	13	—	—	—
loin lean only roasted	3 oz	204	12	—	—	—
loin w/ fat roasted	3 oz	271	21	53	0	—
lungs braised	3 oz	84	3	—	—	—
pancreas braised	3 oz	186	9	—	—	—
rib chop lean only braised	1 chop (1.8 oz)	147	8	—	—	—
rib chop lean only broiled	1 chop (2.1 oz)	162	9	—	—	—
rib chop lean only panfried	1 chop (2oz)	160	9	—	—	—
rib chop lean only roasted	1 chop (2.2 oz)	162	9	—	—	—
rib chop lean & fat braised	1 chop (2.2 oz)	246	18	—	—	—
rib chop lean & fat broiled	1 chop (2.6 oz)	264	20	—	—	—
rib chop lean & fat panfried	1 chop (2.9 oz)	343	29	—	—	—
rib chop lean & fat roasted	1 chop (2.6 oz)	252	19	—	—	—
shoulder arm picnic cured lean & fat roasted	3 oz	238	18	—	—	—
shoulder arm picnic cured lean only roasted	3 oz	145	6	1046	0	—
shoulder arm picnic lean & fat braised	3 oz	293	22	—	—	—
shoulder arm picnic lean & fat roasted	3 oz	281	22	—	—	—
shoulder arm picnic lean only braised	3 oz	211	10	—	—	—
shoulder arm picnic lean only roasted	3 oz	194	11	—	—	—
shoulder blade boston steak lean & fat braised	1 steak (5.6 oz)	594	46	—	—	—
shoulder blade boston steak lean & fat broiled	1 steak (6.5 oz)	647	53	—	—	—
shoulder blade boston steak lean & fat roasted	1 steak (6.5 oz)	594	47	—	—	—
shoulder blade boston steak lean only braised	1 steak (4.6 oz)	382	23	—	—	—

FOOD	PORTION	CAL.	FAT	SOD.	CARB.	FIB.
shoulder blade boston steak lean only broiled	1 steak (5.3 oz)	413	28	—	—	—
shoulder blade boston steak lean only roasted	1 steak (5.5 oz)	404	27	—	—	—
shoulder blade roll cured lean & fat	3 oz	304	25	1412	0	—
shoulder boston blade lean & fat braised	3 oz	316	24	—	—	—
shoulder boston blade lean & fat broiled	3 oz	297	24	—	—	—
shoulder boston blade lean & fat roasted	3 oz	273	21	—	—	—
shoulder boston blade lean only braised	3 oz	250	15	—	—	—
shoulder boston blade lean only broiled	3 oz	233	16	—	—	—
shoulder boston blade lean only roasted	3 oz	218	14	—	—	—
shoulder whole lean only roasted	3 oz	207	13	—	—	—
shoulder whole roasted	3 oz	277	22	58	0	—
sirloin chop lean & fat braised	1 chop (2.4 oz)	250	18	—	—	—
sirloin chop lean & fat broiled	1 chop (2.8 oz)	278	21	—	—	—
sirloin chop lean & fat roasted	1 chop (2.8 oz)	244	17	—	—	—
sirloin chop lean only braised	1 chop (1.9 oz)	149	7	—	—	—
sirloin chop lean only broiled	1 chop (2.3 oz)	165	9	—	—	—
sirloin chop lean only roasted	1 chop (2.5 oz)	175	10	—	—	—
spareribs braised	3 oz	338	26	79	0	—
spleen braised	3 oz	127	3	—	0	—
tail simmered	3 oz	336	30	—	—	—
tenderloin lean only roasted	3 oz	141	4	57	0	—
TAKE-OUT						
pork roast	2 oz	70	3	390	0	—

PORK DISHES
FROZEN
Jimmy Dean

BBQ Pork Rib Sandwich	1 (5.4 oz)	440	23	970	36	1

FOOD	PORTION	CAL.	FAT	SOD.	CARB.	FIB.
TAKE-OUT						
tourtiere	1 piece (4.9 oz)	451	34	—	21	—
POSOLE						
(see HOMINY)						
POT PIE						
FROZEN						
Award Brand						
Beef	1 (7 oz)	350	18	1130	37	3
Chicken	1 (7 oz)	350	19	1140	39	3
Banquet						
Family Entree Chicken Pie	1 serv (8 oz)	450	30	1010	39	6
Macaroni & Cheese	1 pkg (6.5 oz)	200	3	600	35	2
Vegetable & Cheese	1 (7 oz)	390	18	1000	49	3
Vegetable Pie w/ Beef	1 (7 oz)	330	15	1000	38	3
Vegetable Pie w/ Chicken	1 (7 oz)	350	18	950	36	3
Vegetable Pie w/ Turkey	1 (7 oz)	370	20	850	38	3
Empire						
Chicken	1 (8.1 oz)	440	21	960	41	11
Turkey	1 (8.1 oz)	470	23	820	46	11
Great Value						
Beef	1 (7 oz)	390	19	940	38	3
Chicken	1 (7 oz)	380	20	900	39	2
Turkey	1 (7 oz)	400	22	910	42	3
Morton						
Beef	1 (7 oz)	310	17	1380	34	2
Chicken	1 (7 oz)	320	18	1020	32	3
Macaroni & Cheese	1 (6 oz)	160	3	640	30	3
Turkey	1 (7 oz)	300	18	1060	29	2
Ozark Valley						
Chicken	1 (7 oz)	330	19	1010	32	2
Macaroni & Cheese	1 (6.5 oz)	160	3	780	29	0
Turkey	1 (7 oz)	280	16	1030	29	2
Stouffer's						
Beef Pie	1 pkg (10 oz)	450	26	1140	36	3
Chicken Pie	1 pkg (10 oz)	520	33	1000	37	3
Chicken Pie	½ pkg (8 oz)	460	30	850	35	3
Turkey	1 cup (8 oz)	500	31	910	36	3
Turkey	1 pkg (10 oz)	530	33	1040	36	3
Swanson						
Beef	7 oz	370	19	730	36	—
Beef Hungry Man	16 oz	610	31	1360	58	—
Chicken	7 oz	380	22	760	35	—

FOOD	PORTION	CAL.	FAT	SOD.	CARB.	FIB.
Swanson (CONT.)						
Chicken Homestyle	8 oz	410	21	1030	41	—
Hungry Man Chicken	16 oz	630	35	1600	57	—
Hungry Man Turkey	16 oz	650	36	1470	57	—
Turkey	7 oz	380	21	720	36	—
TAKE-OUT						
beef	⅓ of 9 in pie (7.4 oz)	515	30	596	39	—
chicken	⅓ of 9 in pie (8.1 oz)	545	31	594	42	—

POTATO

(*see also* CHIPS, KNISH)

CANNED

FOOD	PORTION	CAL.	FAT	SOD.	CARB.	FIB.
Allen						
Refried Potatoes	½ cup (4.5 oz)	150	3	360	24	11
Butterfield						
Diced	⅔ cup (5.7 oz)	100	0	350	22	3
Sliced	½ cup (5.7 oz)	100	0	390	22	4
Whole	2½ pieces (5.6 oz)	90	0	330	20	2
Del Monte						
New Sliced	⅔ cup (5.4 oz)	60	0	360	13	2
New Whole	⅔ cup (5.5 oz)	60	0	360	13	2
Hormel						
Au Gratin & Bacon	1 can (7.5 oz)	250	14	840	23	2
Scalloped & Ham	1 can (7.5 oz)	260	16	920	20	1
Hunt's						
Whole New	4 oz	70	tr	230	15	tr
Micro Cup Meals						
Scalloped Potatoes With Ham	1 cup (7.5 oz)	260	16	920	20	2
S&W						
New Potatoes Extra Small	½ cup	45	0	310	9	—
Seneca						
Potatoes	½ cup	80	0	264	15	2
Sunshine						
Whole	2½ pieces (5.6 oz)	90	0	330	20	2
potatoes	½ cup	54	tr	—	12	—
FRESH						
Yukon Gold	1 (5.3 oz)	110	0	—	—	—
baked skin only	1 skin (2 oz)	115	tr	12	27	2
baked w/ skin	1 (6.5 oz)	220	tr	16	51	—
baked w/o skin	1 (5 oz)	145	tr	8	34	2

FOOD	PORTION	CAL.	FAT	SOD.	CARB.	FIB.
baked w/o skin	½ cup	57	tr	3	13	1
boiled	½ cup	68	tr	3	16	1
microwaved	1 (7 oz)	212	tr	16	49	—
microwaved w/o skin	½ cup	78	tr	5	18	—
raw w/o skin	1 (3.9 oz)	88	tr	7	20	—
FROZEN						
Budget Gourmet						
Baked With Broccoli And Cheese	1 pkg (10.5 oz)	300	10	740	40	—
Cheddared Potatoes	1 pkg (5.5 oz)	260	16	600	22	—
Cheddared Potatoes With Broccoli	1 pkg (5 oz)	150	7	410	14	—
Three Cheese Potatoes	1 pkg (5.75 oz)	220	11	470	23	—
Empire						
Crinkle Cut French Fries	½ cup (3 oz)	90	2	20	18	7
Latkes Potato Pancakes	1 (2 oz)	80	2	200	15	8
Latkes Mini Potato Pancakes	2 (2 oz)	90	3	160	16	6
Golden						
Potato Pancakes	1 (1.33 oz)	71	3	187	10	—
Green Giant						
One Serve Au Gratin	1 pkg	200	10	560	20	—
One Serve Potatoes & Broccoli In Cheese Sauce	1 pkg	130	5	720	19	—
Healthy Choice						
Cheddar Broccoli Potatoes	1 meal (10.5 oz)	310	5	550	53	8
Garden Potato Casserole	1 meal (9.25 oz)	200	4	520	30	6
Kineret						
Crinkle Cut	18 pieces (3 oz)	120	4	260	20	2
Kugel	1 piece (2.5 oz)	150	10	160	13	1
Latkes	1 (1.5 oz)	90	5	150	9	2
Latkes Mini	10 (3 oz)	160	9	240	18	2
Lean Cuisine						
Deluxe Cheddar	1 pkg (10.4 oz)	270	10	550	30	3
MicroMagic						
French Fries	1 pkg (3 oz)	290	13	30	40	—
Skinny Fries	1 pkg (3 oz)	350	15	40	49	—
Oh Boy!						
Stuffed With Cheddar Cheese	1 (6 oz)	130	4	310	20	4
Stuffed With Real Bacon	1 (6 oz)	120	3	300	20	4

FOOD	PORTION	CAL.	FAT	SOD.	CARB.	FIB.
Ore Ida						
Cheddar Browns	1 patty (3 oz)	90	3	350	14	1
Cottage Fries	14 pieces (3 oz)	130	4	20	21	1
Crispers!	17 pieces (3 oz)	220	13	510	24	2
Crispers! Nacho	10 pieces (3 oz)	170	9	360	21	2
Crispers! Texas	3 oz	170	10	270	19	2
Crispy Crowns!	12 pieces (3 oz)	100	11	450	21	2
Crispy Crunchies	12 pieces (3 oz)	160	9	370	18	2
Deep Fries Crinkle Cuts	18 pieces (3 oz)	160	7	15	23	2
Deep Fries French Fries	22 pieces (3 oz)	160	7	20	22	2
Dinner Fries Country Style	8 pieces (3 oz)	110	3	20	19	1
Fast Fries	23 pieces (3 oz)	140	6	230	20	2
Fast Fries Ranch	22 pieces (3 oz)	150	7	430	21	1
Golden Crinkles	16 pieces (3 oz)	120	4	25	20	2
Golden Fries	16 pieces (3 oz)	120	4	25	20	1
Golden Patties	1 (2.5 oz)	140	7	280	16	1
Golden Twirls	28 pieces (3 oz)	160	7	25	22	2
Hash Browns Country Style	1 cup (2.6 oz)	60	0	10	13	1
Hash Browns Shredded	1 patty (3 oz)	70	0	25	15	1
Hash Browns Southern Style	¾ cup (3 oz)	70	0	25	17	2
Hot Tots	9 pieces (3 oz)	150	6	380	21	2
Mashed Natural Butter	½ cup (2.1 oz)	80	2	140	14	tr
Microwave Crinkle Cuts	1 pkg (3.5 oz)	180	8	10	26	2
Microwave Hash Browns	1 patty (2 oz)	110	6	150	13	tr
Microwave Tater Tots	1 pkg (3.75 oz)	190	10	420	26	2
O'Brien Potatoes	¾ cup (3 oz)	60	0	15	13	2
Pixie Crinkles	33 pieces (3 oz)	140	5	25	21	3
Shoestrings	38 pieces (3 oz)	150	5	20	22	2
Snackin' Fries	1 pkg (5 oz)	180	20	590	36	3
Snackin' Fries Extra Zesty	1 pkg (5 oz)	180	20	510	35	4
Tater ABC's	10 pieces (3 oz)	190	11	310	20	2
Tater Tots	9 pieces (3 oz)	160	8	340	21	2
Tater Tots Bacon	9 pieces (3 oz)	150	7	490	20	1
Tater Tots Onion	9 pieces (3 oz)	150	7	370	20	2
Toaster Hash Browns	2 patties (3.5 oz)	190	12	550	21	1
Topped Broccoli & Cheese	½ (6 oz)	150	4	410	24	4
Topped Salsa & Cheese	½ (5.5 oz)	160	5	430	25	3
Topped Vegetable Primavera	1 (6.13 oz)	160	5	390	23	—

FOOD	PORTION	CAL.	FAT	SOD.	CARB.	FIB.
Ore Ida (CONT.)						
Twice Baked Butter	1 (5 oz)	200	9	350	27	4
Twice Baked Cheddar Cheese	1 (5 oz)	190	8	460	27	3
Twice Baked Ranch	1 (5 oz)	180	6	400	27	3
Twice Bakes Sour Cream & Chives	1 (5 oz)	180	6	370	28	3
Waffle Fries	15 pieces (3 oz)	140	5	35	22	2
Wedges With Skin	9 pieces (3 oz)	110	3	15	19	2
Zesties!	12 pieces (3 oz)	160	9	370	21	1
Stouffer's						
Au Gratin	½ cup (2.25 oz)	130	6	590	15	1
Baked Broccoli & Cheese	1 pkg (10.1 oz)	320	15	770	30	4
Baked Cheddar Cheese & Bacon	1 pkg (9.4 oz)	380	22	900	31	5
Lunch Express Baked Broccoli & Cheese	1 pkg (10.25 oz)	250	9	490	28	6
Scalloped	½ cup (2.25 oz)	130	6	450	17	2
Weight Watchers						
Baked Broccoli & Cheese	10.5 oz	270	6	570	43	—
Baked Broccoli & Ham	11.5 oz	280	17	520	39	—
Baked Chicken Divan	11.25 oz	280	7	480	38	—
Baked Homestyle Turkey	11.75 oz	250	7	510	26	—
french fries	10 strips	111	4	15	17	2
french fries thick cut	10 strips	109	4	23	17	—
hashed brown	½ cup	170	9	27	22	—
potato puffs	½ cup	138	7	462	19	—
potato puffs as prep	1	16	1	52	2	—
HOME RECIPE						
au gratin	½ cup	160	9	528	14	—
mashed	½ cup	111	4	309	18	—
scalloped	½ cup	105	5	409	13	—
MIX						
Betty Crocker						
Au Gratin as prep	½ cup	140	5	580	21	—
Cheddar 'N Bacon as prep	½ cup	140	5	520	21	—
Cheesy Scalloped as prep	½ cup	140	5	560	20	—
Hash Browns as prep	½ cup	160	6	460	24	—
Hash Browns as prep w/o salt	½ cup	160	6	100	24	—
Homestyle American Cheese as prep	½ cup	140	5	610	20	—

FOOD	PORTION	CAL.	FAT	SOD.	CARB.	FIB.
Betty Crocker (CONT.)						
Homestyle Broccoli Au Gratin as prep	½ cup	130	5	540	19	—
Homestyle Cheddar Cheese as prep	½ cup	140	5	530	20	—
Homestyle Cheesy Scalloped as prep	½ cup	140	5	590	20	—
Julienne as prep	½ cup	130	5	580	18	—
Potato Buds as prep	½ cup	130	6	360	17	—
Potato Buds as prep w/o salt	½ cup	130	6	90	17	—
Scalloped as prep	½ cup	140	5	570	20	—
Scalloped & Ham as prep	½ cup	160	6	620	22	—
Smokey Cheddar as prep	½ cup	140	5	680	21	—
Sour Cream 'N Chive as prep	½ cup	140	5	520	21	—
Twice Baked Bacon & Cheddar as prep	½ cup	210	11	600	21	—
Twice Baked Cheddar With Mild Onion as prep	½ cup	190	10	640	20	—
Twice Baked Herbed Butter as prep	½ cup	220	13	540	20	—
Twice Baked Sour Cream & Chive as prep	½ cup	200	11	570	19	—
Country Store						
Mashed not prep	⅓ cup	70	0	10	15	—
French's						
Cheddar & Bacon Casserole	½ cup	130	5	390	18	—
Creamy Italian Scalloped	½ cup	120	3	430	19	—
Creamy Stroganoff	½ cup	130	4	520	20	—
Crispy Top Scalloped With Savory Onion	½ cup	140	5	390	20	—
Real Cheese Scalloped	½ cup	140	5	380	19	—
Real Sour Cream & Chives	½ cup	150	7	550	19	—
Spuds Mashed	½ cup	140	7	380	17	—
Tangy Au Gratin	½ cup	130	5	460	20	—
Hungry Jack						
Mashed Flakes	½ cup	40	7	380	17	—

FOOD	PORTION	CAL.	FAT	SOD.	CARB.	FIB.
Kraft						
Potatoes & Cheese Au Gratin	½ cup	130	5	570	19	—
Potatoes & Cheese Broccoli Au Gratin	½ cup	120	5	530	20	—
Potatoes & Cheese Scalloped	½ cup	140	5	500	20	—
Potatoes & Cheese Scalloped With Ham	½ cup	150	5	510	20	—
au gratin as prep	4½ oz	127	6	601	18	—
instant mashed flakes as prep w/ whole milk & butter	½ cup	118	6	349	16	—
instant mashed flakes not prep	½ cup	78	tr	24	18	—
instant mashed granules as prep w/ whole milk & butter	½ cup	114	5	270	15	—
instant mashed granules not prep	½ cup	372	1	67	86	—
scalloped as prep	4½ oz	127	6	467	18	—
REFRIGERATED						
Simply Potatoes						
Au Gratin	¼ pkg (3 oz)	130	8	370	13	—
Hash Browns	⅕ pkg (4 oz)	100	tr	410	23	—
Hash Browns Onion	⅕ pkg (4 oz)	120	tr	380	26	—
Hash Browns Southwest Style	⅕ pkg (4 oz)	100	tr	410	23	—
Mashed	⅕ pkg (4 oz)	90	2	150	15	—
Scalloped	¼ pkg (3 oz)	100	5	390	11	—
SHELF-STABLE						
Lunch Bucket						
Scalloped	1 pkg (7.5 oz)	160	7	770	20	—
Pantry Express						
Augratin	½ cup	120	5	430	17	2
TAKE-OUT						
au gratin w/ cheese	½ cup	178	10	548	17	—
baked topped w/ cheese sauce	1	475	29	381	47	—
baked topped w/ cheese sauce & bacon	1	451	26	973	44	—
baked topped w/ cheese sauce & broccoli	1	402	14	484	47	—
baked topped w/ cheese sauce & chili	1	481	22	701	56	—

FOOD	PORTION	CAL.	FAT	SOD.	CARB.	FIB.
baked topped w/ sour cream & chives	1	394	22	182	50	—
curry	1 serving (6 oz)	292	16	—	36	4
french fried in beef tallow	1 lg	358	19	187	44	—
french fried in beef tallow	1 reg	237	12	124	29	—
french fried in vegetable oil	1 reg	235	12	124	29	—
french fried in vegetable oil	1 lg	355	19	187	44	—
hash brown	½ cup	163	11	19	17	2
mashed w/ whole milk & margarine	⅓ cup	66	tr	182	13	—
mustard potato salad	3.5 oz	120	6	393	16	—
o'brien	1 cup	157	3	421	30	—
potato dumpling	3½ oz	334	1	1	74	3
potato pancakes	1 (1.3 oz)	101	7	188	11	—
potato salad	½ cup	179	10	661	14	—
potato salad	⅓ cup	108	6	312	13	—
potato salad w/ vegetables	3.5 oz	120	3	390	20	—
scalloped	½ cup	127	5	435	18	—

POTATO STARCH
Manischewitz

Potato Starch	1 cup	570	0	1	137	—
potato starch	3½ oz	335	tr	8	83	—

POUT

ocean baked	3 oz	86	1	66	0	—
ocean fillet baked	4.8 oz	139	2	107	0	—

PRESERVES
(see JAM/JELLY/PRESERVES)

PRETZELS
(see also CHIPS, POPCORN, SNACKS)

A & Eagle

	1 oz	110	2	570	22	—
Beer	1 oz	110	2	610	22	—

Barrel O' Fun

Mini	1 oz	110	1	100	23	1
Sticks	1 oz	110	1	100	23	1
Twists	1 oz	110	1	100	23	1

Estee

Dutch Unsalted	2 (1.1 oz)	130	1	40	26	1
Nuggets Ranch Reduced Sodium	23 (1 oz)	130	2	240	24	tr
Nuggets Reduced Sodium	30 (1 oz)	120	2	180	24	1
Unsalted	23 (1 oz)	120	1	30	25	1

FOOD	PORTION	CAL.	FAT	SOD.	CARB.	FIB.
Formagg						
Pretzel Nuts	1 oz	120	4	390	21	tr
J&J						
Soft	1 (2.25 oz)	170	0	140	37	—
Soft Bites	5 bites	110	0	95	23	—
Lance						
Twist	1 pkg (42 g)	150	1	700	30	—
Manischewitz						
Bagel Pretzels Original	4 (1 oz)	110	0	260	22	1
Mister Salty						
Chips	16 (1 oz)	110	3	620	21	tr
Dutch	2 (1.1 oz)	120	1	580	25	1
Fat Free Chips	16 (1 oz)	100	0	620	22	1
Mini	22 (1 oz)	110	1	440	22	1
Sticks Fat Free	47 (1 oz)	110	0	370	23	1
Twist Fat Free	9 (1 oz)	110	0	380	23	1
Mr. Phipps						
Chips Lower Sodium	16 (1 oz)	120	3	410	21	tr
Chips Original	16 (1 oz)	120	3	630	21	tr
Chips Original Fat Free	16 (1 oz)	100	0	630	22	tr
Planters						
Twists	1 oz	100	1	420	23	1
Twists	1 pkg (1.5 oz)	160	1	640	35	1
Quinlan						
Beers	1 oz	110	2	550	22	1
Hard Sourdough	1 oz	110	2	550	22	1
Logs	1 oz	110	2	550	22	1
Nuggets	1 oz	110	2	550	22	1
Rods	1 oz	110	2	550	22	1
Sticks	1 oz	110	2	550	22	1
Thins	1 oz	110	2	550	22	1
Rold Gold						
Bavarian	3 pieces (1 oz)	120	2	430	22	—
Pretzel Chips	1 oz	110	1	310	22	—
Pretzel Chips Cheese	1 oz	120	3	240	22	—
Rods	3 pieces (1 oz)	110	2	410	23	—
Snack Mix	½ cup (1 oz)	140	6	330	18	—
Sour Dough	1½ pieces (1 oz)	110	2	230	22	—
Sticks	50 pieces (1 oz)	110	2	490	23	—
Thin Twist	10 pieces (1 oz)	110	1	510	23	—
Tiny Twist	15 pieces (1 oz)	110	1	420	23	—
Seyfart's						
Butter Rods	1 oz	110	1	530	21	—

FOOD	PORTION	CAL.	FAT	SOD.	CARB.	FIB.
Snyder's						
Logs	1 oz	310	0	360	22	—
Minis	1 oz	310	0	460	22	—
Minis Unsalted	1 oz	310	0	70	22	—
Nibblers	1 oz	310	0	460	22	—
Oat Bran	1 oz	120	1	300	14	—
Old Fashioned Hard	1 oz	111	0	655	23	—
Old Fashioned Hard Unsalted	1 oz	100	0	89	23	—
Old Tyme	1 oz	310	0	310	22	—
Old Tyme Unsalted	1 oz	110	0	70	22	—
Rods	1 oz	310	0	320	22	—
Sourdough Hard Buttermilk Ranch	1 oz	130	5	250	19	0
Sourdough Hard Cheddar Cheese	1 oz	160	7	320	13	0
Sourdough Hard Honey Mustard & Onion	1 oz	130	5	250	19	0
Stix	1 oz	310	0	900	22	—
Very Thins	1 oz	310	0	720	22	—
Sunshine						
California Pretzels	1 oz	110	2	350	22	1
Ultra Slim-Fast						
Lite N' Tasty	1 oz	100	tr	460	21	4
Wege						
Sourdough	1 oz	102	tr	548	23	—
Unsalted	1 oz	102	tr	60	23	—
Whole Wheat	1 oz	109	1	25	21	—
chocolate covered	1 oz	130	5	—	20	—
chocolate covered	1 (0.4 oz)	50	2	—	8	—
dutch twist	4 (2.1 oz)	229	2	1029	48	2
pretzels	1 oz	108	1	486	23	1
rods	4 (2 oz)	229	2	1029	48	2
sticks	10	10	tr	48	2	—
sticks	120 (2 oz)	229	2	1029	48	2
twist	1 (½ oz)	65	1	258	13	—
twists	10 (2.1 oz)	229	2	1029	48	2
whole wheat	2 med (2 oz)	205	2	115	46	—
whole wheat	2 sm (1 oz)	103	1	58	23	—

PRICKLYPEAR

fresh	1	42	1	6	10	—

PRUNE JUICE

Del Monte	8 fl oz	170	0	20	43	1

FOOD	PORTION	CAL.	FAT	SOD.	CARB.	FIB.
S&W						
Unsweetened	6 oz	120	0	20	31	—
canned	1 cup	181	tr	11	45	3
PRUNES						
CANNED						
Sonoma						
Pitted	3-4 (1.4 oz)	110	0	5	26	2
in heavy syrup	5	90	tr	2	24	—
in heavy syrup	1 cup	245	tr	6	65	—
DRIED						
Del Monte						
Pitted	¼ cup (1.4 oz)	120	0	5	29	3
Unpitted	⅓ cup (1.4 oz)	110	0	5	12	1
Mariani						
Pitted	¼ cup	140	1	—	—	—
Whole	¼ cup	140	1	—	—	—
Sonoma						
Pitted	¼ cup (1.4 oz)	120	0	5	29	3
Sunsweet						
Orange Essence Pitted Prunes	6 (1.4 oz)	100	0	5	26	3
cooked w/ sugar	½ cup	147	tr	2	39	7
cooked w/o sugar	½ cup	113	tr	2	30	6
dried	10	201	tr	3	53	6
dried	1 cup	385	1	6	101	12
PUDDING						
(see also CUSTARD, PUDDING POPS*)*						
HOME RECIPE						
bread pudding	1 recipe 6 serv (26.4 oz)	1266	44	1741	185	—
bread pudding	½ cup (4.4 oz)	212	7	291	31	—
bread w/ raisins	½ cup	180	5	185	31	—
chocolate as prep w/ 2% milk	½ cup (5.5 oz)	206	4	157	41	—
chocolate as prep w/ whole milk	½ cup (5.5 oz)	221	6	137	40	—
corn	⅔ cup	181	9	92	21	—
cornstarch	½ cup (4.4 oz)	137	5	—	20	—
rice	½ cup (5.3 oz)	217	4	85	40	—
yorkshire as prep w/ skim milk	3.5 oz	93	4	—	12	1
yorkshire as prep w/ whole milk	3.5 oz	104	5	—	12	1

FOOD	PORTION	CAL.	FAT	SOD.	CARB.	FIB.
MIX						
Knorr						
Creme Caramel Flan & Sauce as prep	½ cup + 1 tbsp sauce	190	4	70	34	—
*My*T*Fine*						
Butterscotch	mix for 1 serving	90	0	190	22	—
Chocolate	mix for 1 serving	100	0	135	23	0
Chocolate Almond	mix for 1 serving	100	1	135	23	—
Chocolate Fudge	mix for 1 serving	100	0	140	24	1
Lemon	mix for 1 serving	90	0	170	22	—
Vanilla	mix for 1 serving	90	0	120	22	0
Vanilla Tapioca	mix for 1 serving	80	0	160	19	—
Royal						
Banana Cream	mix for 1 serving	80	0	110	20	0
Banana Cream Instant	mix for 1 serving	90	0	390	22	—
Butterscotch	mix for 1 serving	90	0	180	25	0
Butterscotch Instant	mix for 1 serving	90	0	400	22	—
Cherry Vanilla Instant	mix for 1 serving	90	0	300	23	0
Chocolate	mix for 1 serving	90	0	90	22	0
Chocolate Almond Instant	mix for 1 serving	120	1	440	26	—
Chocolate Chocolate Chip Instant	mix for 1 serving	110	1	590	26	0
Chocolate Instant	mix for 1 serving	110	0	450	23	0
Chocolate Peanut Butter Instant	mix for 1 serving	110	1	480	26	0
Chocolate Sugar Free Instant	mix for 1 serving	50	0	420	11	—
Dark'N Sweet Chocolate	mix for 1 serving	90	0	95	22	1
Dark'N Sweet Instant	mix for 1 serving	110	0	460	25	0
Lemon Instant	mix for 1 serving	90	0	320	23	—
Pistachio Instant	mix for 1 serving	90	1	360	22	0
Strawberry Instant	mix for 1 serving	100	0	330	24	—
Toasted Coconut Instant	mix for 1 serving	100	2	450	22	—
Vanilla	mix for 1 serving	80	0	160	20	0
Vanilla Chocolate Chip Instant	mix for 1 serving	90	1	350	22	0
Vanilla Instant	mix for 1 serving	90	0	325	23	—
Weight Watchers						
Chocolate Instant as prep w/ skim milk	½ cup	100	0	430	18	—
Vanilla Instant as prep w/ skim milk	½ cup	90	0	510	19	—
lemon	½ cup (5.1 oz)	163	2	94	36	—

FOOD	PORTION	CAL.	FAT	SOD.	CARB.	FIB.
MIX WITH 2% MILK						
Jell-O						
Banana Instant Sugar Free	½ cup	84	2	392	11	—
Chocolate Instant Sugar Free	½ cup	92	3	381	13	—
Chocolate Sugar Free	½ cup	91	3	164	13	—
Pistachio Instant Sugar Free	½ cup	94	3	393	12	—
Vanilla Instant Sugar Free	½ cup	82	2	199	11	—
banana	½ cup (4.9 oz)	142	2	232	26	—
banana instant	½ cup (5.2 oz)	152	3	435	29	—
chocolate	½ cup (5 oz)	150	3	148	28	—
chocolate instant	½ cup (5.2 oz)	149	3	418	28	—
coconut cream	½ cup (4.9 oz)	148	4	226	25	—
coconut cream instant	½ cup (5.2 oz)	157	3	362	28	—
lemon instant	½ cup (5.2 oz)	155	4	394	30	—
rice	½ cup (5.1 oz)	161	2	159	30	—
tapioca	½ cup (5 oz)	147	2	172	28	—
vanilla	½ cup (4.9 oz)	141	2	224	26	—
vanilla instant	½ cup (5 oz)	147	2	407	28	—
MIX WITH SKIM MILK						
D-Zerta						
Butterscotch	½ cup	68	0	65	12	—
Chocolate	½ cup	65	0	68	11	—
Vanilla	½ cup	69	0	65	12	—
Emes						
Dietetic	½ cup (4 fl oz)	71	1	110	13	—
MIX WITH WHOLE MILK						
Jell-O						
Banana Cream Instant	½ cup	165	4	409	28	—
Butter Pecan Instant	½ cup	170	5	409	28	—
Butterscotch	½ cup	169	4	191	30	—
Butterscotch Instant	½ cup	164	4	447	28	—
Chocolate Fudge Instant	½ cup	175	5	439	31	—
Chocolate Instant	½ cup	176	5	476	31	—
Chocolate Tapioca Americana	½ cup	169	5	168	28	—
Coconut Cream Instant	½ cup	178	6	322	27	—
French Vanilla	½ cup	169	4	185	30	—
French Vanilla Instant	½ cup	165	4	405	28	—
Golden Egg Custard Americana	½ cup	167	6	—	—	—

FOOD	PORTION	CAL.	FAT	SOD.	CARB.	FIB.
Jell-O (CONT.)						
Lemon Instant	½ cup	168	4	362	29	—
Milk Chocolate Instant	½ cup	179	5	468	31	—
Pineapple Cream Instant	½ cup	165	4	361	29	—
Pistachio Instant	½ cup	170	5	408	28	—
Rice Americana	½ cup	175	4	157	30	—
Vanilla	½ cup	156	4	198	26	—
Vanilla Instant	½ cup	168	4	407	29	—
Vanilla Tapioca Americana	½ cup	160	4	170	27	—
banana	½ cup (4.9 oz)	157	4	231	25	—
banana instant	½ cup (5.2 oz)	167	4	434	27	—
chocolate	½ cup (5 oz)	158	5	147	26	—
chocolate instant	½ cup (5.2 oz)	164	5	417	28	—
coconut cream	½ cup (4.9 oz)	160	4	227	25	—
coconut cream instant	½ cup (5.2 oz)	172	5	360	28	—
lemon instant	½ cup (5.2 oz)	169	4	393	30	—
rice	½ cup (5.1 oz)	175	4	158	30	—
tapioca	½ cup (5 oz)	161	4	171	28	—
vanilla	½ cup (4.9 oz)	155	4	223	26	—
vanilla instant	½ cup (5 oz)	181	4	406	28	—
READY-TO-USE						
Del Monte						
Snack Cups Banana	1 serv (4 oz)	140	4	190	25	0
Snack Cups Butterscotch	1 serv (4 oz)	140	4	170	25	0
Snack Cups Chocolate	1 serv (4 oz)	160	4	130	27	0
Snack Cups Chocolate Fudge	1 serv (4 oz)	150	4	190	25	0
Snack Cups Chocolate Peanut Butter	1 serv (4 oz)	160	4	270	28	0
Snack Cups Lite Chocolate	1 serv (4 oz)	100	1	140	19	0
Snack Cups Lite Vanilla	1 serv (4 oz)	90	1	190	18	0
Snack Cups Tapioca	1 serv (4 oz)	140	4	110	23	0
Snack Cups Vanilla	1 serv (4 oz)	150	4	150	26	0
Imagine Foods						
Lemon Dream	1 (4 oz)	120	0	5	30	—
Jell-O						
Chocolate	1 (4 oz)	171	6	121	28	—
Chocolate Caramel Swirl	1 (4 oz)	175	6	122	28	—
Chocolate Vanilla Swirl	1 (5.5 oz)	240	8	173	39	—
Chocolate Vanilla Swirl	1 (4 oz)	175	6	125	28	—
Chocolate Fudge	1 (4 oz)	171	6	121	28	—

FOOD	PORTION	CAL.	FAT	SOD.	CARB.	FIB.
Jell-O (CONT.)						
Chocolate Fudge Milk Chocolate Swirl	1 (4 oz)	171	6	123	29	—
Light Chocolate	1 (4 oz)	104	2	113	21	—
Light Chocolate Fudge	1 (4 oz)	101	1	113	22	—
Light Chocolate Vanilla	1 (4 oz)	104	2	116	21	—
Light Vanilla	1 (4 oz)	104	2	118	20	—
Milk Chocolate	1 (4 oz)	173	6	126	29	—
Tapioca	1 (4 oz)	167	4	135	29	—
Tapioca	1 (5.5 oz)	229	6	186	40	—
Vanilla	1 (4 oz)	182	7	133	28	—
Vanilla	1 (5.5 oz)	250	9	183	38	—
Vanilla Chocolate Swirl	1 (4 oz)	178	6	129	28	—
Matthew Walker						
Plum	3.5 oz	290	7	100	60	1
Snack Pack						
Banana	4.25 oz	145	6	180	22	0
Butterscotch	4.25 oz	170	6	210	27	0
Chocolate	4.25 oz	170	6	120	26	0
Chocolate Fudge	4.25 oz	165	6	125	27	0
Chocolate Marshmallow	4.25 oz	165	6	125	26	0
Lemon	4.25 oz	150	4	75	30	tr
Light Chocolate	4.25 oz	100	2	120	20	0
Light Tapioca	4.25 oz	100	2	105	18	0
Tapioca	4.25 oz	150	5	125	23	0
Vanilla	4.25 oz	170	6	150	27	0
Swiss Miss						
Butterscotch	4 oz	180	6	135	29	0
Chocolate	4 oz	180	6	160	29	0
Chocolate Fudge	4 oz	220	6	180	38	0
Chocolate Sundae	4 oz	220	7	140	36	0
Light Chocolate	4 oz	100	1	120	20	0
Light Chocolate Fudge	4 oz	100	1	120	20	0
Light Vanilla	4 oz	100	1	105	20	0
Light Vanilla Chocolate Parfait	4 oz	100	1	110	20	0
Tapioca	4 oz	160	5	170	27	0
Vanilla	4 oz	190	7	140	30	0
Vanilla Parfait	4 oz	180	6	150	29	0
Vanilla Sundae	4 oz	200	7	180	36	0
Ultra Slim-Fast						
Butterscotch	4 oz	100	tr	230	21	2
Chocolate	4 oz	100	tr	240	21	2
Vanilla	4 oz	100	tr	230	21	2

FOOD	PORTION	CAL.	FAT	SOD.	CARB.	FIB.
banana	1 pkg (5 oz)	180	5	278	30	—
chocolate	1 pkg (5 oz)	189	6	183	32	—
lemon	1 pkg (5 oz)	177	4	199	36	—
rice	1 pkg (5 oz)	231	11	121	31	—
tapioca	1 pkg (5 oz)	169	5	168	28	—
vanilla	1 pkg (4 oz)	146	4	153	25	—
TAKE-OUT						
blancmange	1 serving (4.7 oz)	154	5	—	25	tr
bread pudding	1 serving (6.7 oz)	564	18	—	94	6
bread pudding	½ cup (4.4 oz)	212	7	291	31	—
queen of puddings	1 serving (4.4 oz)	266	10	—	41	tr
rice pudding	1 serving (3 oz)	110	4	—	17	tr
rice w/ raisins	½ cup	246	6	270	42	4
tapioca	½ cup (5.3 oz)	189	7	288	26	—
vanilla	½ cup (4.3 oz)	130	4	113	20	—

PUDDING POPS

(see also ICE CREAM AND FROZEN DESSERTS, PUDDING)

Jell-O

Chocolate	1 pop	79	2	82	13	—
Chocolate Caramel Swirl	1 pop	74	2	63	12	—
Chocolate Fudge	1 pop	79	2	82	13	—
Chocolate Peanut Butter Swirl	1 bar	78	3	70	12	—
Chocolate Swirl	1 pop	80	2	83	13	—
Chocolate Vanilla Swirl	1 pop	78	2	66	13	—
Deluxe Chocolate Covered	1 pop	201	10	212	27	—
Deluxe Peanuts And Chocolate	1 bar	185	9	83	24	—
Milk Chocolate	1 pop	80	2	83	13	—
Vanilla	1 pop	77	2	50	13	—
chocolate	1 (1.6 oz)	72	2	77	12	—
vanilla	1 (1.6 oz)	75	2	50	13	—

PUMMELO

fresh	1	228	tr	7	59	—
sections	1 cup	71	tr	2	18	—

PUMPKIN

CANNED

Libby

Solid Pack	½ cup	60	1	5	15	4

Owatonna

Pumpkin	½ cup	40	1	—	—	—
pumpkin	½ cup	41	tr	6	10	—

FOOD	PORTION	CAL.	FAT	SOD.	CARB.	FIB.
FRESH						
cooked mashed	½ cup	24	tr	2	6	—
flowers cooked	½ cup	10	tr	4	2	—
flowers raw	1	0	0	0	tr	—
leaves cooked	½ cup	7	tr	3	1	—
leaves raw	½ cup	4	tr	2	tr	—
raw cubed	½ cup	15	tr	1	4	—
SEEDS						
dried	1 oz	154	13	5	5	—
roasted	1 cup	1184	96	40	31	—
roasted	1 oz	148	12	5	4	—
salted & roasted	1 cup	1184	96	1294	31	—
salted & roasted	1 oz	148	12	144	4	—
whole roasted	1 cup	285	12	12	34	—
whole roasted	1 oz	127	6	5	15	—
whole salted roasted	1 cup	285	12	268	34	—
whole salted roasted	1 oz	127	6	191	15	—
PURSLANE						
cooked	1 cup	21	tr	51	4	—
raw	1 cup	7	tr	20	1	—
QUAHOGS						
(see CLAMS)						
QUAIL						
breast w/o skin raw	1 (2 oz)	69	2	31	0	—
w/ skin raw	1 quail (3.8 oz)	210	13	58	0	—
w/o skin raw	1 quail (3.2 oz)	123	4	47	0	—
QUICHE						
HOME RECIPE						
lorraine	⅛ of 8 in pie	600	48	653	29	—
TAKE-OUT						
cheese	1 slice (3 oz)	283	20	—	16	1
lorraine	1 slice (3 oz)	352	25	—	18	1
mushroom	1 slice (3 oz)	256	18	—	17	1
QUINCE						
fresh	1	53	tr	4	14	—
QUINOA						
Arrowhead	¼ cup (1.4 oz)	140	2	0	25	4
Eden not prep	¼ cup (1.6 oz)	170	3	0	31	3
quinoa	½ cup	318	5	—	59	—
RABBIT						
domestic w/o bone roasted	3 oz	167	7	40	0	—
wild w/o bone stewed	3 oz	147	3	38	0	—

FOOD	PORTION	CAL.	FAT	SOD.	CARB.	FIB.
RACCOON						
roasted	3 oz	217	12	—	0	—
RADICCHIO						
leaf	3.5 oz	18	tr	—	3	1
raw shredded	½ cup	5	tr	4	1	—
RADISHES						
DRIED						
chinese	½ cup	157	tr	161	37	—
daikon	½ cup	157	tr	161	37	—
FRESH						
Dole	7	20	0	35	3	0
chinese raw	1 (12 oz)	62	tr	71	14	—
chinese raw sliced	½ cup	8	tr	9	2	—
chinese sliced cooked	½ cup	13	tr	10	3	—
daikon raw	1 (12 oz)	62	tr	71	14	—
daikon raw sliced	½ cup	8	tr	9	2	—
daikon sliced cooked	½ cup	13	tr	10	3	—
red raw	10	7	tr	11	2	—
red sliced	½ cup	10	tr	14	2	—
white icicle raw	1 (½ oz)	2	tr	3	tr	—
white icicle raw sliced	½ cup	7	tr	8	1	—
SPROUTS						
raw	½ cup	8	tr	1	1	—
RAISINS						
Del Monte	1 box (1 oz)	90	0	5	22	2
Del Monte	¼ cup (1.4 oz)	130	0	10	31	2
Del Monte	1 box (1.5 oz)	140	0	10	33	3
Del Monte	1 box (0.5 oz)	45	0	0	11	tr
Del Monte						
Golden	¼ cup (1.4 oz)	130	0	10	31	2
Yogurt Raisins Strawberry	1 pkg (0.9 oz)	110	3	25	20	tr
Yogurt Raisins Vanilla	3 tbsp (1 oz)	130	3	30	23	1
Yogurt Raisins Vanilla	1 pkg (0.9 oz)	110	3	25	20	tr
Yogurt Raisins Vanilla	1 pkg (1 oz)	120	3	25	22	tr
Dole						
Golden	½ cup	250	0	25	66	—
Seedless	½ cup	250	0	15	66	—
Sonoma						
Monukka Thompson	¼ cup (1.4 oz)	130	0	10	31	2
Tree Of Life						
Organic	¼ cup (1.4 oz)	130	0	10	31	2

FOOD	PORTION	CAL.	FAT	SOD.	CARB.	FIB.
chocolate coated	10 (0.4 oz)	39	2	4	7	—
chocolate coated	1 cup (6.7 oz)	741	28	68	130	—
golden seedless	1 cup	437	1	17	115	8
seedless	1 tbsp	27	tr	—	7	—
seedless	1 cup	434	1	17	115	8
sultanas	1 oz	88	0	—	23	2

RASPBERRIES
CANNED
in heavy syrup	½ cup	117	tr	4	30	—

FRESH
Dole	1 cup	45	0	0	10	9
raspberries	1 pint	154	2	0	36	—
raspberries	1 cup	61	1	0	14	—

FROZEN
Big Valley						
Raspberries	⅔ cup (4.9 oz)	80	0	0	18	3
Birds Eye						
Whole in Lite Syrup	½ cup	100	1	0	25	4
sweetened	1 cup	256	tr	1	65	—
sweetened	1 pkg (10 oz)	291	tr	1	74	—

RASPBERRY JUICE
After The Fall						
Raspberry Ginger Ale	1 can (12 oz)	150	0	25	36	0
Crystal Geyser						
Juice Squeeze Mountain Raspberry	1 bottle (12 fl oz)	135	0	20	32	—
Kool-Aid						
Sugar Free	8 oz	2	0	24	0	—
Smucker's						
Juice	8 oz	120	0	10	30	—
Juice Sparkler	10 oz	130	tr	5	32	—

MIX
Kool-Aid						
Raspberry	8 oz	98	0	27	25	—

RED BEANS
CANNED
Allen	½ cup (4.5 oz)	160	1	310	19	9
Green Giant	½ cup	90	1	340	19	5
Hunt's						
Small	4 oz	90	tr	560	18	6

DRIED
Bean Cuisine	½ cup	115	1	5	—	5

FOOD	PORTION	CAL.	FAT	SOD.	CARB.	FIB.
MIX						
Bean Cuisine						
Pasta & Beans Barcelona Red With Radiatore	½ cup	170	4	379	170	—
Mahatma						
Red Beans & Rice	1 cup	190	1	790	40	7
RELISH						
Claussen						
Pickle Relish	1 tbsp	14	tr	—	—	—
Del Monte						
Hamburger	1 tbsp (0.5 oz)	20	0	220	6	tr
Hot Dog	1 tbsp (0.5 oz)	15	0	140	4	tr
Sweet Pickle	1 tbsp (0.5 oz)	20	0	125	5	0
Hellman's						
Sandwich Spread	1 tbsp (15 g)	55	5	170	2	—
Old El Paso						
Jalapeno	2 tbsp	5	0	110	1	—
Vlasic						
Dill	1 oz	2	0	415	1	—
Hamburger	1 oz	40	0	255	9	—
Hot Dog	1 oz	40	1	255	8	—
Hot Piccalilli	1 oz	35	0	165	8	—
India	1 oz	30	0	205	8	—
Sweet	1 oz	30	0	220	8	—
cranberry orange	½ cup	246	tr	44	64	—
hamburger	½ cup	158	1	1338	42	—
hamburger	1 tbsp	19	tr	164	5	—
hot dog	½ cup	111	1	1332	28	—
hot dog	1 tbsp	14	tr	164	4	—
piccalilli	1.4 oz	13	tr	—	2	1
sweet	1 tbsp	19	tr	122	5	—
sweet	½ cup	159	1	990	43	—
RENNIN						
tablet	1 (0.9 g)	1	0	234	tr	—
RHUBARB						
fresh	½ cup	13	tr	2	3	—
frzn	½ cup	60	tr	1	3	—
frzn as prep w/ sugar	½ cup	139	tr	2	37	—
RICE						
(see also BRAN, CEREAL, FLOUR, RICE CAKES, WILD RICE)						
BROWN						
Arrowhead						
Basmati	¼ cup (1.5 oz)	150	1	0	33	2

FOOD	PORTION	CAL.	FAT	SOD.	CARB.	FIB.
Arrowhead (CONT.)						
Quick Regular	⅓ cup (1.5 oz)	150	1	0	32	2
Quick Spanish Style	¼ pkg (1.4 oz)	150	1	250	30	2
Quick Vegetable Herb	¼ pkg (1.4 oz)	150	1	160	30	3
Quick Wild Rice & Herb	¼ pkg (1.3 oz)	140	1	220	28	3
Minute						
Precooked as prep	½ cup	121	1	7	26	1
Near East						
Pilaf as prep	1 cup	220	5	710	41	2
S&W						
Quick Natural Long Grain	3.5 oz	110	0	0	25	—
Quick Natural Long Grain cooked	3.5 oz	119	0	0	26	—
long-grain cooked	½ cup	109	tr	5	23	2
medium-grain cooked	½ cup	109	tr	1	23	—
CANNED						
Old El Paso						
Spanish	½ cup	130	1	1340	28	2
Van Camp's						
Spanish	1 cup (9 oz)	180	3	1290	37	3
FROZEN						
Birds Eye						
Rice & Broccoli Au Gratin	½ pkg	150	4	490	24	1
Budget Gourmet						
Oriental Rice With Vegetables	1 pkg (5.75 oz)	230	12	420	28	—
Rice Pilaf With Green Beans	1 pkg (5.5 oz)	230	11	510	30	—
Chun King						
Fried Rice	1 pkg (8 oz)	290	6	1310	48	5
Fried Rice With Chicken	1 pkg (8 oz)	270	6	1330	44	4
Green Giant						
Garden Gourmet Asparagus Pilaf	1 pkg	190	4	610	37	3
Garden Gourmet Sherry Wild Rice	1 pkg	210	4	580	40	3
One Serve Rice 'N Broccoli In Cheese Sauce	1 pkg	180	6	550	25	—
One Serve Rice Peas & Mushrooms With Sauce	1 pkg	130	2	410	27	—

FOOD	PORTION	CAL.	FAT	SOD.	CARB.	FIB.
Green Giant (CONT.)						
Rice Originals Italian Rice 'N Spinach In Cheese Sauce	½ cup	140	4	400	22	—
Rice Originals Pilaf	½ cup	110	1	530	21	—
Rice Originals Rice Medley	½ cup	100	1	310	19	—
Rice Originals Rice 'N Broccoli In Cheese Sauce	½ cup	120	4	510	18	—
Rice Originals White & Wild	½ cup	130	2	540	24	—
Luigino's						
Fried Rice Chicken	1 pkg (8 oz)	250	5	640	38	2
Fried Rice Pork	1 pkg (8 oz)	250	7	830	37	2
Fried Rice Pork & Shrimp	1 pkg (8 oz)	250	5	890	39	2
Fried Rice Shrimp	1 pkg (8 oz)	220	4	730	38	2
Risotto Parmesano	1 pkg (8 oz)	360	20	740	30	2
MIX						
Casbah						
Jambalaya	1 pkg (1.4 oz)	130	0	500	27	1
La Fiesta	1 pkg (1.59 oz)	170	1	400	34	0
Nutted Pilaf as prep	1 cup	220	3	460	40	1
Pilaf as prep	1 cup	200	tr	430	44	tr
Spanish Pilaf as prep	1 cup	200	1	430	44	1
Thai Yum	1 pkg (1.7 oz)	180	3	500	33	1
Goodman's						
Rice & Vermicelli For Beef	¾ cup	160	1	860	33	0
Rice & Vermicelli For Chicken	¾ cup	160	1	920	33	1
Hain						
Rice Almondine	½ cup	130	5	260	17	—
Rice Oriental 3-Grain Goodness	½ cup	120	5	300	15	—
Kikkoman						
Fried Rice Seasoning Mix	1 oz pkg	91	tr	—	—	—
Kitchen Del Sol						
Mediterranean Paella Costa Brave as prep	½ cup (1.2 oz)	130	2	312	23	1
Mediterranean Sunny Lemon Pilaf as prep	½ cup (1.2 oz)	110	1	210	22	1

FOOD	PORTION	CAL.	FAT	SOD.	CARB.	FIB.
Kitchen Del Sol (CONT.)						
Mediterranean Tomato & Basil With Pine Nuts	½ cup (1 oz)	110	4	270	18	1
Knorr						
Risotto Milanese With Saffron	½ cup	130	3	420	24	—
Risotto Tomato	½ cup	110	tr	460	23	—
Risotto With Mushrooms	½ cup	110	tr	430	24	—
Risotto With Onion	½ cup	110	tr	390	24	—
Risotto With Peas And Corn	½ cup	110	1	470	23	—
La Choy						
Chinese Fried Rice	¾ cup	190	1	820	41	tr
Lipton						
Golden Saute Fried Rice Beef	½ cup	124	2	516	24	—
Golden Saute Fried Rice Chicken	½ cup	129	2	509	24	—
Golden Saute Fried Rice Oriental	½ cup	127	2	675	24	—
Rice & Sauce Beef	½ cup	119	1	602	26	0
Rice & Sauce Cajun	½ cup	123	tr	596	26	tr
Rice & Sauce Cheddar Broccoli	½ cup	125	1	487	25	—
Rice & Sauce Chicken	½ cup	124	1	469	25	0
Rice & Sauce Chicken Broccoli	½ cup	129	2	495	25	—
Rice & Sauce Creamy Chicken	½ cup	142	2	417	27	—
Rice & Sauce Herbs & Butter	½ cup	123	2	446	24	0
Rice & Sauce Long Grain & Wild Rice Original	½ cup	121	tr	530	26	0
Rice & Sauce Mushroom	½ cup	123	1	497	26	0
Rice & Sauce Pilaf	½ cup	122	1	410	26	0
Rice & Sauce Skillet Style Spanish	½ cup	104	1	426	21	—
Rice & Sauce Spanish	½ cup	118	1	536	25	0
Rice Asparagus With Hollandaise	½ cup	123	1	462	25	tr
Mahatma						
Broccoli & Cheese	1 cup	200	2	620	41	2

FOOD	PORTION	CAL.	FAT	SOD.	CARB.	FIB.
Mahatma (CONT.)						
Jambalaya	1 cup (2 oz)	190	1	700	43	tr
Long Grain & Wild	1 cup (2 oz)	190	1	1240	41	2
Pilaf	1 cup (2 oz)	190	0	820	43	tr
Spanish	1 cup (2 oz)	180	1	760	42	2
Yellow Rice Mix	1 cup	190	0	970	43	tr
Minute						
Fried Rice With Vermicelli as prep	½ cup	158	5	549	25	—
Microwave Broccoli Almondine	½ cup	143	4	394	24	—
Microwave Cheddar Cheese Broccoli	½ cup	164	5	534	26	—
Microwave French Pilaf	½ cup	133	3	423	24	—
Microwave Long Grain Brown And Wild	½ cup	140	3	312	25	—
Microwave Rice With Savory Cheese Sauce as prep	½ cup	162	5	435	26	—
Rice Drumstick With Vermicelli as prep	½ cup	153	4	686	25	—
Rice Rib Roast With Vermicelli as prep	½ cup	151	4	722	25	—
Near East						
Barley Pilaf as prep	1 cup	220	4	620	41	5
Beef Pilaf as prep	1 cup	220	5	850	42	1
Curry Rice as prep	1 cup	220	4	660	42	1
Lentil Pilaf as prep	1 cup	210	4	650	37	0
Long Grain & Wild as prep	1 cup	220	5	810	42	2
Pilaf Chicken as prep	1 cup	220	5	940	42	1
Pilaf Kosher as prep	1 cup	220	5	870	42	1
Spanish Pilaf as prep	1 cup	230	6	990	42	1
Old El Paso						
Mexican	½ cup	140	2	370	28	—
Pritikin						
Mexican	⅓ cup (2 oz)	200	2	105	43	—
Oriental	⅓ cup (2 oz)	190	2	260	43	—
Rice-A-Roni						
Beef	½ cup	140	4	610	24	—
Beef & Mushroom	½ cup	150	3	740	26	—
Chicken	½ cup	150	3	560	26	—
Chicken & Broccoli	½ cup	150	3	710	25	—
Chicken & Mushroom	½ cup	180	7	840	26	—

FOOD	PORTION	CAL.	FAT	SOD.	CARB.	FIB.
Rice-A-Roni (CONT.)						
Chicken & Vegetables	½ cup	140	3	790	25	—
Fried Rice	½ cup	110	5	700	21	—
Herb & Butter	½ cup	130	4	790	22	—
Long Grain & Wild Chicken w/ Almonds	½ cup	140	4	690	24	—
Long Grain & Wild Original	½ cup	130	3	660	23	—
Long Grain & Wild Pilaf	½ cup	130	3	550	23	—
Pilaf	½ cup	150	4	620	25	—
Risotto	½ cup	200	6	1130	32	—
Spanish	½ cup	150	4	1090	25	—
Stroganoff	½ cup	200	8	810	27	—
Yellow Rice	½ cup	140	4	780	25	—
Success						
Beef Oriental	½ cup	190	1	920	43	2
Broccoli & Cheese	½ cup	200	2	690	41	2
Brown & Wild	½ cup	190	1	830	40	3
Classic Chicken	½ cup	150	1	720	32	1
Long Grain & Wild	½ cup	190	0	890	42	1
Pilaf	½ cup	200	0	630	44	2
Spanish	½ cup	190	1	780	43	1
Ultra Slim-Fast						
Oriental Style	2.3 oz	240	1	900	58	4
Rice & Chicken Sauce	2.3 oz	240	1	1080	56	4
Uncle Ben						
Brown & Wild Fast Cooking	1 serv (1.3 oz)	120	1	383	26	1
Country Inn Broccoli Almondine	1 serv (1.2 oz)	124	2	367	25	1
Country Inn Broccoli & White Cheddar	1 serv (1.2 oz)	131	3	288	24	1
Country Inn Broccoli Au Gratin	1 serv (1.1 oz)	116	2	342	22	1
Country Inn Chicken With Wild Rice	1 serv (1.1 oz)	108	1	359	23	1
Country Inn Creamy Chicken & Mushroom	1 serv (1.3 oz)	138	3	380	24	1
Country Inn Creamy Chicken & Wild Rice	1 serv (1.3 oz)	135	1	340	27	1
Country Inn Green Bean Almondine	1 serv (1.2 oz)	128	2	280	25	1
Country Inn Herbed Au Gratin	1 serv (1.2 oz)	119	2	361	24	1

FOOD	PORTION	CAL.	FAT	SOD.	CARB.	FIB.
Uncle Ben (CONT.)						
Country Inn Homestyle Chicken & Vegetables	1 serv (1.3 oz)	139	3	298	24	1
Country Inn Rice Florentine	1 serv (1.2 oz)	212	2	354	24	1
Country Inn Vegetable Pilaf	1 serv (1.2 oz)	115	1	357	25	1
Country Inn Chicken Stock	1 serv (1.2 oz)	123	1	269	24	1
Long Grain & Wild Chicken Stock Sauce	1 serv (1.3 oz)	133	2	601	25	1
Long Grain & Wild Fast Cooking	1 serv (1 oz)	101	tr	450	22	1
Long Grain & Wild Garden Vegetable Blend	1 serv (1.3 oz)	128	1	601	26	1
Long Grain & Wild Original	1 serv (1 oz)	96	tr	363	21	1
Watkins						
Brown & Wild	¼ cup (1.6 oz)	160	0	10	34	3
Calico Medley	¼ cup (1.6 oz)	160	0	30	37	4
East/West Medley	¼ cup (1.6 oz)	160	0	0	33	5
Heartland Medley	¼ cup (1.6 oz)	160	0	10	35	4
Minnesota Medley	¼ cup (1.6 oz)	160	0	10	34	2
White & Wild	¼ cup (1.6 oz)	160	0	5	34	1
TAKE-OUT						
pilaf	½ cup	84	3	362	11	3
risotto	6.6 oz	426	18	—	65	3
spanish	¾ cup	363	27	1339	19	—
WHITE						
Arrowhead						
Basmati	¼ cup (1.5 oz)	150	0	0	34	tr
Casbah						
Basmati as prep	1 cup	158	tr	—	36	—
Minute						
Boil In Bag Long Grain as prep	½ cup	94	0	4	21	—
Long Grain as prep	⅔ cup	150	3	31	27	1
Rice as prep	⅔ cup	141	2	21	27	1
Rice Long Grain & Wild as prep	½ cup	149	4	574	25	—
S&W						
Long Grain cooked	3.5 oz	106	0	0	23	—
Superfino						
Arborio Rice	½ cup	100	0	5	22	—

FOOD	PORTION	CAL.	FAT	SOD.	CARB.	FIB.
Uncle Ben						
Boil-In-Bag	1 serv (0.9 oz)	94	tr	9	22	tr
Converted	1 serv (1.2 oz)	123	tr	1	27	tr
In An Instant	1 serv (1.1 oz)	111	tr	10	25	tr
glutinous cooked	½ cup	116	tr	6	25	—
long-grain cooked	½ cup	131	tr	2	28	tr
long-grain instant cooked	½ cup	80	tr	2	17	tr
long-grain parboiled cooked	½ cup	100	tr	3	22	tr
medium-grain cooked	½ cup	132	tr	0	29	—
short-grain cooked	½ cup	133	tr	0	29	—
starch	3½ oz	343	0	61	85	—

RICE CAKES
(*see also* POPCORN CAKES)

FOOD	PORTION	CAL.	FAT	SOD.	CARB.	FIB.
Hain						
5-Grain	1	40	tr	10	8	—
Mini Apple Cinnamon	½ oz	60	tr	10	12	0
Mini Barbeque	½ oz	70	3	50	10	0
Mini Cheese	½ oz	60	2	100	10	0
Mini Honey Nut	½ oz	60	tr	30	11	0
Mini Nacho Cheese	½ oz	70	2	90	10	—
Mini Plain	½ oz	60	tr	20	12	0
Mini Plain No Salt Added	½ oz	60	tr	5	12	0
Mini Ranch	½ oz	70	3	90	9	0
Mini Teriyaki	½ oz	50	tr	75	12	0
Plain	1	40	tr	10	8	—
Plain No Salt Added	1	40	tr	<5	8	—
Sesame	1	40	tr	10	8	—
Sesame No Salt	1	40	tr	<5	8	—
Ka-Me						
Cheese	16 pieces (1 oz)	120	2	180	24	0
Onion	16 pieces (1 oz)	120	1	75	25	0
Plain	16 pieces (1 oz)	120	2	15	25	0
Seaweed	16 pieces (1 oz)	120	2	100	25	0
Sesame	16 pieces (1 oz)	120	2	85	24	0
Unsalted	16 pieces (1 oz)	120	1	0	26	0
Lundberg						
Organic Lightly Salted	1	60	1	120	14	—
Organic Unsalted	1	60	1	3	14	—
Premium Lightly Salted	1	60	1	120	14	—
Premium Unsalted	1	60	1	3	14	—
Sesame Lightly Salted	1	59	0	6	16	—
Mother's						
Mini Apple	5 (0.5 oz)	50	0	40	12	0

FOOD	PORTION	CAL.	FAT	SOD.	CARB.	FIB.
Mother's (CONT.)						
Mini Caramel	5 (0.5 oz)	50	0	40	12	0
Mini Cinnamon	5 (0.5 oz)	50	0	40	12	0
Mini Plain Unsalted	7 (0.5 oz)	60	0	0	12	0
Multigrain Lightly Salted	1 (0.3 oz)	35	0	30	7	0
Rye Unsalted	1 (0.3 oz)	35	0	0	7	1
Wheat Unsalted	1 (0.3 oz)	35	0	0	7	1
Pritikin						
Mini Apple Crisp	5 (0.5 oz)	50	0	20	12	—
Multigrain	1 (0.3 oz)	35	0	20	7	—
Multigrain Unsalted	1 (0.3 oz)	35	0	0	7	—
Plain	1 (0.3 oz)	35	0	20	7	—
Plain Unsalted	1 (0.3 oz)	35	0	0	7	—
Sesame Low Sodium	1 (0.3 oz)	35	0	20	7	—
Sesame Unsalted	1 (0.3 oz)	35	0	0	7	—
Quaker						
Apple Cinnamon	1 (0.5 oz)	50	0	0	11	—
Banana Crunch	1 (0.5 oz)	50	0	45	11	—
Cinnamon Crunch	1 (0.5 oz)	50	0	25	11	—
Mini Apple Cinnamon	5 (0.5 oz)	50	0	0	12	—
Mini Banana Nut	5 (0.5 oz)	50	0	40	12	—
Mini Butter Popped Corn	6 (0.5 oz)	50	0	120	12	—
Mini Caramel Corn	5 (0.5 oz)	50	0	25	12	—
Mini Chocolate Crunch	5 (0.5 oz)	50	0	10	12	—
Mini Cinnamon Crunch	5 (0.5 oz)	50	0	25	12	—
Mini Honey Nut	5 (0.5 oz)	50	0	25	12	—
Mini Monterey Jack	6 (0.5 oz)	50	0	100	11	—
Mini White Cheddar	6 (0.5 oz)	50	0	120	11	—
Salt-Free	1 (0.3 oz)	35	0	0	7	—
Salted	1 (0.3 oz)	35	0	15	7	—
Tree Of Life						
Fat Free Mini Apple Cinnamon	15	60	0	5	13	0
Fat Free Mini Caramel	15	60	0	10	13	0
Fat Free Mini Honey Nut	15	60	0	0	13	0
Fat Free Mini Jalapeno	15	60	0	25	13	0
Fat Free Mini Plain	15	50	0	45	12	0
brown rice	1 (0.3 oz)	35	tr	29	7	tr
brown rice & buckwheat	1 (0.3 oz)	34	tr	10	7	tr
brown rice & buckwheat unsalted	1 (0.3 oz)	34	tr	tr	7	tr
brown rice & corn	1 (0.3 oz)	35	tr	26	7	—
brown rice & rye	1 (0.3 oz)	35	tr	10	7	tr
brown rice & sesame seed	1 (0.3 oz)	35	tr	20	7	—

FOOD	PORTION	CAL.	FAT	SOD.	CARB.	FIB.
brown rice multigrain	1 (0.3 oz)	35	tr	23	7	—
brown rice multigrain unsalted	1 (0.3 oz)	35	tr	tr	7	—
brown rice unsalted	1 (0.3 oz)	35	tr	3	7	tr
ROCKFISH						
pacific cooked	1 fillet (5.2 oz)	180	3	114	0	—
pacific cooked	3 oz	103	2	65	0	—
pacific raw	3 oz	80	1	51	0	—
ROE						
(see individual fish names)						
fish	3.5 oz	39	2	—	tr	—
fresh baked	1 oz	58	2	—	1	—
fresh baked	3 oz	173	7	—	2	—
ROLL						
(see also BISCUIT, CROISSANT, ENGLISH MUFFIN, MUFFIN, POPOVER, SCONE)						
FROZEN						
Pepperidge Farm						
Cinnamon Roll	1 (2¼ oz)	220	14	190	34	—
Sara Lee						
All Butter Cinnamon Roll w/ Icing	1	280	11	220	43	—
All Butter Cinnamon Roll w/o Icing	1	230	11	220	31	—
Weight Watchers						
Cinnamon Rolls	1 (2.1 oz)	180	5	170	31	—
HOME RECIPE						
dinner as prep w/ 2% milk	1 (2½ in)	111	3	145	19	—
dinner as prep w/ whole milk	1 (2½ in)	112	3	145	19	—
raisin & nut	1 (2 oz)	196	7	185	30	—
MIX						
Dromedary						
Hot Roll Mix	2	239	5	410	41	—
Natural Ovens						
German Hard	1 (2.1 oz)	138	1	140	36	1
Gourmet Dinner	1 (1 oz)	50	1	140	15	2
Hearty Sandwich	1 (1.8 oz)	110	1	140	30	2
Pillsbury						
Hot Roll Mix	2	240	4	430	42	—
READY-TO-EAT						
Alvarado St. Bakery						
Burger Buns	1 (2.2 oz)	140	2	290	27	3

FOOD	PORTION	CAL.	FAT	SOD.	CARB.	FIB.
Alvarado St. Bakery (CONT.)						
Hot Dog Buns	1 (2.2 oz)	140	2	290	28	3
Arnold						
8-inch Francisco	1 (2.5 oz)	210	3	260	39	—
Augusto Pan Cubano	1	230	3	500	43	2
Bakery Light	1 (1.5 oz)	80	<2	190	21	4
Bran'nola Buns	1 (1.5 oz)	100	1	160	20	3
Deli Kaiser	1	170	2	—	34	—
Deli Onion	1	170	2	—	34	—
Dinner Plain	1 (0.7 oz)	50	1	80	9	1
Dinner Sesame	1 (0.7 oz)	50	1	80	9	1
Dutch Egg	1	130	3	180	21	2
French Francisco	1 (2.5 oz)	210	3	260	39	—
French Mini Francisco	1	130	2	140	24	—
Hamburger	1	120	2	190	20	2
Hot Dog	1 (1.5 oz)	110	2	160	21	1
Hot Dog Bran'nola	1 (1.5 oz)	110	2	170	18	1
Hot Dog New England Style	1	110	2	160	20	1
Italian 8-inch Savoni	1	210	3	—	38	3
Kaiser Francisco	1 (2 oz)	180	—	230	34	—
Onion Premium	1 (2.6 oz)	180	1	340	38	2
Onion Soft	1	140	—	200	28	2
Party Petite	2	70	2	70	10	1
Potato	1	140	2	210	25	2
Sandwich Soft Sesame	1	130	3	220	23	2
Sourdough Brown N' Serve	1 (1 oz)	100	1	120	19	—
Sourdough Francisco	1 (1 oz)	100	1	120	19	—
Wheat Old Fashioned	2	80	3	98	11	—
August Bros.						
Dinner	1	90	1	170	18	—
Kaiser	1	170	1	310	35	2
Onion	1	160	1	310	33	2
Sesame Cubano	1	170	1	310	35	2
Bread Du Jour						
Bavarian Cracked Wheat	1 (1.2 oz)	90	1	190	17	1
Crusty Italian	1 (1.2 oz)	80	1	190	16	tr
French Petite	1 (3.5 oz)	230	2	530	47	2
Rye	1 (1.2 oz)	90	2	230	16	1
Sourdough	1 (2.2 oz)	140	2	230	29	2
Country Kitchen						
Frankfurt	1	120	2	—	—	—

FOOD	PORTION	CAL.	FAT	SOD.	CARB.	FIB.
Dicarlo's						
Extra Sourdough	1 (1.6 oz)	100	1	230	20	1
French	1 (1 oz)	70	1	150	14	tr
Hollywood						
Dark Bread	1	40	tr	—	—	—
Dinner Light Pan Special Formula	1	60	tr	—	—	—
Sliced Light Special Formula	1	80	tr	—	—	—
Home Pride						
Dinner Wheat	1 (1.9 oz)	160	4	270	26	2
Hamburger Potato Bun	1 (1.9 oz)	130	2	270	27	2
Hot Dog Potato Bun	1 (1.9 oz)	130	2	270	27	2
Sandwich Roll Wheat	1 (1.9 oz)	160	4	270	26	2
White	2 (1.6 oz)	130	4	230	22	1
Levy						
Sub Old Country	1	180	2	230	34	—
Martin's						
Big Marty Poppy	1	170	2	320	31	3
Big Marty Sesame	1	170	2	320	31	3
Hoagie	1	240	3	430	41	3
Hoagie Sesame	1	240	3	430	41	4
Potato Dinner	1	100	1	135	18	1
Potato Long	1	140	1	200	27	2
Potato Party	1	50	1	70	10	1
Potato Sandwich	1	140	1	200	26	2
Sandwich Whole Wheat 100% Stoneground	1	160	2	290	28	5
Matthew's						
Salad Roll	1	110	2	190	19	2
Sandwich	1	110	2	180	19	2
Pepperidge Farm						
Brown 'N Serve Club	1	100	1	190	19	1
Brown 'N Serve French	½ roll	180	2	380	36	1
Brown 'N Serve Hearth	1	50	1	100	10	tr
Dinner	1	60	2	95	8	tr
Dinner Country Style Classic	1	50	1	90	9	0
Finger Poppy Seed	1	50	2	80	8	tr
Finger Sesame Seed	1	60	2	85	9	tr
Frankfurter Dijon	1	160	5	230	23	2
Frankfurter Side Sliced	1	140	3	270	24	1
Frankfurter Top Sliced	1	140	3	270	24	1
Frankfurter w/ Poppy Seeds	1	130	2	280	23	1

FOOD	PORTION	CAL.	FAT	SOD.	CARB.	FIB.
Pepperidge Farm (CONT.)						
French Style	1	100	1	230	20	1
Hamburger	1	130	2	240	22	1
Heat & Serve Butter Crescent	1	110	6	150	13	tr
Heat & Serve Golden Twist	1	110	5	150	14	tr
Hoagie Soft	1	210	5	320	34	1
Old Fashioned	1	50	2	85	7	tr
Parker House	1	60	1	80	9	tr
Party	1	30	1	50	5	tr
Potato Sandwich	1	160	4	260	28	1
Sandwich Onion w/ Poppy Seeds	1	150	3	260	26	1
Sandwich Salad	1	110	4	150	16	—
Sandwich w/ Sesame Seeds	1	140	3	230	23	1
Soft Family	1	100	2	190	18	1
Sourdough French	1	100	1	240	19	1
Roman Meal						
Brown & Serve	2 (2 oz)	140	3	275	24	2
Dinner	2 (2 oz)	136	2	282	24	2
Hamburger	1 (1.6 oz)	111	2	229	19	2
Hotdog	1 (1.5 oz)	103	2	214	18	2
Sandwich	1 (2.7 oz)	181	3	392	31	3
The Baker						
Honey Cinnamon Raisin	1 (2 oz)	150	2	115	31	4
Wonder						
Brown N' Serve Buttermilk	1 (1 oz)	70	1	160	13	tr
Brown 'N Serve Wheat	1 (1 oz)	70	1	135	14	tr
Brown 'N Serve White	1 (1 oz)	70	1	135	14	tr
Dinner White Light	1 (1 oz)	60	1	150	9	4
Hamburger	1 (1.5 oz)	110	2	250	21	tr
Hamburger Light	1 (1.5 oz)	80	2	210	13	5
Hamburger Wheat	1 (2.2 oz)	170	3	370	31	1
Hot Dog	1 (1.5 oz)	110	2	250	21	tr
Hot Dog Light	1 (1.5 oz)	80	2	210	13	5
Tea Dinner Rolls	1 (1.5 oz)	80	1	210	19	5
brown & serve	1 (1 oz)	85	2	148	14	—
cheese	1 (2.3 oz)	238	12	236	29	—
cinnamon raisin	1 (2¾ in)	223	10	229	31	4
dinner	1 (1 oz)	85	2	148	14	—
egg	1 (2½ in)	107	2	191	18	1

FOOD	PORTION	CAL.	FAT	SOD.	CARB.	FIB.
french	1 (1.3 oz)	105	2	232	19	—
hamburger	1 (1½ oz)	123	2	241	22	—
hamburger multi-grain	1 (1½ oz)	113	2	197	19	2
hamburger reduced calorie	1 (1½ oz)	84	1	190	18	3
hard	1 (3½ in)	167	2	310	30	—
hot cross bun	1	202	4	—	38	1
hot dog	1 (1½ oz)	123	2	241	22	—
hot dog multi-grain	1 (1½ oz)	113	2	197	19	2
hot dog reduced calorie	1 (1½ oz)	84	1	190	18	3
kaiser	1 (3½ in)	167	2	310	30	—
oat bran	1 (1.2 oz)	78	2	136	13	1
rye	1 (1 oz)	81	1	253	15	—
submarine	1 (4.7 oz)	155	2	313	30	—
wheat	1 (1 oz)	77	2	96	13	—
whole wheat	1 (1 oz)	75	1	135	15	—
REFRIGERATED						
Pillsbury						
Best Quick Cinnamon Rolls w/ Icing	1	110	5	260	17	—
Butterflake	1	140	5	530	20	—
Crescent	1	100	6	230	11	—
cinnamon w/ frosting	1	109	4	250	17	—
crescent	1 (1 oz)	98	4	341	14	—

ROMAN BEANS

FOOD	PORTION	CAL.	FAT	SOD.	CARB.	FIB.
Progresso	½ cup	110	tr	420	18	12

ROSE APPLE

FOOD	PORTION	CAL.	FAT	SOD.	CARB.	FIB.
fresh	3½ oz	32	tr	—	7	—

ROSE HIP

FOOD	PORTION	CAL.	FAT	SOD.	CARB.	FIB.
fresh	3½ oz	91	0	146	19	—

ROSELLE

FOOD	PORTION	CAL.	FAT	SOD.	CARB.	FIB.
fresh	1 cup	28	tr	3	6	—

ROSEMARY

FOOD	PORTION	CAL.	FAT	SOD.	CARB.	FIB.
dried	1 tsp	4	tr	1	1	—

ROUGHY

FOOD	PORTION	CAL.	FAT	SOD.	CARB.	FIB.
orange baked	3 oz	75	1	69	0	—

RUTABAGA

FOOD	PORTION	CAL.	FAT	SOD.	CARB.	FIB.
CANNED						
Sunshine						
Diced	½ cup (4.2 oz)	30	0	220	7	3
FRESH						
cooked mashed	½ cup	41	tr	22	9	—
raw cubed	½ cup	25	tr	14	6	—

FOOD	PORTION	CAL.	FAT	SOD.	CARB.	FIB.
SABLEFISH						
baked	3 oz	213	17	61	0	—
fillet baked	5.3 oz	378	30	108	0	—
smoked	1 oz	72	6	206	0	—
smoked	3 oz	218	17	626	0	—
SAFFLOWER						
seeds dried	1 oz	147	11	—	10	—
SAFFRON						
saffron	1 tsp	2	tr	1	tr	—
SAGE						
Watkins	¼ tsp (0.5 g)	0	0	0	0	0
ground	1 tsp	2	tr	tr	tr	—
SALAD						
(*see also* LETTUCE, PASTA SALAD)						
MIX						
Dole						
Caesar Salad	⅓ pkg (3.5 oz)	170	14	480	9	1
Classic Blend	3.5 oz	25	1	20	4	1
Coleslaw Blend	3.5 oz	30	1	35	5	2
French Blend	3.5 oz	25	1	15	4	1
Italian Blend	3.5 oz	25	1	45	3	1
Salad-In-A-Minute Oriental	3.5 oz	110	7	290	12	2
Salad-In-A-Minute Spinach	3.5 oz	180	9	660	19	3
Fresh Express						
American Salad	1½ cups (3 oz)	20	0	10	3	1
Caesar Salad	1½ cups (3 oz)	140	11	320	8	1
European Salad	1½ cups (3 oz)	20	0	10	3	1
Garden Salad	1½ cups (3 oz)	20	0	10	3	1
Italian Salad	1½ cups (3 oz)	20	0	0	3	1
Oriental Salad	1½ cups (3 oz)	120	8	330	11	1
Riviera Salad	1½ cups (3 oz)	10	0	0	2	1
Spinach Salad	1½ cups (3 oz)	130	3	430	23	3
Suddenly Salad						
Caesar as prep	½ cup	170	8	450	20	—
Ranch & Bacon as prep	½ cup	210	11	320	22	—
Ranch & Bacon as prep low fat recipe	½ cup	160	5	350	23	—
TAKE-OUT						
chef w/o dressing	1½ cups	386	28	279	9	—
tossed w/o dressing	1½ cups	32	tr	53	7	—

FOOD	PORTION	CAL.	FAT	SOD.	CARB.	FIB.
tossed w/o dressing	¾ cup	16	0	27	3	—
tossed w/o dressing w/ cheese & egg	1½ cups	102	6	119	5	—
tossed w/o dressing w/ chicken	1½ cups	105	2	209	4	—
tossed w/o dressing w/ pasta & seafood	1½ cups (14.6 oz)	380	21	1572	32	—
tossed w/o dressing w/ shrimp	1½ cups	107	2	487	7	—
waldorf	½ cup	79	6	49	6	1

SALAD DRESSING
HOME RECIPE

french	1 tbsp	88	10	92	1	—
vinegar & oil	1 tbsp	72	8	tr	tr	—

MIX
Good Seasons

Blue Cheese & Herbs as prep	1 tbsp	72	8	148	1	—
Buttermilk Farm as prep	1 tbsp	58	6	137	1	—
Cheese Garlic as prep	1 tbsp	72	8	167	1	—
Cheese Italian as prep	1 tbsp	72	8	127	1	—
Classic Dill	1 pkg	28	tr	2273	5	—
Garlic & Herbs as prep	1 tbsp	71	8	187	1	—
Italian as prep	1 tbsp	71	8	172	1	—
Italian Lite as prep	1 tbsp	27	3	177	1	—
Italian No Oil as prep	1 tbsp	7	0	32	2	—
Lemon & Herbs as prep	1 tbsp	71	8	143	1	—
Lite Cheese Italian as prep	1 tbsp	27	3	137	1	—
Lite Ranch as prep	1 tbsp	29	2	115	2	—
Lite Zesty Italian as prep	1 tbsp	26	3	133	1	—
Mild Italian as prep	1 tbsp	73	8	192	1	—
Ranch as prep	1 tbsp	57	6	112	1	—
Zesty Italian as prep	1 tbsp	71	8	121	1	—

Hain

No Oil 1000 Island	1 tbsp	12	0	150	3	—
No Oil Bleu Cheese	1 tbsp	14	1	190	1	—
No Oil Buttermilk	1 tbsp	11	tr	150	1	—
No Oil Caesar	1 tbsp	6	tr	200	1	—
No Oil French	1 tbsp	12	0	340	3	—
No Oil Garlic & Cheese	1 tbsp	6	tr	180	1	—
No Oil Herb	1 tbsp	2	0	140	1	—

FOOD	PORTION	CAL.	FAT	SOD.	CARB.	FIB.
Hain (CONT.)						
No Oil Italian	1 tbsp	2	0	170	1	—
READY-TO-USE						
Estee						
Blue Cheese	2 tbsp (1 oz)	15	1	80	1	—
Creamy French	2 tbsp (1 oz)	10	0	80	2	—
Creamy French Fat Free	1 pkg (0.5 oz)	5	0	40	1	—
Creamy Garlic	2 tbsp (1 oz)	60	0	80	2	—
Creamy Garlic Fat Free	1 pkg (0.5 oz)	5	0	40	1	—
Creamy Italian	2 tbsp (1 oz)	15	1	80	2	—
Fat Free Thousand Island	1 pkg (0.5 oz)	5	0	40	1	—
Italian	2 tbsp (1 oz)	5	0	80	1	—
Italian Fat Free	1 pkg (0.5 oz)	0	0	40	tr	—
Low Fat Blue Cheese	1 pkg (0.5 oz)	5	0	40	tr	—
Thousand Island	2 tbsp (1 oz)	10	0	80	2	—
Hain						
1000 Island	1 tbsp	50	5	85	0	—
Canola Garden Tomato	1 tbsp	60	6	150	1	—
Canola Italian	1 tbsp	50	5	150	1	—
Canola Spicy French Mustard	1 tbsp	50	5	190	1	—
Canola Tangy Citrus	1 tbsp	50	5	75	1	—
Creamy Caesar	1 tbsp	60	6	220	1	—
Creamy Caesar Low Salt	1 tbsp	60	6	15	1	—
Creamy French	1 tbsp	60	6	80	1	—
Creamy Italian	1 tbsp	80	8	100	0	—
Creamy Italian No Salt Added	1 tbsp	80	8	25	1	—
Cucumber Dill	1 tbsp	80	8	210	0	—
Dijon Vinaigrette	1 tbsp	50	5	180	1	—
Garlic & Sour Cream	1 tbsp	70	7	100	0	—
Honey & Sesame	1 tbsp	60	5	210	2	—
Italian Cheese Vinaigrette	1 tbsp	55	6	130	0	—
Old Fashioned Buttermilk	1 tbsp	70	7	100	0	—
Poppyseed Rancher's	1 tbsp	60	7	105	0	—
Savory Herb No Salt Added	1 tbsp	90	10	45	0	—
Swiss Cheese Vinaigrette	1 tbsp	60	7	160	0	—
Traditional Italian	1 tbsp	80	8	330	0	—
Traditional Italian No Salt Added	1 tbsp	60	6	20	1	—

FOOD	PORTION	CAL.	FAT	SOD.	CARB.	FIB.
Healthy Sensation						
Blue Cheese	1 tbsp	19	1	144	4	—
French	1 tbsp	21	1	121	4	—
Honey Dijon	1 tbsp	26	1	142	5	—
Italian	1 tbsp	7	tr	141	1	—
Ranch	1 tbsp	15	tr	138	3	—
Thousand Island	1 tbsp	20	tr	134	4	—
Hollywood						
Caesar	1 tbsp	70	7	65	2	0
Creamy French	1 tbsp	70	7	45	2	0
Creamy Italian	1 tbsp	90	9	140	2	0
Dijon Vinaigrette	1 tbsp	60	6	40	2	0
Italian	1 tbsp	90	9	300	1	0
Italian Cheese	1 tbsp	80	8	60	2	0
Old Fashion Buttermilk	1 tbsp	75	8	40	1	0
Poppy Seed Rancher's	1 tbsp	75	8	35	1	0
Thousand Island	1 tbsp	60	6	15	3	0
Kraft						
Bacon & Tomato	2 tbsp (1.1 oz)	140	14	260	2	0
Buttermilk Ranch	2 tbsp (1 oz)	150	16	230	2	0
Caesar	2 tbsp (1.1 oz)	130	13	370	2	0
Caesar Ranch	2 tbsp (1 oz)	140	15	300	1	0
Catalina With Honey	2 tbsp (1.2 oz)	140	12	310	8	0
Catalina French	2 tbsp (1.2 oz)	140	11	390	8	0
Chunky Blue Cheese	2 tbsp (1.2 oz)	90	7	470	5	0
Coleslaw	2 tbsp (1.2 oz)	150	12	420	8	0
Creamy Caesar	2 tbsp (1 oz)	140	15	200	1	0
Creamy Garlic	2 tbsp (1.1 oz)	110	11	350	2	0
Creamy Italian	2 tbsp (1.1 oz)	110	11	230	3	0
Cucumber Ranch	2 tbsp (1.1 oz)	150	15	220	2	0
Deliciously Right Bacon & Tomato	2 tbsp (1.1 oz)	60	5	300	3	0
Deliciously Right Caesar	2 tbsp (1.1 oz)	50	5	560	2	0
Deliciously Right Catalina French	2 tbsp (1.2 oz)	80	4	400	9	0
Deliciously Right Creamy Italian	2 tbsp (1.1 oz)	50	5	250	3	0
Deliciously Right Cucumber Ranch	2 tbsp (1.1 oz)	60	5	450	2	0
Deliciously Right French	2 tbsp (1.2 oz)	50	3	260	6	0
Deliciously Right Italian	2 tbsp (1.1 oz)	70	7	240	3	0
Deliciously Right Ranch	2 tbsp (1.1 oz)	110	11	310	2	0
Deliciously Right Thousand Island	2 tbsp (1.2 oz)	70	4	320	8	0

FOOD	PORTION	CAL.	FAT	SOD.	CARB.	FIB.
Kraft (CONT.)						
Free Blue Cheese	2 tbsp (1.2 oz)	50	0	340	12	1
Free Catalina	2 tbsp (1.2 oz)	45	0	360	11	tr
Free French	2 tbsp (1.2 oz)	50	0	300	12	tr
Free Honey Dijon	2 tbsp (1.2 oz)	50	0	330	11	1
Free Italian	2 tbsp (1.1 oz)	10	0	290	2	0
Free Peppercorn Ranch	2 tbsp (1.2 oz)	50	0	360	11	1
Free Ranch	1 tbsp (1.2 oz)	50	0	310	11	tr
Free Red Wine Vinegar	2 tbsp (1.1 oz)	15	0	400	3	0
Free Thousand Island	2 tbsp (1.2 oz)	45	0	300	11	1
French	2 tbsp (1.1 oz)	120	12	260	4	0
Honey Dijon	2 tbsp (1.1 oz)	150	15	200	4	0
House Italian	2 tbsp (1.1 oz)	120	12	240	3	0
Oil-Free Italian	2 tbsp (1.1 oz)	5	0	450	2	0
Peppercorn Ranch	2 tbsp (1 oz)	170	18	340	1	0
Pesto Italian	2 tbsp (1.1 oz)	140	15	290	2	0
Ranch	2 tbsp (1 oz)	170	18	270	2	0
Roka Blue Cheese	2 tbsp (1.2 oz)	90	7	470	5	0
Russian	2 tbsp (1.2 oz)	130	10	280	10	0
Salsa Ranch	2 tbsp (1 oz)	130	13	320	1	0
Salsa Zesty Garden	2 tbsp (1.1 oz)	70	6	280	3	tr
Sour Cream & Onion Ranch	2 tbsp (1 oz)	170	18	240	1	0
Thousand Island	2 tbsp (1.1 oz)	110	10	310	5	0
Thousand Island With Bacon	2 tbsp (1 oz)	120	12	190	5	0
Zesty Italian	2 tbsp (1.1 oz)	110	11	530	2	0
Marzetti						
Bacon Spinach Salad	2 tbsp	80	15	260	16	15
Blue Cheese	2 tbsp	160	17	230	0	0
Buttermilk & Herb	2 tbsp	180	20	260	1	0
Buttermilk Bacon Ranch	2 tbsp	180	19	270	1	0
Buttermilk Blue Cheese	2 tbsp	160	18	220	1	0
Buttermilk Parmesan Pepper	2 tbsp	170	18	310	1	0
Buttermilk Parmesan Ranch	2 tbsp	160	17	240	1	0
Buttermilk Ranch	2 tbsp	180	20	250	1	0
Buttermilk Veggie Dip	2 tbsp	170	18	240	1	0
Caesar	2 tbsp	150	16	390	1	0
Caesar Ranch	2 tbsp	190	20	300	2	0
California French	2 tbsp	160	13	240	11	0
Celery Seed	2 tbsp	160	13	180	10	0
Chunky Blue Cheese	2 tbsp	150	16	300	1	0

FOOD	PORTION	CAL.	FAT	SOD.	CARB.	FIB.
Marzetti (CONT.)						
Classic Caesar Ranch	2 tbsp	190	20	300	2	0
Country French	2 tbsp	150	13	220	7	0
Cracked Peppercorn	2 tbsp	140	14	280	1	0
Creamy Garlic Italian	2 tbsp	160	17	140	1	0
Creamy Italian	2 tbsp	150	16	170	1	0
Crispy Celery Seed	2 tbsp	160	13	190	11	0
Dijon Honey Mustard	2 tbsp	140	13	180	6	0
Dijon Ranch	2 tbsp	170	18	190	2	0
Dutch Sweet'N Sour	2 tbsp	160	13	200	10	0
Fat Free California French	2 tbsp	45	0	330	11	0
Fat Free Honey Dijon	2 tbsp	60	0	190	14	1
Fat Free Honey French	2 tbsp	45	0	330	11	0
Fat Free Italian	2 tbsp	15	0	450	3	0
Fat Free Peppercorn Ranch	2 tbsp	30	0	420	7	1
Fat Free Ranch	2 tbsp	30	0	430	7	1
Fat Free Raspberry	2 tbsp	70	0	150	18	0
Fat Free Slaw	2 tbsp	45	0	390	11	0
Fat Free Sweet & Sour	2 tbsp	45	0	290	14	0
Fat Free Thousand Island	2 tbsp	35	0	370	9	0
Garden Ranch	2 tbsp	180	19	250	1	0
Gusto Italian	2 tbsp	120	13	740	1	0
Honey Dijon	2 tbsp	140	13	170	6	0
Honey Dijon Ranch	2 tbsp	150	15	200	2	0
Honey French	2 tbsp	160	14	230	11	0
Honey French Blue Cheese	2 tbsp	160	13	260	11	0
House Caesar	2 tbsp	150	16	340	1	0
Italian With Olive Oil	2 tbsp	120	13	480	1	0
Light Slaw	2 tbsp	60	7	380	10	0
Light Blue Cheese	2 tbsp	60	6	650	4	0
Light Buttermilk Ranch	2 tbsp	90	9	280	3	0
Light California French	2 tbsp	80	6	360	8	0
Light Chunky Blue Cheese	2 tbsp	80	7	330	4	0
Light French	2 tbsp	40	2	320	6	0
Light Honey French	2 tbsp	80	4	250	12	0
Light Italian	2 tbsp	60	5	570	3	0
Light Ranch	2 tbsp	90	8	430	3	0
Light Red Wine Vinegar & Oil	2 tbsp	20	1	490	3	0
Light Sweet & Sour	2 tbsp	100	6	260	11	0

FOOD	PORTION	CAL.	FAT	SOD.	CARB.	FIB.
Marzetti (CONT.)						
Light Thousand Island	2 tbsp	70	5	350	6	0
Old Fashioned Poppyseed	2 tbsp	140	11	220	10	0
Olde Venice Italian	2 tbsp	130	13	490	2	0
Olde World Caesar	2 tbsp	150	16	340	1	0
Parmesan Pepper	2 tbsp	160	17	260	1	0
Peppercorn Ranch	2 tbsp	180	19	220	1	0
Poppyseed	2 tbsp	160	13	310	10	0
Potato Salad Dressing	2 tbsp	120	13	300	7	0
Ranch	2 tbsp	180	20	260	1	0
Red Wine Vinegar & Oil	2 tbsp	130	14	460	2	0
Romano Cheese Caesar	2 tbsp	150	16	370	1	0
Romano Italian	2 tbsp	160	17	390	1	0
Savory Italian	2 tbsp	110	12	520	3	0
Slaw	2 tbsp	170	16	370	6	0
Southern Slaw	2 tbsp	100	11	210	14	0
Sweet & Saucy	2 tbsp	140	12	290	9	0
Sweet & Sour	2 tbsp	160	13	210	10	0
Thousand Island	2 tbsp	150	15	230	5	0
Vintage Champagne	2 tbsp	150	16	460	2	0
Wilde Raspberry	2 tbsp	150	12	65	12	0
Newman's Own						
Italian Light	1 tbsp (0.5 fl oz)	10	tr	170	tr	—
Olive Oil & Vinegar	1 tbsp (0.5 fl oz)	80	9	80	tr	—
Ranch	1 tbsp (0.5 fl oz)	90	9	80	1	—
Pfeiffer						
1000 Island	2 tbsp	140	14	220	4	0
California French	2 tbsp	140	12	290	9	0
French	2 tbsp	150	13	220	7	0
Honey Dijon	2 tbsp	140	13	170	6	0
Lite Italian	2 tbsp	50	5	410	3	0
Ranch	2 tbsp	180	20	260	1	0
Savory Italian	2 tbsp	110	12	520	3	0
Pritikin						
Dijon Balsamic Vinaigrette	2 tbsp (1 oz)	3	0	125	6	—
French	2 tbsp (1 oz)	35	0	130	8	—
Honey Dijon	2 tbsp (1 oz)	45	0	130	11	—
Honey French	2 tbsp (1 oz)	40	0	135	11	—
Italian	2 tbsp (1 oz)	20	0	115	5	—
Raspberry Vinaigrette	2 tbsp (1 oz)	45	0	70	11	—
Red Wing						
"K" Dressing	1 tbsp (0.5 oz)	70	7	90	4	0

FOOD	PORTION	CAL.	FAT	SOD.	CARB.	FIB.
Red Wing (CONT.)						
Chunky Blue Cheese	2 tbsp (1 oz)	130	13	290	3	0
Creamy Ranch	2 tbsp (1 oz)	150	15	280	2	0
French Traditional	2 tbsp (1 oz)	130	11	250	8	0
Italian Traditional	2 tbsp (1 oz)	100	9	550	4	0
Spicy Sweet French	2 tbsp (1 oz)	130	11	370	8	0
Thousand Island Thick & Rich	2 tbsp (1 oz)	110	9	270	8	0
S&W						
Blue Cheese Low Calorie	1 tbsp	25	2	200	2	—
Creamy Cucumber Low Calorie	1 tbsp	25	2	190	2	—
Creamy Italian Low Calorie	1 tbsp	10	1	180	1	—
French Low Calorie	1 tbsp	18	0	120	3	—
Italian No-Oil	1 tbsp	2	0	290	0	—
Russian Low Calorie	1 tbsp	25	1	120	4	—
Thousand Island Low Calorie	1 tbsp	25	2	105	2	—
Seven Seas						
Creamy Italian	2 tbsp (1.1 oz)	110	12	510	2	0
Free Italian	2 tbsp (1.1 oz)	10	0	480	2	0
Free Ranch	2 tbsp (1.2 oz)	50	0	330	12	1
Free Red Wine Vinegar	2 tbsp (1.1 oz)	15	0	400	3	0
Green Goddess	2 tbsp (1 oz)	120	13	260	1	0
Herbs & Spices	2 tbsp (1.1 oz)	120	12	320	1	0
Ranch	2 tbsp (1 oz)	150	16	250	2	0
Red Wine Vinegar & Oil	2 tbsp (1.1 oz)	110	11	510	2	0
Reduced Calorie Creamy Italian	2 tbsp (1.1 oz)	60	5	490	2	0
Reduced Calorie Italian With Olive Oil	2 tbsp (1.1 oz)	50	5	450	2	0
Reduced Calorie Ranch	2 tbsp (1.1 oz)	100	9	320	5	0
Reduced Calorie Red Wine Vinegar & Oil	2 tbsp (1.1 oz)	60	5	310	2	0
Two Cheese Italian	2 tbsp (1.1 oz)	70	7	240	3	0
Viva Buttermilk	2 tbsp (1.1)	150	16	230	3	0
Viva Caesar	2 tbsp (1.1 oz)	120	12	500	2	0
Viva Italian	2 tbsp (1.1 oz)	110	11	580	2	0
Viva Reduced Calorie Italian	2 tbsp (1.1 oz)	45	4	390	2	0
Tree Of Life						
Cafe Venice	2 tbsp (1 oz)	100	12	170	2	0
Fat Free Blue Cheese	2 tbsp (1 oz)	15	1	260	2	—

FOOD	PORTION	CAL.	FAT	SOD.	CARB.	FIB.
Tree Of Life (CONT.)						
Fat Free Honey French	2 tbsp (1 oz)	35	0	150	8	—
Fat Free Italian Garlic	2 tbsp (1 oz)	20	0	260	4	—
Fat Free Oriental Ginger	2 tbsp (1 oz)	15	0	310	3	—
Frisco's Raspberry	2 tbsp (1 oz)	120	11	80	5	0
Maison Caesar	2 tbsp (1 oz)	70	6	115	1	0
Shanghai Palace	2 tbsp (1 oz)	80	7	310	3	0
Ultra Slim-Fast						
French	1 tbsp	20	tr	150	4	0
Italian	1 tbsp	6	tr	170	1	0
W.J. Clark						
Ginger Orange Vinaigrette	1 tbsp	73	7	134	tr	0
Herbs & Romano	1 tbsp	67	6	111	2	0
Lemon Peppercorn	1 tbsp	72	7	135	tr	0
Lime Cilantro Vinaigrette	1 tbsp	73	8	147	tr	0
Poppy Seed	1 tbsp	75	6	106	3	0
Sweet Pepper Basil	1 tbsp	69	7	127	2	0
Tarragon Honey Mustard	1 tbsp	66	6	139	2	0
Walden Farms						
Bleu Cheese Fat Free	2 tbsp (1 oz)	25	0	240	4	0
Creamy Italian With Parmesan Fat Free	1 tbsp (1 oz)	25	0	360	4	0
Fat Free Balsamic Vinaigrette	2 tbsp (1 oz)	15	0	360	3	0
Fat Free Caesar	2 tbsp (1 oz)	25	0	360	4	0
Fat Free Italian	2 tbsp (1 oz)	10	0	290	2	0
Fat Free Raspberry Vinaigrette	2 tbsp (1 oz)	20	0	290	4	0
Fat Free Russian	2 tbsp (1 oz)	30	0	240	6	0
French Style Fat Free	2 tbsp (1 oz)	25	0	360	4	0
Honey Dijon Fat Free	2 tbsp (1 oz)	25	0	240	6	0
Italian Sodium Free Fat Free	2 tbsp (1 oz)	10	0	0	2	0
Italian Sugar Free Fat Free	2 tbsp (1 oz)	0	0	290	0	0
Italian With Sun Dried Tomato	2 tbsp (1 oz)	15	0	290	3	0
Ranch Fat Free	2 tbsp (1 oz)	25	0	290	4	0
Ranch With Sun Dried Tomato	2 tbsp (1 oz)	25	0	290	4	0
Thousand Island Fat Free	2 tbsp (1 oz)	35	0	240	7	0
Weight Watchers						
Caesar	1 tbsp	4	0	200	1	—

FOOD	PORTION	CAL.	FAT	SOD.	CARB.	FIB.
Weight Watchers (CONT.)						
Caesar	1 pkg (¾ oz)	6	0	280	1	—
Cucumber Creamy	1 tbsp	18	0	85	4	—
Italian	1 pkg (¾ oz)	8	tr	270	2	—
Italian	1 tbsp	6	tr	200	1	—
Italian Creamy	1 tbsp	12	0	85	3	—
Peppercorn Creamy	1 tbsp	8	0	85	2	—
Ranch Creamy	1 pkg (¾ oz)	35	tr	130	8	—
Ranch Creamy	1 tbsp	25	tr	100	6	—
Russian	1 tbsp	50	5	80	2	—
Thousand Island	1 tbsp	50	5	80	2	—
Wishbone						
Blue Cheese Chunky	1 tbsp	73	8	148	1	—
Blue Cheese Chunky Lite	1 tbsp	40	4	197	2	0
Classic Lite Dijon Vinaigrette	1 tbsp	30	3	176	1	—
Classic Lite Olive Oil Italian	1 tbsp	20	2	155	1	—
Classic Olive Oil Italian	1 tbsp	33	3	190	2	—
Creamy Italian	1 tbsp	54	6	149	1	—
Deluxe French	1 tbsp	57	5	83	2	0
Dijon Vinaigrette Classic	1 tbsp	57	6	159	1	0
French Fat Free	1 tbsp	6	tr	249	1	—
French Lite	1 tbsp	30	3	67	4	0
French Red	1 tbsp	64	6	170	4	—
French Sweet 'N Spicy	1 tbsp	613	6	156	3	—
French Sweet 'N Spicy Lite	1 tbsp	17	tr	134	4	—
Italian	1 tbsp	45	5	281	1	—
Italian Cream Lite	1 tbsp	26	2	148	2	—
Italian Lite	1 tbsp	6	tr	249	1	—
Lite Caesar With Olive Oil	1 tbsp	26	3	172	1	—
Lite French Red	1 tbsp	17	tr	155	3	—
Lite Olive Oil Vinaigrette	1 tbsp	16	1	133	2	—
Lite Red Wine Vinaigrette Olive Oil	1 tbsp	20	2	151	1	—
Olive Oil Vinaigrette	1 tbsp	30	3	126	2	—
Ranch	1 tbsp	76	8	103	1	—
Ranch Lite	1 tbsp	42	4	148	3	0
Red Wine Olive Oil Vinaigrette	1 tbsp	34	3	191	2	—
Robusto Italian	1 tbsp	46	5	288	2	0
Russian	1 tbsp	54	3	173	7	tr

FOOD	PORTION	CAL.	FAT	SOD.	CARB.	FIB.
Wishbone (CONT.)						
Russian Lite	1 tbsp	21	tr	142	5	—
Thousand Island	1 tbsp	66	6	168	3	—
Thousand Island Lite	1 tbsp	22	1	135	5	—
blue cheese	1 tbsp	77	8	—	1	—
french	1 tbsp	67	6	214	3	—
french reduced calorie	1 tbsp	22	1	128	4	—
italian	1 tbsp	69	7	116	2	—
italian reduced calorie	1 tbsp	16	2	118	1	—
russian	1 tbsp	76	8	133	2	—
russian reduced calorie	1 tbsp	23	1	141	5	—
sesame seed	1 tbsp	68	7	153	1	—
thousand island	1 tbsp	59	6	109	2	—
thousand island reduced calorie	1 tbsp	24	2	153	3	—
SALMON						
CANNED						
Bumble Bee						
Keta	3.5 oz	160	8	490	0	—
Pink	3.5 oz	160	8	490	0	—
Pink Skinless & Boneless	3.25 oz	120	5	420	0	—
Red	3.5 oz	180	10	490	0	—
Red Skinless & Boneless	3.25 oz	130	6	420	0	—
Deming's						
Alaska Keta	½ cup	140	5	450	0	—
Alaska Pink	½ cup	140	6	450	0	—
Alaska Red Sockeye	½ cup	170	9	450	0	—
Double Q						
Alaska Pink	½ cup	140	6	450	0	—
Humpty Dumpty						
Alaska Chum	½ cup	140	2	450	0	—
Libby						
Keta	½ can (3.8 oz)	140	6	—	—	—
Pink	½ can (3.8 oz)	150	7	—	—	—
S&W						
Bluepack Fancy Diet	½ cup	188	11	45	0	—
Red Fancy Sockeye Bluepack	½ cup	190	10	590	0	—
chum w/ bone	3 oz	120	5	414	0	—
chum w/ bone	1 can (13.9 oz)	521	20	1797	0	—
pink w/ bone	3 oz	118	5	471	0	—
pink w/ bone	1 can (15.9 oz)	631	27	2514	0	—

FOOD	PORTION	CAL.	FAT	SOD.	CARB.	FIB.
sockeye w/ bone	3 oz	130	6	458	0	—
sockeye w/ bone	1 can (12.9 oz)	566	27	1987	0	—
FRESH						
atlantic baked	3 oz	155	7	48	0	—
chinook baked	3 oz	196	11	51	0	—
chum baked	3 oz	131	4	54	0	—
coho cooked	3 oz	157	6	50	0	—
coho cooked	½ fillet (5.4 oz)	286	12	91	0	—
coho raw	3 oz	124	5	39	0	—
pink baked	3 oz	127	4	73	0	—
roe raw	3.5 oz	207	10	—	1	—
sockeye cooked	3 oz	183	9	102	0	—
sockeye cooked	½ fillet (5.4 oz)	334	17	102	0	—
sockeye raw	3 oz	143	7	40	0	—
SMOKED						
chinook	1 oz	33	1	220	0	—
chinook	3 oz	99	4	666	0	—
TAKE-OUT						
salmon cake	1 (3 oz)	241	15	602	6	—

SALSA
(see also KETCHUP, SAUCE)

FOOD	PORTION	CAL.	FAT	SOD.	CARB.	FIB.
Casa Fiesta						
Chili Salsa	1 oz	9	tr	117	2	—
Chi-Chi's						
Hot	2 tbsp (1 oz)	10	0	160	1	0
Medium	1 tbsp (1 oz)	10	0	140	1	0
Mild	2 tbsp (1 oz)	10	0	150	1	0
Verde Medium	2 tbsp (1.2 oz)	15	0	180	3	0
Verde Mild	2 tbsp (1.2 oz)	15	0	180	3	0
Del Monte						
Mexicana	2 tbsp (1.1 oz)	5	0	200	2	1
Taquera	2 tbsp (1.1 oz)	5	0	220	2	1
Verde	2 tbsp (1.1 oz)	10	0	280	2	tr
Frito Lay						
Hot	1 oz	12	0	180	2	—
Medium	1 oz	12	0	150	2	—
Mild	1 oz	12	0	200	2	—
Hain						
Hot	¼ cup	22	0	480	4	—
Mild	¼ cup	20	0	410	4	—
Haluva Good Cheese						
Cheese & Salsa	2 tbsp (1.1 oz)	80	6	210	3	0
Thick & Chunky Hot	2 tbsp (1.2 oz)	10	0	180	2	0

FOOD	PORTION	CAL.	FAT	SOD.	CARB.	FIB.
Heluva Good Cheese (CONT.)						
Thick & Chunky Mild	2 tbsp (1.2 oz)	10	0	180	2	0
Hot Cha Cha						
Medium	2 tbsp (1 oz)	5	0	0	2	—
Louise's						
Fat Free BBQ Black Bean	1 oz	10	0	110	2	0
Fat Free Black Bean	1 oz	10	0	110	2	0
Fat Free Medium	1 oz	10	0	80	3	1
Fat Free Mild	1 oz	10	0	80	3	1
Fat Free Nacho Queso	1 oz	15	0	45	3	0
Muir Glen						
Organic Fat Free Hot	2 tbsp (1.1 oz)	10	0	160	2	0
Organic Fat Free Medium	2 tbsp (1.1 oz)	10	0	160	2	0
Organic Fat Free Mild	2 tbsp (1.1 oz)	10	0	160	2	0
Newman's Own						
Bandito Hot	1 tbsp (0.7 oz)	6	tr	120	tr	—
Bandito Medium	1 tbsp (0.7 oz)	6	tr	45	tr	—
Bandito Mild	1 tbsp (0.7 oz)	6	tr	40	tr	—
Old El Paso						
Homestyle Chunky Mild	2 tbsp	5	0	110	1	—
Medium	2 tbsp	5	0	110	1	—
Picante Salsa Hot	2 tbsp	10	tr	160	2	—
Picante Salsa Medium	2 tbsp	10	tr	160	2	—
Picante Salsa Mild	2 tbsp	10	tr	160	2	—
Thick'n Chunky Green Chili	2 tbsp	3	0	270	1	—
Thick'n Chunky Hot	2 tbsp	10	0	130	2	—
Thick'n Chunky Medium	2 tbsp	10	0	140	2	—
Thick'n Chunky Mild	2 tbsp	10	0	140	2	—
Thick'n Chunky Salsa Verde	2 tbsp	10	tr	135	2	1
Ortega						
Hot Green Chili	1 tbsp	6	0	190	2	—
Medium Green Chili	1 tbsp	6	0	190	1	—
Mild Green Chili	1 tbsp	8	0	190	2	—
Pace						
Thick & Chunky	2 tbsp (1 fl oz)	12	0	321	2	1
Roserita						
Chunky Hot	3 tbsp (1.5 oz)	25	tr	300	6	tr
Chunky Medium	3 tbsp (1.5 oz)	25	tr	350	6	tr
Chunky Mild	3 tbsp (1.5 oz)	25	tr	340	6	tr
Taco Salsa Chunky Medium	3 tbsp (1.5 oz)	25	tr	310	6	tr
Taco Salsa Chunky Mild	3 tbsp (1.5 oz)	25	tr	300	6	tr

FOOD	PORTION	CAL.	FAT	SOD.	CARB.	FIB.
Tree Of Life						
Hot	2 tbsp (1 oz)	10	0	30	2	—
Medium	2 tbsp (1 oz)	10	0	30	2	—
Mild	2 tbsp (1 oz)	10	0	30	2	—
No Salt	2 tbsp (1 oz)	10	0	20	2	—
Watkins						
Salsa Seasoning Blend	⅛ tsp (0.5 g)	0	0	5	0	0
Tropical	2 tbsp (1 oz)	60	0	430	13	0
SALSIFY						
fresh sliced cooked	½ cup	46	tr	11	10	—
raw sliced	½ cup	55	tr	13	12	—
SALT SUBSTITUTES						
Morton	1 tsp	2	tr	—	—	—
Papa Dash						
Lite Lite Lite Salt	¼ tsp (0.5 g)	1	0	87	tr	—
Salt Lover's Blend	¼ tsp (0.7 g)	tr	0	231	tr	—
SALT/SEASONED SALT						
(see also SALT SUBSTITUTES)						
Hain						
Sea Salt	1 tsp	0	0	2255	0	—
Sea Salt Iodized	1 tsp	0	0	2255	0	—
Morton						
Garlic	1 tsp	3	tr	—	—	—
Iodized	1 tsp	tr	0	—	—	—
Kosher	1 tsp	0	0	—	—	—
Lite	1 tsp	tr	0	—	—	—
Nature's Season Seasoning Blend	1 tsp	3	tr	—	—	—
Non-Iodized	1 tsp	0	0	—	—	—
Seasoned	1 tsp	4	tr	—	—	—
Watkins						
Bacon Cheese Salt	¼ tbsp (1 g)	0	0	280	0	0
Butter Salt	¼ tbsp (1 g)	0	0	330	0	0
Cheese Salt	¼ tbsp (1 g)	0	0	290	0	0
Garlic Salt	¼ tsp (1 g)	0	0	270	0	0
Salt & Vinegar Seasoning	¼ tsp (1 g)	0	0	105	0	0
Seasoning Salt	¼ tsp (1 g)	0	0	270	0	0
Sour Cream & Onion Salt	¼ tbsp (1 g)	0	0	270	0	0
salt	1 tbsp (18 g)	0	0	6976	0	—
salt	1 tsp (6 g)	0	0	2325	0	—

FOOD	PORTION	CAL.	FAT	SOD.	CARB.	FIB.
SAPODILLA						
fresh	1	140	2	20	34	—
fresh cut up	1 cup	199	3	29	48	—
SAPOTES						
fresh	1	301	1	21	76	—
SARDINES						
CANNED						
Del Monte						
In Tomato Sauce	1 fish (1.4 oz)	50	3	130	1	tr
Empress						
Skinless & Boneless Olive Oil	1 can (3.8 oz)	420	38	530	2	—
Skinless & Boneless Soy Oil	1 can (4.4 oz)	500	45	630	2	—
Port Clyde						
In Louisiana Hot Sauce	1 can (3.75 oz)	170	9	760	1	0
In Mustard Sauce	1 can (3.75 oz)	150	9	450	1	1
In Soybean Oil drained	1 can (3.3 oz)	220	17	360	0	0
In Soybean Oil Select Small	1 can (3.3 oz)	220	17	360	0	0
In Soybean Oil With Hot Chilies	1 can (3.3 oz)	155	9	310	0	0
In Spring Water	1 can (3.3 oz)	170	10	240	0	0
In Tomato Sauce	1 can (3.75 oz)	150	9	480	0	0
S&W						
Norwegian Brisling	1.5 oz	130	10	220	0	—
Underwood						
Brisling In Olive Oil	3.75 oz	260	20	450	1	—
In Mustard Sauce	3.75 oz	220	16	560	2	—
In Sild Oil drained	3.75 oz	460	42	120	1	—
In Soya Oil drained	3 oz	230	18	400	1	—
In Tomato Sauce	3.75 oz	220	16	500	2	—
With Tabasco Pepper Sauce drained	3 oz	220	16	400	1	—
Viking's Delight						
Brisling In Olive Oil	1 can (3.75 oz)	460	42	450	1	—
Brisling In Olive Oil drained	1 can (3.75 oz)	260	20	450	1	—
atlantic in oil w/ bone	1 can (3.2 oz)	192	11	465	0	—
atlantic in oil w/ bone	2	50	3	121	0	—
pacific in tomato sauce w/ bone	1	68	5	157	0	—
pacific in tomato sauce w/ bone	1 can (13 oz)	658	44	1532	0	—

FOOD	PORTION	CAL.	FAT	SOD.	CARB.	FIB.
FRESH						
raw	3½ oz	135	5	100	0	—
SAUCE						
(see also BARBECUE SAUCE, GRAVY, PIZZA, SALSA, SPAGHETTI SAUCE, TOMATO)						
DRY						
Cajun King						
Etoufee Seasoning Mix	3.5 oz	383	6	1087	70	—
Jambalaya Seasoning Mix	3.5 oz	375	9	2855	61	—
Kikkoman						
Marinade For Meat	1 oz pkg	64	tr	—	—	—
Sweet & Sour	2⅛ oz pkg	228	tr	—	—	—
Teriyaki	1½ oz pkg	125	tr	—	—	—
Knorr						
Au Jus as prep	2 oz	8	tr	160	1	—
Bearnaise as prep	2 oz	170	17	340	5	—
Classic Brown Gravy as prep	2 oz	25	1	300	3	—
Demi-Glace as prep	2 oz	30	1	310	4	—
Hollandaise as prep	2 oz	170	18	310	5	—
Hunter as prep	2 oz	25	tr	340	4	—
Lyonnaise as prep	2 oz	20	tr	360	3	—
Mushroom as prep	2 oz	60	3	240	5	—
Napoli as prep	4 oz	100	3	960	17	—
Pepper as prep	2 oz	20	1	380	3	—
bearnaise as prep w/ milk & butter	1 cup	701	68	1265	18	—
cheese as prep w/ milk	1 cup	307	17	1566	23	—
curry as prep w/ milk	1 cup	270	15	1276	26	—
mushroom as prep w/ milk	1 cup	228	10	1533	24	—
sour cream as prep w/ milk	1 cup	509	30	1007	45	—
stroganoff as prep	1 cup	271	11	1829	34	—
sweet & sour as prep	1 cup	294	tr	779	73	—
teriyaki as prep	1 cup	131	1	4791	28	—
white as prep w/ milk	1 cup	241	13	796	21	—
JARRED						
Armour						
Chili Hot Dog	¼ cup (2.2 oz)	120	9	310	6	—
Meatless Sloppy Joe Sauce	¼ cup (2.2 oz)	30	0	430	7	—
Best Foods						
Tartar	1 tbsp (14 g)	70	8	190	tr	—

FOOD	PORTION	CAL.	FAT	SOD.	CARB.	FIB.
Bright Day						
Tartar	1 tbsp	50	5	—	—	—
Casa Fiesta						
Taco Mild	1 oz	9	tr	117	2	—
Chi-Chi's						
Taco Thick & Chunky	1 tbsp (0.5 oz)	10	0	75	1	0
Contadina						
Sweet 'n Sour	2 tbsp	40	1	110	8	—
Del Monte						
Cocktail	¼ cup (2.7 oz)	100	0	910	24	0
Sloppy Joe Hickory Flavor	¼ cup (2.4 oz)	70	0	700	18	0
Sloppy Joe Italian Style	¼ cup (2.4 oz)	70	0	700	16	0
Sloppy Joe Original	¼ cup (2.4 oz)	70	0	680	16	0
El Molino						
Taco Red Mild	2 tbsp	10	0	170	2	—
Escoffier						
Diable	1 tbsp	20	0	160	4	—
Gebhardt						
Enchilada Sauce	3 tbsp (1.5 oz)	25	1	170	2	tr
Hot Dog Chili Sauce	2 tbsp	30	1	180	4	tr
Hot Sauce	½ tsp	tr	tr	55	tr	tr
Gold's						
Rib	1 oz	60	0	250	14	—
Golden Dipt						
Cajun Style	1 oz	90	8	360	5	—
Creole	1 oz	20	1	190	2	—
Dijonaisse	1 oz	52	4	130	2	—
French White	1 oz	55	4	210	3	—
Ginger Teriyaki Marinade	1 oz	120	7	920	12	—
Lemon Butter Dill	1 oz	100	9	190	4	—
Lemon Herb Marinade	1 oz	130	14	210	2	—
Seafood Cocktail	1 tbsp	20	0	210	5	—
Seafood Cocktail Extra Hot	1 tbsp	20	0	210	5	—
Tartar	1 tbsp	70	7	100	2	—
Tartar Lite	1 tbsp	50	4	40	4	—
Guiltless Gourmet						
Picante Hot	1 oz	6	0	133	1	tr
Picante Medium	1 oz	6	0	133	1	tr
Heinz						
Worcestershire	1 tbsp	6	0	170	1	—
Hellman's						
Tartar	1 tbsp (14 g)	70	8	190	tr	—

FOOD	PORTION	CAL.	FAT	SOD.	CARB.	FIB.
Heluva Good Cheese						
Cocktail	¼ cup (1.6 oz)	40	0	410	10	—
Hormel						
Not-So-Sloppy-Joe Sauce	¼ cup (2.2 oz)	70	0	720	15	1
House Of Tsang						
Bangkok Padang	1 tbsp (0.6 oz)	45	3	240	4	0
Hoisin	1 tsp (6 g)	15	0	105	3	0
Mandarin Marinade	1 tbsp (0.6 oz)	25	0	680	6	0
Saigon Sizzle	1 tbsp (0.6 oz)	40	1	350	8	0
Spicy Brown Bean	1 tsp (6 g)	15	0	125	3	0
Stir Fry Classic	1 tbsp (0.6 oz)	25	1	570	4	0
Stir Fry Sweet & Sour	1 tbsp (0.6 oz)	35	0	50	8	0
Stir Fry Szechuan Spicy	1 tbsp (0.6 oz)	20	1	490	4	0
Sweet & Sour Concentrate	1 tsp (6 g)	10	0	15	3	0
Teriyaki Korean	1 tbsp (0.6 oz)	30	1	430	6	0
Just Rite						
Hot Dog	2 oz	60	3	220	6	tr
Ka-Me						
Black Bean Sauce	1 tbsp (0.5 oz)	10	0	550	2	1
Chili Sauce Hot Garlic	1 tbsp (0.5 oz)	15	0	115	4	1
Duck Sauce	2 tbsp (1 oz)	80	0	480	20	0
Fish Sauce	1 tbsp (0.5 fl oz)	10	0	1300	1	0
Hoisin Sauce	2 tbsp (1 oz)	45	0	620	10	1
Hot Sauce	1 tsp (5 g)	0	0	80	1	0
Lemon Sauce	1 tbsp (0.5 oz)	45	0	125	11	0
Mandarin Orange Sauce	2 tbsp (1 oz)	80	0	430	21	0
Oyster Sauce	1 tbsp (0.5 fl oz)	10	0	460	3	0
Plum	2 tbsp (1 fl oz)	80	0	420	19	0
Stir Fry Sauce	1 tbsp	10	0	570	1	0
Sweet & Sour	2 tbsp (1 fl oz)	50	0	270	13	0
Szechuan	1 tbsp (0.5 oz)	20	1	410	2	2
Tamari	1 tbsp (0.5 fl oz)	10	1	930	1	0
Tempura Sauce	2 tbsp (1 fl oz)	15	0	1790	3	0
Teriyaki Sauce	1 tbsp (0.5 fl oz)	10	0	480	2	0
Kikkoman						
Stir-Fry	1 tbsp	16	tr	369	3	1
Sweet & Sour	1 tbsp	19	tr	97	4	tr
Teriyaki	1 tbsp	15	0	626	3	0
Knorr						
Grilling And Broiling Chardonnay	1.6 oz	50	4	630	4	—

FOOD	PORTION	CAL.	FAT	SOD.	CARB.	FIB.
Knorr (CONT.)						
Grilling And Broiling Tequilla Lime	1.6 oz	50	3	690	6	—
Grilling And Broiling Spicy Plum	1.7 oz	60	2	790	11	—
Grilling And Broiling Tuscan Herb	1.6 oz	50	4	600	5	—
Microwave Hollandaise	1 oz	50	5	190	1	—
Microwave Mandarin Ginger	1.6 oz	50	4	690	5	—
Microwave Parmesano	1.6 oz	50	4	680	3	—
Microwave Vera Cruz	3.3 oz	70	3	580	9	—
Kraft						
Sandwich Spread & Burger Sauce	1 tbsp (0.5 oz)	50	5	100	3	0
Sweet'n Sour	2 tbsp (1.3 oz)	80	1	180	19	0
Tartar Sauce Nonfat	2 tbsp (1.1 oz)	25	0	210	5	tr
La Choy						
Duck Sauce Sweet & Sour	1 tbsp	25	tr	40	7	tr
Sweet & Sour	1 tbsp	25	tr	40	7	tr
Lawry's						
Marinade Lemon Pepper	1 tbsp (0.5 oz)	10	1	380	1	—
Teriyaki Marinade	2 tbsp	72	tr	7100	11	tr
Lea & Perrins						
Steak	1 oz	40	tr	220	10	—
Worcestershire	1 tsp	5	tr	55	1	—
Worcestershire White Wine	1 tsp	4	tr	40	1	—
Manwich						
Mexican	2.5 oz	35	1	460	9	1
Sloppy Joe	2.5 oz	40	tr	390	10	1
Marzetti						
Teriyaki Stir-Fry	2 tbsp	80	2	820	14	0
McIlhenny						
7 Spice Chili	2 tbsp (1.1 fl oz)	16	tr	191	3	1
Tabasco	1 tsp	1	tr	30	tr	tr
Mrs. Dash						
Steak	1 tbsp	17	tr	10	4	—
Newman's Own						
Bandito Diavalo Spicy	4 oz	70	2	530	11	—
Old El Paso						
Enchilada Green	2 tbsp	11	1	200	3	—
Enchilada Hot	¼ cup	30	1	250	4	—

FOOD	PORTION	CAL.	FAT	SOD.	CARB.	FIB.
Old El Paso (CONT.)						
Enchilada Mild	¼ cup	25	1	250	4	—
Picante Thick'n Chunky Hot	2 tbsp	10	0	160	2	—
Picante Thick'n Chunky Medium	2 tbsp	10	0	140	2	—
Picante Thick'n Chunky Mild	2 tbsp	10	0	130	2	—
Taco Hot	1 tbsp	5	0	90	1	—
Taco Medium	1 tbsp	5	0	70	1	—
Taco Mild	1 tbsp	5	0	85	1	—
Tomatoes & Green Chilies	¼ cup	10	0	310	2	—
Tomatoes & Jalapenos	¼ cup	11	0	290	3	1
Ortega						
Taco Thick & Smooth Hot	1 tbsp	8	0	105	2	0
Taco Thick & Smooth Mild	1 tbsp	8	0	115	2	0
Taco Western Style	1 oz	8	0	—	—	—
Pace						
Picante	2 tbsp (1 fl oz)	7	0	294	2	tr
Progresso						
Alfredo	½ cup	340	30	1080	6	—
Primavera Creamy	½ cup	190	17	410	8	1
Red Wing						
Chili Sauce	1 tbsp (0.6 oz)	20	0	220	5	0
Seafood Cocktail	¼ cup (2 oz)	90	1	830	22	0
Sauceworks						
Cocktail	¼ cup (2.3 oz)	60	1	800	13	tr
Sweet'n Sour	2 tbsp (1.2 oz)	60	0	125	14	0
Tartar	2 tbsp (1.1 oz)	100	10	180	4	0
Tartar Natural Lemon & Herb	2 tbsp (1 oz)	150	16	170	tr	0
Simmer Chef						
Golden Honey Mustard	½ cup (4 fl oz)	150	2	400	30	1
Hearty Onion & Mushroom	½ cup (4 fl oz)	50	1	670	9	1
Snow's						
Newburg With Sherry	⅓ cup	120	8	520	10	—
Welsh Rarebit Cheese	½ cup	170	11	460	10	—
Tabasco						
Picante	2 tbsp (1.5 oz)	17	tr	313	3	1

FOOD	PORTION	CAL.	FAT	SOD.	CARB.	FIB.
Trappey						
Indi-Pep West Indian Style Pepper Sauce	1 tsp (0.1 oz)	1	tr	41	tr	tr
Mexi Pep Louisiana Hot Sauce	1 tsp (0.1 oz)	tr	tr	59	tr	tr
Pepper Sauce	1 tsp (0.2 oz)	1	tr	85	tr	tr
Red Devil Buffalo Style Hot Sauce	1 tsp (0.1 oz)	1	tr	59	tr	tr
Red Devil Cayenne Pepper Sauce	1 tsp (0.1 oz)	1	tr	44	tr	tr
Worcestershire Chef Magic	1 tsp (0.1 oz)	3	tr	39	1	tr
Watkins						
Beef Marinade	¼ tbsp (2 g)	5	0	160	1	0
Calypso Hot Pepper Sauce	1 tsp (5 g)	10	0	25	3	0
Caribbean Red Pepper Sauce	1 tsp (5 g)	10	0	25	3	0
Chicken & Pork Marinade	¼ tbsp (2 g)	5	0	280	2	0
Fish & Seafood Marinade	¼ tbsp (2 g)	10	0	100	1	0
Inferno Hot Pepper Sauce	2 tbsp (1 oz)	35	0	930	8	1
Meat Magic	1 tsp (6 g)	10	0	190	2	0
Steak Sauce	1 tbsp (0.5 oz)	20	0	220	4	0
Weight Watchers						
Tartar	1 tbsp	35	3	80	3	—
Wise						
Picante	2 tbsp	12	0	130	3	—
Wolf Brand						
Hot Dog	1.25 oz	44	2	199	4	—
teriyaki	1 tbsp	15	0	690	3	—
teriyaki	1 oz	30	0	1380	6	—
SHELF-STABLE						
Cheez Whiz						
Cheese Sauce With Mild Salsa Zap-A-Pack	2 tbsp (1.2 oz)	90	8	580	3	0
Zap-A-Pack	2 tbsp (1.2 oz)	90	8	580	3	0
Fresh Gourmet						
Stir 'n Sauce Italian	1 tbsp (0.5 oz)	30	1	230	5	—
SAUERKRAUT						
CANNED						
Claussen						
Sauerkraut	½ cup	17	tr	—	—	—

FOOD	PORTION	CAL.	FAT	SOD.	CARB.	FIB.
Eden						
Organic	½ cup (3.9 oz)	25	0	580	4	3
Hebrew National						
Gallon Kraut	½ cup	25	0	800	4	—
New Kraut	½ cup (3.1 oz)	50	1	550	11	—
Schorr's						
New Kraut	½ cup (3.2 oz)	50	1	550	11	—
Seneca						
Sauerkraut	2 tbsp	5	0	192	0	1
SnowFloss						
Kraut	4 oz	28	0	780	4	1
Kraut Bavarian Style	4 oz	64	0	780	12	1
Vlasic						
Old Fashioned	1 oz	4	0	280	1	—
canned	½ cup	22	tr	780	5	—

SAUERKRAUT JUICE
S&W

FOOD	PORTION	CAL.	FAT	SOD.	CARB.	FIB.
Juice	4 oz	14	0	1120	3	—

SAUSAGE
(*see also* HOT DOG, SAUSAGE SUBSTITUTES)
Aidells

FOOD	PORTION	CAL.	FAT	SOD.	CARB.	FIB.
Andouille Cajun Cooked	1 (3.5 oz)	220	17	770	1	—
Burmese Curry Cooked	1 (3.5 oz)	220	15	730	3	—
Chicken & Apple Fresh	1 (1.9 oz)	110	8	250	1	—
Chicken & Apple Smoked	1 (3.5 oz)	220	16	730	0	0
Chicken & Turkey New Mexico Smoked	1 (3.5 oz)	220	16	600	2	—
Chicken & Turkey Thai Fresh	1 (3.5 oz)	200	16	600	0	—
Chicken & Turkey Thai Smoked	1 (3.5 oz)	220	16	770	0	—
Chicken & Turkey With Sun-Dried Tomatoes & Basil Fresh	1 (3.5 oz)	200	15	550	1	—
Chicken & Turkey With Sun-Dried Tomatoes & Basil Smoked	1 (3.5 oz)	200	14	730	0	—
Creole Hot Cooked	1 (3.5 oz)	220	16	600	2	—
Duck & Turkey Smoked	1 (3.5 oz)	220	16	700	1	—
Hunter's Cooked	1 (3.5 oz)	240	19	720	0	—

FOOD	PORTION	CAL.	FAT	SOD.	CARB.	FIB.
Aidells (CONT.)						
Italian Hot Fresh	1 (3.5 oz)	230	18	550	0	—
Italian Mild Fresh	1 (3.5 oz)	230	18	550	0	—
Lamb & Beef With Rosemary Fresh	1 (3.5 oz)	220	16	600	2	—
Lemon Chicken Cooked	1 (3.5 oz)	220	16	700	1	—
Mexican Chorizo Beef Fresh	1 (3.5 oz)	400	37	550	3	—
Whiskey Fennel Cooked	1 (3.5 oz)	230	18	730	1	—
Armour						
Country Sausage Lower Salt	1 oz	110	11	—	—	—
Country Sausage Lower Salt Links	1 oz	110	11	—	—	—
Country Sausage Lower Salt Patties	1.5 oz	160	16	—	—	—
Pork	1 oz	110	11	—	—	—
Pork Links	1 oz	110	11	—	—	—
Pork Patties	1.5 oz	160	16	—	—	—
Vienna Sausage 25% Less Fat	3 (1.9 oz)	130	11	420	1	—
Vienna Sausage In BBQ Sauce	3 (2.1 oz)	160	14	550	4	—
Vienna Sausage In Beef Stock	3 (1.9 oz)	170	16	420	1	—
Vienna Sausage In Hot Sauce	3 (2.1 oz)	170	15	630	3	—
Vienna Sausage Smoked	3 (1.9 oz)	170	16	420	1	—
Banner						
Sausage Tripe	2 oz	90	5	430	2	—
Bilinski's						
Chicken & Vegetable	1 (3 oz)	80	2	530	2	tr
Chicken Italian With Peppers & Onions	1 (3 oz)	120	4	800	1	—
Golden Brown						
Beef	1	80	7	160	tr	—
Mild	1	100	10	150	tr	—
Spicy	1	100	9	150	tr	—
Healthy Choice						
Low Fat Smoked	2 oz	70	2	590	4	1
Low Fat Smoked Polska Kielbasa	2 oz	70	2	590	4	1
Hebrew National						
Beef Knocks	1 (3 oz)	260	25	670	—	—

FOOD	PORTION	CAL.	FAT	SOD.	CARB.	FIB.
Hebrew National (CONT.)						
Polish Beef	1 link	240	22	680	—	—
Hillshire						
Beer Bratwurst	1 (2 oz)	190	17	500	2	—
Bratwurst Fresh	1 (2 oz)	190	17	410	1	—
Bratwurst Light Fresh	1 (2 oz)	150	11	620	2	—
Bratwurst Spicy	1 (2 oz)	180	17	490	1	—
Flavorseal Kielbasa	2 oz	190	17	540	2	—
Polska						
Flavorseal Kielbasa	2 oz	190	17	550	2	—
Polska Beef						
Flavorseal Kielbasa	2 oz	130	11	512	1	—
Polska Lite						
Flavorseal Kielbasa	2 oz	190	17	530	2	—
Polska Mild						
Flavorseal Kielbasa	2 oz	90	5	500	2	—
Polska Turkey						
Flavorseal Smoked	2 oz	190	17	500	2	—
Flavorseal Smoked Beef	2 oz	180	16	490	2	—
Flavorseal Smoked	2 oz	190	15	500	1	—
Beef & Cheddar						
Flavorseal Smoked	2 oz	180	16	490	2	—
Country Recipe						
Flavorseal Smoked Hot	2 oz	180	16	510	2	—
Flavorseal Smoked Lite	2 oz	130	11	512	1	—
Flavorseal Smoked	2 oz	90	5	500	2	—
Turkey						
Flavorseal Smoked	2 oz	200	18	500	1	—
w/ Italian Seasoning						
Italian Mild	1 (2 oz)	190	17	490	2	—
Italian Mild Light	1 (2 oz)	150	11	620	2	—
Italian Hot	1 (2 oz)	180	17	500	1	—
Italian Hot Light	1 (2 oz)	150	11	620	2	—
Kielbasa Fresh Polska	1 (2 oz)	190	17	410	1	—
Kielbasa Fresh Polska	1 (2 oz)	150	11	620	2	—
Lower Fat						
Links 80% Fat Free	2 oz	150	12	640	1	—
Cheddar Hots						
Links 80% Fat Free	2 oz	130	10	630	2	—
Kielbasa						
Links 80% Fat Free	2 oz	130	10	640	2	—
Smokies						
Links Brats Fully Cooked	2 oz	170	16	380	1	—
Links Bratwurst Smoked	2 oz	190	17	540	1	—

FOOD	PORTION	CAL.	FAT	SOD.	CARB.	FIB.
Hillshire (CONT.)						
Links Bun Size Cheddarwurst	2 oz	200	18	480	1	—
Links Bun Size Kielbasa	2 oz	180	16	570	2	—
Links Bun Size Smoked	2 oz	180	16	570	2	—
Links Bun Size Smoked Beef	2 oz	180	16	570	2	—
Links Cheddarwurst	2 oz	190	17	480	1	—
Links Cheddarwurst Lite	1 link (2.7 oz)	190	15	680	2	—
Links Hot	2 oz	190	16	530	2	—
Links Hot Beef	2 oz	190	17	560	1	—
Links Hot Lite	1 link (2.7 oz)	190	15	690	2	—
Links Keilbasa Polska	2 oz	190	17	530	2	—
Links Keilbasa Polska Lite	1 link (2.7 oz)	190	15	610	2	—
Links Knockwurst Lite	2 oz	180	16	460	1	—
Links Lit'l Polskas	2 oz	180	16	600	2	—
Links Lit'l Smokies	2 oz	180	16	600	2	—
Links Lit'l Smokies Beef	2 oz	180	16	600	2	—
Links Lit'l Smokies Cheddar	2 oz	180	16	600	2	—
Links Lit'l Smokies Light	2 oz	120	8	600	1	—
Links Polish	2 oz	190	17	520	2	—
Links Smoked	2 oz	190	18	520	1	—
Mexican Style	1 (2 oz)	190	17	410	1	—
Mexican Style Lower Fat	1 (2 oz)	150	11	620	2	—
Hormel						
Light & Lean 97 Dinner Smoked	2 oz	60	2	640	2	0
Pickled Hot	6 (2 oz)	140	11	380	1	0
Pickled Smoked	6 (2 oz)	140	11	380	1	0
Vienna	2 oz	140	13	420	1	0
Vienna Chicken	2 oz	90	10	420	1	0
Jimmy Dean						
Brick Sausage	2.5 oz	270	25	550	0	0
Bulk	2.5 oz	300	28	490	0	0
Hickory Smoked Dinner Sausage	2 oz	170	14	500	2	0
Pattie Pre-Cooked	1 (1.9 oz)	230	22	520	0	0
Polska Kielbaska	2 oz	170	15	500	1	0
Sage Pattie	1 (2 oz)	200	19	340	0	0
Sausage Pattie Raw	1 (2 oz)	200	19	400	0	0
Skinless Link	4 (2 oz)	200	19	440	0	0
Skinless Link	2 (2 oz)	200	19	440	0	0

FOOD	PORTION	CAL.	FAT	SOD.	CARB.	FIB.
Jones						
Brown & Serve Bacon	1	90	8	140	tr	—
Brown & Serve Beef	1	90	9	190	tr	—
Brown & Serve Light	1	60	5	140	1	—
Brown & Serve Regular	1	100	10	150	tr	—
Cello Beef	1 slice (1 oz)	130	13	160	tr	—
Cello Hot Country	1 slice (1 oz)	110	10	170	tr	—
Cello Original	1 slice (1 oz)	100	10	180	tr	—
Dinner Link	1	280	28	310	tr	—
Golden Brown Light Links	1	60	5	130	1	—
Golden Brown Mild Pattie	1	150	14	220	tr	—
Italian	1	160	14	420	tr	—
Light Link	1	70	6	210	1	—
Little Link	1	140	14	170	tr	—
Patties	1	150	14	270	tr	—
Scrapple	1 slice (1½ oz)	90	6	230	5	—
Little Sizzlers						
Brown & Serve	3 links (2.1 oz)	190	22	670	1	0
Brown & Serve	2 patties (1.4 oz)	190	18	560	1	0
Cooked	2 patties (2 oz)	250	23	680	0	0
Cooked	3 links (1.4 oz)	210	20	570	0	0
Heat & Serve Pork cooked	3 links (1.4 oz)	210	20	570	0	0
Louis Rich						
Polska Kielbasa	2 oz	80	5	510	1	0
Smoked Sausage With Cheese cooked	1 (1 oz)	47	3	269	1	—
Turkey	2.5 oz	110	6	580	3	0
Turkey & Cheese Smoked	2 oz	90	5	550	2	0
Turkey Links	2 (2 oz)	90	6	470	1	0
Turkey Smoked	2 oz	90	5	510	2	0
Mr. Turkey						
Breakfast	2.5 oz	130	9	460	0	—
Hearty Blend Polish Kielbasa	1 oz	70	6	260	1	—
Hearty Blend Smoked	1 oz	70	6	260	1	—
Hot Smoked	1 oz	45	3	250	2	—
Italian Smoked	1 oz	45	3	250	2	—
Polish Kielbasa	1 oz	45	3	250	2	—
Smoked	1 oz	45	3	250	2	—

FOOD	PORTION	CAL.	FAT	SOD.	CARB.	FIB.
Old Smokehouse						
Summer Sausage	1 oz	110	10	400	1	0
Oscar Mayer						
Pork cooked	2 links (1.7 oz)	170	15	410	1	0
Smokies Beef	1 (1.5 oz)	120	11	430	1	0
Smokies Cheese	1 (1.5 oz)	130	12	450	1	0
Smokies Links	1 (1.5 oz)	130	12	430	1	0
Smokies Little	6 (2 oz)	170	16	580	1	0
Perdue						
Breakfast Links Turkey cooked	1 (1.3 oz)	40	3	106	tr	—
Breakfast Patties Turkey cooked	1 (1.3 oz)	61	4	175	tr	—
Hot Italian Turkey cooked	1 (2 oz)	94	6	348	0	—
Sweet Italian Turkey cooked	1 (2 oz)	94	6	348	0	—
Rudy's Farm						
Italian Hot	2.5 oz	240	22	570	0	0
Italian Mild	2.5 oz	240	22	500	0	0
Italian Mild Natural Casing	1 (2 oz)	190	17	410	0	0
Morning Right Link	3 (2.9 oz)	150	10	260	0	0
Morning Right Pattie	2 (2.9 oz)	150	10	260	0	0
Pattie Pre-Cooked	1 (1.4 oz)	100	6	200	0	1
Smoked	4 (2.1 oz)	200	18	590	1	0
Sweet Link	1 (3.9 oz)	380	35	820	1	0
Shofar						
Knockwurst Beef	1 (3 oz)	260	23	620	tr	0
Tyson						
Country Pork	3.5 oz	320	29	905	1	—
Wampler Longacre						
Breakfast Links	1 (2.8 oz)	170	12	525	2	—
Italian Links	1 (2.8 oz)	170	12	520	2	—
Tinderlings Garlic & Pepper	1 (3.5 oz)	143	5	500	3	—
Turkey	1 pattie (2 oz)	120	8	380	4	—
Turkey	1 link (1 oz)	60	4	190	1	—
bierschinken	3.5 oz	174	11	753	tr	—
bierwurst	3.5 oz	258	21	—	0	—
blutwurst uncooked	3½ oz	424	39	680	0	—
bockwurst	3.5 oz	276	25	700	0	—
bockwurst pork & veal raw	1 link (2.3 oz)	200	18	—	tr	—
bratwurst pork	1 oz	92	8	315	1	—

FOOD	PORTION	CAL.	FAT	SOD.	CARB.	FIB.
bratwurst pork & beef	1 link (2.5 oz)	226	19	778	2	—
bratwurst pork cooked	1 link (3 oz)	256	22	473	2	—
country-style pork cooked	1 link (½ oz)	48	4	168	tr	—
country-style pork cooked	1 patty (1 oz)	100	8	349	tr	—
fleischwurst	3.5 oz	305	29	829	0	—
gelbwurst uncooked	3½ oz	363	33	640	0	—
italian pork cooked	1 (3 oz)	268	21	765	1	—
italian pork cooked	1 (2.4 oz)	216	17	618	1	—
jagdwurst	3.5 oz	211	16	818	0	—
kielbasa pork	1 oz	88	8	305	1	—
knockwurst pork & beef	1 (2.4 oz)	209	19	687	1	—
knockwurst pork & beef	1 oz	87	8	286	1	—
mettwurst uncooked	3½ oz	483	45	1090	0	—
plockwurst uncooked	3½ oz	312	45	—	0	—
polish pork	1 (8 oz)	739	65	1989	4	—
polish pork	1 oz	92	8	248	tr	—
pork & beef cooked	1 patty (1 oz)	107	10	217	1	—
pork & beef cooked	1 link (½ oz)	52	5	105	tr	—
pork cooked	1 patty (1 oz)	100	8	349	tr	—
pork cooked	1 link (½ oz)	48	4	168	tr	—
regensburger uncooked	3½ oz	354	31	—	0	—
smoked beef cooked	1 sausage (1.4 oz)	134	12	—	—	—
smoked pork	1 sm link (½ oz)	62	5	240	tr	—
smoked pork	1 link (2.4 oz)	265	22	1020	1	—
smoked pork & beef	1 sm link (½ oz)	54	5	151	tr	—
smoked pork & beef	1 link (2.4 oz)	229	21	151	1	—
vienna canned	7 (4 oz)	315	28	1077	2	—
vienna canned	1 (½ oz)	45	4	152	tr	—
weisswurst uncooked	3½ oz	305	27	620	0	—
zungenwurst (tongue)	3.5 oz	285	24	—	0	—
TAKE-OUT						
pork	1 link (0.5 oz)	48	4	168	tr	—
pork	1 patty (1 oz)	100	8	349	tr	—

SAUSAGE DISHES
FROZEN
Jimmy Dean

Italian Sausage & Mozzarella Sandwich	1 (4.5 oz)	380	22	1030	28	2

Ovenstuffs

French Roll Italian Sausage	1 (4.75 oz)	390	22	910	29	—
French Roll Pepperoni	1 (4.75 oz)	370	20	870	30	—
TAKE-OUT						
sausage roll	1 (2.3 oz)	311	24	—	22	1

FOOD	PORTION	CAL.	FAT	SOD.	CARB.	FIB.
SAUSAGE SUBSTITUTES						
Knox Mountain Farm						
No-So-Sausage	1 serv (1/10 pkg)	120	1	696	6	2
LaLoma						
Linketts	2 (71 g)	140	8	320	2	—
Little Links	2 (46 g)	90	5	180	2	—
Lightlife						
Lean Links Breakfast	1.25 oz	69	3	250	4	—
Lean Links Italian	1.5 oz	83	3	300	5	—
Morningstar Farms						
Breakfast Links	2 (45 g)	90	5	300	3	—
Breakfast Patties	2 (76 g)	190	12	710	7	—
Country Crisp Patties	1 (71 g)	220	15	620	13	—
Grillers	1 (64 g)	180	12	350	5	—
White Wave						
Meatless Healthy Links	2 (1.6 oz)	140	10	450	5	3
Worthington						
Leanies	1 link (40 g)	100	6	440	2	—
Prosage Links	2 (45 g)	130	9	460	3	—
Saucettes	2 links (67 g)	150	11	430	3	—
Super-Links	1 (48 g)	100	7	440	3	—
Veja-Links	2 (62 g)	140	10	330	4	—
SAVORY						
ground	1 tsp	4	tr	tr	1	—
SCALLOP						
FRESH						
raw	3 oz	75	1	137	2	—
FROZEN						
Mrs. Paul's						
Fried	2 oz	160	7	320	18	—
HOME RECIPE						
breaded & fried	2 lg	67	3	144	3	—
TAKE-OUT						
breaded & fried	6 (5 oz)	386	19	919	38	—
SCONE						
Finnegan's						
Irish Raisin	1 (2.7 oz)	90	2	176	20	1
HOME RECIPE						
apricot scone	1	232	7	201	39	—
TAKE-OUT						
cheese	1 (1.75 oz)	182	9	—	22	1
fruit	1 (1.75 oz)	158	5	—	27	2
plain	1 (1.75 oz)	181	7	—	27	1

FOOD	PORTION	CAL.	FAT	SOD.	CARB.	FIB.

SCROD
FROZEN
Gorton's

FOOD	PORTION	CAL.	FAT	SOD.	CARB.	FIB.
Microwave Entree Baked	1 pkg	320	18	420	18	—

SCUP
fresh baked

FOOD	PORTION	CAL.	FAT	SOD.	CARB.	FIB.
	3 oz	115	3	46	0	—

SEA BASS
(*see* BASS)

SEA TROUT
(*see* TROUT)

SEAWEED
Eden

FOOD	PORTION	CAL.	FAT	SOD.	CARB.	FIB.
Agar Agar Bars	1 tbsp (2.5 oz)	10	0	10	2	2
Agar Agar Flakes	1 tbsp (2.5 oz)	10	0	10	2	2
Arame	½ cup (0.3 oz)	30	0	120	7	7
Hiziki	½ cup (0.3 oz)	30	0	160	6	6
Kombu	3.5 in piece (3.3 g)	10	0	90	2	1
Nori	1 sheet (2.5 g)	10	0	5	1	1
Sushi Nori	1 sheet (2.5 g)	10	0	5	1	1
Wakame	½ cup (0.3 oz)	25	0	660	4	4
Wakame Flakes	½ cup (0.3 oz)	25	0	720	4	4

Maine Coast

FOOD	PORTION	CAL.	FAT	SOD.	CARB.	FIB.
Alaria	⅓ cup (7 g)	18	0	301	3	2
Dulse	⅓ cup (7 g)	18	0	122	3	2
Dulse Flakes	1 oz	75	1	493	13	9
Kelp	⅓ cup (7 g)	17	0	312	3	3
Kelp Crunch	1 bar (1 oz)	129	6	109	14	2
Kelp Crunch Peanut-Raisin	1 bar (1 oz)	129	6	109	14	2
Laver	⅓ cup (7 g)	22	0	113	3	3
Sea Seasoning Dulse	1 g	3	0	17	1	—
Sea Seasoning Dulse With Celery	1 g	3	0	17	1	—
Sea Seasoning Dulse With Garlic	1 g	3	0	13	1	—
Sea Seasoning Dulse With Sesame	1 g	3	0	6	1	—
Sea Seasoning Kelp	1 g	3	0	35	1	—
Sea Seasoning Kelp With Cayenne	1 g	3	0	35	1	—
Sea Seasoning Nori	1 g	3	0	8	1	—
Sea Seasoning Nori With Ginger	1 g	3	0	3	1	—

FOOD	PORTION	CAL.	FAT	SOD.	CARB.	FIB.
agar dried	1 oz	87	tr	29	23	—
agar fresh	1 oz	tr	tr	3	2	—
irishmoss fresh	1 oz	14	tr	19	4	—
kelp fresh	1 oz	12	tr	66	3	—
kombu fresh	1 oz	12	tr	66	3	—
laver fresh	1 oz	10	tr	14	1	—
nori fresh	1 oz	10	tr	14	1	—
spirulina dried	1 oz	83	2	309	7	—
spirulina fresh	1 oz	7	tr	28	1	—
tangle fresh	1 oz	12	tr	66	3	—
wakame fresh	1 oz	13	tr	249	3	—

SEITAN
(see WHEAT)

SEMOLINA

dry	½ cup	303	tr	1	61	3

SESAME
Arrowhead

Sesame Tahini	1 oz	170	17	5	4	—
Casbah						
Tahini Sauce Mix as prep	¼ cup	160	13	160	10	tr
Eden						
Sesame Shake	½ tsp (1.5 g)	10	1	40	0	tr
Sesame Shake Garlic	½ tsp (1.5 g)	10	1	35	0	tr
Sesame Shake Organic Seaweed	½ tsp (1.5 g)	10	1	35	0	tr
Erewhon						
Sesame Butter	2 tbsp (32 g)	190	17	20	3	—
Sesame Tahini	2 tbsp (32 g)	200	18	65	3	—
Joyva						
Tahini	2 tbsp (1 oz)	200	18	25	3	1
Planters						
Nut Mix	1 oz	150	12	240	9	2
Stone-Buhr						
Seeds Raw	4 tsp (1 oz)	180	16	10	3	1
seeds	1 tsp	16	2	1	tr	—
seeds dried	1 cup	825	72	16	34	—
seeds dried	1 tbsp	52	5	1	2	—
seeds roasted & toasted	1 oz	161	14	3	7	—
sesame butter	1 tbsp	95	8	2	4	1
sesame crunch candy	1 oz	146	9	—	14	—
sesame crunch candy	20 pieces (1.2 oz)	181	12	—	18	—
sesame sticks	1 oz	153	10	422	13	—

FOOD	PORTION	CAL.	FAT	SOD.	CARB.	FIB.
sesame sticks unsalted	1 oz	153	10	8	13	—
tahini from roasted & toasted kernels	1 tbsp	89	8	17	3	—
tahini from stone ground kernels	1 tbsp	86	7	11	4	—
tahini from unroasted kernels	1 tbsp	85	8	0	3	—

SESBANIA

flower	1	1	0	0	tr	—
flowers	1 cup	5	tr	3	1	—
flowers cooked	1 cup	23	tr	11	5	—

SHAD

american baked	3 oz	214	15	56	0	—
roe baked w/ butter & lemon	3.5 oz	126	3	73	2	—
roe raw	3½ oz	130	2	—	2	—

SHALLOTS

dried	1 tbsp	3	0	1	1	—
raw chopped	1 tbsp	7	tr	1	2	—

SHARK

batter-dipped & fried	3 oz	194	12	103	5	—
raw	3 oz	111	4	67	0	—

SHEEPSHEAD FISH

cooked	1 fillet (6.5 oz)	234	3	136	0	—
cooked	3 oz	107	1	62	0	—
raw	3 oz	92	2	61	0	—

SHELLFISH
(*see individual names*, SHELLFISH SUBSTITUTES)

SHELLFISH SUBSTITUTES

Louis Kemp

Crab Delights Chunk Style	2 oz	54	tr	320	5	—
Lobster Delights	2 oz	60	tr	470	6	—
Maryland Style Cakes	2.5 oz	154	9	780	10	—

Ocean Magic

Imitation King Crab	3 oz	80	tr	740	11	—
crab imitation	3 oz	87	1	715	1	—
scallop imitation	3 oz	84	tr	676	9	—
shrimp imitation	3 oz	86	1	599	8	—
surimi	1 oz	28	tr	40	2	—
surimi	3 oz	84	1	122	6	—

FOOD	PORTION	CAL.	FAT	SOD.	CARB.	FIB.
SHELLIE BEANS						
shellie beans	½ cup	37	tr	408	8	—
SHERBET						
(see also ICES AND ICE POPS)						
Borden						
Orange	½ cup	110	1	40	25	—
Bresler's						
All Flavors	3.5 oz	140	2	—	30	—
Hood						
Lime Orange Lemon	½ cup (3.1 oz)	120	1	35	26	0
Orange	½ cup (3.1 oz)	120	1	35	26	0
Rainbow Swirl	½ cup (3.1 oz)	120	1	30	26	0
Raspberry Orange Lime	½ cup (3.1 oz)	120	1	30	26	0
Sealtest						
Lime	½ cup (3 oz)	130	1	30	28	0
Orange	½ cup (3 oz)	130	1	30	28	0
Rainbow Orange Red Raspberry Lime	½ cup (3 oz)	130	1	25	28	0
Red Raspberry	½ cup (3 oz)	130	1	25	28	0
orange	½ gal	2158	31	706	469	—
orange	1 bar (2.75 fl oz)	91	1	30	20	—
orange	½ cup (4 fl oz)	132	2	44	29	—
orange home recipe	½ cup	120	2	30	24	—
SHRIMP						
CANNED						
Robinson						
Canned Shrimp	2 oz	58	1	—	—	—
S&W						
Deveined Medium Whole Shrimp	2 oz	65	0	—	1	—
canned	3 oz	102	2	143	1	—
canned	1 cup	154	3	216	1	—
FRESH						
cooked	3 oz	84	1	190	0	—
cooked	4 large	22	tr	49	0	—
raw	4 large	30	tr	42	tr	—
raw	3 oz	90	1	126	1	—
FROZEN						
Cajun Cookin'						
Shrimp Creole	12 oz	390	11	1130	55	—
Shrimp Etouffee	17 oz	360	9	1170	52	—
Shrimp Jambalaya	12 oz	450	20	800	43	—

FOOD	PORTION	CAL.	FAT	SOD.	CARB.	FIB.
Gorton's						
Butterfly Shrimp	4 oz	160	tr	540	16	—
Microwave Crunchy Shrimp	5 oz	380	20	870	35	—
Microwave Entree Shrimp Scampi	1 pkg	390	30	470	21	—
Shrimp Crisps	4 oz	280	15	740	26	—
Mrs. Paul's						
Entrees Light Seafood & Clams With Linguini	10 oz	240	5	750	36	—
READY-TO-USE						
American Original Foods						
Fried	4 oz	253	12	—	23	—
TAKE-OUT						
breaded & fried	4 large	73	4	103	3	—
breaded & fried	3 oz	206	10	292	10	—
breaded & fried	6 to 8 (6 oz)	454	25	1447	40	—
jambalaya	¾ cup	188	5	83	26	8
SMELT						
rainbow cooked	3 oz	106	3	65	0	—
rainbow raw	3 oz	83	2	51	0	—
SNACKS						
(*see also* CHIPS, FRUIT SNACKS, NUTS MIXED, POPCORN, PRETZELS)						
Bakem-ets	21 pieces (1 oz)	160	10	850	2	—
Hot'N Spicy	21 pieces (1 oz)	150	9	750	1	—
Bugles						
Nacho Cheese	1 oz	160	9	250	17	—
Ranch	1 oz	150	9	290	16	—
Cheetos						
Cheddar Valley	26 pieces (1 oz)	160	9	240	16	1
Crunchy	26 pieces (1 oz)	150	9	310	17	1
Curls	15 pieces (1 oz)	150	9	270	17	1
Flamin' Hot	26 pieces (1 oz)	150	9	240	16	1
Light	38 pieces (1 oz)	140	6	280	19	1
Paws	16 pieces (1 oz)	160	10	310	15	1
Puffed Ball	38 pieces (1 oz)	160	10	360	16	1
Puffs	33 pieces (1 oz)	160	9	330	16	1
Cheez Doodles						
Crunchy	1 oz	160	10	230	16	—
Puffed	1 oz	150	9	360	16	—
Chex						
Snack Mix Barbeque	½ cup (1.1 oz)	130	5	330	20	1
Snack Mix Cool Sour Cream And Onion	½ cup (1 oz)	130	4	310	21	2

FOOD	PORTION	CAL.	FAT	SOD.	CARB.	FIB.
Chex (CONT.)						
Snack Mix Golden Cheddar	½ cup (1 oz)	130	4	310	20	1
Snack Mix Traditional	⅔ cup (1.2 oz)	150	5	410	23	2
Combos						
Cheddar Cheese Cracker	1 pkg (1.7 oz)	250	13	520	28	1
Cheddar Cheese Cracker	1 oz	140	8	300	16	0
Cheddar Cheese Pretzel	1 pkg (1.8 oz)	240	9	560	33	1
Cheddar Cheese Pretzel	1 oz	130	5	310	18	0
Chili Cheese w/ Corn Shell	1 pkg (1.7 oz)	230	11	710	29	2
Chili Cheese w/ Corn Shell	1 oz	140	6	420	17	1
Mustard Pretzel	1 pkg (1.8 oz)	230	8	500	35	1
Mustard Pretzel	1 oz	130	4	270	19	1
Nacho Cheese Pretzel	1 pkg (1.7 oz)	230	8	580	34	1
Nacho Cheese Pretzel	1 oz	130	5	320	19	1
Nacho Cheese w/ Tortilla Shell	1 pkg (1.7 oz)	230	11	640	30	1
Nacho Cheese w/ Tortilla Shell	1 oz	140	6	380	17	1
Peanut Butter Cracker	1 oz	140	8	260	15	1
Pepperoni & Cheese Pizza	1 pkg (1.7 oz)	240	11	480	30	1
Pepperoni & Cheese Pizza	1 oz	140	7	280	17	0
Pizzeria Pretzel	1 oz	130	5	290	19	1
Pizzeria Pretzel	1 pkg (1.8 oz)	230	8	520	35	1
Tortilla Ranch	1 bag (1.7 oz)	240	12	610	29	1
Tortilla Ranch	1 oz	140	7	350	17	1
Cornnuts						
Barbecue	1 oz	120	4	270	22	2
Nacho Cheese	1 oz	120	4	180	22	2
Original	1 pkg (2 oz)	260	8	340	40	4
Original	1 oz	120	4	170	22	2
Picante	1 oz	120	4	260	22	2
Ranch	1 oz	120	4	190	20	2
Eagle						
Cheese Crunch	1 oz	160	10	310	16	—
Energy Food Factory						
Poprice Cheddar Cheese	½ oz	60	3	110	8	—
Poprice Herb & Garlic	½ oz	50	2	70	10	—
Poprice Lite	½ oz	50	2	70	9	—
Poprice Original No Salt	½ oz	45	0	1	11	—

FOOD	PORTION	CAL.	FAT	SOD.	CARB.	FIB.
Estee						
Snack Crisps Apple Cinnamon	27 crisps (1 oz)	130	3	110	24	1
Snack Crisps Apple Cinnamon	1 pkg (0.66 oz)	90	2	70	16	tr
Snack Crisps Chocolate	30 crisps (1 oz)	130	3	110	23	2
Snack Crisps Chocolate	1 pkg (0.66 oz)	90	2	70	15	1
Snack Crisps Lemon	1 pkg (0.66 oz)	90	2	70	16	tr
Snack Crisps Lemon	30 (1 oz)	130	3	110	23	tr
Snack Crisps Ranch	30 (1 oz)	130	3	200	22	tr
Snack Crisps Ranch	1 pkg (0.6 oz)	90	2	135	15	0
Snack Crisps White Cheddar	1 pkg (0.6 oz)	90	2	135	14	tr
Snack Crisps White Cheddar	27 crisps (1 oz)	130	3	200	22	tr
Frito Lay						
Corn Nuggets Toasted	1.38 oz	170	5	265	29	—
Funyums						
Onion Rings	11 pieces (1 oz)	140	7	265	18	1
Handi-Snacks						
Peanut Butter'n Crackers	1 pkg (1.1 oz)	180	12	150	12	1
Peanut Butter'n Grahamsticks	1 pkg (1.1 oz)	170	10	130	14	1
Hapi						
Chili Bits	½ cup (1 oz)	110	0	180	25	1
Health Valley						
Cheddar Lites	0.75 oz	40	2	35	4	tr
Cheddar Lites With Green Onion	0.75 oz	40	2	35	4	tr
Lance						
Cheese Balls	1 pkg (32 g)	190	13	420	16	—
Crunchy Cheese Twists	1 pkg (42 g)	260	16	290	25	—
Gold-N-Chees	1 pkg (39 g)	180	9	410	23	—
Pork Skins	1 pkg (14 g)	80	5	270	0	—
Pork Skins BBQ	1 pkg (14 g)	80	5	400	0	—
Mr. Peanut						
Peanut Butter Crisps Graham	12 pieces (1.1 oz)	150	8	100	18	2
Planters						
Cheez Balls	1 pkg (1 oz)	150	10	330	15	1
Cheez Balls	1 oz	150	10	300	15	1
Cheez Curls	1 pkg (1.2 oz)	190	12	380	19	1
Cheez Curls	1 oz	150	10	310	15	1
Heat Snack Mix	1 oz	140	8	230	13	2

FOOD	PORTION	CAL.	FAT	SOD.	CARB.	FIB.
Snyder's						
Cheddar Cheese Twists	1 oz	150	8	200	17	—
Kruncheez	1 oz	160	10	170	15	—
Onion Toasters	1 oz	150	8	280	17	3
Snack Mix	1 oz	170	8	410	11	tr
Sopaipillas Apple & Cinnamon	1 oz	150	8	15	18	1
Ultra Slim-Fast						
Lite N' Tasty Cheese Curls	1 oz	110	3	360	20	3
Weight Watchers						
Cheese Curls	½ oz	70	2	45	10	—
oriental mix	1 oz	155	12	235	9	—
pork skins	1 oz	154	9	521	0	—
pork skins	½ oz	77	4	261	0	—
pork skins barbecue	1 oz	152	9	756	1	—
pork skins barbecue	½ oz	76	5	378	tr	—
trail mix	1 oz	131	8	65	13	—
trail mix	1 cup (5.3 oz)	693	44	343	67	—
trail mix tropical	1 oz	115	5	3	19	—
trail mix w/ chocolate chips	1 oz	137	9	34	13	—
trail mix w/ chocolate chips	1 cup (5.1 oz)	707	47	177	66	—

SNAIL

cooked	3 oz	233	1	350	13	—
raw	3 oz	117	tr	175	7	—

SNAP BEANS

FOOD	PORTION	CAL.	FAT	SOD.	CARB.	FIB.
CANNED						
green	½ cup	13	tr	170	3	1
green low sodium	½ cup	13	tr	1	3	1
italian	½ cup	13	tr	170	3	1
italian low sodium	½ cup	13	tr	1	3	1
yellow	½ cup	13	tr	170	3	1
yellow low sodium	½ cup	13	tr	1	3	1
FRESH						
green cooked	½ cup	22	tr	2	5	—
green raw	½ cup	17	tr	3	4	1
yellow cooked	½ cup	22	tr	2	5	—
yellow raw	½ cup	17	tr	3	4	—
FROZEN						
green cooked	½ cup	18	tr	9	4	—
italian cooked	½ cup	18	tr	9	4	—
yellow cooked	½ cup	18	tr	9	4	—

FOOD	PORTION	CAL.	FAT	SOD.	CARB.	FIB.
SNAPPER						
cooked	1 fillet (6 oz)	217	3	96	0	—
cooked	3 oz	109	1	48	0	—
raw	3 oz	85	1	54	0	—
SODA						
(*see also* DRINK MIXERS, MINERAL/BOTTLED WATER)						
7 Up	1 oz	12	0	—	—	—
Cherry	1 oz	13	0	—	—	—
Cherry Diet	1 oz	tr	0	—	—	—
Diet	1 oz	tr	0	—	—	—
Gold	1 oz	13	0	—	—	—
Gold Diet	1 oz	tr	0	—	—	—
Canada Dry						
Birch Beer Brown	8 fl oz	110	0	40	27	0
Birch Beer Clear	8 fl oz	110	0	40	27	0
Black Cherry Wishniak	8 fl oz	130	0	40	32	0
Cactus Cooler	8 fl oz	110	0	40	27	0
California Strawberry	8 fl oz	110	0	45	27	0
Club	8 fl oz	0	0	60	0	0
Club Sodium Free	8 fl oz	0	0	0	0	0
Concord Grape	8 fl oz	120	0	45	29	0
Diet Ginger Ale	8 fl oz	0	0	60	0	0
Diet Ginger Ale Cherry	8 fl oz	0	0	60	0	0
Diet Ginger Ale Cranberry	8 fl oz	0	0	50	tr	0
Diet Ginger Ale Lemon	8 fl oz	5	0	60	0	0
Diet Tonic Water	8 fl oz	0	0	35	0	0
Diet Tonic Water Twist Of Lime	8 fl oz	0	0	45	0	0
Ginger Ale	8 fl oz	100	0	20	25	0
Ginger Ale Cherry	8 fl oz	110	0	25	27	0
Ginger Ale Cranberry	8 fl oz	100	0	15	25	0
Ginger Ale Golden	8 fl oz	100	0	10	24	0
Ginger Ale Lemon	8 fl oz	100	0	20	25	0
Half & Half	8 fl oz	110	0	25	27	0
Hi-Spot	8 fl oz	110	0	50	28	0
Island Lime	8 fl oz	140	0	15	33	0
Jamaica Cola	8 fl oz	110	0	10	27	0
Lemon Sour	8 fl oz	100	0	15	21	0
Peach	8 fl oz	120	0	40	30	0
Pina Pineapple	8 fl oz	110	0	40	26	0
Seltzer	8 fl oz	0	0	10	0	0
Seltzer Cherry	8 fl oz	0	0	10	0	0

FOOD	PORTION	CAL.	FAT	SOD.	CARB.	FIB.
Canada Dry (CONT.)						
Seltzer Cranberry Lime	8 fl oz	0	0	10	0	0
Seltzer Grapefruit	8 fl oz	0	0	10	0	0
Seltzer Lemon Lime	8 fl oz	0	0	10	0	0
Seltzer Mandarin Orange	8 fl oz	0	0	10	0	0
Seltzer Peach	8 fl oz	0	0	10	0	0
Seltzer Raspberry	8 fl oz	0	0	10	0	0
Seltzer Strawberry	8 fl oz	0	0	10	0	0
Seltzer Tropical	8 fl oz	0	0	10	0	0
Sunripe Orange	8 fl oz	140	0	45	35	0
Tahitian Treat	8 fl oz	150	0	45	36	0
Tonic Water	8 fl oz	100	0	15	24	0
Tonic Water Twist Of Lime	8 fl oz	100	0	20	24	0
Vanilla Cream	8 fl oz	120	0	40	30	0
Vichy Water	8 fl oz	0	0	490	0	0
Wild Cherry	8 fl oz	110	0	40	28	0
Clearly 2						
Black Cherry	8 fl oz	2	0	9	0	—
Key Lime	8 fl oz	2	0	9	0	—
Clearly Canadian						
Alpine Fruit & Berries	8 fl oz	90	0	9	23	—
Boysenberry Mist	8 fl oz	2	0	9	0	—
Coastal Cranberry	8 fl oz	90	0	9	22	—
Country Raspberry	8 fl oz	80	0	9	19	—
Green Apple	8 fl oz	80	0	9	19	—
Mountain Blackberry	8 fl oz	100	0	9	24	—
Orchard Peach Strawberry	8 fl oz	90	0	9	22	—
Summer Strawberry	8 fl oz	80	0	9	19	—
Western Longanberry	8 fl oz	80	0	9	19	—
Wild Cherry	8 fl oz	90	0	9	23	—
Coca-Cola						
Cherry	8 fl oz	104	0	4	28	—
Classic	8 fl oz	97	0	9	27	—
Classic Caffeine-Free	8 fl oz	97	0	9	27	—
Coke II	8 fl oz	105	0	4	29	—
Diet Cherry	8 fl oz	1	0	4	tr	—
Diet Coke	8 fl oz	1	0	4	tr	—
Diet Coke Caffeine-Free	6 fl oz	tr	0	—	—	—
Diet Coke Caffeine-free	8 fl oz	1	0	4	tr	—
Cott						
Cola	8 fl oz	110	0	10	27	0
Ginger Ale	8 fl oz	90	0	20	20	0

FOOD	PORTION	CAL.	FAT	SOD.	CARB.	FIB.
Cott (CONT.)						
Grape	8 fl oz	130	0	25	30	0
Orange	8 fl oz	140	0	25	33	0
Pineapple	8 fl oz	130	0	25	32	0
Punch	8 fl oz	130	0	25	32	0
Seltzer	8 fl oz	0	0	0	0	0
Crush						
Cherry	8 fl oz	140	0	30	35	0
Grape	8 fl oz	110	0	—	—	0
Orange	8 fl oz	140	0	—	—	0
Orange Diet	8 fl oz	0	0	—	0	0
Pineapple	8 fl oz	140	0	30	35	0
Strawberry	8 fl oz	130	0	—	—	0
Tropical Fruit Punch	1 can (11.5 fl oz)	200	0	—	—	0
Tropical Fruit Punch	1 bottle (10 fl oz)	180	0	20	44	0
Diet Rite						
Black Cherry Salt/ Sodium Free	8 fl oz	2	0	0	1	—
Cola	8 fl oz	1	0	0	tr	—
Cola Caffeine/Sugar Free	8 fl oz	1	0	7	tr	—
Cola Salt/Sodium Free	8 fl oz	1	0	tr	tr	—
Fruit Punch Salt/Sodium Free	8 fl oz	2	0	0	tr	—
Golden Peach Salt/ Sodium Free	8 fl oz	2	0	0	tr	—
Key Lime Salt/Sodium Free	8 fl oz	7	0	0	2	—
Pink Grapefruit Salt/ Sodium Free	8 fl oz	2	0	0	1	—
Red Raspberry Salt/ Sodium Free	8 fl oz	3	0	tr	1	—
Tangerine Salt/Sodium Free	8 fl oz	2	0	0	tr	—
White Grape Salt/ Sodium Free	8 fl oz	1	0	0	tr	—
Dr Pepper						
Diet	1 oz	tr	0	—	—	—
Free	1 oz	12	0	—	—	—
Free Diet	1 oz	tr	0	—	—	—
Fanta						
Ginger Ale	8 fl oz	86	0	4	23	—
Grape	8 fl oz	117	0	9	31	—
Orange	8 fl oz	118	0	9	32	—
Root Beer	8 fl oz	111	0	4	29	—

FOOD	PORTION	CAL.	FAT	SOD.	CARB.	FIB.
Health Valley						
Ginger Ale	12 oz	153	1	30	35	0
Rootbeer Old Fashioned	12 oz	120	1	12	26	—
Sarsaparilla Rootbeer	12 oz	153	1	27	35	—
Wild Berry	12 oz	142	1	27	33	—
Hires						
Cream	8 fl oz	130	0	30	0	0
Cream Soda Diet	8 fl oz	0	0	35	0	0
Original Mocha	8 fl oz	100	0	45	24	0
Original Mocha Diet	8 fl oz	5	0	45	0	0
Root Beer	8 fl oz	130	0	45	31	0
Root Beer Diet	8 fl oz	0	0	70	0	0
Like						
Cola	1 oz	13	0	—	—	—
Cola Sugar Free	1 oz	tr	0	—	—	—
Manischewitz						
Seltzer No Salt Added No Calories	8 fl oz	0	0	9	0	—
Mello Yellow						
Diet	8 fl oz	4	0	tr	tr	—
Minute Maid						
Berry	8 fl oz	111	0	9	30	—
Diet Orange	8 fl oz	2	0	0	0	—
Fruit Punch	8 fl oz	117	0	10	32	—
Grape	8 fl oz	121	0	9	32	—
Grapefruit	8 fl oz	108	0	9	29	—
Orange	8 fl oz	118	0	0	32	—
Peach	8 fl oz	110	0	9	29	—
Pineapple	8 fl oz	109	0	9	30	—
Raspberry	8 fl oz	111	0	9	30	—
Strawberry	8 fl oz	122	0	9	33	—
Mountain Dew						
Diet	8 fl oz	2	0	0	tr	—
Mr. PiBB						
Diet	8 fl oz	1	0	2	tr	—
Mug						
Cream	8 fl oz	122	0	21	32	—
Diet Cream	8 fl oz	2	0	29	0	—
Diet Root Beer	8 fl oz	1	0	26	tr	—
Root Beer	8 fl oz	141	0	26	29	—
Nehi						
Cream	8 fl oz	120	0	0	32	—
Fruit Punch	8 fl oz	120	0	35	34	—
Ginger Ale	8 fl oz	90	0	35	24	—

FOOD	PORTION	CAL.	FAT	SOD.	CARB.	FIB.
Nehi (CONT.)						
Grape	8 fl oz	120	0	35	32	—
Orange	8 fl oz	130	0	35	35	—
Peach	8 fl oz	130	0	35	34	—
Pineapple	8 fl oz	130	0	0	36	—
Quinine Water	8 fl oz	90	0	35	23	—
Root Beer	8 fl oz	120	0	35	32	—
Strawberry	8 fl oz	120	0	35	32	—
Wild Red	8 fl oz	120	0	33	32	—
Old Colony						
Grape	8 fl oz	140	0	40	32	0
Pepsi						
Diet	8 fl oz	1	0	tr	tr	—
Diet Caffeine Free	8 fl oz	1	0	tr	tr	—
Ramblin' Root Beer	8 fl oz	120	0	4	33	—
Razing Razberry						
Cola	8 fl oz	117	0	0	31	—
Royal Crown						
Caffeine Free Cola	8 fl oz	110	0	35	29	—
Cherry	8 fl oz	110	0	35	29	—
Cola	8 fl oz	100	0	35	28	—
Diet	8 fl oz	1	0	tr	tr	—
Diet Caffeine Free	8 fl oz	1	0	tr	tr	—
Diet Cranberry Apple Salt/Sodium Free	8 fl oz	2	0	1	tr	—
Diet Cranberry Salt/ Sodium Free	8 fl oz	2	0	1	tr	—
Royal Mistic						
Caribbean Fruit Punch	16 fl oz	230	0	5	57	—
Grape Strawberry	16 fl oz	230	0	5	57	—
'N Juice Black Cherry	12 fl oz	146	0	26	36	—
'N Juice Peach Vanilla	12 fl oz	146	0	18	36	—
'N Juice Tangerine Orange	12 fl oz	146	0	30	36	—
'N Juice Tropical Supreme	12 fl oz	152	0	14	38	—
'N Juice Wild Berry	12 fl oz	156	0	30	38	—
Sparkling Diet With Lime Kiwi	11.1 fl oz	0	0	<90	0	—
Sparkling Diet With Raspberry Boysenberry	11.1 fl oz	0	0	<90	0	—
Sparkling Diet With Royal Peach	11.1 fl oz	0	0	<90	0	—

FOOD	PORTION	CAL.	FAT	SOD.	CARB.	FIB.
Royal Mistic (cont.)						
Sparkling Diet With Wild Cherry	11.1 fl oz	0	0	<90	0	—
Sparkling With Lime Kiwi	11.1 fl oz	112	0	38	28	—
Sparkling With Mandarin Orange Pineappple	11.1 fl oz	120	0	18	30	—
Sparkling With Mango Passion	11.1 fl oz	112	0	34	28	—
Sparkling With Raspberry Boysenberry	11.1 fl oz	112	0	24	28	—
Sparkling With Royal Peach	11.1 fl oz	112	0	30	28	—
Sparkling With Wild Cherry	11.1 fl oz	112	0	28	28	—
Schweppes						
Bitter Lemon	8 fl oz	110	0	45	28	0
Club	8 fl oz	0	0	70	0	0
Club Sodium Free	8 fl oz	0	0	0	0	0
Diet Ginger Ale Dry Grape	8 fl oz	2	0	90	0	0
Diet Ginger Ale Raspberry	8 fl oz	0	0	75	0	0
Ginger Ale	8 fl oz	90	0	50	22	0
Ginger Ale Diet	8 fl oz	0	0	75	0	0
Ginger Ale Dry Grape	8 fl oz	100	0	50	26	0
Ginger Ale Raspberry	8 fl oz	100	0	50	26	0
Ginger Beer	8 fl oz	100	0	90	25	0
Grape	8 fl oz	130	0	55	33	0
Grapefruit	8 fl oz	110	0	75	27	0
Lemon Sour	8 fl oz	110	0	25	26	0
Lemon-Lime	8 fl oz	100	0	75	25	0
Seltzer Black Berry	8 fl oz	0	0	10	0	0
Seltzer Lemon	8 fl oz	0	0	10	0	0
Seltzer Lemon Lime	8 fl oz	0	0	10	0	0
Seltzer Lime	8 fl oz	0	0	10	0	0
Seltzer Orange	8 fl oz	0	0	10	0	0
Seltzer Peaches & Cream	8 fl oz	0	0	10	0	0
Seltzer Raspberry	8 fl oz	0	0	0	0	0
Tonic Citrus	8 fl oz	90	0	25	20	0
Tonic Cranberry	8 fl oz	90	0	25	20	0
Tonic Raspberry	8 fl oz	90	0	25	20	0

FOOD	PORTION	CAL.	FAT	SOD.	CARB.	FIB.
Schweppes (CONT.)						
Tonic Water Diet	8 fl oz	0	0	85	0	0
Shasta						
Black Cherry	12 oz	162	0	—	—	—
Cherry Cola	12 oz	140	0	—	—	—
Citrus Mist	12 oz	170	0	—	—	—
Club	12 oz	0	0	—	—	—
Cola	8 oz	98	0	—	—	—
Cola	12 oz	147	0	—	—	—
Collins	12 oz	118	0	—	—	—
Creme	12 oz	154	0	—	—	—
Diet Birch Beer	12 oz	4	0	—	—	—
Diet Cola	8 oz	0	0	—	—	—
Diet Ginger Ale	8 oz	0	0	—	—	—
Diet Lemon Lime	8 oz	0	0	—	—	—
Dr. Diablo	12 oz	140	0	—	—	—
Free Cola	12 oz	151	0	—	—	—
Fruit Punch	12 oz	173	0	—	—	—
Ginger Ale	8 oz	80	0	—	—	—
Ginger Ale	12 oz	120	0	—	—	—
Grape	12 oz	177	0	—	—	—
Lemon Lime	8 oz	97	0	—	—	—
Lemon Lime	12 oz	146	0	—	—	—
Orange	12 oz	177	0	—	—	—
Red Berry	12 oz	158	0	—	—	—
Red Pop	12 oz	158	0	—	—	—
Root Beer	12 oz	154	0	—	—	—
Strawberry	12 oz	147	0	—	—	—
Tonic Water	12 oz	0	0	—	—	—
Slice						
Diet Lemon Lime	8 fl oz	5	0	1	tr	—
Diet Mandarin	8 fl oz	5	0	10	tr	—
Lemon Lime	8 fl oz	100	0	10	26	—
Mandarin Orange	8 fl oz	128	0	10	33	—
Red	8 fl oz	128	0	10	33	—
Snapple						
Amazin' Grape	8 fl oz	120	0	5	28	—
Cherry Lime Ricky	8 fl oz	110	0	0	27	—
Creme D'Vanilla	8 fl oz	130	0	0	33	—
French Cherry	8 fl oz	120	0	0	29	—
Kiwi Peach	8 fl oz	120	0	0	29	—
Kiwi Strawberry	8 fl oz	130	0	5	33	—
Mango Madness	8 fl oz	130	0	5	33	—
Passion Supreme	8 fl oz	120	0	0	29	—

FOOD	PORTION	CAL.	FAT	SOD.	CARB.	FIB.
Snapple (CONT.)						
Peach Melba	8 fl oz	120	0	0	31	—
Raspberry	8 fl oz	120	0	0	31	—
Seltzer Black Cherry	8 fl oz	0	0	0	0	—
Seltzer Lemon Lime	8 fl oz	0	0	0	0	—
Seltzer Original	8 fl oz	0	0	0	0	—
Seltzer Tangerine	8 fl oz	0	0	0	0	—
Tru Root Beer	8 fl oz	110	0	0	29	—
Sprite						
Diet	8 fl oz	3	0	0	0	—
Sundrop						
Cherry	8 fl oz	130	0	15	21	0
Diet	8 fl oz	5	0	65	0	0
Sunkist						
Cactus Cooler	8 fl oz	110	0	40	27	0
Cherry	8 fl oz	140	0	35	35	0
Diet Citrus	8 fl oz	0	0	90	0	0
Diet Orange	8 fl oz	5	0	75	0	0
Fruit Punch	8 fl oz	130	0	35	33	0
Orange	8 fl oz	140	0	40	35	0
Peach	8 fl oz	120	0	40	30	0
Pineapple	8 fl oz	140	0	35	35	0
Strawberry	8 fl oz	140	0	35	34	0
Tropical Chill						
Cola	8 fl oz	117	0	0	31	—
Diet	8 fl oz	1	0	0	tr	—
Upper 10						
Diet	8 fl oz	3	0	0	1	—
Diet Salt/Sodium Free	8 fl oz	3	0	0	1	—
Salt Free	8 fl oz	100	0	0	29	—
Welch's						
Sparkling Apple	12 oz	180	0	—	—	—
Sparkling Grape	12 oz	180	0	—	—	—
Sparkling Orange	12 oz	180	0	—	—	—
Sparkling Strawberry	12 oz	180	0	—	—	—
Wink						
Diet	8 fl oz	5	0	95	1	0
club	12 oz	0	0	75	0	—
cola	12 oz	151	tr	14	39	—
cream	12 oz	191	0	43	49	—
diet cola	12 oz	2	0	21	tr	—
diet cola w/ Nutrasweet	12 oz	2	0	21	tr	—
diet cola w/ saccharin	12 oz	2	0	57	tr	—
ginger ale	12 oz can	124	0	25	32	—

FOOD	PORTION	CAL.	FAT	SOD.	CARB.	FIB.
grape	12 oz	161	0	57	42	—
lemon lime	12 oz	149	0	41	38	—
orange	12 oz	177	0	49	46	—
pepper type	12 oz	151	tr	38	38	—
quinine	12 oz	125	0	15	32	—
root beer	12 oz	152	0	49	39	—
tonic water	12 oz	125	0	15	32	—

SOLDIER BEANS
DRIED
Bean Cuisine	½ cup	115	1	5	—	5

SOLE
FRESH
cooked	3 oz	99	1	89	0	—
cooked	1 fillet (4.5 oz)	148	2	133	0	—
lemon raw	3½ oz	85	1	80	0	—
raw	3½ oz	90	1	100	0	—

FROZEN
Gorton's						
Fishmarket Fresh	5 oz	110	1	140	1	—
Microwave Entree In Lemon Butter	1 pkg	380	24	560	17	—
Microwave Entree In Wine Sauce	1 pkg	180	8	770	3	—
Mrs. Paul's						
Light Fillets	1 fillet	240	10	450	20	—
Van De Kamp's						
Light Fillets	1 piece	250	12	480	18	—
Natural Fillets	4 oz	100	2	105	0	—

TAKE-OUT
battered & fried	3.2 oz	211	11	484	15	—
breaded & fried	3.2 oz	211	11	484	15	—

SORBET
(*see* ICES AND ICE POPS)

SORGHUM
sorghum	½ cup	325	3	—	72	—

SOUFFLE
HOME RECIPE
cheese	3.5 oz	253	20	—	10	tr
grand marnier	1 cup	109	4	58	14	—
lemon chilled	1 cup	176	tr	108	34	—
raspberry chilled	1 cup	173	tr	108	34	—
spinach	1 cup	218	18	763	3	—

FOOD	PORTION	CAL.	FAT	SOD.	CARB.	FIB.
SOUP						
CANNED						
American Original						
New England Chowder	4 oz	64	1	—	8	—
New England Chowder as prep w/ milk	4 oz	145	6	—	14	—
Campbell						
Asparagus Cream Of as prep	8 oz	80	4	820	10	—
Bean Homestyle as prep	8 oz	130	1	700	25	—
Bean With Bacon as prep	8 oz	140	4	840	21	—
Beef as prep	8 oz	80	2	830	10	—
Beef Broth as prep	8 oz	16	0	820	1	—
Beef Noodle as prep	8 oz	70	3	830	7	—
Beef Noodle Homestyle as prep	8 oz	80	4	810	7	—
Beefy Mushroom as prep	8 oz	60	3	960	5	—
Broccoli Cream Of as prep	8 oz	80	5	790	8	—
Broccoli Cream Of as prep w/ 2% milk	8 oz	140	7	850	14	—
Celery Cream Of as prep	8 oz	100	7	820	8	—
Cheddar Cheese as prep	8 oz	110	6	810	10	—
Chicken Alphabet as prep	8 oz	80	3	800	10	—
Chicken & Stars as prep	8 oz	60	2	870	7	—
Chicken Barley as prep	8 oz	70	2	850	10	—
Chicken Broth as prep	8 oz	30	2	710	2	—
Chicken Broth & Noodles as prep	8 oz	45	1	860	8	—
Chicken Cream Of as prep	8 oz	110	7	810	9	—
Chicken Gumbo as prep	8 oz	60	2	900	8	—
Chicken Mushroom Creamy as prep	8 oz	120	8	920	8	—
Chicken 'n Dumplings as prep	8 oz	80	3	960	9	—
Chicken Noodle as prep	8 oz	60	2	900	8	—
Chicken Noodle Homestyle as prep	8 oz	70	3	880	8	—
Chicken Noodle-O's as prep	8 oz	70	2	820	9	—

FOOD	PORTION	CAL.	FAT	SOD.	CARB.	FIB.
Campbell (CONT.)						
Chicken Vegetable as prep	8 oz	70	3	850	8	—
Chicken With Rice as prep	8 oz	60	3	790	7	—
Chili Beef as prep	8 oz	140	5	840	20	—
Chunky Chicken Nuggets w/ Vegetables & Noodles	10¾ oz	190	6	1060	24	—
Clam Chowder Manhattan Style as prep	8 oz	70	2	820	10	—
Clam Chowder New England as prep	8 oz	80	3	870	12	—
Clam Chowder New England as prep w/ whole milk	8 oz	150	7	930	17	—
Consomme as prep	8 oz	25	0	750	2	—
Curly Noodle With Chicken as prep	8 oz	80	3	800	11	—
French Onion as prep	8 oz	60	2	900	9	—
Green Pea as prep	8 oz	160	3	820	25	—
Healthy Request Bean With Bacon as prep	8 oz	140	4	470	22	—
Healthy Request Chicken Noodle as prep	8 oz	60	2	460	8	—
Healthy Request Chicken With Rice as prep	8 oz	60	3	480	7	—
Healthy Request Cream Of Chicken	8 oz	70	2	490	11	—
Healthy Request Cream Of Mushroom as prep	8 oz	60	2	460	9	—
Healthy Request Hearty Chicken Vegetable	8 oz	120	2	460	16	—
Healthy Request Ready-To-Serve Chicken Broth	8 oz	10	0	400	1	—
Healthy Request Ready-To-Serve Hearty Chicken Noodle	8 oz	80	2	470	7	—
Healthy Request Ready-To-Serve Hearty Chicken Rice	8 oz	110	2	400	15	—

FOOD	PORTION	CAL.	FAT	SOD.	CARB.	FIB.
Campbell (CONT.)						
Healthy Request Ready-To-Serve Hearty Minestrone	8 oz	90	3	430	13	—
Healthy Request Ready-To-Serve Hearty Vegetable	8 oz	110	3	480	17	—
Healthy Request Ready-To-Serve Hearty Vegetable Beef	8 oz	120	3	490	15	—
Healthy Request Tomato as prep	8 oz	90	2	430	17	—
Healthy Request Tomato as prep w/ skim milk	8 oz	130	2	490	22	—
Healthy Request Vegetable as prep	8 oz	90	2	500	14	—
Healthy Request Vegetable Beef as prep	8 oz	70	2	490	9	—
Home Cookin' Bean & Ham	10¾ oz	210	4	1000	29	—
Home Cookin' Beef With Vegetables & Pasta	10¾ oz	140	2	1060	18	—
Home Cookin' Chicken Minestrone	10¾ oz	180	6	950	17	—
Home Cookin' Chicken Gumbo With Sausages	10¾ oz	140	4	1090	15	—
Home Cookin' Chicken Rice	10¾ oz	150	6	1090	10	—
Home Cookin' Chicken With Noodles	10¾ oz	140	4	1150	12	—
Home Cookin' Country Vegetable	10¾ oz	120	2	1070	20	—
Home Cookin' Garden Tomato	10¾ oz	150	3	930	29	—
Home Cookin' Hearty Lentil	10¾ oz	170	2	930	28	—
Home Cookin' Minestrone	10¾ oz	140	3	1220	22	—
Home Cookin' Split Pea With Ham	10¾ oz	230	1	1310	38	—
Home Cookin' Vegetable Beef	10¾ oz	140	3	1160	17	—

FOOD	PORTION	CAL.	FAT	SOD.	CARB.	FIB.
Campbell (CONT.)						
Minestrone as prep	8 oz	80	2	900	13	—
Mushroom Cream Of as prep	8 oz	100	7	820	8	—
Mushroom Golden as prep	8 oz	70	3	870	9	—
Nacho Cheese as prep	8 oz	110	8	740	8	—
Nacho Cheese as prep w/ milk	8 oz	180	12	800	13	—
Noodles & Ground Beef as prep	8 oz	90	4	820	10	—
Onion Cream Of as prep	8 oz	100	5	830	12	—
Onion Cream Of as prep w/ whole milk & water	8 oz	140	7	860	15	—
Oyster Stew as prep	8 oz	70	5	840	5	—
Oyster Stew as prep w/ whole milk	8 oz	140	9	890	10	—
Pepper Pot as prep	8 oz	90	4	970	9	—
Potato Cream Of as prep	8 oz	80	3	870	12	—
Potato Cream Of as prep w/ whole milk & water	8 oz	120	4	900	15	—
Ready-To-Serve Chunky Beef	10¾ oz	200	5	1100	24	—
Ready-To-Serve Chunky Beef Stroganoff	10¾ oz	320	16	1230	28	—
Ready-To-Serve Chunky Chicken Corn Chowder	10¾ oz	340	21	1200	23	—
Ready-To-Serve Chunky Chicken Noodle	10¾ oz	200	7	1140	20	—
Ready-To-Serve Chunky Chicken Vegetable	9½ oz	170	6	1080	19	—
Ready-To-Serve Chunky Chicken With Rice	9½ oz	140	4	1060	16	—
Ready-To-Serve Chunky Chili Beef	11 oz	290	7	1120	37	—
Ready-To-Serve Chunky Creamy Chicken Mushroom	10½ oz	270	19	1280	13	—
Ready-To-Serve Chunky Creole Style	10¾ oz	240	8	910	31	—
Ready-To-Serve Chunky Ham 'n Butter Bean	10¾ oz	280	10	1180	34	—
Ready-To-Serve Chunky Manhattan Style Clam Chowder	10¾ oz	160	4	1110	24	—

FOOD	PORTION	CAL.	FAT	SOD.	CARB.	FIB.
Campbell (CONT.)						
Ready-To-Serve Chunky Mediterranean Vegetable	9½ oz	170	6	1010	24	—
Ready-To-Serve Chunky Minestrone	9½ oz	160	4	870	24	—
Ready-To-Serve Chunky New England Clam Chowder	10¾ oz	290	17	1200	26	—
Ready-To-Serve Chunky Old Fashioned Bean w/ Ham	11 oz	290	9	1110	38	—
Ready-To-Serve Chunky Old Fashioned Chicken	10¾ oz	180	5	1220	21	—
Ready-To-Serve Chunky Old Fashioned Vegetable Beef	10¾ oz	190	5	1100	20	—
Ready-To-Serve Chunky Pepper Steak	10¾ oz	180	3	1050	24	—
Ready-To-Serve Chunky Sirloin Burger	10¾ oz	220	9	1240	23	—
Ready-To-Serve Chunky Split Pea w/ Ham	10¾ oz	230	6	1080	33	—
Ready-To-Serve Chunky Steak & Potato	10¾ oz	200	5	1140	24	—
Ready-To-Serve Chunky Turkey Vegetable	9⅜ oz	150	6	1060	16	—
Ready-To-Serve Chunky Vegetable	10¾ oz	160	4	1100	28	—
Ready-To-Serve Low Sodium Chicken Vegetable Beef	10¾ oz	180	5	90	19	—
Ready-To-Serve Low Sodium Chicken Broth	10½ oz	30	1	85	2	—
Ready-To-Serve Low Sodium Chicken With Noodles	10¾ oz	170	5	90	17	—
Ready-To-Serve Low Sodium Mushroom Cream Of	10½ oz	210	14	55	18	—
Ready-To-Serve Low Sodium Split Pea	10¾ oz	230	4	30	37	—
Ready-To-Serve Low Sodium Tomato With Tomato Pieces	10½ oz	190	6	45	30	—

FOOD	PORTION	CAL.	FAT	SOD.	CARB.	FIB.
Campbell (CONT.)						
Scotch Broth as prep	8 oz	80	3	870	9	—
Shrimp Cream Of as prep	8 oz	90	6	810	8	—
Shrimp Cream Of as prep w/ whole milk	8 oz	160	10	860	13	—
Split Pea With Bacon as prep	8 oz	160	4	780	24	—
Teddy Bear as prep	8 oz	70	2	790	11	—
Tomato as prep	8 oz	90	2	680	17	—
Tomato as prep w/ 2% milk	8 oz	150	4	740	22	—
Tomato Bisque as prep	8 oz	120	3	820	22	—
Tomato Homestyle Cream Of as prep	8 oz	110	3	810	20	—
Tomato Homestyle Cream Of as prep w/ whole milk	8 oz	180	7	860	25	—
Tomato Rice Old Fashioned as prep	8 oz	110	2	730	22	—
Tomato Zesty as prep	8 oz	100	2	760	20	—
Turkey Noodle as prep	8 oz	70	2	880	9	—
Turkey Vegetable as prep	8 oz	70	3	710	8	—
Vegetable as prep	8 oz	90	2	830	14	—
Vegetable Beef as prep	8 oz	70	2	780	10	—
Vegetable Homestyle as prep	8 oz	60	2	880	9	—
Vegetable Old Fashioned as prep	8 oz	60	2	880	9	—
Vegetarian Vegetable as prep	8 oz	80	2	790	13	—
Won Ton as prep	8 oz	40	1	850	5	—
College Inn						
Beef Broth	½ can (7 oz)	16	0	960	1	—
Chicken Broth	½ can (7 oz)	35	3	990	0	0
Chicken Broth Lower Salt	½ can (7 oz)	20	2	550	0	0
Gold's						
Borscht	8 oz	100	0	1280	21	—
Borscht Lo-Cal	8 oz	20	tr	1160	5	—
Schav	8 oz	25	0	1380	4	—
Gorton's						
New England Clam Chowder as prep w/ whole milk	¼ can	140	5	740	17	—

FOOD	PORTION	CAL.	FAT	SOD.	CARB.	FIB.
Goya						
Black Bean	7.5 oz	160	4	720	29	9
Hain						
Chicken Broth	8¾ fl oz	70	6	870	0	—
Chicken Broth No Salt Added	8¾ fl oz	60	5	75	0	—
Chicken Noodle	9½ fl oz	120	4	980	11	—
Chicken Noodle No Salt Added	9½ fl oz	120	4	90	12	—
Creamy Mushroom	9¼ fl oz	110	4	740	16	—
Italian Vegetable Pasta	9½ fl oz	160	5	910	25	—
Italian Vegetable Pasta Low Sodium	9½ fl oz	140	6	90	22	—
Minestrone	9½ fl oz	170	2	1060	27	—
Minestrone No Salt Added	9½ fl oz	160	4	35	28	—
Mushroom Barley	9½ fl oz	100	2	600	17	—
New England Clam Chowder	9¼ fl oz	180	4	780	26	—
Split Pea	9½ fl oz	170	1	970	28	—
Split Pea No Salt Added	9½ fl oz	170	1	40	29	—
Turkey Rice	9½ fl oz	100	3	970	10	—
Turkey Rice No Salt Added	9½ fl oz	120	4	85	13	—
Vegetable Broth	9½ fl oz	45	0	1180	10	—
Vegetable Broth Low Sodium	9½ fl oz	40	tr	85	8	—
Vegetable Chicken	9½ fl oz	120	4	930	14	—
Vegetable Chicken No Salt Added	9½ fl oz	130	4	100	14	—
Vegetable Split Pea	9½ fl oz	170	1	970	28	—
Vegetable Split Pea No Salt Added	9½ fl oz	170	1	70	27	—
Vegetarian Lentil	9½ fl oz	160	3	690	25	—
Vegetarian Lentil No Salt Added	9½ fl oz	160	3	65	24	—
Vegetarian Vegetable	9½ fl oz	140	4	920	22	—
Vegetarian Vegetable No Salt Added	9½ fl oz	150	5	45	23	—
Health Valley						
Beef Broth	7.5 oz	10	tr	420	2	0
Beef Broth No Salt Added	7.5 oz	10	tr	5	2	0
Black Bean	7.5 oz	150	2	280	24	16

FOOD	PORTION	CAL.	FAT	SOD.	CARB.	FIB.
Health Valley (CONT.)						
Black Bean No Salt Added	7.5 oz	150	2	20	24	16
Chicken Broth	7.5 oz	35	2	410	1	0
Chicken Broth No Salt Added	7.5 oz	35	2	0	1	0
Chunky Chicken Vegetable	7.5 oz	125	2	290	20	4
Chunky Five Bean Vegetable	7.5 oz	110	2	290	21	11
Chunky Five Bean Vegetable No Salt Added	7.5 oz	110	2	60	21	11
Chunky Vegetable Chicken No Salt Added	7.5 oz	125	2	60	20	4
Green Split Pea	7.5 oz	180	tr	290	34	15
Green Split Pea No Salt Added	7.5 oz	180	tr	25	34	15
Lentil	7.5 oz	220	4	290	33	10
Lentil No Salt Added	7.5 oz	220	4	25	4	10
Manhattan Clam Chowder	7.5 oz	110	2	290	15	2
Manhattan Clam Chowder No Salt Added	7.5 oz	110	2	60	15	2
Minestrone	7.5 oz	130	3	290	19	13
Minestrone No Salt Added	7.5 oz	130	3	90	19	13
Mushroom Barley	7.5 oz	100	2	290	2	9
Mushroom Barley No Salt Added	7.5 oz	100	2	20	16	9
Potato Leek	7.5 oz	130	2	290	23	7
Potato Leek No Salt Added	7.5 oz	130	2	20	23	7
Tomato	7.5 oz	130	3	290	21	1
Tomato No Salt Added	7.5 oz	130	3	40	21	1
Vegetable	7.5 oz	110	1	300	20	8
Vegetable No Salt Added	7.5 oz	110	1	40	20	8
Healthy Choice						
Bean & Ham	1 cup (8.7 oz)	180	3	460	34	10
Beef & Potato	1 cup (8.5 oz)	120	2	440	18	3
Chicken Corn Chowder	1 cup (8.8 oz)	150	3	430	27	7
Chicken With Pasta	1 cup (8.6 oz)	120	3	490	18	1

FOOD	PORTION	CAL.	FAT	SOD.	CARB.	FIB.
Healthy Choice (CONT.)						
Chicken With Rice	1 cup (8.4 oz)	100	3	470	13	3
Chili Beef	1 cup (9 oz)	190	1	490	33	18
Country Vegetable	1 cup (8.6 oz)	100	1	420	22	6
Garden Vegetable	1 cup (8.6 oz)	110	1	450	22	6
Hearty Chicken	1 cup (8.7 oz)	140	3	480	20	3
Lentil	1 cup (8.7 oz)	140	1	460	30	5
Minestrone	1 cup (8.6 oz)	110	2	470	21	3
New England Clam Chowder	1 cup (8.8 oz)	130	3	480	19	7
Old Fashioned Chicken Noodle	1 cup (8.8 oz)	130	2	460	21	2
Split Pea With Ham	1 cup (8.8 oz)	160	2	470	26	5
Tomato Garden	1 cup (8.6 oz)	110	2	430	19	3
Turkey With White & Wild Rice	1 cup (8.4 oz)	110	3	410	18	3
Vegetable Beef	1 cup (8.8 oz)	170	2	430	32	8
Hormel						
Bean & Ham	1 cup (7.5 oz)	190	4	650	28	7
Beef Vegetable	1 cup (7.5 oz)	90	1	740	14	2
Broccoli Cheese With Ham	1 cup (7.5 oz)	170	13	700	10	1
Chicken & Rice	1 cup (7.5 oz)	110	3	900	17	1
Chicken Noodle	1 cup (7.5 oz)	110	3	690	13	1
New England Clam Chowder	1 cup (7.5 oz)	130	5	820	16	1
Potato Cheese With Ham	1 cup (7.5 oz)	190	13	730	16	1
Manischewitz						
Borscht Low Calorie	8 fl oz	20	0	725	4	—
Borscht With Beets	8 fl oz	80	0	660	20	—
Schav	1 cup	11	tr	4	—	—
Old El Paso						
Black Bean With Bacon	1 cup	160	2	960	26	7
Chicken Vegetable	1 cup	110	3	620	13	0
Chicken With Rice	1 cup	90	3	680	10	0
Garden Vegetable	1 cup	110	3	710	17	0
Hearty Beef	1 cup	120	3	690	14	0
Hearty Chicken Noodle	1 cup	110	3	720	10	0
Pritikin						
Chicken & Rice	1 cup (8.8 oz)	80	1	250	13	—
Chicken Broth	1 cup (8.5 oz)	15	0	290	1	—
Chicken Pasta	1 cup (8.6 oz)	100	1	290	18	—
Hearty Vegetable	1 cup (8.8 oz)	90	1	290	20	—
Lentil	1 cup (8.4 oz)	130	1	280	24	—

FOOD	PORTION	CAL.	FAT	SOD.	CARB.	FIB.
Pritikin (CONT.)						
Minestrone	1 cup (8.8 oz)	90	1	290	19	—
Split Pea	1 cup (9.2 oz)	140	1	290	29	—
Three Bean Chili	½ cup (4.5 oz)	90	1	170	19	—
Vegetable Broth	1 cup (8.3 oz)	20	0	250	3	—
Vegetarian Vegetables	1 cup (9 oz)	100	0	290	23	—
Progresso						
Beef	1 can (10.5 fl oz)	180	6	840	17	—
Beef Barley	1 can (10.5 fl oz)	150	5	870	16	—
Beef Minestrone	1 can (10.5 fl oz)	180	6	1000	18	—
Beef Noodle	9.5 fl oz	170	4	1030	18	—
Beef Vegetable	1 can (10.5 fl oz)	170	3	880	18	—
Chickarina	9.5 fl oz	130	5	820	13	—
Chicken Barley	9.25 fl oz	100	2	710	12	4
Chicken Broth	4 fl oz	8	0	360	0	—
Chicken Cream Of	9.5 fl oz	190	11	970	12	—
Chicken Minestrone	1 can (10.5 fl oz)	140	4	1060	14	—
Chicken Noodle	1 can (10.5 fl oz)	120	4	970	8	—
Chicken Rice	1 can (10.5 fl oz)	120	4	990	12	—
Chicken Vegetable	1 can (10.5 fl oz)	150	4	790	18	—
Corn Chowder	9.25 fl oz	200	10	840	22	—
Escarole In Chicken Broth	9.25 fl oz	30	1	1100	2	—
Green Split Pea	1 can (10.5 fl oz)	201	3	920	31	—
Ham & Bean	9.5 fl oz	140	2	950	28	8
Hearty Beef	9.5 fl oz	160	4	820	15	—
Hearty Chicken	1 can (10.5 fl oz)	130	4	960	9	—
Hearty Minestrone	9.25 fl oz	110	2	740	16	—
Homestyle Chicken	9.5 fl oz	110	3	740	12	—
Lentil	1 can (10.5 fl oz)	140	4	1000	24	—
Lentil With Sausage	9.5 fl oz	170	8	840	21	5
Macaroni & Bean	1 can (10.5 fl oz)	150	4	1020	27	—
Manhattan Clam Chowder	9.5 fl oz	120	2	800	13	—
Minestrone	1 can (10.5 fl oz)	120	3	930	25	—
Mushroom Cream Of	9.25 fl oz	160	10	1120	14	—
New England Style Clam Chowder	1 can (10.5 fl oz)	220	12	1050	21	—
Seasoned Beef Broth	4 fl oz	40	tr	380	tr	—
Split Pea With Ham	1 can (10.5 fl oz)	160	5	980	24	6
Tomato	9.5 fl oz	120	3	1000	20	—
Tomato Beef With Rotini	9.5 fl oz	170	6	930	18	—
Tomato Tortellini	9.5 fl oz	130	5	1040	16	—
Tortellini	9.5 fl oz	90	3	930	11	—

FOOD	PORTION	CAL.	FAT	SOD.	CARB.	FIB.
Progresso (CONT.)						
Tortellini Creamy	9.25 fl oz	240	16	910	17	—
Vegetable	1 can (10.5 fl oz)	80	2	1190	15	—
Zesty Minestrone	9.5 fl oz	150	8	1130	19	—
Snow's						
Manhattan Clam Chowder as prep w/ water	7.5 fl oz	70	2	630	9	—
New England Clam Chowder as prep w/ milk	7.5 fl oz	140	6	670	13	—
New England Corn Chowder as prep w/ milk	7.5 fl oz	150	6	640	18	—
New England Fish Chowder as prep w/ milk	7.5 fl oz	130	6	620	11	—
New England Seafood Chowder as prep w/ milk	7.5 fl oz	130	6	690	11	—
Swanson						
Beef Broth	7¼ oz	18	1	750	1	—
Chicken Broth	7¼ oz	30	2	900	2	—
Natural Goodness Clear Chicken Broth	7¼ oz	20	1	580	1	—
Vegetable Broth	7.25 fl oz	20	1	920	3	—
Weight Watchers						
Chicken Noodle	10.5 oz	80	2	1230	9	—
Mushroom Cream Of	10.5 oz	90	2	1250	14	—
asparagus cream of as prep w/ milk	1 cup	161	8	1041	16	—
asparagus cream of as prep w/ water	1 cup	87	4	981	11	—
beef broth ready-to-serve	1 can (14 oz)	27	1	1294	tr	—
beef broth ready-to-serve	1 cup	16	1	782	tr	—
beef noodle as prep w/ water	1 cup	84	3	952	9	—
black bean as prep w/water	1 cup	116	2	1198	20	—
black bean turtle soup	1 cup	218	1	922	40	—
celery cream of as prep w/ milk	1 cup	165	10	1010	15	—
celery cream of as prep w/ water	1 cup	90	6	949	9	—
celery cream of not prep	1 can (10¾ oz)	219	14	2308	21	—

FOOD	PORTION	CAL.	FAT	SOD.	CARB.	FIB.
cheese as prep w/ milk	1 cup	230	15	1020	16	—
cheese as prep w/ water	1 cup	155	10	959	11	—
cheese not prep	1 can (11 oz)	377	25	2331	26	—
chicken broth as prep w/ water	1 cup	39	1	776	1	—
chicken cream of as prep w/ milk	1 cup	191	11	1046	15	—
chicken cream of as prep w/ water	1 cup	116	7	986	9	—
chicken gumbo as prep w/ water	1 cup	56	1	955	8	—
chicken noodle as prep w/ water	1 cup	75	2	1107	9	—
chicken rice as prep w/ water	1 cup	251	2	814	7	—
clam chowder manhattan as prep w/ water	1 cup	77	2	1029	12	—
clam chowder new england as prep w/ water	1 cup	95	3	914	12	—
clam chowder new england as prep w/ milk	1 cup	163	7	992	17	—
consomme w/ gelatin as prep w/ water	1 cup	29	0	637	2	—
consomme w/ gelatin not prep	1 can (10½ oz)	71	0	1550	4	—
escarole ready-to-serve	1 cup	27	2	3865	2	—
french onion as prep w/ water	1 cup	57	2	1053	8	—
gazpacho ready-to-serve	1 cup	57	2	1183	1	—
minestrone as prep w/ water	1 cup	83	3	911	11	—
mushroom cream of as prep w/ milk	1 cup	203	14	1076	15	—
mushroom cream of as prep w/ water	1 cup	129	9	1031	9	—
oyster stew as prep w/ milk	1 cup	134	8	1040	10	—
oyster stew as prep w/ water	1 cup	59	4	980	4	—
pepperpot as prep w/ water	1 cup	103	5	970	9	—
potato cream of as prep w/ milk	1 cup	148	6	1060	17	—
potato cream of as prep w/ water	1 cup	73	2	1000	11	—
scotch broth as prep w/ water	1 cup	80	3	1012	9	—

FOOD	PORTION	CAL.	FAT	SOD.	CARB.	FIB.
split pea w/ ham as prep w/ water	1 cup	189	4	1008	28	—
tomato as prep w/ milk	1 cup	160	6	932	22	—
tomato as prep w/water	1 cup	86	2	872	17	—
vegetarian vegetable as prep w/ water	1 cup	72	2	823	12	—
vichyssoise	1 cup	148	6	1060	17	—
DRY						
4C						
Noodle	8 oz	50	2	960	7	—
Onion Reduced Salt	8 oz	30	1	760	5	—
Armour						
Bouillon Cubes Beef	1 (4 g)	5	0	920	1	—
Bouillon Cubes Chicken	1 (4 g)	5	0	910	1	—
Arrowhead						
Bean & Barley	¼ cup (1.9 oz)	170	0	0	35	7
Bean Cuisine						
Bean Bouillabaisse	1 cup (7.5 fl oz)	174	tr	5	18	5
Island Black Bean	1 cup (8.6 fl oz)	202	tr	7	24	8
Lots of Lentil	1 cup (7.7 oz)	166	tr	7	19	6
Mesa Maize	1 cup (9.2 fl oz)	179	tr	9	21	6
Rocky Mountain Red Bean	1 cup (8.6 oz)	202	tr	7	24	8
Sante Fe Corn Chowder	1 cup (9.2 oz)	179	tr	9	21	6
Thick As Fog Split Pea	1 cup (8.6 fl oz)	189	tr	13	21	1
Ultima Pasta E Fagioli	1 cup (8.6 fl oz)	179	tr	8	22	4
White Bean Provencal	1 cup (7.7 fl oz)	166	tr	7	19	6
Campbell						
Bean With Bacon 'n Ham Microwave	7½ oz	230	5	830	38	—
Chicken Noodle as prep	8 oz	100	2	710	16	—
Chicken Noodle Microwave	7½ oz	100	4	870	11	—
Chicken With Rice Microwave	7½ oz	100	4	820	14	—
Chili Beef Microwave	7½ oz	190	4	870	32	—
Hearty Noodle as prep	8 oz	90	1	840	15	—
Noodle as prep	8 oz	110	2	700	19	—
Onion as prep	8 oz	30	0	700	7	—
Vegetable as prep	8 oz	40	0	710	8	—
Vegetable Beef Microwave	7½ oz	100	2	830	16	—
Campbell's Cup						
Beef Noodle	1 (1.35 oz)	130	2	1270	23	—

FOOD	PORTION	CAL.	FAT	SOD.	CARB.	FIB.
Campbell's Cup (CONT.)						
Chicken Noodle	1 (1.35 oz)	140	3	1340	22	—
Chicken Noodle w/ White Meat as prep	6 oz	90	2	770	12	—
Creamy Chicken w/ White Meat as prep	6 oz	90	4	1020	12	—
Hearty Noodles With Vegetables	1 (1.7 oz)	180	2	1320	32	—
Noodle With Chicken Broth as prep	6 oz	90	2	910	15	—
Casbah						
Black Bean	1 pkg (1.7 oz)	170	2	530	30	9
Split Pea	1 pkg (2.3 oz)	230	1	500	40	10
Sweet Corn Chowder	1 pkg (1.2 oz)	125	1	440	26	2
Vegetarian Chili	1 pkg (1.8 oz)	170	2	430	31	7
Cup-A-Ramen						
Beef With Vegetables as prep	8 oz	270	10	1530	38	—
Beef With Vegetables Low Fat as prep	8 oz	220	2	1600	44	—
Chicken With Vegetables as prep	8 oz	270	10	1470	38	—
Chicken With Vegetables Low Fat as prep	8 oz	220	2	1500	44	—
Oriental With Vegetables as prep	8 oz	270	10	1210	38	—
Oriental With Vegetables Low Fat as prep	8 oz	220	2	1400	44	—
Shrimp With Vegetables as prep	8 oz	280	10	1190	40	—
Shrimp With Vegetables Low Fat as prep	8 oz	230	2	1290	45	—
Cup-A-Soup						
Chicken Broth	6 oz	19	1	605	3	0
Chicken Vegetable	6 oz	47	1	566	8	—
Creamy Broccoli And Cheese	6 oz	70	3	595	10	—
Green Pea	6 oz	113	4	553	14	tr
Hearty Chicken And Noodles	6 oz	110	2	587	20	—
Hearty Creamy Chicken Lots-A-Noodles	7 oz	179	8	639	21	0
Mushroom Cream Of	6 oz	71	3	756	9	0
Onion	6 oz	27	1	665	5	tr

FOOD	PORTION	CAL.	FAT	SOD.	CARB.	FIB.
Cup-A-Soup (CONT.)						
Tomato	6 oz	103	1	524	21	0
Emes						
Beef Base	1 tsp	18	tr	10	2	—
Chicken Base	1 tsp	18	tr	10	2	—
Fantastic						
Cha-Cha Chili Low Fat	1 pkg	220	1	470	37	13
George Washington						
Broth & Brown Seasoning	1 serv	6	0	—	—	—
Broth & Golden Seasoning	1 serv	6	0	—	—	—
Broth & Onion Seasoning	1 serv	12	0	—	—	—
Broth & Vegetable Seasoning	1 serv	12	0	—	—	—
Golden Dipt						
Lobster Bisque	¼ pkg	30	1	560	5	—
Manhattan Clam Chowder	¼ pkg	80	2	700	13	—
New England Clam Chowder	¼ pkg	24	2	680	12	—
Seafood Chowder	¼ pkg	70	2	730	12	—
Shrimp Bisque	¼ pkg	30	1	570	5	—
Goodman's						
Cup Of Soup Beef	1 pkg (1½ cups)	180	3	1640	32	2
Cup Of Soup Chicken Noodle	1 pkg (1½ cups)	180	3	1360	31	2
Cup Of Soup Vegetable	1 pkg (1½ cups)	180	3	1500	32	2
Matzo Ball & Soup	1 cup	40	1	1040	9	1
Matzo Ball & Soup 50% Less Salt	1 serv	50	1	640	10	1
Noodleman	1 cup	45	1	990	9	0
Noodleman Low Sodium	1 cup	50	1	95	9	1
Onion	1 cup	30	1	1280	5	1
Onion Low Sodium	1 cup	30	1	115	6	1
Hain						
Cheese & Broccoli	¾ cup	310	22	980	19	—
Cheese Savory	¾ cup	250	16	890	20	—
Savory Lentil	¾ cup	130	2	810	20	—
Savory Minestrone	¾ cup	110	1	870	20	—
Savory Mushroom	¾ cup	210	15	710	11	—
Savory Mushroom No Salt Added	¾ cup	250	20	180	15	—

FOOD	PORTION	CAL.	FAT	SOD.	CARB.	FIB.
Hain (CONT.)						
Savory Onion	¾ cup	50	2	900	6	—
Savory Onion No Salt Added	¾ cup	50	1	470	9	—
Savory Potato Leek	¾ cup	260	18	690	20	—
Savory Split Pea	¾ cup	310	10	940	16	—
Savory Tomato	¾ cup	220	14	770	19	—
Savory Vegetable	¾ cup	80	1	730	13	—
Savory Vegetable No Salt Added	¾ cup	80	1	330	13	—
Herb-Ox						
Beef Bouillon	1 cube (3.5 g)	10	0	700	1	0
Beef Instant Bouillon Powder	1 tsp (4 g)	10	0	750	1	0
Beef Instant Broth & Seasoning Pack	1 pkg (4.5 g)	10	0	900	1	0
Beef Instant Broth & Seasoning Pack Low Sodium	1 pkg (4 g)	15	0	5	2	0
Chicken Bouillon	1 cube (4 g)	10	0	1040	1	0
Chicken Instant Bouillon Powder	1 tsp (4 g)	10	0	1040	1	0
Chicken Instant Broth & Seasoning Pack	1 pkg (5 g)	10	0	760	1	0
Chicken Instant Broth & Seasoning Pack Low Sodium	1 pkg (4 g)	15	0	20	1	0
Vegetable Bouillon	1 cube (4 g)	10	0	1000	1	0
Hodgson Mill						
13 Bean not prep	1.5 oz	100	1	0	14	12
Hurst						
15 Bean Soup Beef	1 serv (1.7 oz)	160	1	360	27	1
15 Bean Soup Cajun	1 serv (1.7 oz)	160	1	140	27	9
15 Bean Soup Chicken	1 serv (1.7 oz)	160	1	380	27	1
15 Bean Soup Chili	1 serv (1.7 oz)	160	1	240	27	1
15 Bean Soup Ham	1 serv (1.7 oz)	160	1	90	26	1
Spanish-American Black Bean	1 serv (1.3 oz)	120	1	280	22	8
Ka-Me						
Won Ton Chicken not prep	1 pkg (1.25 oz)	180	11	770	18	1
Won Ton Pork not prep	1 pkg (1.25 oz)	180	11	770	18	1
Knorr						
Black Bean Cup-A-Soup as prep	1 pkg	200	1	690	37	9

FOOD	PORTION	CAL.	FAT	SOD.	CARB.	FIB.
Knorr (CONT.)						
Broccoli as prep	8 fl oz	160	8	1050	16	—
Cauliflower as prep	8 fl oz	100	3	750	13	—
Chef's Series Wild Mushroom as prep	8 fl oz	100	3	800	14	—
Chick 'N Pasta as prep	8 fl oz	90	2	850	16	—
Chicken Bouillon as prep	8 fl oz	16	1	1200	tr	—
Chicken Flavored Noodle as prep	8 fl oz	100	2	710	18	—
Chicken Noodle Instant as prep	6 fl oz	25	tr	870	4	—
Fine Herb as prep	8 fl oz	130	6	990	15	—
Fish Bouillon as prep	8 fl oz	10	tr	1130	tr	—
French Onion as prep	8 fl oz	50	1	970	9	—
Hearty Minestrone Cup-A-Soup as prep	1 pkg	150	1	720	29	1
Lentil Cup-A-Soup as prep	1 pkg	220	0	900	40	6
Mushroom as prep	8 fl oz	100	4	870	12	—
Navy Bean Cup-A-Soup as prep	1 pkg	140	0	870	27	5
Oriental Hot And Sour as prep	8 fl oz	50	1	670	9	—
Oxtail Hearty Beef as prep	8 fl oz	70	2	1120	10	—
Potato Leek Cup-A-Soup as prep	1 pkg	120	0	970	24	1
Spinach as prep	8 fl oz	100	5	890	11	—
Spring Vegetable With Herbs as prep	8 fl oz	30	tr	710	6	—
Tomato Basil as prep	8 fl oz	90	3	940	14	—
Tortellini In Brodo as prep	8 fl oz	60	1	820	11	—
Vegetable as prep	8 fl oz	35	1	840	7	—
Vegetable Cup-A-Soup as prep	1 pkg	100	0	840	21	0
Vegetarian Vegetable Bouillon as prep	8 fl oz	16	1	990	1	—
Kojel						
Hearty Potato With Vegetables Instant	1 serv (6 fl oz)	60	0	650	15	2
Noodle Soup Chicken Flavor Instant	1 serv (6 fl oz)	70	1	590	11	2
Split Pea Instant	1 serv (6 fl oz)	60	tr	380	14	3

FOOD	PORTION	CAL.	FAT	SOD.	CARB.	FIB.
Kojel (CONT.)						
Tomato Instant	1 serv (6 fl oz)	50	0	540	15	1
Vegetable Chicken Couscous Instant	1 serv (6 fl oz)	80	1	530	18	2
Lipton						
Beef Mushroom	8 oz	38	1	763	7	—
Beefy Onion	8 oz	27	1	635	5	—
Chicken Noodle	8 oz	82	2	702	12	—
Chicken Noodle Hearty	8 oz	81	1	766	14	—
Country Vegetable	8 oz	80	1	803	16	—
Giggle Noodle	8 oz	72	2	708	12	—
Hearty Noodles With Vegetables	8 oz	75	2	687	12	—
Instant Oriental Noodle Beef	8 oz	177	1	912	34	—
Instant Oriental Noodle Chicken	8 oz	180	2	785	33	—
Onion	8 oz	20	tr	632	4	—
Onion Golden	8 oz	62	2	716	11	—
Onion Mushroom	8 oz	41	1	684	7	0
Ring-O-Noodle	8 oz	67	2	708	11	—
Vegetable	8 oz	37	1	640	7	tr
Lite Line						
Beef Bouillon Instant Low Sodium	1 tsp	12	tr	5	2	—
Chicken Bouillon Instant Low Sodium	1 tsp	12	tr	5	2	—
Manischewitz						
Minestrone as prep	6 fl oz	50	tr	160	9	—
Split Pea as prep	6 fl oz	45	tr	320	9	—
Vegetable as prep	6 fl oz	50	tr	65	9	—
Maruchan						
Instant Lunch Oriental Noodles Beef	1 pkg (2.25 oz)	290	13	1260	37	—
Instant Lunch Oriental Noodles Chicken	1 pkg (2.25 oz)	290	13	1270	36	2
Instant Lunch Oriental Noodles Chicken Mushroom	1 pkg (2.25 oz)	280	13	1380	34	—
Instant Lunch Oriental Noodles Mushroom	1 pkg (2.25 oz)	290	13	1310	35	—
Instant Lunch Oriental Noodles Pork	1 pkg (2.25 oz)	290	13	1390	35	—
Instant Lunch Oriental Noodles Shrimp	1 pkg (2.25 oz)	290	13	1260	37	—

FOOD	PORTION	CAL.	FAT	SOD.	CARB.	FIB.
Maruchan (CONT.)						
Instant Lunch Oriental Noodles Toast Onion	1 pkg (2.25 oz)	270	12	1290	34	—
Instant Lunch Oriental Noodles Vegetable Beef	1 pkg (2.25 oz)	290	12	1340	34	—
Instant Wonton Chicken	1 pkg (1.49 oz)	200	12	1440	19	—
Instant Wonton Hot & Sour	1 pkg (1.49 oz)	200	11	1070	21	—
Instant Wonton Oriental	1 pkg (1.49 oz)	190	12	1340	19	—
Instant Wonton Pork	1 pkg (1.49 oz)	200	12	1450	19	—
Instant Wonton Shrimp	1 pkg (1.49 oz)	200	12	1120	19	—
Oriental Noodle Picante Style Beef	1 pkg (2.25 oz)	290	15	950	37	—
Oriental Noodle Picante Style Chicken	1 pkg (2.25 oz)	290	15	920	38	—
Oriental Noodle Picante Style Shrimp	1 pkg (2.25 oz)	300	16	1120	36	—
Ramen Beef	½ pkg (1.5 oz)	190	9	770	26	—
Ramen Chicken	½ pkg (1.5 oz)	190	8	780	20	—
Ramen Chicken Mushroom	½ pkg (1.5 oz)	190	8	780	25	—
Ramen Chili	½ pkg (1.5 oz)	190	9	710	26	—
Ramen Mushroom	½ pkg (1.5 oz)	190	9	910	25	—
Ramen Oriental	½ pkg (1.5 oz)	190	9	990	26	—
Ramen Pork	½ pkg (1.5 oz)	190	9	890	25	—
Ramen Shrimp	½ pkg (1.5 oz)	190	9	820	26	—
Wonton Beef	⅓ pkg (0.68 oz)	90	5	890	8	—
Wonton Chicken	⅓ pkg (0.67 oz)	90	5	810	8	—
Wonton Pork	⅓ pkg (0.68 oz)	90	5	930	9	—
Wonton Vegetable	⅓ pkg (0.7 oz)	90	6	980	9	—
Nile Spice						
Couscous Almondine	1 pkg	200	3	490	37	2
Couscous Garbanzo	1 pkg	220	3	500	39	2
Couscous Lentil Curry	1 pkg	200	2	730	36	4
Couscous Minestrone	1 pkg	180	2	590	34	2
Couscous Parmesan	1 pkg	200	3	570	34	2
Homestyle Black Bean	1 pkg	190	2	570	34	2
Homestyle Chicken Flavored Vegetable	1 pkg	120	2	600	20	4
Homestyle Lentil	1 pkg	180	2	500	31	3
Homestyle Minestrone	1 pkg	160	2	550	29	4
Homestyle Red Beans & Rice	1 pkg	190	2	560	36	3

FOOD	PORTION	CAL.	FAT	SOD.	CARB.	FIB.
Nile Spice (CONT.)						
Homestyle Split Pea	1 pkg	200	2	710	35	6
Homestyle Sweet Corn Chowder	1 pkg	120	3	420	20	0
Italian Tomato	1 pkg	140	4	670	21	2
Potato Leek	1 pkg	150	6	490	21	2
Potato Romano	1 pkg	140	5	550	19	3
Ramen Noodle						
Beef as prep	8 oz	190	8	1010	26	—
Beef Low Fat as prep	8 oz	160	1	890	32	—
Chicken as prep	8 oz	190	8	970	26	—
Chicken Low Fat as prep	8 oz	160	1	940	32	—
Oriental as prep	8 oz	190	8	930	26	—
Oriental Low Fat as prep	8 oz	150	1	940	31	—
Pork as prep	8 oz	200	8	860	26	—
Pork Low Fat as prep	8 oz	150	1	1140	31	—
Ultra Slim-Fast						
Beef Noodle	6 oz	45	tr	700	7	2
Chicken Leek	6 oz	50	tr	1070	7	2
Chicken Noodle	6 oz	45	tr	970	6	2
Creamy Broccoli	6 oz	75	tr	800	14	2
Creamy Tomato	6 oz	60	tr	800	10	2
Hearty Vegetable	6 oz	50	tr	750	7	2
Onion	6 oz	45	tr	930	7	2
Potato Leek	6 oz	80	tr	780	15	2
Weight Watchers						
Beef Broth Instant	1 pkg	8	0	910	1	—
Chicken Broth Instant	1 pkg	8	0	900	1	—
Chicken Noodle	7.5 oz	90	1	450	13	—
Chunky Beef Stew	7.5 oz	120	2	450	14	—
New England Clam Chowder	7.5 oz	90	0	450	16	—
Vegetable Beef	7.5 oz	90	1	450	13	—
Wylers						
Beef Bouillon Instant	1 tsp	6	tr	930	1	—
Beef Bouillon Instant Cube	1	6	tr	930	1	—
Chicken Bouillon Instant	1 tsp	8	tr	900	1	—
Chicken Bouillon Instant Cube	1	8	tr	900	1	—
Onion Bouillon Instant	1 tsp	10	tr	910	1	—
Vegetable Bouillon Instant	1 tsp	6	tr	910	1	—
asparagus cream of as prep w/ water	1 cup	59	2	801	9	—

FOOD	PORTION	CAL.	FAT	SOD.	CARB.	FIB.
beef broth	1 pkg (0.2 oz)	14	1	1019	1	—
beef broth as prep w/ water	1 cup	19	1	1368	2	—
beef broth cube	1 cube (3.6 g)	6	tr	864	1	—
beef broth cube as prep w/ water	1 cup	8	tr	1152	1	—
celery cream of as prep w/ water	1 cup	63	2	839	10	—
chicken broth	1 pkg (0.2 oz)	16	1	1116	1	—
chicken broth as prep w/ water	1 cup	21	1	1484	1	—
chicken broth cube	1 cube (4.8 g)	9	tr	1152	1	—
chicken broth cube as prep w/ water	1 cup	13	tr	792	2	—
chicken cream of as prep w/ water	1 cup	107	5	1184	13	—
chicken noodle as prep w/ water	1 cup	53	1	1284	7	—
french onion not prep	1 pkg (1.4 oz)	115	2	3493	21	—
leek as prep w/ water	1 cup	71	2	966	11	—
onion as prep w/ water	1 cup	28	1	848	5	—
tomato as prep w/ water	1 cup	102	2	943	19	—
FROZEN						
Jaclyn's						
Barley & Mushroom	7.5 fl oz	90	1	234	16	—
Split Pea	7.5 fl oz	180	2	183	31	—
Vegetable	7.5 fl oz	90	1	195	18	—
Kettle Ready						
Asparagus Cream Of	6 oz	62	5	415	5	—
Black Bean With Ham	6 oz	154	6	567	23	—
Boston Clam Chowder	6 oz	131	7	420	13	0
Broccoli Cream Of	6 oz	94	7	487	6	0
Cauliflower Cream Of	6 oz	93	7	432	6	—
Cheddar Broccoli Cream Of	6 oz	137	11	595	5	—
Chicken Cream Of	6 oz	98	6	676	5	—
Chicken Gumbo	6 oz	94	4	380	12	—
Chicken Noodle	6 oz	94	3	599	12	—
Chili	6 oz	161	7	425	14	—
Corn & Broccoli Chowder	6 oz	102	5	451	13	0
Creamy Cheddar	6 oz	158	13	625	7	—
French Onion	6 oz	42	2	508	5	—
Garden Vegetable	6 oz	85	3	460	12	0
Hearty Beef Vegetable	6 oz	85	3	353	11	—

FOOD	PORTION	CAL.	FAT	SOD.	CARB.	FIB.
Kettle Ready (CONT.)						
Hearty Minestrone	6 oz	104	4	352	15	—
Manhattan Clam Chowder	6 oz	69	3	564	8	—
Mushroom Cream Of	6 oz	85	6	422	6	—
New England Clam Chowder	6 oz	116	7	336	11	tr
Potato Cream Of	6 oz	121	5	404	17	0
Savory Bean With Ham	6 oz	113	4	404	20	—
Split Pea With Ham	6 oz	155	4	351	25	0
Tomato Florentine	6 oz	106	4	389	15	—
Tortellini In Tomato	6 oz	122	5	548	15	—
Tabatchnick						
Barley Mushroom	1 serv (7.5 oz)	70	0	540	13	3
Barley Mushroom No Salt Added	1 serv (7.5 oz)	70	0	98	13	3
Broccoli Cream Of	1 serv (7.5 oz)	90	4	740	12	3
Cabbage	1 serv (7.5 oz)	60	0	160	14	2
Chicken With Dumplings	1 serv (7.5 oz)	70	2	830	13	1
Corn Chowder	1 serv (7.5 oz)	150	6	650	22	1
Minestrone	1 serv (7.5 oz)	150	1	550	27	10
New England Potato	1 serv (7.5 oz)	150	6	540	21	2
New York Chicken	1 serv (7.5 oz)	35	0	850	6	0
Old Fashion Potato	1 serv (7.5 oz)	70	0	540	16	2
Pea	1 serv (7.5 oz)	180	2	520	31	11
Pea No Salt Added	1 serv (7.5 oz)	180	2	79	31	11
Spinach Cream Of	1 serv (7.5 oz)	90	4	630	11	2
Vegetable	1 serv (7.5 oz)	110	1	580	20	4
Vegetable No Salt Added	1 serv (7.5 oz)	110	1	77	20	4
Wisconsin Cheddar Vegetable	1 serv (7.5 oz)	140	9	930	12	1
Yankee Bean	1 serv (7.5 oz)	160	2	570	27	11
SHELF-STABLE						
Lunch Bucket						
Chicken Noodle	1 pkg (7.25 oz)	90	2	810	13	—
Country Vegetable	1 pkg (7.25 oz)	70	1	740	15	—
TAKE-OUT						
beef stew soup	1 cup (8.8 oz)	221	5	461	20	—
black bean turtle soup	1 cup	241	1	6	45	—
brunswick stew soup	1 cup (8.5 oz)	232	6	438	17	—
corn & cheese chowder	¾ cup	215	12	386	21	3
gazpacho	1 cup	46	tr	63	5	—
greek	¾ cup	63	2	386	7	2
hot & sour	1 serv (14 oz)	173	8	475	8	1

FOOD	PORTION	CAL.	FAT	SOD.	CARB.	FIB.
hot & sour	1 cup	74	2	—	—	—
oxtail	5 oz	64	3	—	7	—
pasta e fagiolo	1 cup (8.8 oz)	194	5	790	30	—
ratatouille	1 cup (7.5 oz)	266	25	329	12	—

SOUR CREAM
(see also SOUR CREAM SUBSTITUTES)

FOOD	PORTION	CAL.	FAT	SOD.	CARB.	FIB.
Breakstone	2 tbsp (1 oz)	60	5	15	1	0
Free	2 tbsp (1.1 oz)	35	0	25	6	0
Half & Half	2 tbsp (1.1 oz)	45	4	20	2	0
Cabot						
Light	1 oz	33	2	72	2	—
Friendship						
Light	2 tbsp (1 oz)	35	3	30	2	0
Sour Cream	2 tbsp (1 oz)	60	5	15	2	0
Heluva Good Cheese						
Fat-Free	2 tbsp (1.1 oz)	20	0	45	3	0
Light	2 tbsp (1.1 oz)	40	3	20	3	0
Sour Cream	2 tbsp (1.1 oz)	60	5	15	2	0
Hood						
Fat Free	2 tbsp (1 oz)	20	0	25	3	0
Light	2 tbsp (1 oz)	40	3	20	2	0
Knudsen						
Free	2 tbsp (1.1 oz)	35	0	25	6	0
Hampshire	2 tbsp (1 oz)	60	6	15	1	0
Light	2 tbsp (1.1 oz)	40	3	20	2	0
Naturally Yours						
No Fat	2 tbsp (1 fl oz)	15	0	15	1	—
Sealtest						
Free	2 tbsp (1.1 oz)	35	0	25	6	0
Light	2 tbsp (1.1 oz)	40	3	20	2	0
Weight Watchers						
Light Sour	2 tbsp	35	2	40	2	—
sour cream	1 tbsp	26	3	6	1	—
sour cream	1 cup	493	48	123	10	—

SOUR CREAM SUBSTITUTES

FOOD	PORTION	CAL.	FAT	SOD.	CARB.	FIB.
Pet						
Imitation	1 tbsp	25	2	25	tr	—
Tofutti						
Better Than Sour Cream Sour Supreme	1 oz	50	5	120	1	—
nondairy	1 oz	59	6	29	2	—
nondairy	1 cup	479	45	235	15	—

FOOD	PORTION	CAL.	FAT	SOD.	CARB.	FIB.
SOURSOP						
fresh	1	416	2	87	105	—
fresh cut up	1 cup	150	1	31	38	—
SOY						
(*see also* ICE CREAM AND FROZEN DESSERTS, MILK SUBSTITUTES, MISO, SOY SAUCE, SOYBEANS, TEMPEH, TOFU)						
Eden						
Tamari Organic Domestic	1 tbsp (0.5 oz)	15	0	970	2	0
Tamari Organic Imported	1 tbsp (0.5 oz)	15	0	1130	2	0
LaLoma						
Soyagen All Purpose	¼ cup	130	6	150	14	—
Soyagen Carob	¼ cup	140	6	160	16	—
Soyagen No Sucrose	¼ cup	130	6	210	14	—
Tree Of Life						
Shoyu	1 tbsp (0.5 oz)	15	0	960	1	—
Tamari Reduced Sodium	1 tbsp (0.5 oz)	20	0	700	1	—
Tamari Wheat Free	1 tbsp (0.5 oz)	15	0	940	1	—
Worthington						
Soyamel	1 oz	130	7	150	11	—
lecithin	1 tbsp	104	14	—	0	—
roasted & toasted	1 cup	490	26	4	33	—
soy milk	1 cup	79	5	30	4	—
soya cheese	1.4 oz	128	11	—	tr	0
SOY SAUCE						
(*see also* SAUCE, SOY)						
Eden						
Shoyu Organic	1 tbsp (0.5 oz)	15	0	1040	2	0
Shoyu Traditional	1 tbsp (0.5 oz)	15	0	1010	2	0
House Of Tsang						
Dark	1 tbsp (0.6 oz)	10	0	860	1	0
Ginger Flavored	1 tbsp (0.6 oz)	20	0	730	4	0
Ginger Flavored Low Sodium	1 tbsp (0.6 oz)	10	0	280	2	0
Light	1 tbsp (0.6 oz)	5	0	900	0	0
Low Sodium	1 tbsp (0.6 oz)	5	0	280	0	0
Mushroom Flavored Low Sodium	1 tbsp (0.6 oz)	10	0	280	2	0
Ka-Me						
Chinese Dark	1 tbsp (0.5 fl oz)	10	0	1020	3	0
Chinese Light	1 tbsp (0.5 fl oz)	5	0	1170	1	0
Dark	1 tbsp (0.5 fl oz)	10	0	1020	3	0
Japanese	1 tbsp (0.5 fl oz)	5	0	520	1	0

FOOD	PORTION	CAL.	FAT	SOD.	CARB.	FIB.
Ka-Me (CONT.)						
Light	1 tbsp (0.5 fl oz)	5	0	1170	1	0
Mild	1 tbsp (0.5 fl oz)	5	0	490	0	0
Kikkoman						
Lite	1 tbsp	13	0	564	2	—
Soy Sauce	1 tbsp	12	0	938	2	0
La Choy						
Lite	½ tsp	1	tr	110	tr	tr
Trappey						
Chef Magic	1 tbsp (0.5 oz)	23	tr	952	4	tr
shoyu	1 tbsp	9	tr	1029	2	—
soy sauce	1 tbsp	7	tr	1024	1	—
tamari	1 tbsp	11	tr	1005	1	—

SOYBEANS

(*see also* MILK SUBSTITUTES, MISO, SOY, TEMPEH, TOFU)

FOOD	PORTION	CAL.	FAT	SOD.	CARB.	FIB.
dried cooked	1 cup	298	15	1	17	—
dry-roasted	½ cup	387	19	2	28	—
green cooked	½ cup	127	6	13	10	4
roasted	½ cup	405	22	140	29	—
roasted & toasted	1 oz	129	7	1	9	—
roasted & toasted salted	1 cup	490	26	176	33	—
roasted & toasted salted	1 oz	129	7	54	9	—
sprouts raw	½ cup	43	2	5	3	—
sprouts steamed	½ cup	38	2	5	3	—
sprouts stir fried	1 cup	125	7	14	9	—

SPAGHETTI

(*see* PASTA, PASTA DINNERS, PASTA SALAD, SPAGHETTI SAUCE)

SPAGHETTI SAUCE

(*see also* PIZZA, TOMATO)

JARRED

FOOD	PORTION	CAL.	FAT	SOD.	CARB.	FIB.
Classico						
Beef & Pork	4 fl oz	80	4	540	7	—
Four Cheese	4 fl oz	70	4	440	7	—
Ripe Olives & Mushrooms	4 fl oz	50	2	470	7	—
Spicy Red Pepper	4 fl oz	50	2	250	6	—
Sweet Peppers & Onions	4 fl oz	50	4	360	7	—
Tomato & Basil	4 fl oz	60	3	340	6	—
Contadina						
Italian	¼ cup	20	0	280	4	tr
Thick & Zesty	¼ cup	15	0	320	4	1
Del Monte	¼ cup	15	0	330	4	1
Traditional	½ cup (4.4 oz)	80	1	470	15	tr

FOOD	PORTION	CAL.	FAT	SOD.	CARB.	FIB.
Del Monte (CONT.)						
Traditional No Sugar Added	½ cup (4.4 oz)	60	1	470	11	tr
With Garlic & Onion	½ cup (4.4 oz)	70	1	440	15	tr
With Green Peppers & Mushrooms	½ cup (4.4 oz)	70	1	320	13	tr
With Meat	½ cup (4.4 oz)	40	2	390	13	tr
With Mushrooms	½ cup (4.4 oz)	80	2	520	15	tr
Eden						
Organic	½ cup (4.4 oz)	80	3	320	12	3
Organic No Salt Added	½ cup (4.4 oz)	80	3	10	12	3
Enrico's						
Fat Free Organic Basil	½ cup (4 oz)	50	0	220	8	4
Fat Free Organic Garlic	½ cup (4 oz)	50	0	340	9	5
Fat Free Organic Hot Pepper	½ cup (4 oz)	50	0	350	8	5
Fat Free Organic Mushroom	½ cup (4 oz)	60	0	400	10	7
Fat Free Organic Traditional	½ cup (4 oz)	45	0	280	4	6
Healthy Choice						
Extra Chunky Garlic & Onions	½ cup (4.4 oz)	50	1	390	11	2
Extra Chunky Italian Style Vegetable	½ cup (4.4 oz)	50	1	390	11	2
Extra Chunky Mushrooms	½ cup (4.4 oz)	50	1	390	10	2
Original Garlic & Herbs	½ cup (4.4 oz)	50	1	390	10	2
Original Mushrooms	½ cup (4.4 oz)	50	1	390	10	2
Original Traditional	½ cup (4.4 oz)	50	1	390	10	2
Original With Meat	½ cup (4.4 oz)	50	1	390	8	2
Super Chunky Mushrooms & Sweet Peppers	½ cup (4.4 oz)	50	1	390	11	2
Super Chunky Vegetable Primavera	½ cup (4.4 oz)	50	1	390	11	2
Hunt's						
Chunky	¼ cup (2.2 fl oz)	30	1	290	4	1
Classic Italian With Parmesan	½ cup (4.4 fl oz)	50	2	630	8	2
Homestyle Traditional No Sugar Added	½ cup (4.4 fl oz)	60	3	600	7	2
Traditional	4 oz	70	2	530	12	2
Traditional Light	½ cup (4 oz)	40	1	420	7	3

FOOD	PORTION	CAL.	FAT	SOD.	CARB.	FIB.
Hunt's (CONT.)						
With Meat	4 oz	70	2	570	12	2
With Mushrooms	4 oz	70	2	560	12	2
Mama Rizzo's						
Mushroom Onion	½ cup (4.3 oz)	60	2	290	9	1
Pepper Mushroom Onion	½ cup (4.3 oz)	60	2	290	9	1
Pepper Primavera Vegetable	½ cup (4.2 oz)	50	2	220	8	2
Pepper Tomato Basil Garlic	½ cup (4.7 oz)	60	2	490	10	1
Primavera Vegetable	½ cup (4.2 oz)	50	2	220	8	2
Tomato Basil Garlic	½ cup (4.6 oz)	60	2	500	8	2
Muir Glen						
Organic Cabernet Marinara	½ cup (4.4 oz)	45	0	350	10	2
Organic Chunky Style	½ cup (4.5 oz)	80	2	300	13	3
Organic Fat Free Tomato Basil	½ cup (4.3 oz)	50	0	300	10	2
Organic Garlic Onion	½ cup (4.3 oz)	50	0	300	11	3
Organic Garlic Roasted Garlic	½ cup (4.4 oz)	45	0	350	10	2
Organic Green Pepper & Mushroom	½ cup (4.5 oz)	70	2	360	10	4
Organic Italian Herb	½ cup (4.5 oz)	60	0	300	13	2
Organic Romano Cheese	½ cup (4.5 oz)	90	3	300	14	4
Organic Sun Dried Tomato	½ cup (4.4 oz)	40	0	360	9	2
Organic Sweet Pepper Onion	½ cup (4.4 oz)	40	0	300	8	1
Organic Tomato Basil	½ cup (4.3 oz)	50	0	300	10	2
Newman's Own						
Marinara	4 oz	70	2	560	11	—
Marinara With Mushrooms	4 oz	70	2	560	11	—
Sockarooni	4 oz	70	2	560	11	—
Prego						
Chunky Sausage & Green Peppers	4 oz	160	8	500	19	—
Extra Chunky Garden Combination	4 oz	80	2	420	14	—
Extra Chunky Mushroom & Green Pepper	4 oz	100	4	410	14	—

FOOD	PORTION	CAL.	FAT	SOD.	CARB.	FIB.
Prego (CONT.)						
Extra Chunky Mushroom & Onion	4 oz	100	4	490	13	—
Extra Chunky Mushroom & Tomato	4 oz	110	5	500	14	—
Extra Chunky Mushroom With Extra Spice	4 oz	100	3	450	17	—
Extra Chunky Tomato & Onion	4 oz	110	5	490	14	—
Marinara	4 oz	100	6	620	10	—
Meat Flavored	4 oz	140	6	660	20	—
Mushroom	4 oz	130	5	630	20	—
Onion & Garlic	4 oz	110	4	510	16	—
Regular	4 oz	130	5	630	20	—
Three Cheese	4 oz	100	2	410	17	—
Tomato & Basil	4 oz	100	2	370	18	—
Pritikin						
Chunky Garden	½ cup (4 oz)	50	1	30	12	—
Marinara	½ cup (4 oz)	60	0	260	13	—
Original	½ cup (4 oz)	60	1	30	13	—
Progresso						
Bolognese	½ cup	150	12	520	12	3
Marinara	½ cup	90	5	520	9	—
Meat Flavored	½ cup	110	5	660	13	—
Mushroom	½ cup	110	5	630	13	—
Sicilian	½ cup	30	3	660	2	tr
Ragu						
Fino Italian Garlic & Basil	½ cup (4.5 oz)	90	3	580	15	2
Fino Italian Garden Medley	½ cup (4.5 oz)	90	3	580	14	2
Fino Italian Parmesan	½ cup (4.5 oz)	100	3	580	15	2
Fino Italian Sliced Mushroom	½ cup (4.5 oz)	90	3	580	14	2
Fino Italian Tomato & Herb	½ cup (4.5 oz)	90	3	580	15	2
Fino Italian Zesty Tomato	½ cup (4.5 oz)	90	3	580	14	2
Gardenstyle Chunky Garden Combination	½ cup (4.5 oz)	120	4	540	18	3
Gardenstyle Chunky Green & Red Pepper	½ cup (4.5 oz)	120	4	570	19	2
Gardenstyle Chunky Mushroom & Green Pepper	½ cup (4.5 oz)	120	4	570	18	3
Gardenstyle Chunky Mushroom & Onion	½ cup (4.5 oz)	120	4	560	19	3

FOOD	PORTION	CAL.	FAT	SOD.	CARB.	FIB.
Ragu (CONT.)						
Gardenstyle Chunky Tomato Garlic & Onion	½ cup (4.5 oz)	120	4	550	19	3
Gardenstyle Super Mushroom	½ cup (4.5 oz)	120	4	540	19	3
Gardenstyle Super Vegetable Primavera	½ cup (4.5 oz)	110	4	480	17	4
Homestyle Mushroom	½ cup (4.5 oz)	120	4	650	18	3
Homestyle Tomato & Herb	½ cup (4.5 oz)	120	4	650	18	3
Homestyle With Meat	½ cup (4.5 oz)	130	4	650	18	3
Light Chunky Mushroom	½ cup (4.4 oz)	50	0	410	10	2
Light Garden Harvest	½ cup (4.4 oz)	50	0	410	11	2
Light No Sugar Added	½ cup (4.4 oz)	60	0	410	9	3
Light Tomato & Herb	½ cup (4.4 oz)	50	0	410	10	2
Old World Style Marinara	½ cup (4.4 oz)	90	5	820	9	3
Old World Style Mushrooms	½ cup (4.4 oz)	80	3	820	10	3
Old World Style Traditional	½ cup (4.4 oz)	80	3	820	10	3
Old World Style With Meat	½ cup (4.4 oz)	90	5	820	9	3
Sauce	4 fl oz	80	4	740	9	—
Thick & Hearty Mushroom	½ cup (4.5 oz)	120	3	580	19	3
Thick & Hearty Spaghetti Sauce	4 oz	100	3	460	15	—
Thick & Hearty Tomato & Herb	½ cup (4.5 oz)	120	3	580	19	3
Thick & Hearty With Meat	1.2 cup (4.5 oz)	130	5	580	19	3
Tree Of Life						
Pasta Sauce	½ cup (4 oz)	50	2	290	9	—
Pasta Sauce Calabrese	½ cup (3.9 oz)	60	3	310	9	—
Pasta Sauce Fat Free Classic	½ cup (3.9 oz)	40	0	250	8	0
Pasta Sauce Fat Free Mushroom & Basil	½ cup (3.9 oz)	30	0	300	7	0
Pasta Sauce Fat Free Onion & Garlic	½ cup (3.9 oz)	30	0	240	7	0
Pasta Sauce Fat Free Sweet Pepper	½ cup (3.9 oz)	30	0	280	7	0
Pasta Sauce No Salt	½ cup (3.9 oz)	50	2	0	9	—

FOOD	PORTION	CAL.	FAT	SOD.	CARB.	FIB.
Weight Watchers						
With Meat	⅓ cup	45	1	310	7	—
With Mushrooms	⅓ cup	35	0	300	7	—
marinara sauce	1 cup	171	8	1572	25	—
spaghetti sauce	1 cup	272	12	1236	40	—
REFRIGERATED						
Contadina						
Alfredo	½ cup (4.2 fl oz)	400	38	510	8	0
Four Cheese Sauce With White Wine & Shallots	½ cup (4.2 fl oz)	320	25	480	8	0
Light Alfredo	½ cup (4.2 fl oz)	190	13	560	10	0
Light Chunky Tomato	½ cup (4.4 fl oz)	45	0	470	8	3
Light Garden Vegetable	½ cup (4.4 fl oz)	45	1	540	8	3
Marinara	½ cup (4.4 fl oz)	80	4	470	8	2
Pesto With Basil	¼ cup (2 oz)	310	30	440	5	0
Pesto With Sun Dried Tomatoes	¼ cup (2 oz)	250	24	520	6	3
Plum Tomato With Basil	½ cup (4.4 fl oz)	70	3	450	8	3
Spicy Italian Sausage & Bell Pepper	½ cup (4.4 fl oz)	100	5	540	9	3
Di Giorno						
Alfredo	¼ cup (2.2 oz)	230	22	550	2	0
Four Cheese	¼ cup (2.2 oz)	200	19	410	2	0
Light Chunky Tomato With Basil	½ cup (4.5 oz)	70	0	290	16	2
Light Reduced Fat Alfredo	¼ cup (2.4 oz)	170	10	600	16	0
Marinara	½ cup (4.5 oz)	100	5	530	12	3
Olive Oil & Garlic With Grated Cheese	¼ cup (2.1 oz)	370	36	540	3	0
Pesto	¼ cup (2.2 oz)	320	31	500	3	0
Plum Tomato & Mushroom	½ cup (4.4 oz)	70	0	310	15	2
Traditional Meat	½ cup (4.5 oz)	120	6	610	12	3
TAKE-OUT						
bolognese	5 oz	195	15	—	4	tr

SPANISH FOOD

(*see also* BEANS, CHIPS, DINNER, PEPPERS, SALSA, SNACKS, SAUCE, TORTILLA)

FOOD	PORTION	CAL.	FAT	SOD.	CARB.	FIB.
CANNED						
Casa Fiesta						
Picante Mild	1 oz	9	tr	117	2	—
Chi-Chi's						
Picante Hot	2 tbsp (1 oz)	10	0	270	2	0

FOOD	PORTION	CAL.	FAT	SOD.	CARB.	FIB.
Chi-Chi's (CONT.)						
Picante Medium	2 tbsp (1 oz)	10	0	200	2	0
Picante Mild	2 tbsp (1 oz)	10	0	210	2	0
Pico De Gallo	2 tbsp (1.2 oz)	10	0	170	2	0
Derby						
Tamales	2	160	7	570	15	1
El Molino						
Enchilada Sauce Hot	2 tbsp	16	1	100	2	—
Green Chili Sauce Mild	2 tbsp	10	0	210	2	—
Gebhardt						
Enchiladas	2	310	24	460	20	2
Tamales	2	290	22	730	19	2
Tamales Jumbo	2	400	30	1025	26	3
Guiltless Gourmet						
Picante Mild	1 oz	6	0	133	1	tr
Queso Mild Cheddar	1 oz	22	tr	150	5	tr
Hormel						
Tamales Beef	1 can (7.5 oz)	290	21	1030	20	3
Tamales Beef	3 (7.5 oz)	280	21	1010	20	3
Tamales Chicken	3 (7.5 oz)	210	10	1040	23	2
Tamales Hot Spicy Beef	3 (7.5 oz)	280	21	1010	20	3
Tamales Jumbo Beef	2 (6.9 oz)	270	20	940	18	3
Old El Paso						
Tamales	2	190	12	380	16	—
Rosarita						
Enchilada Sauce Mild	2.5 oz	25	1	230	3	tr
Picante Chunky Hot	3 tbsp (2 fl oz)	18	tr	515	4	tr
Picante Chunky Medium	3 tbsp (2 fl oz)	16	tr	650	4	tr
Picante Chunky Mild	3 tbsp (2 oz)	25	tr	630	5	tr
Van Camp's						
Tamales	2 (5.1 oz)	210	13	610	20	3
Wolf Brand						
Tamales	7.5 oz	328	25	1181	25	—
FROZEN						
Banquet						
Beef Enchilada	1 pkg (11 oz)	320	12	1330	54	10
Chimichanga Meal	1 pkg (9.5 oz)	470	23	1180	56	9
Enchilada Cheese	1 pkg (11 oz)	350	6	1500	56	9
Enchilada Chicken	1 pkg (11 oz)	360	10	1580	54	9
Family Entree Beef Enchilada w/ Cheese	1 serv (4.67 oz)	130	4	690	19	3
El Charrito						
Enchiladas 4 Grande Beef	1 pkg (16.5 oz)	890	47	—	—	—

FOOD	PORTION	CAL.	FAT	SOD.	CARB.	FIB.
Healthy Choice						
Beef Burrito Ranchero Medium	1 (5.4 oz)	290	7	500	44	6
Beef Burrito Ranchero Mild	1 (5.4 oz)	300	7	480	45	7
Beef Enchilada Rio Grande	1 meal (13.4 oz)	410	8	480	70	9
Burrito Chicken Con Queso	1 (5.4 oz)	280	6	600	43	5
Chicken Enchilada Supreme	1 meal (13.4 oz)	390	9	390	60	8
Enchiladas Suiza Chicken	1 meal (10 oz)	270	4	440	43	5
Feista Chicken Fajitas	1 meal (7 oz)	260	4	410	36	5
Jimmy Dean						
Burrito Breakfast Bacon	1 (4 oz)	260	8	680	37	1
Burrito Breakfast Sausage	1 (4 oz)	250	8	580	36	2
Le Menu						
Entree LightStyle Enchiladas Chicken	8 oz	280	8	530	32	—
Lean Cuisine						
Enchanadas Chicken	1 meal (9.9 oz)	220	6	390	29	4
Enchilada Suiza Chicken	1 meal (9 oz)	290	5	530	48	5
Life Choice						
Burrito Black Bean	1 meal (13.2 oz)	410	2	570	86	13
Vegetable Enchilada Sonora	1 meal (14 oz)	420	2	600	89	11
Lightlife						
Vegetarian Taco	2 oz	51	1	280	4	—
Old El Paso						
Burrito Beef & Bean Hot	1	320	10	850	45	—
Burrito Beef & Bean Medium	1	320	10	800	46	—
Burrito Beef & Bean Mild	1	330	9	690	48	—
Burrito Beef & Cheese	1	290	9	840	44	3
Chimichangas Beef	1	310	20	470	37	—
Chimichangas Chicken	1	350	16	460	39	—
Patio						
Burrito Bean & Cheese	1 (5 oz)	270	5	530	46	7
Burrito Beef & Bean	1 (5 oz)	280	7	660	45	7
Burrito Beef & Bean Green Chili	1 (5 oz)	260	5	890	44	7
Burrito Beef & Bean Red Chili	1 (5 oz)	260	5	640	42	7

FOOD	PORTION	CAL.	FAT	SOD.	CARB.	FIB.
Patio (CONT.)						
Burrito Chicken	1 (5 oz)	260	4	740	44	3
Burrito Red Chili	1 (5 oz)	270	6	850	42	6
Enchilada Beef Dinner	1 meal (12 oz)	320	8	1810	52	9
Enchilada Cheese Dinner	1 meal (12 oz)	330	8	1570	52	10
Enchilada Chicken	1 pkg (12 oz)	380	9	1470	58	9
Family Entree Beef Enchilada	2 (5.7 oz)	170	4	940	27	5
Family Entree Enchilada Beef	2 (5.3 oz)	250	7	1350	35	8
Family Entree Enchilada Beef & Cheese	2 (5.3 oz)	250	6	1130	35	9
Family Entree Enchilada Cheese	2 (5.7 oz)	170	4	880	26	4
Fiesta Dinner	1 meal (12 oz)	340	9	1760	51	11
Mexican Dinner	1 meal (13.25 oz)	440	15	1840	59	13
Salis Con Queso	1 pkg (11 oz)	390	20	1570	33	10
Patio Britos						
Beef & Bean	10 (6 oz)	420	19	800	51	7
Nacho Beef	10 (6 oz)	410	18	1050	48	5
Nacho Cheese	10 (6 oz)	360	13	500	52	3
Spicy Chicken	10 (6 oz)	400	16	640	52	3
Rudy's Farm						
Burrito Beef/Bean	1 (5 oz)	326	12	765	43	5
Burrito Hot Beef/Bean	1 (5 oz)	305	9	844	44	5
Senor Felix's						
Burrito Black Bean	1 (10 oz)	540	18	510	70	7
Burrito Black Bean Soy	1 (5 oz)	240	7	360	36	3
Burrito Charbroiled Chicken	1 + 4 tsp sauce (6.7 oz)	320	11	910	40	7
Burrito Chicken	1 (10 oz)	520	20	1240	51	3
Burrito Hot Potato	1 (10 oz)	560	24	470	67	5
Burrito Sonora Style	1 + 4 tsp sauce (6.7 oz)	280	8	240	45	3
Burrito Soy Hot	1 (10 oz)	520	20	470	70	5
Burrito Yucatan Style	1 + 4 tsp sauce (6.7 oz)	310	9	500	46	5
Empanadas Chicken	1 (4.7 oz)	340	15	650	41	13
Empanadas Corn & Rice	1 (4.7 oz)	280	13	530	37	6
Empanadas Pumpkin & Mushroom	1 (4.7 oz)	260	11	520	32	6
Empanadas Spinach & Ricotta	1 (4.7 oz)	260	12	520	32	6
Enchilada Red Pepper	1 (10 oz)	420	19	640	51	8

FOOD	PORTION	CAL.	FAT	SOD.	CARB.	FIB.
Senor Felix's (CONT.)						
Enchilada Soy Verda	1 (10 oz)	430	24	1230	41	6
Enchilada Supreme Soy Cheese	1 (10 oz)	460	23	490	48	6
Enchilada Verde	1 (5 oz)	423	23	1140	41	6
Tamales Blue Corn & Soy Cheese	2 + 4 tsp sauce (5.7 oz)	240	10	830	28	3
Tamales Chicken	2 + 4 tsp sauce (5.7 oz)	240	9	480	30	8
Tamales Gourmet Vegetarian	2 + 4 tsp sauce	240	9	480	30	8
Taquitos Blue Corn Soy	3 + 4 tsp sauce (5.2 oz)	230	11	560	27	3
Taquitos Chicken	2 + 4 tsp sauce (5.7 oz)	240	10	830	28	3
Stouffer's						
Cheese Enchilada	1 pkg (9.75 oz)	370	14	890	48	5
Chicken Enchilada	1 pkg (10 oz)	370	14	970	45	3
Swanson						
Enchiladas Beef	13¾ oz	480	21	1350	55	—
Mexican Style Combination	14¼ oz	490	18	1760	62	—
Mexican Style Hungry Man	20¼ oz	820	41	2080	88	—
Today's Tamales						
Cheese & Chili	1 pkg (7 oz)	390	21	630	38	6
Del Sol	1 pkg (6.5 oz)	310	15	650	40	15
Original Bean	1 pkg (7 oz)	330	11	520	49	10
Spicy Taco	1 pkg (7 oz)	310	15	570	41	10
Tyson						
Fajita Kit Beef	3.84 oz	160	4	240	21	—
Fajita Kit Chicken	4 oz	80	2	240	2	—
Van De Kamp's						
Mexican Holiday Enchilada Dinner Beef	12 oz	390	15	—	—	—
Mexican Holiday Enchilada Dinner Cheese	12 oz	450	20	—	—	—
Weight Watchers						
Enchiladas Ranchero Beef	9.12 oz	190	5	500	18	—
Enchiladas Ranchero Cheese	8.87 oz	260	10	550	25	—
Enchiladas Suiza Chicken	9 oz	230	7	530	25	—

FOOD	PORTION	CAL.	FAT	SOD.	CARB.	FIB.
Weight Watchers (CONT.)						
Fajitas Chicken	6.75 oz	210	5	490	24	—
MIX						
Gebhardt						
Menudo Mix	1 tsp	5	tr	310	1	tr
Hain						
Taco Seasoning Mix	1/10 pkg	10	0	200	2	—
Old El Paso						
Burrito Seasoning Mix	1/8 pkg	17	0	275	3	1
Burrito Dinner (with filling)	1 serv	299	13	430	36	4
Enchilada Seasoning Mix	1/18 pkg	6	0	80	1	0
Guacamole Seasoning Mix	1/2 pkg	7	0	240	2	0
Taco Seasoning Mix	1/12 pkg	8	tr	240	2	—
Ortega						
Taco Meat Seasoning Mix Mild	1 filled taco	90	1	999	18	—
Quaker						
Masa Harina De Maiz	2 tortillas	137	2	5	28	3
Masa Trigo	2 tortillas	149	4	794	25	1
READY-TO-USE						
Casa Fiesta						
Taco Shells	3.5 oz	480	23	10	60	—
Chi-Chi's						
Taco Shells White Corned	2 (1 oz)	130	6	0	17	2
Gebhardt						
Taco Shells	1	50	2	tr	7	tr
Old El Paso						
Taco Shells	1	55	3	50	6	1
Taco Shells Mini	3	70	4	60	7	1
Taco Shells Super	1	100	6	95	11	2
Taco Shells White Corn	1	60	3	10	6	—
Tastaco Shells	1	100	5	10	11	1
Tostada Shells	1	55	3	65	6	1
Rosarita						
Taco Shells	1 shell (11 g)	50	2	tr	7	tr
Tostada Shells	1 shell (14 g)	60	3	tr	8	tr
taco shell baked	1 med (1/2 oz)	61	3	48	8	tr
taco shell baked w/o salt	1 med (1/2 oz)	61	3	2	8	tr
TAKE-OUT						
burrito w/ apple	1 lg (5.4 oz)	484	20	443	73	—
burrito w/ apple	1 sm (2.6 oz)	231	10	211	35	—

FOOD	PORTION	CAL.	FAT	SOD.	CARB.	FIB.
burrito w/ beans	2 (7.6 oz)	448	14	986	71	—
burrito w/ beans & cheese	2 (6.5 oz)	377	12	1166	55	—
burrito w/ beans & chili peppers	2 (7.2 oz)	413	15	1043	58	—
burrito w/ beans & meat	2 (8.1 oz)	508	18	1335	66	—
burrito w/ beans cheese & beef	2 (7.1 oz)	331	13	990	40	—
burrito w/ beans cheese & chili peppers	2 (11.8 oz)	663	23	2060	85	—
burrito w/ beef	2 (7.7 oz)	523	21	1492	59	—
burrito w/ beef & chili peppers	2 (7.1 oz)	426	17	1116	49	—
burrito w/ beef cheese & chili peppers	2 (10.7 oz)	634	25	2091	64	—
burrito w/ cherry	1 sm (2.6 oz)	231	10	211	35	—
burrito w/ cherry	1 lg (5.4 oz)	484	20	443	73	—
chimichanga w/ beef	1 (6.1 oz)	425	20	910	43	—
chimichanga w/ beef & cheese	1 (6.4 oz)	443	23	956	39	—
chimichanga w/ beef & red chili peppers	1 (6.7 oz)	424	19	1169	46	—
chimichanga w/ beef cheese & red chili peppers	1 (6.3 oz)	364	18	895	38	—
enchilada w/ cheese	1 (5.7 oz)	320	19	784	29	—
enchilada w/ cheese & beef	1 (6.7 oz)	324	18	1320	30	—
enchirito w/ cheese beef & beans	1 (6.8 oz)	344	16	1251	34	—
enchilada w/ eggplant	1	142	5	—	—	—
frijoles w/ cheese	1 cup (5.9 oz)	226	8	882	29	—
nachos w/ cheese	6 to 8 (4 oz)	345	19	816	36	—
nachos w/ cheese & jalapeno peppers	6 to 8 (7.2 oz)	607	34	1736	60	—
nachos w/ cheese beans ground beef & peppers	6 to 8 (8.9 oz)	568	31	1800	56	—
nachos w/ cinnamon & sugar	6 to 8 (3.8 oz)	592	36	439	63	—
taco	1 sm (6 oz)	370	21	802	27	—
taco salad	1½ cups	279	15	763	24	—
taco salad w/ chili con carne	1½ cups	288	13	886	27	—
tostada w/ beans & cheese	1 (5.1 oz)	223	10	543	27	—
tostada w/ beans beef & cheese	1 (7.9 oz)	334	17	870	30	—

FOOD	PORTION	CAL.	FAT	SOD.	CARB.	FIB.
tostada w/ beef & cheese	1 (5.7 oz)	315	16	896	23	—
tostada w/ guacamole	2 (9.2 oz)	360	23	789	32	—

SPARE RIBS
(see PORK)

SPELT
Arrowhead	1 oz	83	1	1	20	4

SPICES
(see HERBS/SPICES, INDIVIDUAL NAMES)

SPINACH
CANNED
Del Monte

50% Less Salt	½ cup (4 oz)	30	0	180	4	2
Chopped	½ cup (4 oz)	30	0	360	4	2
No Salt Added	½ cup (4 oz)	30	0	85	4	2
Whole Leaf	½ cup (4 oz)	30	0	360	4	2
Popeye						
Chopped	½ cup (4.1 oz)	40	1	310	6	4
Leaf	½ cup (4.2 oz)	45	1	310	7	4
Low Sodium	½ cup (4.2 oz)	35	1	35	4	3
S&W						
Northwest Premium	½ cup	25	0	395	3	—
Sunshine						
Chopped	½ cup (4.1 oz)	40	1	310	6	4
spinach	½ cup	25	1	29	4	—
FRESH						
Dole	3 oz	9	tr	107	tr	8
Fresh Express	1½ cups (3 oz)	40	0	160	10	5
cooked	½ cup	21	tr	63	3	2
mustard chopped cooked	½ cup	14	tr	—	3	—
mustard raw chopped	½ cup	17	tr	—	3	—
new zealand chopped cooked	½ cup	11	tr	97	2	—
new zealand raw	½ cup	4	tr	36	1	—
raw chopped	½ cup	6	tr	22	1	1
raw chopped	1 pkg (10 oz)	46	1	160	7	—
FROZEN						
Birds Eye						
Chopped	½ cup	20	0	90	3	3
Creamed	½ cup	90	5	320	9	1
Leaf	½ cup	20	0	90	4	3
Budget Gourmet						
Au Gratin	1 pkg (5.5 oz)	160	11	600	9	—

FOOD	PORTION	CAL.	FAT	SOD.	CARB.	FIB.
Fresh Like						
Cut Leaf	3.5 oz	21	tr	81	4	1
Green Giant						
Creamed	½ cup	70	3	480	10	—
Cut Leaf In Butter Sauce	½ cup	40	2	380	6	4
Harvest Fresh	½ cup	25	0	170	5	3
Stouffer's						
Creamed	½ cup (2.25 oz)	150	12	380	8	2
Souffle	½ cup (4 oz)	150	10	480	9	—
Tabatchnick						
Creamed	7.5 oz	60	2	270	8	2
cooked	½ cup	27	tr	82	5	—

SPINACH JUICE

juice	3½ oz	7	0	73	1	—

SPORTS DRINKS

(*see also* NUTRITIONAL SUPPLEMENTS)

FOOD	PORTION	CAL.	FAT	SOD.	CARB.	FIB.
Gatorade						
Citrus Cooler	1 cup (8 oz)	50	0	110	14	—
Fruit Punch	1 cup (8 oz)	50	0	110	14	—
Grape	1 cup (8 oz)	50	0	110	14	—
Iced Tea Cooler	1 cup (8 oz)	50	0	110	14	—
Lemon-Lime	1 cup (8 oz)	50	0	110	14	—
Lemonade	1 cup (8 oz)	50	0	110	14	—
Orange	1 cup (8 oz)	50	0	110	14	—
Tropical Fruit	1 cup (8 oz)	50	0	110	14	—
PowerAde						
Fruit Punch	8 fl oz	72	0	28	19	—
Grape	8 fl oz	73	0	28	19	—
Lemon-Lime	8 fl oz	72	0	28	19	—
Orange	8 fl oz	72	0	28	19	—
Slice						
All Sport Diet Lemon Lime	8 fl oz	1	0	40	0	—
All Sport Lemon Lime	8 fl oz	72	0	55	19	—
All Sport Orange	8 fl oz	74	0	55	19	—
All Sport Punch	8 fl oz	81	0	55	22	—
Snapple						
Sport Fruit	1 bottle	80	0	60	20	—
Sport Lemon	1 bottle	80	0	60	20	—
Sport Lemon Lime	1 bottle	80	0	60	20	—
Sport Orange	1 bottle	80	0	60	20	—

SPOT

baked	3 oz	134	5	32	0	—

FOOD	PORTION	CAL.	FAT	SOD.	CARB.	FIB.
SQUAB						
breast w/o skin raw	1 (3.5 oz)	135	5	—	0	—
w/ skin raw	1 squab (6.9 oz)	584	47	—	0	—
w/o skin raw	1 squab (5.9 oz)	239	13	—	0	—
SQUASH						
(see also ZUCCHINI*)*						
CANNED						
Allen						
Yellow	½ cup (4.2 oz)	25	0	160	5	2
Sunshine						
Yellow	½ cup (4.2 oz)	25	0	160	5	2
crookneck sliced	½ cup	14	tr	5	3	—
FRESH						
Nature's Pasta						
Spaghetti Squash	1 cup (5.5 oz)	20	0	30	4	2
acorn cooked mashed	½ cup	41	tr	3	11	3
acorn cubed baked	½ cup	57	tr	4	15	2
butternut baked	½ cup	41	tr	4	11	2
crookneck raw sliced	½ cup	12	tr	1	3	1
crookneck sliced cooked	½ cup	18	tr	1	4	1
hubbard baked	½ cup	51	tr	8	11	3
hubbard cooked mashed	½ cup	35	tr	6	8	3
scallop raw sliced	½ cup	12	tr	1	3	1
scallop sliced cooked	½ cup	14	tr	1	3	1
spaghetti cooked	½ cup	23	tr	14	5	2
FROZEN						
Birds Eye						
Winter Cooked	½ cup	45	0	0	11	2
Southland						
Butternut	4 oz	45	0	—	—	—
Prepared Squash	3.6 oz	80	2	—	—	—
butternut cooked mashed	½ cup	47	tr	2	12	3
crookneck sliced cooked	½ cup	24	tr	6	5	—
SEEDS						
dried	1 oz	154	13	5	5	—
dried	1 cup	747	63	24	25	—
roasted	1 oz	148	12	5	4	—
roasted	1 cup	1184	96	40	31	—
salted & roasted	1 oz	148	12	5	4	—
salted & roasted	1 cup	1184	96	1294	31	—
whole roasted	1 oz	127	6	5	15	—
whole roasted	1 cup	285	12	5	34	—
whole salted roasted	1 cup	285	12	368	34	—
whole salted roasted	1 oz	127	6	191	15	—

FOOD	PORTION	CAL.	FAT	SOD.	CARB.	FIB.
SQUID						
fried	3 oz	149	6	260	7	—
raw	3 oz	78	1	37	3	—
SQUIRREL						
roasted	3 oz	147	4	102	0	—
STAR FRUIT						
Sonoma						
Dried	7-9 pieces (1.4 oz)	140	0	0	34	0
STRAWBERRIES						
CANNED						
in heavy syrup	½ cup	117	tr	5	30	—
FRESH						
Dole	8	50	0	0	13	3
strawberries	1 pint	97	1	4	22	—
strawberries	1 cup	45	1	2	10	4
FROZEN						
Big Valley	⅔ cup (4.9 oz)	50	0	0	12	2
Birds Eye						
Halved In Delicious Syrup	½ cup	120	0	0	30	2
Halved In Lite Syrup	½ cup	90	0	5	22	2
Whole In Lite Syrup	½ cup	80	0	0	20	2
sweetened sliced	1 cup	245	tr	8	66	—
sweetened sliced	1 pkg (10 oz)	273	tr	9	74	—
unsweetened	1 cup	52	tr	3	14	—
whole sweetened	1 cup	200	tr	3	54	—
whole sweetened	1 pkg (10 oz)	223	tr	3	60	—
STRAWBERRY JUICE						
Juice Works	6 oz	100	0	—	—	—
Kern's						
Nectar	6 fl oz	110	0	0	28	—
Kool-Aid						
Koolers	1 (8.45 oz)	136	0	3	36	—
Libby						
Nectar	1 can (11.5 fl oz)	210	0	10	52	—
Smucker's						
Juice	8 oz	130	0	10	31	—
Tang						
Strawberry	8.45 fl oz	121	0	1	32	—

FOOD	PORTION	CAL.	FAT	SOD.	CARB.	FIB.
Wylers						
Drink Mix Unsweetened Strawberry Split	8 oz	2	0	28	1	—
MIX						
Kool-Aid						
Strawberry	8 oz	98	0	27	25	—

STUFFING/DRESSING
HOME RECIPE

FOOD	PORTION	CAL.	FAT	SOD.	CARB.	FIB.
bread as prep w/ water & fat	½ cup	251	15	627	25	—
bread as prep w/ water egg & fat	½ cup	107	7	319	9	—
MIX						
Arnold						
All Purpose Seasoned	½ oz	50	0	200	9	1
Corn	½ oz	50	1	140	9	1
Herb Seasoned	½ oz	50	tr	150	2	1
Sage & Onion	½ oz	50	tr	230	9	1
Betty Crocker						
Chicken	½ cup	180	9	620	21	—
Traditional Herb	½ cup	180	8	640	22	—
Brownberry						
Corn	1 oz	103	2	350	19	2
Herb	1 oz	100	1	297	19	2
Sage & Onion	1 oz	97	1	450	18	2
Golden Grain						
Bread Stuffing Chicken	½ cup	180	9	730	20	—
Bread Stuffing Corn Bread	½ cup	180	9	870	21	—
Bread Stuffing Herb & Butter	½ cup	180	9	810	20	—
Bread Stuffing With Wild Rice	½ cup	180	9	710	21	—
Kellogg's						
Croutettes	1 cup (1.2 oz)	120	0	460	25	0
Pepperidge Farm						
Corn Bread	1 oz	110	1	320	22	—
Country Style	1 oz	100	1	400	21	—
Cube	1 oz	110	1	400	22	—
Distinctive Apple Raisin	1 oz	110	1	410	21	—
Distinctive Classic Chicken	1 oz	110	1	410	20	—

FOOD	PORTION	CAL.	FAT	SOD.	CARB.	FIB.
Pepperidge Farm (cont.)						
Distinctive Country Garden Herb	1 oz	120	4	300	18	—
Distinctive Vegetable & Almond	1 oz	110	3	250	19	—
Distinctive Wild Rice & Mushroom	1 oz	130	5	310	17	—
Herb Seasoned	1 oz	110	1	380	22	—
Stove Top						
Beef as prep	½ cup	178	9	586	22	—
Chicken as prep	½ cup	176	8	561	21	—
Chicken With Rice as prep	½ cup	182	9	557	22	—
Cornbread as prep	½ cup	175	8	557	22	—
Flex Serve Chicken as prep	½ cup	173	9	577	20	—
Flex Serve Cornbread as prep	½ cup	181	9	591	22	—
Flex Serve Homestyle Herb as prep	½ cup	173	9	515	20	—
Long Grain & Wild Rice as prep	½ cup	182	9	553	22	—
Select Wild Rice & Mushroom	½ cup	172	9	—	—	—
Wonder						
Seasoned Stuffing	1 cup (0.9 oz)	60	1	135	12	tr
bread dry as prep	½ cup	178	9	543	22	3
cornbread as prep	½ cup	179	9	455	22	—
TAKE-OUT						
bread	½ cup (3½ oz)	195	8	534	26	3
sausage	½ cup	292	11	258	40	1
STURGEON						
cooked	3 oz	115	4	—	0	—
raw	3 oz	90	3	—	0	—
roe raw	3.5 oz	207	10	—	1	—
smoked	3 oz	147	4	—	0	—
smoked	1 oz	48	1	—	0	—
SUCKER						
white baked	3 oz	101	3	44	0	—
SUGAR						
(see also FRUCTOSE, SUGAR SUBSTITUTES, SYRUP)						
C&H						
White	1 tsp	16	0	—	4	—

FOOD	PORTION	CAL.	FAT	SOD.	CARB.	FIB.
Domino						
White	1 tsp	16	0	0	4	—
Hain						
Turbinado	1 tbsp	50	0	0	12	—
Hollywood						
Turbinado	1 tbsp	50	0	0	12	—
brown packed	1 cup (7.7 oz)	828	0	86	214	—
brown unpacked	1 cup (5.1 oz)	546	0	57	141	—
maple	1 piece (1 oz)	100	tr	3	26	—
powdered	1 tbsp (0.3 oz)	31	0	0	8	—
powdered unsifted	1 cup (4.2 oz)	467	tr	2	119	—
white	1 tsp (4 g)	15	0	0	4	—
white	1 tbsp	45	0	tr	12	—
white	1 packet (6 g)	25	0	tr	6	—
white	1 cup (7 oz)	773	0	3	200	—

SUGAR SUBSTITUTES
(see also FRUCTOSE*)*

FOOD	PORTION	CAL.	FAT	SOD.	CARB.	FIB.
Equal	1 pkg	4	0	0	tr	—
NatraTaste	1 pkg (1 g)	0	0	0	1	—
S&W						
Liquid Table Sweetener	⅛ tsp	0	0	0	0	—
Sprinkle Sweet	1 tsp	2	0	1	tr	—
SugarTwin	1 pkg (0.8 g)	3	0	5	1	—
Brown	1 tsp (0.4 g)	2	0	3	tr	—
Sweet One	1 pkg (1 g)	4	0	0	1	—
Sweet*10	⅛ tsp	0	0	2	0	—
Sweet'N Low						
Granulated	1 pkg (1g)	4	0	1	—	—
Weight Watchers						
Sweet'ner	1 pkg	4	0	20	1	—

SUGAR-APPLE

FOOD	PORTION	CAL.	FAT	SOD.	CARB.	FIB.
fresh	1	146	tr	15	37	—
fresh cut up	1 cup	236	1	24	59	—

SUNDAE TOPPINGS
(see ICE CREAM TOPPINGS*)*

SUNFISH

FOOD	PORTION	CAL.	FAT	SOD.	CARB.	FIB.
pumpkinseed baked	3 oz	97	1	87	0	—

SUNFLOWER

FOOD	PORTION	CAL.	FAT	SOD.	CARB.	FIB.
Erewhon						
Sunflower Seed Butter	2 tbsp (32 g)	200	18	20	3	—
Fisher						
Seeds Oil Roasted	1 oz	170	15	170	6	—

FOOD	PORTION	CAL.	FAT	SOD.	CARB.	FIB.
Fisher (CONT.)						
Seeds Salted In Shell shelled	1 oz	160	14	100	6	—
Seeds Salted In Shell unshelled	1 oz	170	15	110	6	—
Planters						
Kernels	1 pkg (1.7 oz)	290	25	260	9	7
Kernels	1 pkg (2 oz)	340	29	310	11	8
Kernels Barbecue	1 pkg (1.7 oz)	290	25	180	10	6
Kernels Honey Roasted	1 pkg (1.7 oz)	280	22	105	15	6
Kernels Salted	1 oz	170	14	140	4	4
Munch'N Go Singles Dry Roasted	1 pkg	120	11	70	4	1
Nuts Dry Roasted	¼ cup (1.1 oz)	190	17	230	6	4
Original With Shell Dry Roasted	¾ cup	160	15	35	5	2
Stone-Buhr						
Seeds Raw	4 tsp (1 oz)	170	14	10	6	6
dried	1 cup	821	71	4	27	—
dried	1 oz	162	14	1	5	—
dry roasted	1 oz	165	14	1	7	—
dry roasted	1 cup	745	64	4	31	—
dry roasted salted	1 oz	165	14	195	7	—
dry roasted salted	1 cup	745	64	975	31	—
oil roasted	1 cup	830	78	4	20	—
oil roasted salted	1 cup	830	78	804	20	—
oil roasted salted	1 oz	175	16	201	4	—
sunflower butter	1 tbsp	93	8	82	4	—
sunflower butter w/o salt	1 tbsp	93	8	1	4	—
toasted	1 oz	176	16	1	6	—
toasted	1 cup	826	76	4	28	—
toasted salted	1 cup	826	76	817	28	—
toasted salted	1 oz	176	16	204	6	—

SURF

CANNED

| *American Original* | 4 oz | 100 | tr | — | 7 | — |

FRESH

| *American Original* | 4 oz | 90 | tr | — | 2 | — |

SUSHI

TAKE-OUT

california roll	1 piece (0.8 oz)	28	1	37	4	—
kim chi	⅛ cup (5.8 oz)	18	tr	2143	4	—
sashimi	1 serving (6 oz)	198	7	718	4	—

FOOD	PORTION	CAL.	FAT	SOD.	CARB.	FIB.
tuna roll	1 piece (0.7 oz)	23	tr	33	3	—
vegetable roll	1 piece (1.2 oz)	27	1	47	5	—
vinegared ginger	⅓ cup (1.6 oz)	48	tr	6	12	—
wasabi	2 tsp (0.3 oz)	5	tr	124	1	—
yellowtail roll	1 piece (0.6 oz)	25	1	32	3	—

SWAMP CABBAGE

chopped cooked	½ cup	10	tr	60	2	—
raw chopped	1 cup	11	tr	63	2	—

SWEET POTATO
(see also YAM)
CANNED
Princella

Mashed	⅔ cup (5.1 oz)	120	1	30	28	3

Royal Prince

Candied	½ cup (4.9 oz)	210	1	50	50	2
Halves	3 pieces (5.7 oz)	190	1	40	46	4
Orange Pineapple	½ cup (4.8 oz)	210	1	30	43	3

Sugary Sam

Mashed	⅔ cup (5.1 oz)	120	1	30	28	3
in syrup	½ cup	106	tr	38	25	—
pieces	1 cup	183	tr	107	42	—

FRESH

baked w/ skin	1 (3½ oz)	118	tr	12	28	3
leaves cooked	½ cup	11	tr	4	2	—
mashed	½ cup	172	tr	21	40	3

FROZEN
Mrs. Paul's

Candied Sweet Potatoes	4 oz	170	0	40	42	—
Candied Sweets 'N Apples	4 oz	160	0	60	38	—
cooked	½ cup	88	tr	7	21	—

TAKE-OUT

candied	3½ oz	144	3	73	29	—

SWEETBREADS

beef braised	3 oz	230	15	51	0	—
lamb braised	3 oz	199	13	44	0	—
veal braised	3 oz	218	12	—	0	—

SWISS CHARD

cooked	½ cup	18	tr	158	4	—
raw chopped	½ cup	3	tr	38	1	—

SWORDFISH

cooked	3 oz	132	4	98	0	—
raw	3 oz	103	3	76	0	—

FOOD	PORTION	CAL.	FAT	SOD.	CARB.	FIB.

SYRUP
(see also ICE CREAM TOPPINGS, PANCAKE/WAFFLE SYRUP)

FOOD	PORTION	CAL.	FAT	SOD.	CARB.	FIB.
Eden						
Barley Malt Organic Syrup	1 tbsp (0.7 fl oz)	60	0	0	14	0
Estee						
Blueberry Lite	¼ cup (2.4 oz)	80	0	70	20	—
Home Brands						
Maple Rich	1 oz	110	0	—	—	—
Karo						
Corn Syrup Dark	1 cup (331 g)	975	0	610	243	—
Corn Syrup Dark	1 tbsp (21 g)	60	0	40	15	—
Corn Syrup Light	1 cup (331 g)	960	0	480	241	—
Corn Syrup Light	1 tbsp (21 g)	60	0	30	15	—
McIlhenny						
Cane	2 tbsp (1.4 oz)	130	0	20	32	tr
Quik						
Strawberry	1⅔ tbsp	100	0	0	24	—
Red Wing						
Strawberry	2 tbsp (1.4 oz)	110	0	5	28	0
S&W						
Blueberry Diet	1 tbsp	4	0	25	1	—
Maple Flavored Diet	1 tbsp	4	0	25	1	—
Strawberry Diet	1 tbsp	4	0	25	1	—
Smucker's						
All Flavors Fruit Syrup	2 tbsp	100	0	<10	26	—
Tree Of Life						
Maple	¼ cup (2.1 oz)	200	0	7	53	—
Rice Syrup	2 tbsp (1 oz)	120	1	5	29	—
Whistling Wings						
Blueberry	1 oz	45	tr	1	10	tr
Raspberry	1 oz	60	tr	2	14	0
corn	2 tbsp	122	0	19	32	—
corn dark	1 tbsp (0.7 oz)	56	0	31	15	—
corn dark	1 cup (11.5 oz)	925	tr	608	251	—
corn light	1 cup (11.5 oz)	925	tr	395	251	—
corn light	1 tbsp (0.7 oz)	56	0	24	15	—
malt	1 tbsp (0.8 oz)	76	0	8	17	—
malt	1 cup (13 oz)	1222	tr	134	274	—
maple	1 tbsp (0.8 oz)	52	0	2	13	—
maple	1 cup (11.1 oz)	824	1	27	212	—
raspberry	3.5 oz	267	0	2	66	—
rose hip	3.5 oz	33	0	—	8	0

FOOD	PORTION	CAL.	FAT	SOD.	CARB.	FIB.
sorghum	1 tbsp (0.7 oz)	61	0	2	16	—
sorghum	1 cup (11.6 oz)	957	0	28	247	—

TACO
(see SPANISH FOOD)

TAHINI
(see SESAME)

TAMARIND
fresh	1	5	tr	1	1	—
fresh cut up	1 cup	287	1	33	75	—

TANGERINE
CANNED
in light syrup	½ cup	76	tr	8	20	—
juice pack	½ cup	46	tr	7	12	—

FRESH
Dole	2	70	1	2	19	2
sections	1 cup	86	tr	3	22	—
tangerine	1	37	tr	1	9	—

TANGERINE JUICE
After The Fall
After The Fall	1 can (12 oz)	170	0	35	40	0

Dole
Mandarin frzn as prep	8 fl oz	140	0	30	35	0

Minute Maid
Frozen	8 fl oz	120	0	0	29	—
canned sweetened	1 cup	125	1	2	30	—
fresh	1 cup	106	tr	2	25	—
frzn sweetened as prep	1 cup	110	tr	2	27	—
frzn sweetened not prep	6 oz	344	1	7	83	—

TAPIOCA
General Foods
Minute Tapioca	1 tbsp	32	tr	—	8	—
pearl dry	⅓ cup	174	0	0	45	1
starch	3½ oz	344	tr	4	85	—

TARO
chips	1 oz	141	7	97	19	—
chips	10 (0.8 oz)	115	6	79	16	—
leaves cooked	½ cup	18	tr	2	3	—
raw sliced	½ cup	56	tr	6	14	—
shoots sliced cooked	½ cup	10	tr	1	2	—
sliced cooked	½ cup (2.3 oz)	94	tr	10	23	—
tahitian sliced cooked	½ cup	30	tr	37	5	—

FOOD	PORTION	CAL.	FAT	SOD.	CARB.	FIB.
TARRAGON						
ground	1 tsp	5	tr	1	1	—
TEA/HERBAL TEA						
(see also ICED TEA)						
HERBAL						
Bigelow						
Almond Orange	5 fl oz	tr	tr	tr	tr	—
Apple Orchard	5 fl oz	5	tr	tr	1	—
Apple Spice	5 fl oz	tr	tr	1	tr	—
Chamomile	5 fl oz	tr	tr	2	—	—
Chamomile Mint	5 fl oz	tr	tr	tr	tr	—
Cinnamon Orange	5 fl oz	tr	tr	tr	tr	—
Early Riser	5 fl oz	3	tr	tr	1	—
Feeling Free	5 fl oz	1	tr	1	tr	—
Fruit & Almond	5 fl oz	1	tr	tr	tr	—
Hibiscus & Rose Hips	5 fl oz	1	tr	1	tr	—
I Love Lemon	5 fl oz	1	tr	tr	tr	—
Lemon & C	5 fl oz	tr	tr	tr	tr	—
Looking Good	5 fl oz	1	tr	1	tr	—
Mint Blend	5 fl oz	tr	tr	3	tr	—
Mint Medley	5 fl oz	1	tr	3	tr	—
Orange & C	5 fl oz	tr	tr	tr	tr	—
Orange & Spice	5 fl oz	1	tr	1	tr	—
Peppermint	5 fl oz	tr	tr	2	tr	—
Roasted Grains & Carob	5 fl oz	3	tr	1	1	—
Spearmint	5 fl oz	tr	tr	tr	tr	—
Sweet Dreams	5 fl oz	1	tr	1	tr	—
Take-A-Break	5 fl oz	3	tr	1	1	—
Celestial Seasonings						
Almond Sunset	8 fl oz	3	tr	2	1	—
Bengal Spice	8 fl oz	5	tr	3	1	—
Caffeine Free	8 fl oz	2	tr	5	1	—
Chamomile	8 fl oz	2	tr	1	1	—
Cinnamon Apple Spice	8 fl oz	<3	tr	1	tr	—
Cinnamon Rose	8 fl oz	<4	tr	1	1	—
Country Peach Spice	8 fl oz	3	tr	1	1	—
Cranberry Cove	8 fl oz	2	tr	1	1	—
Emperor's Choice	8 fl oz	4	tr	2	1	—
Ginseng Plus	8 fl oz	3	tr	4	1	—
Grandma's Tummy Mint	8 fl oz	2	tr	7	tr	—
Lemon Mist	8 fl oz	3	tr	3	tr	—
Lemon Zinger	8 fl oz	4	tr	1	1	—
Mama Bear's Cold Care	8 fl oz	6	tr	2	tr	—

FOOD	PORTION	CAL.	FAT	SOD.	CARB.	FIB.
Celestial Seasonings (CONT.)						
Mandarin Orange Spice	8 fl oz	5	tr	2	1	—
Mellow Mint	8 fl oz	2	tr	5	tr	—
Mint Magic	8 fl oz	1	tr	13	tr	—
Orange Zinger	8 fl oz	6	tr	1	1	—
Peppermint	8 fl oz	2	tr	9	1	—
Raspberry Patch	8 fl oz	4	tr	1	1	—
Red Zinger	8 fl oz	4	tr	2	1	—
Roastaroma	8 fl oz	10	tr	3	2	—
Sleepytime	8 fl oz	4	tr	2	1	—
Spearmint	8 fl oz	5	1	6	tr	—
Strawberry Fields	8 fl oz	4	tr	1	1	—
Sunburst C	8 fl oz	3	tr	6	1	—
Tropical Escape	8 fl oz	1	tr	7	1	—
Wild Forest Blackberry	8 fl oz	2	tr	1	1	—
REGULAR						
Bigelow						
Chinese Fortune	5 fl oz	1	tr	tr	tr	—
Cinnamon Stick	5 fl oz	1	tr	tr	tr	—
Constant Comment	5 fl oz	1	tr	tr	tr	—
Darjeeling Blend	5 fl oz	1	tr	tr	tr	—
Earl Gray	5 fl oz	1	tr	tr	tr	—
English Teatime	5 fl oz	1	tr	tr	tr	—
Lemon Lift	5 fl oz	1	tr	tr	tr	—
Orange Pekoe	5 fl oz	1	tr	tr	tr	—
Peppermint Stick	5 fl oz	1	tr	1	tr	—
Plantation Mint	5 fl oz	1	tr	1	tr	—
Raspberry Royale	5 fl oz	1	tr	tr	tr	—
Celestial Seasonings						
Cinnamon Vienna	8 fl oz	2	tr	1	1	—
Earl Grey Extraordinary	8 fl oz	3	tr	tr	1	—
English Breakfast Classic	8 fl oz	3	tr	tr	tr	—
Lemon	8 fl oz	7	tr	1	1	—
Mint	8 fl oz	4	tr	1	1	—
Morning Thunder	8 fl oz	3	tr	1	tr	—
Naturally Decaffeinated	8 fl oz	10	1	1	tr	—
Orange Spice	8 fl oz	7	tr	1	1	—
Orange Spice Decaff	8 fl oz	7	tr	1	1	—
Organically Grown	8 fl oz	12	tr	1	1	—
Raspberry	8 fl oz	7	tr	1	1	—
Natural Touch						
Kaffree	8 fl oz	0	0	<1	0	—
Nestea						
Tea Bag as prep	6 oz	0	0	0	0	—

FOOD	PORTION	CAL.	FAT	SOD.	CARB.	FIB.
brewed tea	6 oz	2	0	5	tr	—
instant unsweetened as prep w/ water	8 oz	2	0	8	tr	—
TEFF						
Arrowhead						
Whole Grain	¼ cup (1.6 oz)	160	1	5	32	6
TEMPEH						
Lightlife	4 oz	182	6	10	9	—
Garden Vege	4 oz	142	4	125	9	2
White Wave						
Burger	1 patty (3 oz)	110	3	270	10	6
Lemon Broil	1 patty (2 oz)	130	6	340	11	4
Organic Wild Rice	⅓ block (2.7 oz)	140	4	10	12	6
Teriyaki Burger	1 patty (3 oz)	110	2	340	11	6
tempeh	½ cup	165	6	5	14	—
THYME						
Watkins	¼ tsp (0.5 oz)	0	0	0	0	0
ground	1 tsp	4	tr	1	1	—
TILEFISH						
cooked	½ fillet (5.3 oz)	220	7	88	0	—
cooked	3 oz	125	4	50	0	—
raw	3 oz	81	2	45	0	—
TOFU						
Azumaya						
Blue Label	3.5 oz	46	1	2	4	—
Green Label	3.5 oz	68	2	2	4	—
Name Age Fried	3.5 oz	144	4	2	9	—
Red Label	3.5 oz	68	1	3	5	—
Casbah						
Gyro as prep w/ tofu	1 patty (2 oz)	105	3	480	15	tr
Jaclyn's						
Grilled In Black Bean Sauce	10.75 oz	270	8	170	45	—
Grilled In Peanut Sauce	10.75 oz	260	9	145	44	—
Mori-Nu						
Extra Firm	1 in slice (3 oz)	55	2	60	2	—
Firm	1 in slice (3 oz)	50	3	30	2	—
Lite Extra Firm	1 in slice (3 oz)	35	1	80	1	—
Lite Firm	1 in slice (3 oz)	35	1	70	1	—
Soft	1 in slice (3 oz)	45	3	5	2	—
Nasoya						
Extra Firm	⅕ block (3 oz)	90	5	10	1	0

FOOD	PORTION	CAL.	FAT	SOD.	CARB.	FIB.
Nasoya (CONT.)						
Firm	⅕ block (3 oz)	80	4	10	2	0
Silken	⅙ block (3 oz)	50	2	10	2	0
Soft	⅕ block (3 oz)	60	3	5	2	0
Spring Creek						
Baked Barbeque	2 oz	88	4	234	7	—
Baked Cajun	2 oz	87	4	228	5	—
Baked Teriyaki	2 oz	84	4	393	3	—
Great Balls Of Tofu!	2 (3 oz)	107	5	485	5	—
Nigari Firm	4 oz	140	8	30	tr	3
Tofu Salads !Onion Dip	2 oz	46	14	155	6	—
Tofu Salads !Taco Dip	2 oz	46	14	175	6	—
Tofu Salads Missing Egg	2 oz	49	14	167	6	—
Tree Of Life						
Baked	⅕ block (3.2 oz)	150	8	310	5	0
Firm	⅕ block (3.2 oz)	100	5	5	2	0
Raw Firm	⅕ block (3.2 oz)	100	5	5	2	0
Ready Ground Hot & Spicy	⅓ pkg (3 oz)	60	4	10	2	0
Ready Ground Original	⅓ pkg (3 oz)	60	4	10	2	0
Ready Ground Savory Garlic	⅓ pkg (3 oz)	60	4	10	2	0
Reduced Fat	⅕ block (3.2 oz)	90	4	5	4	2
Savory Baked	⅕ block (3.2 oz)	140	8	310	4	0
Smoked Hot'N Spicy	½ block (3 oz)	120	5	120	3	0
Smoked Original	½ block (3 oz)	120	5	120	3	0
White Wave						
Baked Tofus Teriyaki Oriental Style	¼ block (2 oz)	120	6	240	3	1
Hard	4 oz	120	7	15	1	—
International Baked Italian Garlic Herb	¼ pkg (2 oz)	120	6	240	3	1
International Baked Mexican Jalapeno	¼ pkg (2 oz)	120	6	240	3	1
International Baked Oriental Teriyaki	¼ pkg (2 oz)	120	6	240	3	1
International Baked Thai Sesame Peanut	¼ pkg (2 oz)	120	6	240	3	1
Soft	4 oz	120	7	15	1	—
firm	¼ block (3 oz)	118	7	11	3	1
firm	½ cup	183	11	17	5	2
fresh fried	1 piece (½ oz)	35	3	2	1	tr
fuyu salted & fermented	1 block (⅓ oz)	13	1	316	1	tr
koyadofu dried frozen	1 piece (½ oz)	82	5	1	2	tr

FOOD	PORTION	CAL.	FAT	SOD.	CARB.	FIB.
okara	½ cup	47	1	6	8	1
regular	½ cup	94	6	9	2	1
regular	¼ block (4 oz)	88	6	8	2	1
YOGURT						
Stir Fruity						
Black Cherry	6 oz	141	2	51	25	—
Blueberry	6 oz	140	1	43	26	—
Lemon Chiffon	6 oz	152	3	43	26	—
Mixed Berry	6 oz	149	2	34	26	—
Orange	6 oz	143	2	51	26	—
Peach	6 oz	160	3	34	27	—
Pina Colada	6 oz	162	3	43	28	—
Raspberry	6 oz	155	2	34	29	—
Spiced Apple	6 oz	167	2	43	31	—
Strawberry	6 oz	140	2	51	25	—
Tropical Fruit	6 oz	170	2	43	32	—

TOFUTTI
(*see* ICE CREAM AND FROZEN DESSERTS)

TOMATILLO
fresh	1 (1.2 oz)	11	tr	0	2	—
fresh chopped	½ cup	21	1	1	4	—

TOMATO
(*see also* PIZZA, SPAGHETTI SAUCE)
CANNED
Claussen

Kosher	1	9	tr	—	—	—
Contadina						
California Sliced	½ cup	40	tr	—	—	—
Crushed	¼ cup	20	0	150	4	1
Italian Paste	2 tbsp	40	1	320	7	1
Italian Style Pear	½ cup	25	0	220	4	1
Italian Style Stewed	½ cup	40	0	260	8	1
Mexican Style Stewed	½ cup	40	0	220	9	1
Pasta Ready Primavera	½ cup	50	2	600	8	1
Pasta Ready Tomatoes	½ cup	50	2	550	7	1
Pasta Ready With Crushed Red Pepper	½ cup	60	3	690	8	1
Pasta Ready With Mushrooms	½ cup	50	2	640	9	1
Pasta Ready With Olives	½ cup	60	3	640	8	1
Pasta Ready With Three Cheeses	½ cup	70	4	650	8	tr

FOOD	PORTION	CAL.	FAT	SOD.	CARB.	FIB.
Contadina (CONT.)						
Paste	2 tbsp	30	0	20	6	1
Peeled Whole	½ cup	25	0	220	4	1
Puree	¼ cup	20	0	15	4	tr
Recipe Ready	½ cup	25	0	200	5	3
Stewed	½ cup	40	0	250	9	1
Del Monte						
Paste	2 tbsp (1.2 oz)	30	0	25	7	2
Peeled Diced	½ cup (4.4 oz)	25	0	160	6	2
Puree	¼ cup (2.2 oz)	30	0	25	7	1
Sauce	¼ cup (2.1 oz)	20	0	340	4	tr
Sauce No Salt Added	¼ cup (2.1 oz)	20	0	20	4	tr
Stewed Cajun Style	½ cup (4.4 oz)	35	0	460	9	2
Stewed Chunky Chili	½ cup (4.5 oz)	30	0	600	8	2
Stewed Chunky Pasta	½ cup (4.5 oz)	45	0	560	11	2
Stewed Chunky Pizza	½ cup (4.5 oz)	35	0	670	9	2
Stewed Chunky Salsa	½ cup (4.5 oz)	35	0	560	8	2
Stewed Italian Style	½ cup (4.4 oz)	30	0	420	8	2
Stewed Mexican Style	½ cup (4.4 oz)	35	0	400	9	2
Stewed Original	½ cup (4.4 oz)	35	0	360	9	2
Stewed Original No Salt Added	½ cup (4.4 oz)	35	0	50	9	2
Wedges	½ cup (4.4 oz)	35	0	380	9	2
Whole Peeled	½ cup (4.4 oz)	25	0	160	6	2
Eden						
Crushed Organic	¼ cup (2.1 oz)	20	0	0	3	1
Sauce Lightly Seasoned	¼ cup (2.1 oz)	25	0	45	5	1
Health Valley						
Sauce	1 cup	70	1	460	13	tr
Sauce Low Sodium	1 cup	70	1	35	13	1
Hebrew National						
Pickled	⅓ tomato (1 oz)	4	0	280	1	—
Hunt's						
All Natural Sauce	¼ cup (2.2 fl oz)	15	0	360	3	tr
Crushed Angela Mia	4 oz	35	tr	260	7	tr
Crushed Italian	4 oz	40	tr	460	9	tr
Italian Pear Shaped	4 oz	20	tr	320	5	tr
Paste	1 oz	25	0	80	5	1
Paste Italian Style	2 oz	50	tr	430	11	2
Paste No Salt Added	2 oz	45	tr	25	11	2
Paste With Garlic	2 oz	50	tr	440	11	2
Peeled Choice-Cut	4 oz	20	tr	460	5	1
Puree	4 oz	45	tr	150	10	2
Sauce Herb	4 oz	70	2	470	12	2

FOOD	PORTION	CAL.	FAT	SOD.	CARB.	FIB.
Hunt's (CONT.)						
Sauce Italian	4 oz	60	2	460	10	2
Sauce Meatloaf Fixin's	4 oz	20	tr	580	5	tr
Sauce No Salt Added	4 oz	35	tr	20	8	2
Sauce Special	4 oz	35	tr	280	8	2
Sauce With Bits	4 oz	30	tr	620	7	2
Sauce With Garlic	4 oz	70	2	480	10	2
Sauce With Mushrooms	4 oz	25	tr	710	6	2
Stewed	4 oz	35	tr	400	8	tr
Stewed Italian	4 oz	40	tr	370	9	tr
Stewed No Salt Added	4 oz	35	tr	20	8	tr
Whole	4 oz	20	tr	330	5	tr
Whole Italian	4 oz	25	tr	420	6	tr
Whole No Salt Added	4 oz	20	tr	15	5	tr
Muir Glen						
Organic Chunky Sauce	¼ cup (2.3 oz)	20	0	160	4	1
Organic Crushed With Basil	¼ cup (2.3 oz)	25	0	85	4	1
Organic Diced	½ cup (4.5 oz)	25	0	290	4	1
Organic Diced No Salt Added	½ cup (4.5 oz)	25	0	45	4	1
Organic Ground Peeled	¼ cup (2.3 oz)	10	0	100	2	1
Organic Italian Style Diced	½ cup (4.4 oz)	25	0	290	4	1
Organic Paste	2 tbsp (1.2 oz)	30	0	20	6	1
Organic Puree	¼ cup (2.2 oz)	20	0	20	5	1
Organic Sauce	¼ cup (2.2 oz)	20	0	190	5	1
Organic Sauce No Salt Added	¼ cup (2.2 oz)	20	0	30	5	1
Organic Stewed	½ cup (4.5 oz)	30	0	290	7	tr
Organic Stewed Italian Style	½ cup (4.4 oz)	30	0	290	7	tr
Organic Stewed Mexican Style	½ cup (4.4 oz)	30	0	290	7	tr
Organic Whole Peeled	½ cup (4.6 oz)	30	0	260	5	1
Rosoff's						
Pickled	⅓ tomato (1 oz)	5	0	290	1	—
S&W						
Aspic Supreme	½ cup	60	0	860	16	—
Diced In Rich Puree	½ cup	35	0	290	8	—
Italian Stewed Sliced	½ cup	35	0	355	9	—
Italian Style w/ Basil	½ cup	25	0	220	5	—
Paste	6 oz	150	0	100	35	—
Peeled Ready Cut	½ cup	25	0	220	6	—

FOOD	PORTION	CAL.	FAT	SOD.	CARB.	FIB.
S&W (CONT.)						
Puree	½ cup	60	0	35	14	—
Sauce	½ cup	40	0	620	9	—
Sauce Chunky	½ cup	45	0	615	10	—
Stewed 50% Salt Reduced	½ cup	35	0	180	7	—
Stewed Mexican Style	½ cup	40	0	360	8	—
Stewed Sliced	½ cup	35	0	355	9	—
Whole Diet	½ cup	25	0	20	5	—
Whole Peeled	½ cup	25	0	220	6	—
Schorr's						
Pickled	⅓ tomato (1 oz)	4	0	280	1	—
Sonoma						
Dried Spice Medley oil drained	1 tbsp (0.5 oz)	50	4	200	3	1
Pesto	¼ cup (2 oz)	110	9	125	6	1
Tapenade	1 tbsp (0.7 oz)	70	6	5	4	1
Tree Of Life						
Sauce	¼ cup (2 oz)	20	0	9	4	—
paste	½ cup	110	1	86	25	6
puree	1 cup	102	tr	532	25	6
puree w/o salt	1 cup	102	tr	49	25	6
red whole	½ cup	24	tr	195	5	—
sauce	½ cup	37	tr	738	9	2
sauce spanish style	½ cup	40	tr	—	9	2
sauce w/ mushrooms	½ cup	42	tr	552	10	—
sauce w/ onion	½ cup	52	tr	672	12	—
stewed	½ cup	34	tr	325	8	—
w/ green chiles	½ cup	18	tr	481	4	—
wedges in tomato juice	½ cup	34	tr	285	8	—
DRIED						
Sonoma						
Bits	2-3 tsp (5 g)	15	0	5	3	1
Halves	2-3 halves (5 g)	15	0	5	3	1
Julienne	7-9 pieces (5 g)	15	0	5	3	1
Pasta Toss	½ cup (0.7 oz)	70	0	75	13	3
Season It	2-3 tsp (5 g)	20	0	25	3	1
sun dried	1 piece	5	tr	42	1	—
sun dried	1 cup	140	2	1131	30	—
sun dried in oil	1 cup (4 oz)	235	15	293	26	—
sun dried in oil	1 piece (3 g)	6	tr	8	1	—
FRESH						
cooked	½ cup	32	1	13	7	—
green	1	30	tr	16	6	—

FOOD	PORTION	CAL.	FAT	SOD.	CARB.	FIB.
red	1 (4½ oz)	26	tr	11	6	2
red chopped	1 cup	35	tr	16	8	2
TAKE-OUT						
stewed	1 cup	80	3	460	13	—

TOMATO JUICE

FOOD	PORTION	CAL.	FAT	SOD.	CARB.	FIB.
Campbell	6 oz	40	0	540	8	—
Del Monte						
Snap-E-Tom	10 fl oz	60	0	840	13	2
Snap-E-Tom	6 fl oz	40	0	500	8	1
Snap-E-Tom	8 fl oz	50	0	670	11	2
Hunt's						
No Salt Added	6 oz	35	tr	25	8	2
Mott's						
Beefamato	8 fl oz	80	0	780	20	1
Clamato	8 fl oz	100	0	720	24	2
Clamato Caesar	8 fl oz	100	0	780	24	0
Muir Glen						
Organic	8 oz	40	0	550	7	tr
S&W						
California	6 oz	35	0	600	8	—
Diet	½ cup	35	0	20	8	—
beef broth & tomato	5½ oz	61	tr	220	14	—
clam & tomato	1 can (5½ oz)	77	tr	664	18	—
tomato juice	½ cup	21	tr	441	5	—
tomato juice	6 oz	32	tr	658	8	—

TONGUE

FOOD	PORTION	CAL.	FAT	SOD.	CARB.	FIB.
beef simmered	3 oz	241	18	51	tr	—
lamb braised	3 oz	234	17	57	0	—
pork braised	3 oz	230	16	93	0	—

TOPPINGS
(*see* ICE CREAM TOPPINGS)

TORTILLA
(*see also* CHIPS TORTILLA, SPANISH FOOD)

FOOD	PORTION	CAL.	FAT	SOD.	CARB.	FIB.
Alvarado St. Bakery						
Burrito Size	1 (2.2 oz)	170	4	480	30	1
Fajita Size	1 (1.6 oz)	130	3	370	23	1
El Charrito						
Corn	2	95	1	—	—	—
Flour	2	170	4	—	—	—
Old El Paso						
Flour	1	150	3	360	27	—

FOOD	PORTION	CAL.	FAT	SOD.	CARB.	FIB.
Tyson						
Burrito Style Flour	1	170	4	40	29	—
Burrito Style Hand Stretched Small Flour	1	106	2	50	19	—
Burrito Style Heat Pressed Large Flour	1	182	4	90	33	—
Enchilada Style Corn	1	54	tr	4	11	—
Fajito Style Flour	1	89	2	21	15	—
Soft Taco Flour	1	121	3	28	20	—
Whole Wheat	1	120	3	32	20	—
Wonder						
Low Fat Wheat	1 (1.4 oz)	120	2	280	24	1
Low Fat White	1 (1.4 oz)	110	2	280	22	1
corn	1 (6 in diam)	56	1	40	12	1
corn w/o salt	1, 6 in diam (.9 oz)	56	1	3	12	1
flour w/o salt	1, 8 in diam (1.2 oz)	114	3	167	20	1

TORTILLA CHIPS
(*see* CHIPS)

TREE FERN

FOOD	PORTION	CAL.	FAT	SOD.	CARB.	FIB.
chopped cooked	½ cup	28	tr	3	8	—

TRITICALE

FOOD	PORTION	CAL.	FAT	SOD.	CARB.	FIB.
dry	½ cup	323	2	5	69	17
triticale not prep	3.5 oz	329	2	26	64	7

TROUT

FOOD	PORTION	CAL.	FAT	SOD.	CARB.	FIB.
Clear Springs						
Rainbow	3.5 oz	140	7	35	tr	—
baked	3 oz	162	7	57	0	—
rainbow cooked	3 oz	129	4	29	0	—
sea trout baked	3 oz	113	4	63	0	—

TRUFFLES

FOOD	PORTION	CAL.	FAT	SOD.	CARB.	FIB.
fresh	3½ oz	25	1	77	17	—

TUNA
(*see also* TUNA DISHES)
CANNED

FOOD	PORTION	CAL.	FAT	SOD.	CARB.	FIB.
Bumble Bee						
Chunk Light In Oil	2 oz	160	12	250	0	—
Chunk Light In Water	2 oz	60	1	250	0	—
Chunk White In Oil	2 oz	160	12	250	0	—
Chunk White In Water	2 oz	70	2	250	0	—
Chunk White In Water Diet	2 oz	60	1	30	0	—

FOOD	PORTION	CAL.	FAT	SOD.	CARB.	FIB.
Bumble Bee (CONT.)						
Solid White In Oil	2 oz	130	8	250	0	—
Solid White In Water	2 oz	70	2	250	0	—
Empress						
Chunk Light	2 oz	60	1	310	0	—
Chunk Light Tongol	2 oz	50	1	55	0	—
Solid White	2 oz	70	2	310	0	—
S&W						
Chunk Light Fancy In Oil	2 oz	140	10	450	0	—
Chunk Light Fancy In Water	2 oz	60	1	500	0	—
Fancy White Albacore in Oil	2 oz	160	12	450	0	—
Tree Of Life						
Tongol In Spring Water	2 oz	60	0	310	0	0
Tongol In Spring Water No Salt Water	2 oz	70	0	95	0	0
light in oil	3 oz	169	7	301	0	—
light in oil	1 can (6 oz)	399	14	606	0	—
light in water	1 can (5.8 oz)	192	1	558	0	—
light in water	3 oz	99	1	287	0	—
white in oil	3 oz	158	7	336	0	—
white in oil	1 can (6.2 oz)	331	14	704	0	—
white in water	1 can (6 oz)	234	4	673	0	—
white in water	3 oz	116	2	333	0	—
FRESH						
bluefin cooked	3 oz	157	5	43	0	—
bluefin raw	3 oz	122	4	33	0	—
skipjack baked	3 oz	112	1	40	0	—
yellowfin baked	3 oz	118	1	40	0	—
TUNA DISHES						
FROZEN						
Chefwich						
Tuna Melt	5 oz	360	14	—	—	—
Mrs. Paul's						
Microwave Tuna Sandwich	1	200	6	590	23	—
MIX						
Bumble Bee						
Tuna Mix-ins Classic Italian	⅓ pkg (0.17 oz)	25	0	5	5	—
Tuna Mix-ins Garden & Herb	⅓ pkg (0.17 oz)	25	0	5	5	—

FOOD	PORTION	CAL.	FAT	SOD.	CARB.	FIB.
Bumble Bee (CONT.)						
Tuna Mix-ins Lemon Herb	⅓ pkg (0.17 oz)	25	0	5	6	—
Tuna Mix-ins Zesty Tomato	⅓ pkg (0.17 oz)	25	0	5	5	—
Tuna Helper						
Au Gratin as prep	⅕ pkg (6 oz)	280	11	980	30	—
Buttery Rice as prep	⅕ pkg (6 oz)	280	11	1040	32	—
Cheesy Noodles as prep	⅕ pkg (7.75 oz)	240	8	980	27	—
Creamy Mushroom as prep	⅕ pkg (7 oz)	220	6	740	29	—
Creamy Noodles as prep	⅕ pkg (8 oz)	300	14	960	29	—
Fettucine Alfredo as prep	⅕ pkg (7 oz)	300	13	1000	30	—
Romanoff as prep	⅕ pkg (8 oz)	290	8	820	38	—
Tetrazzini as prep	⅕ pkg (6 oz)	240	8	780	27	—
Tuna Pot Pie as prep	⅙ pkg (5.1 oz)	420	27	890	31	—
Tuna Salad as prep	⅕ pkg (5.5 oz)	420	27	870	29	—
READY-TO-USE						
The Spreadables						
Tuna Salad	¼ can	90	6	—	—	—
Wampler Longacre						
Salad	1 oz	60	4	130	3	—
TAKE-OUT						
tuna salad	1 cup	383	19	824	19	—
tuna salad	3 oz	159	8	342	8	—
tuna salad submarine sandwich w/ lettuce & oil	1	584	28	1294	55	—

TURBOT
european baked	3 oz	104	3	163	0	—

TURKEY
(*see also* DINNER, HOT DOG, TURKEY DISHES, TURKEY SUBSTITUTES)

FOOD	PORTION	CAL.	FAT	SOD.	CARB.	FIB.
CANNED						
Armour						
Turkey Loaf	2 oz	110	8	390	1	—
Hormel						
Chunk	2 oz	70	3	340	0	0
Chunk Turkey Ham	2 oz	70	4	600	0	0
Chunk White	2 oz	60	1	320	0	0
Swanson						
White	2½ oz	80	1	260	1	—
Underwood						
Chunky Light	2.08 oz	75	2	330	2	—
w/ broth	½ can (2.5 oz)	116	5	332	0	—
w/ broth	1 can (5 oz)	231	10	663	0	—

FOOD	PORTION	CAL.	FAT	SOD.	CARB.	FIB.
FRESH						
Butterball						
Ground All White Meat	3 oz	100	3	55	tr	—
Louis Rich						
Ground	3 oz	140	9	105	0	0
Mr. Turkey						
Ground 85% Fat Free	3.5 oz	210	16	90	0	—
Ground 91% Fat Free	3.5 oz	170	10	90	1	—
Perdue						
Breast Cutlets Thin-Sliced Skinless & Boneless	1 oz	28	tr	13	0	—
Breast Fillets Skinless & Boneless Fit 'n Easy cooked	1 oz	28	tr	13	0	—
Breast Hotel Style Prime w/ Skin cooked	1 oz	43	2	12	0	—
Breast Skinless Boneless Fit 'n Easy cooked	1 oz	28	tr	13	0	—
Breast Tenderloins Skinless & Boneless cooked	1 oz	29	tr	12	0	—
Breast w/ Skin Fresh Young cooked	1 oz	44	2	14	0	—
Drumsticks w/ Skin Fresh Young cooked	1 oz	36	2	19	0	—
Ground cooked	1 oz	35	2	17	0	—
Ground Breast Meat cooked	1 oz	28	tr	13	0	—
Thighs Skinless & Boneless Fit 'n Fresh cooked	1 oz	36	2	15	0	—
Thighs w/ Skin Fresh Young cooked	1 oz	48	3	20	0	—
Whole Dark Meat w/ skin cooked	1 oz	48	3	18	0	—
Whole White Meat Fresh Young w/ Skin cooked	1 oz	44	2	13	0	—
Wings Drummettes w/ Skin Fresh Young cooked	1 oz	43	2	18	0	—
Wings Portions w/ Skin Fresh Young cooked	1 oz	51	3	18	0	—
Wings w/ Skin Fresh Young cooked	1 oz	45	2	20	0	—

FOOD	PORTION	CAL.	FAT	SOD.	CARB.	FIB.
Shady Brook						
Breast Prime Young	3 oz	140	7	—	—	—
Wings	3 oz	130	6	—	—	—
Swift-Eckrich						
Ground All White	3 oz	100	3	55	tr	—
Wampler Longacre						
Ground raw	1 oz	60	4	20	0	—
back w/ skin roasted	½ back (9 oz)	637	38	191	0	—
breast w/ skin roasted	4 oz	212	8	70	0	—
dark meat w/ skin roasted	3.6 oz	230	12	79	0	—
dark meat w/o skin roasted	1 cup (5 oz)	262	10	110	0	—
dark meat w/o skin roasted	3 oz	170	7	72	0	—
ground cooked	3 oz	188	11	68	0	—
leg w/ skin roasted	2.5 oz	147	7	55	0	—
leg w/ skin roasted	1 (1.2 lbs)	1133	54	420	0	—
light meat w/ skin roasted	from ½ turkey (2.3 lbs)	2069	87	658	0	—
light meat w/ skin roasted	4.7 oz	268	11	85	0	—
light meat w/o skin roasted	4 oz	183	4	75	0	—
neck simmered	1 (5.3 oz)	274	11	84	0	—
skin roasted	1 oz	141	13	17	0	—
skin roasted	from ½ turkey (9 oz)	1096	98	132	0	—
w/ skin roasted	8.4 oz	498	23	164	0	—
w/ skin roasted	½ turkey (4 lbs)	3857	181	1269	0	—
w/ skin neck & giblets roasted	½ turkey (8.8 lbs)	4123	190	1358	1	—
w/o skin roasted	7.3 oz	354	10	147	0	—
w/o skin roasted	1 cup (5 oz)	238	7	99	0	—
wing w/ skin roasted	1 (6.5 oz)	426	23	114	0	—
FROZEN						
roast boneless seasoned light & dark meat roasted	1 pkg (1.7 lbs)	1213	45	5320	24	—
FROZEN PREPARED						
Empire						
Patties	1 (3.1 oz)	200	10	280	14	1
READY-TO-USE						
Alpine Lace						
Breast Fat Free	2 oz	50	0	290	0	—
Carl Buddig						
Honey Turkey	1 oz	40	2	360	1	—
Turkey	1 oz	50	3	340	1	0
Turkey Ham	1 oz	40	2	430	1	0

FOOD	PORTION	CAL.	FAT	SOD.	CARB.	FIB.
Empire						
Barbecue Whole	5 oz	250	12	320	0	0
Bologna	3 slices (1.8 oz)	90	6	430	3	0
Oven Prepared Breast Slices	3 slices (1.8 oz)	50	1	200	1	0
Pastrami	3 slices (1.8 oz)	60	2	270	0	1
Salami	3 slices (1.8 oz)	70	4	350	1	0
Smoked Breast Slices	3 slices (1.8 oz)	40	0	350	0	0
Falls						
BBQ	3 oz	140	8	300	—	—
Gourmet Breast	3 oz	80	1	320	—	—
Premium Cooked Breast	3 oz	100	2	240	—	—
Hansel n' Gretel						
Breast Gourmet	1 oz	28	1	170	1	—
Breast Gourmet Smoked	1 oz	31	1	170	tr	—
Breast Honey	1 oz	28	1	170	1	—
Breast Lessalt Cooked	1 oz	25	1	140	tr	—
Breast Oven Cooked	1 oz	26	tr	180	tr	—
Doubledecker Turkey Corned Beef	1 oz	30	1	195	1	—
Doubledecker Turkey Ham	1 oz	30	1	185	1	—
Healthy Choice						
Deli-Thin Honey Roast & Smoked	6 slices (2 oz)	70	2	410	2	0
Deli-Thin Roasted Breast	6 slices (2 oz)	60	2	550	1	0
Deli-Thin Smoked Breast	6 slices (2 oz)	60	2	420	1	0
Deli-Thin Turkey Ham	6 slices (2 oz)	60	2	550	1	0
Fresh-Trak Honey Roast & Smoked Breast	1 slice (1 oz)	35	1	200	1	0
Fresh-Trak Oven Roasted Breast	1 slice (1 oz)	35	1	270	1	0
Honey Roasted & Smoked	1 slice (1 oz)	35	1	220	1	0
Oven Roasted Breast	1 slice (1 oz)	35	1	270	1	0
Smoked Breast	1 slice (1 oz)	30	1	230	0	0
Variety Pack Regular	3 slices (2.2 oz)	70	2	530	2	0
Hebrew National						
Deli Thin Hickory Smoked	1.8 oz	55	1	310	—	—
Deli Thin Lemon Garlic	1.8 oz	50	1	400	—	—
Deli Thin Oven Roasted	1.8 oz	80	1	420	—	—

FOOD	PORTION	CAL.	FAT	SOD.	CARB.	FIB.
Hillshire						
Deli Select Honey Roasted Breast	1 slice	10	tr	90	tr	—
Deli Select Oven Roasted Breast	1 slice	10	tr	105	tr	—
Deli Select Smoked Breast	1 slice	10	tr	100	tr	—
Deli Select Turkey Ham	1 slice	10	tr	95	tr	—
Flavor Pack 90-99% Fat Free Honey Roasted Breast	1 slice (0.75 oz)	20	tr	200	1	—
Flavor Pack 90-99% Fat Free Oven Roasted Breast	1 slice (0.75 oz)	20	tr	230	1	—
Flavor Pack 90-99% Fat Free Smoked Breast	1 slice (0.75 oz)	20	tr	220	tr	—
Honey Cured Breast	1 oz	35	1	340	2	—
Lunch 'N Munch Smoked Turkey/ Cheddar	1 pkg (4.5 oz)	350	21	1130	20	—
Lunch 'N Munch Smoked Turkey/ Cheddar/ Brownie	1 pkg (4.5 oz)	400	22	1240	34	—
Lunch 'N Munch Turkey/ Cheddar/ Brownie/ Hi-C	1 pkg (4.5 oz + 6 fl oz)	500	22	1260	58	—
Smoked Breast	1 oz	35	1	340	1	—
Hormel						
Light & Lean 97 Breast Sliced	1 slice (1 oz)	30	1	360	0	0
Light & Lean 97 Breast Smoked	3 oz	80	1	780	1	0
Light & Lean 97 Cuts	16 pieces (1 oz)	30	1	460	1	0
Light & Lean 97 Cuts Smoked	16 pieces (1 oz)	30	1	460	1	0
Louis Rich						
Bologna	1 slice (28 g)	50	4	250	1	0
Breaded Nuggets	4 (3.2 oz)	260	15	640	15	0
Breaded Patties	1 (3 oz)	220	13	550	13	0
Breaded Sticks	3 (3 oz)	230	15	580	12	0
Carving Board Oven Roasted Breast	2 slices (1.6 oz)	40	1	560	0	0
Carving Board Oven Roasted Thin Carved Breast	6 slices (2.1 oz)	60	1	740	0	0

FOOD	PORTION	CAL.	FAT	SOD.	CARB.	FIB.
Louis Rich (CONT.)						
Carving Board Smoked Breast	2 slices (1.6 oz)	40	1	560	0	0
Chopped Ham	1 slice (1 oz)	46	3	290	0	0
Cotto Salami	1 slice (28 g)	40	3	290	0	0
Deli-Thin Smoked Breast	4 slices (1.8 oz)	50	1	490	1	0
Fat Free Hickory Smoked Breast	1 slice (1 oz)	25	0	300	1	0
Fat Free Oven Roasted Breast	1 slice (28 g)	25	0	310	1	0
Ham Round	1 slice (28 g)	34	1	300	0	0
Ham Square	3 slices (2.2 oz)	70	3	710	1	0
Hickory Smoked Dinner Slices Breast	1 slice (2.8 oz)	80	1	1060	2	0
Honey Cured Turkey Ham	3 slices (2.2 oz)	70	2	660	2	0
Honey Roasted Breast	1 slice (1 oz)	30	1	320	1	0
Honey Roasted Dinner Slices Breast	1 slice (2.8 oz)	80	1	940	3	0
Oven Roasted Breast	2 oz	60	2	640	2	0
Oven Roasted Breast	1 slice (1 oz)	30	1	310	1	0
Oven Roasted Deli-Thin Breast	4 slices (1.8 oz)	50	1	580	2	0
Oven Roasted Dinner Slices Breast	1 slice (2.8 oz)	70	1	910	2	0
Pastrami	2 slices (1.6 oz)	45	2	520	0	0
Salami	1 slice (28 g)	45	3	290	0	0
Skinless Barbecued Breast	2 oz	60	1	680	2	0
Skinless Hickory Smoked Breast	2 oz	60	1	760	1	0
Skinless Honey Roasted Breast	2 oz	60	1	690	2	0
Skinless Oven Roasted Breast	2 oz	50	1	650	1	0
Smoked Breast	1 slice (1 oz)	25	1	260	0	0
Smoked White	1 slice (1 oz)	30	1	290	0	0
Turkey Ham	4 slices (1.8 oz)	60	2	580	0	0
Mr. Turkey						
Deli Cuts Hardwood Smoked Breast	3 slices	30	1	340	1	—
Deli Cuts Honey Roasted Breast	3 slices	30	1	310	2	—
Deli Cuts Oven Roasted Breast	3 slices	30	1	270	2	—

FOOD	PORTION	CAL.	FAT	SOD.	CARB.	FIB.
Mr. Turkey (CONT.)						
Deli Cuts Turkey Ham	3 slices	35	2	310	1	—
Deli Cuts Turkey Pastrami	3 slices	35	1	255	1	—
Hardwood Smoked Breast	1 slice	30	1	280	2	—
Hardwood Smoked Turkey Ham	1 slice	35	2	320	0	—
Honey Cured Turkey Ham	1 slice	30	1	320	1	—
Oven Roasted Breast	1 slice	30	1	270	2	—
Smoked Breakfast Turkey Ham	1 oz	30	1	325	1	—
Turkey Bologna	1 slice	70	5	370	1	—
Turkey Cotto Salami	1 slice	50	4	240	1	—
Turkey Ham	1 slice	35	2	320	0	—
Turkey Pastrami	1 slice	30	1	290	1	—
Oscar Mayer						
Deli-Thin Roast	4 slices (1.8 oz)	50	1	560	2	0
Deli-Thin Smoked Honey Roasted	4 slices (1.8 oz)	60	1	520	2	0
Free Oven Roasted Breast	4 slices (1.8 oz)	40	0	610	2	—
Free Smoked Breast	4 slices (1.8 oz)	40	0	550	2	—
Healthy Favorites Oven Roasted Breast	4 slices (1.8 oz)	40	0	610	2	0
Healthy Favorites Smoked Breast	4 slices (1.8 oz)	40	0	550	2	0
Lunchables Fun Pack Turkey/Pacific Cooler	1 pkg (11.2 oz)	460	21	1310	53	tr
Lunchables Fun Pack Turkey/Surfer Cooler	1 pkg (11.2 oz)	440	16	1220	60	0
Lunchables Turkey/Cheddar	1 pkg (4.5 oz)	360	22	1650	20	1
Lunchables Turkey Oven Roasted/ Green Onion Cheese	1 pkg (4.5 oz)	380	20	1270	36	1
Lunchables Turkey Smoked/ Ranch & Herb Cheese	1 pkg (4.5 oz)	380	20	1280	36	1
Perdue						
Nuggets	1 (0.67 oz)	54	3	112	3	—
Sara Lee						
Hardwood Smoked Breast Of Turkey	2 oz	60	1	550	0	—

FOOD	PORTION	CAL.	FAT	SOD.	CARB.	FIB.
Sara Lee (CONT.)						
Hardwood Smoked Turkey Ham	2 oz	60	2	620	1	—
Honey Roasted Breast Of Turkey	2 oz	60	0	550	2	—
Honey Roasted Turkey Ham	2 oz	70	3	660	3	—
Mesquite Smoked Breast Of Turkey	2 oz	60	2	510	0	—
Oven Roasted Breast Of Turkey	2 oz	60	2	370	0	—
Peppered Breast Of Turkey	2 oz	50	0	420	2	—
Seasoned Breast Of Turkey Pastrami	2 oz	60	1	510	2	—
Tyson						
Breast	1 slice	20	tr	136	tr	—
Ham	1 slice	23	tr	182	1	—
Wampler Longacre						
Bologna	1 oz	60	5	260	tr	—
Breast Chops	1 serv (4 oz)	120	1	90	0	—
Breast Sliced	1 slice (1 oz)	35	tr	310	1	—
Breast Sliced Smoked	1 slice (0.75 oz)	20	tr	210	1	—
Burger	1 (4 oz)	230	17	90	0	—
Burger	1 (3 oz)	170	13	70	0	—
Burger Barbecue	1 (4 oz)	240	17	280	4	—
Chef Select Breast Skinless	1 oz	35	tr	220	tr	—
Chef Select Breast Smoked	1 oz	35	1	240	1	—
Chunk Dark Smoked Cured	1 oz	45	3	300	1	—
Chunk Ham 12% Water Smoked	1 oz	45	3	200	tr	—
Chunk Ham 20% Water	1 oz	40	2	370	2	—
Chunk Pastrami	1 oz	35	2	280	tr	—
Cook-In-The-Bag Breast	1 oz	30	1	125	1	—
Cook-In-The-Bag Breast Mini	1 oz	30	1	105	tr	—
Cook-In-The-Bag Combo Roast	1 oz	35	1	125	tr	—
Cook-In-The-Bag Thigh Roast	1 oz	40	2	130	1	—
Dark Smoked Cured	1 oz	45	3	3000	1	—

FOOD	PORTION	CAL.	FAT	SOD.	CARB.	FIB.
Wampler Longacre (CONT.)						
Deli Chef Breast And White Meat No Skin	1 oz	40	2	240	1	—
Gourmet Breast	1 oz	35	1	300	1	—
Gourmet Breast Mini	1 oz	35	1	300	1	—
Gourmet Breast Mini Smoked	1 oz	35	1	240	1	—
Gourmet Breast Smoked	1 oz	30	tr	230	1	—
Gourmet Brown & Glazed Breast	1 oz	35	1	240	1	—
Gourmet Brown & Roasted Breast	1 oz	35	1	260	1	—
Gourmet Honey Cured Breast	1 oz	30	1	210	1	—
Lean-Lite Breast Skinless	1 oz	35	tr	160	0	—
Lean-Lite Deli Breast	1 oz	35	1	160	0	—
Lean-Lite Deli Breast Smoked	1 oz	35	1	170	1	—
Old Fashioned Brown & Roasted Breast	1 oz	35	tr	160	tr	—
Pastrami	1 oz	35	2	280	tr	—
Premium Breast Skinless	1 oz	30	tr	250	1	—
Premium Brown & Roasted Breast Skinless	1 oz	16	1	300	1	—
Roll Combo	1 oz	44	3	187	tr	—
Roll Sliced Breast	1 slice (0.75 oz)	30	tr	250	1	—
Roll White	1 oz	45	3	200	tr	—
Salami	1 oz	50	3	280	1	—
Salt Watchers Breast Skinless	1 oz	35	1	20	0	—
Seasoned Roast	1 oz	40	2	90	0	—
Sliced Salami	1 slice (0.8 oz)	45	3	240	1	—
Tenderlings BBQ	1 serv (4 oz)	110	tr	520	0	—
Tenderlings Cajun	1 serv (4 oz)	110	tr	560	0	—
Tenderlings Garlic & Pepper	1 serv (4 oz)	110	tr	600	0	—
Tenderlings Original	1 serv (4 oz)	110	tr	480	0	—
Turkey Ham 12% Water Baked	1 oz	45	3	200	tr	—
Turkey Ham 20% Water Baked	1 oz	40	2	370	1	—

FOOD	PORTION	CAL.	FAT	SOD.	CARB.	FIB.
Wampler Longacre (CONT.)						
Unseasoned Roast	1 oz	40	2	15	0	—
Whole Browned & Roasted	1 oz	60	3	100	tr	—
Weight Watchers						
Deli Thin Smoked Breast	5 slices (⅓ oz)	10	tr	80	tr	—
Oven Roasted Breast	2 slices (¾ oz)	25	1	200	tr	—
Oven Roasted Turkey Ham	2 slices (¾ oz)	25	1	210	tr	—
Roasted & Smoked Breast	2 slices (¾ oz)	25	1	170	tr	—
bologna	1 oz	57	4	249	tr	—
breast	1 slice (¾ oz)	23	tr	301	0	—
diced light & dark seasoned	½ lb	313	14	1928	2	—
diced light & dark seasoned	1 oz	39	2	241	tr	—
ham thigh meat	1 pkg (8 oz)	291	12	2260	1	—
ham thigh meat	2 oz	73	3	565	tr	—
pastrami	2 oz	80	4	698	1	—
pastrami	1 pkg (8 oz)	320	14	2372	4	—
patties battered & fried	1 (3.3 oz)	266	17	752	15	—
patties battered & fried	1 (2.3 oz)	181	12	512	10	—
patties breaded & fried	1 (3.3 oz)	266	17	752	15	—
patties breaded & fried	1 (2.3 oz)	181	12	512	10	—
poultry salad sandwich spread	1 oz	238	4	107	2	—
poultry salad sandwich spread	1 tbsp	109	2	49	1	—
prebasted breast w/ skin roasted	½ breast (1.9 lbs)	1087	30	3434	0	—
prebasted breast w/ skin roasted	1 breast (3.8 lbs)	2175	60	6868	0	—
prebasted thigh w/ skin roasted	1 thigh (11 oz)	494	27	1371	0	—
roll light & dark meat	1 oz	42	2	166	1	—
roll light meat	1 oz	42	2	139	2	—
salami cooked	2 oz	111	8	569	tr	—
salami cooked	1 pkg (8 oz)	446	31	2278	1	—
turkey loaf breast meat	2 slices (1.5 oz)	47	1	608	0	—
turkey loaf breast meat	1 pkg (6 oz)	187	3	2433	0	—
turkey sticks battered & fried	1 stick (2.3 oz)	178	11	536	11	—

FOOD	PORTION	CAL.	FAT	SOD.	CARB.	FIB.
turkey sticks breaded & fried	1 stick (2.3 oz)	178	11	536	11	—

TURKEY DISHES
(see also DINNER, TURKEY SUBSTITUTES)

CANNED

Dinty Moore

American Classics Chicken With Mashed Potatoes	1 bowl (10 oz)	250	7	1040	27	3
American Classics Turkey & Dressing With Gravy	1 bowl (10 oz)	280	7	1120	32	4

FROZEN

Hot Pocket

Stuffed Sandwich Turkey & Ham With Cheese	1 (4.5 oz)	320	13	680	38	1

Lean Pockets

Stuffed Sandwich Turkey & Ham With Cheddar	1 (4.5 oz)	260	7	810	35	4
Stuffed Sandwich Turkey Broccoli & Cheese	1 (4.5 oz)	260	8	710	35	4

Luigino's

Gravy Dressing & Turkey	1 pkg (8 oz)	340	15	910	36	2

Ovenstuffs

Turkey Turnover	1 (4.75 oz)	350	16	700	35	—
gravy & turkey	1 cup (8.4 oz)	160	6	1328	11	—
gravy & turkey	1 pkg (5 oz)	95	4	786	7	—

READY-TO-USE

Spreadables

Turkey Salad	¼ can	100	6	—	—	—

Wampler Longacre

Meatloaf Italian	1 serv (4 oz)	114	5	640	5	—
Meatloaf Mexican	1 serv (4 oz)	114	5	680	4	—
Meatloaf Original	1 serv (4 oz)	126	5	620	10	—
Salad	1 oz	60	4	140	3	—
Salad Turkey Ham	1 oz	50	4	190	3	—
Teriyaki	1 serv (4 oz)	112	tr	640	14	—

TURKEY SUBSTITUTES

Harvest Direct

TVP Poultry Chunks	3.5 oz	280	1	15	32	18
TVP Poultry Ground	3.5 oz	280	1	15	32	18

FOOD	PORTION	CAL.	FAT	SOD.	CARB.	FIB.
White Wave						
Meatless Sandwich Slices	2 slices (1.6 oz)	80	0	400	7	1
Worthington						
Smoked Turkey Slices	4 slices (76 g)	180	12	820	5	—
Turkey Slices	2 slices (63 g)	130	9	430	3	—
TURMERIC						
ground	1 tsp	8	tr	1	1	—
TURNIPS						
CANNED						
Allen						
Chopped Greens And Diced Turnip	½ cup (4.2 oz)	30	1	20	5	tr
Greens	½ cup (4.2 oz)	25	1	15	3	2
Luck's						
Turnip Greens w/ Diced Turnips Seasoned w/ Pork	7.5 oz	90	6	—	—	—
Sunshine						
Chopped Greens And Diced Turnip	½ cup (4.2 oz)	30	1	20	5	tr
Greens	½ cup (4.2 oz)	25	1	15	3	2
greens	½ cup	17	tr	325	3	—
FRESH						
cooked mashed	½ cup (4.2 oz)	47	tr	25	10	—
cubed cooked	½ cup (3 oz)	33	tr	17	7	—
greens chopped cooked	½ cup	15	tr	21	3	—
greens raw chopped	½ cup	7	tr	11	2	1
raw cubed	½ cup (2.4 oz)	25	tr	14	6	—
FROZEN						
Southland						
Mashed	3.6 oz	90	6	—	—	—
Rutabaga Yellow Turnips	4 oz	50	0	—	—	—
greens cooked	½ cup	24	tr	12	4	2
TURTLE						
raw	3½ oz	85	1	—	0	—
TUSK FISH						
raw	3½ oz	79	tr	113	0	—
VANILLA						
Hershey						
Vanilla Milk Chips	¼ cup	240	14	65	25	—

FOOD	PORTION	CAL.	FAT	SOD.	CARB.	FIB.
Virginia Dare						
Vanilla Extract	1 tsp	10	0	—	—	—

VEAL
(*see also* BEEF, DINNER, VEAL DISHES)
FRESH

FOOD	PORTION	CAL.	FAT	SOD.	CARB.	FIB.
cutlet lean only braised	3 oz	172	4	57	0	—
cutlet lean only fried	3 oz	156	4	65	0	—
ground broiled	3 oz	146	6	70	0	—
loin chop w/ bone lean & fat braised	1 chop (2.8 oz)	227	14	64	0	—
loin chop w/ bone lean only braised	1 chop (2.4 oz)	155	6	58	0	—
shoulder w/ bone lean only braised	3 oz	169	5	83	0	—
sirloin w/ bone lean & fat roasted	3 oz	171	9	71	0	—
sirloin w/ bone lean only roasted	3 oz	143	5	72	0	—

VEAL DISHES
TAKE-OUT

FOOD	PORTION	CAL.	FAT	SOD.	CARB.	FIB.
parmigiana	4.2 oz	279	18	545	6	2

VEGETABLE JUICE
Mott's

FOOD	PORTION	CAL.	FAT	SOD.	CARB.	FIB.
Vegetable Juice as prep	8 fl oz	60	0	800	13	2
Muir Glen						
Organic	8 oz	70	0	620	15	3
Organic Reduced Sodium	8 oz	70	0	465	15	3
Odwalla						
Vegetable Cocktail	8 fl oz	70	0	290	18	2
Smucker's						
Vegetable Juice Hearty	8 fl oz	58	tr	714	13	—
Vegetable Juice Hot & Spicy	8 fl oz	58	tr	650	13	—
V8						
No Salt Added	6 fl oz	35	0	45	8	—
Original	6 fl oz	35	0	560	8	—
Spicy Hot	6 fl oz	35	0	650	8	—
vegetable juice cocktail	6 fl oz	34	tr	664	8	—
vegetable juice cocktail	½ cup	22	tr	442	6	—

FOOD	PORTION	CAL.	FAT	SOD.	CARB.	FIB.

VEGETABLES MIXED
(see also individual vegetables, VEGETABLE JUICE)

CANNED

Allen

FOOD	PORTION	CAL.	FAT	SOD.	CARB.	FIB.
Green Beans And Potatoes	½ cup (4.2 oz)	35	0	220	7	2
Okra & Tomatoes	½ cup (4 oz)	25	0	380	5	3
Okra Tomatoes & Corn	½ cup (4.1 oz)	30	0	280	6	4
Chi-Chi's						
Diced Tomatoes & Green Chilies	¼ cup (2.5 oz)	20	0	340	4	0
Del Monte						
Mixed	½ cup (4.4 oz)	40	0	360	8	2
Peas And Carrots	½ cup (4.5 oz)	60	0	360	11	2
Green Giant						
Garden Medley	½ cup	40	tr	290	9	1
Hanover						
Mixed	½ cup	110	0	—	—	—
Vegetable Salad	½ cup	90	0	—	—	—
House Of Tsang						
Vegetables & Sauce Cantonese Classic	½ cup (4.2 oz)	70	1	930	13	1
Vegetables & Sauce Hong Kong Sweet & Sour	½ cup (4.5 oz)	160	0	580	40	0
Vegetables & Sauce Szechuan Hot & Spicy	½ cup (4.2 oz)	70	1	1090	14	1
Vegetables & Sauce Tokyo Teriyaki	½ cup (4.4 oz)	100	0	1240	22	0
Ka-Me						
Stir Fry	½ cup (4.5 oz)	20	0	10	4	2
La Choy						
Chop Suey Vegetables	½ cup	10	tr	320	2	tr
S&W						
Garden Salad Marinated	½ cup	60	0	670	11	—
Mixed Vegetables Old Fashion Harvest Time	½ cup	35	0	380	6	—
Peas & Carrots Water Pack	½ cup	35	0	5	7	—
Succotash Country Style	½ cup	80	1	250	16	—
Sweet Peas & Diced Carrots	½ cup	50	0	310	9	—
Sweet Peas w/ Tiny Pearl Onions	½ cup	60	1	490	10	—

FOOD	PORTION	CAL.	FAT	SOD.	CARB.	FIB.
Seneca						
Peas & Carrots	½ cup	60	0	408	9	4
Succotash	½ cup	90	0	240	18	2
Sunshine						
Green Beans And Potatoes	½ cup (4.2 oz)	35	0	220	7	2
Trappey						
Okra & Tomatoes	½ cup (4 oz)	25	0	380	5	3
Okra Tomatoes & Corn	½ cup (4.1 oz)	30	0	280	6	4
mixed vegetables	½ cup	39	tr	122	8	—
peas & carrots	½ cup	48	tr	332	11	—
peas & carrots low sodium	½ cup	48	tr	332	11	—
peas & onions	½ cup	30	tr	265	5	—
succotash	½ cup	102	1	325	23	—
FROZEN						
Big Valley						
California Blend	¾ cup (3 oz)	25	0	20	6	3
Italian Blend	¾ cup (3 oz)	30	0	20	5	2
Oriental Blend	¾ cup (3 oz)	25	0	10	5	3
Stew Vegetables	⅔ cup (3 oz)	40	0	30	10	2
Winter Blend	¾ cup (3 oz)	25	0	15	4	2
Birds Eye						
Broccoli Cauliflower And Carrots With Cheese Sauce	½ pkg	80	4	390	7	4
Farm Fresh Broccoli And Cauliflower	¾ cup	30	0	25	5	3
Farm Fresh Broccoli Carrots And Water Chestnuts	¾ cup	40	0	35	8	3
Farm Fresh Broccoli Cauliflower And Carrots	¾ cup	35	0	40	7	3
Farm Fresh Broccoli Cauliflower And Red Peppers	¾ cup	30	0	25	5	3
Farm Fresh Broccoli Corn And Red Peppers	⅔ cup	60	1	15	14	3
Farm Fresh Broccoli Green Beans Pearl Onions and Red Peppers	¾ cup	35	0	15	7	3

FOOD	PORTION	CAL.	FAT	SOD.	CARB.	FIB.
Birds Eye (CONT.)						
Farm Fresh Broccoli Red Peppers Onions And Mushrooms	¾ cup	30	0	20	6	3
Farm Fresh Brussels Sprouts Cauliflower And Carrots	¾ cup	40	0	30	8	4
Farm Fresh Cauliflower Carrots And Snow Peas	⅔ cup	35	0	30	8	4
In Butter Sauce Broccoli Cauliflower And Carrots	½ cup	40	2	180	6	2
In Sauce Peas And Pearl Onions With Seasonings	½ cup	70	0	440	13	3
Internationals Austrian	3.3 oz	70	3	390	6	1
Internationals Bavarian	3.3 oz	90	5	260	11	2
Internationals California	3.3 oz	90	4	200	10	3
Internationals French Country	3.3 oz	70	4	230	6	2
Internationals Italian	3.3 oz	80	5	250	8	2
Internationals Japanese	3.3 oz	60	3	270	6	2
Internationals New England	3.3 oz	100	5	280	12	2
Mixed	½ cup	60	0	40	13	2
Peas And Potatoes With Cream Sauce	½ cup	100	3	420	16	1
Polybag	½ cup	60	0	40	12	2
Budget Gourmet						
Mandarin Vegetables	1 pkg (5.25 oz)	160	11	440	13	—
New England Recipe Vegetables	1 pkg (5.5 oz)	230	13	380	21	—
Spring Vegetables In Cheese Sauce	1 pkg (5 oz)	130	8	370	9	—
Fresh Like						
California Blend	3.5 oz	31	tr	21	7	1
Chuckwagon Blend	3.5 oz	71	1	5	17	1
Italian Blend	3.5 oz	33	tr	21	7	1
Midwestern Blend	3.5 oz	42	tr	32	9	1
Mixed	3.5 oz	69	tr	48	14	1
Oriental Blend	3.5 oz	26	tr	11	5	1
Peas & Carrots	3.5 oz	63	tr	63	12	1
Winter Blend	3.5 oz	26	tr	26	5	1

FOOD	PORTION	CAL.	FAT	SOD.	CARB.	FIB.
Green Giant						
American Mixtures California	½ cup	25	0	40	6	2
American Mixtures Heartland	½ cup	25	0	35	6	2
American Mixtures New England	½ cup	70	1	75	14	4
American Mixtures San Francisco	½ cup	25	0	35	7	2
American Mixtures Sante Fe	½ cup	70	1	0	16	2
American Mixtures Seattle	½ cup	25	0	35	7	2
Broccoli Cauliflower And Carrots In Butter Sauce	½ cup	30	1	240	4	—
Broccoli Cauliflower And Carrots In Cheese Sauce	½ cup	60	2	490	9	2
Harvest Fresh Mixed Vegetables	½ cup	40	0	125	9	2
Mixed	½ cup	40	0	40	9	2
Mixed In Butter Sauce	½ cup	60	2	300	11	2
One Serve Broccoli Carrots & Rotini In Cheese Sauce	1 pkg	120	3	520	20	—
One Serve Broccoli Cauliflower And Carrots	1 pkg	25	0	45	7	3
Valley Combinations Broccoli & Cauliflower	½ cup	60	2	340	9	—
Hanover						
Broccoli Cut & Cauliflower Cut	½ cup	20	0	—	—	—
Caribbean Blend	½ cup	20	0	—	—	—
Garden Medley	½ cup	20	0	—	—	—
Mixed	½ cup	50	0	—	—	—
Oriental Blend	½ cup	25	0	—	—	—
Succotash	½ cup	80	0	—	—	—
Summer Vegetables	½ cup	35	0	—	—	—
Vegetables For Soup	½ cup	60	0	—	—	—
La Choy						
Mixed Fancy	½ cup	12	tr	30	2	1

FOOD	PORTION	CAL.	FAT	SOD.	CARB.	FIB.
Ore Ida						
Stew Vegetables	⅔ cup (3 oz)	50	0	50	11	tr
Soglowek						
Golden Vegetarian Nuggets	4 pieces (2.5 oz)	190	11	220	9	1
Southland						
Peppers & Onions	2 oz	15	0	—	—	—
Soup Mix Vegetables	3.2 oz	50	0	—	—	—
Stew Vegetables	4 oz	60	0	—	—	—
Tree Of Life						
Mixed	½ cup (3 oz)	65	0	60	13	3
Veg-All						
Country Wisconsin Blend	3.5 oz	52	tr	16	13	1
Scandinavian Blend	3.5 oz	48	tr	32	9	1
Vegetables For Soup (Eight)	3.5 oz	34	tr	44	12	1
Vegetables For Soup (Nine)	3.5 oz	52	tr	43	11	1
Vegetables For Soup (Potatoes)	3.5 oz	53	tr	44	12	1
Vegetables For Stew 4-Way	3.5 oz	51	tr	42	12	1
Vegetables For Stew 5-Way	3.5 oz	54	tr	42	12	1
mixed vegetables cooked	½ cup	54	tr	32	12	2
peas & carrots cooked	½ cup	38	tr	55	8	—
peas & onions cooked	½ cup	40	tr	—	8	—
succotash cooked	½ cup	79	1	38	17	—
SHELF-STABLE						
Pantry Express						
Corn Green Beans Carrots Pasta In Tomato Sauce	½ cup	80	2	330	17	3
Green Beans Potatoes And Mushrooms In A Seasoned Sauce	½ cup	50	2	430	9	2
Mixed Vegetables	½ cup	35	tr	300	8	1
TAKE-OUT						
caponata	¼ cup	28	1	—	—	—
curry	1 serving (7.7 oz)	398	33	—	22	—
pakoras	1 (2 oz)	108	5	—	12	3
ratatouille	8.8 oz	190	16	—	10	5
samosa	2 (4 oz)	519	46	—	25	3
succotash	½ cup	111	1	16	23	—

FOOD	PORTION	CAL.	FAT	SOD.	CARB.	FIB.
VENISON						
Broken Arrow Ranch						
Antelope Chili Meat	3.5 oz	115	2	76	1	—
Antelope Ground Venison	3.5 oz	110	2	69	tr	—
Antelope Stew Meat	3.5 oz	110	2	54	2	—
Nilgai Chili Meat	3.5 oz	115	2	76	1	—
Nilgai Leg	3.5 oz	100	1	55	1	—
Nilgai Stew Meat	3.5 oz	110	2	54	2	—
Venison & Beef Smoked Sausage	6 oz	432	30	—	4	—
Venison Meat Chunks	6 oz	175	2	—	0	—
Venison Salami	6 oz	252	8	—	0	—
roasted	3 oz	134	3	46	0	—
VINEGAR						
Hain						
Cider	1 tbsp	2	0	1	4	—
Ka-Me						
Chinese Seasoned	1 tbsp (0.5 fl oz)	5	0	60	1	0
Rice Wine Chinese	1 tbsp (0.5 fl oz)	5	0	0	1	0
Rice Wine Japanese	1 tbsp (0.5 oz)	0	0	0	1	0
Seasoned Rice Japanese	1 tbsp (0.5 fl oz)	10	0	180	3	0
Nakano						
Rice	1 tbsp	0	0	1	0	—
Regina						
Red Wine	1 oz	4	0	0	0	—
Tree Of Life						
Apple Cider Organic	1 tbsp (0.5 oz)	0	0	0	tr	—
Brown Rice	1 tbsp (0.5 oz)	2	0	45	0	—
White House						
Apple Cider	2 tbsp	2	0	0	1	0
Red Wine	2 tbsp	4	0	5	2	—
cider	1 tbsp	tr	0	tr	1	—
WAFFLES						
FROZEN						
Aunt Jemima						
Blueberry	2 (2.5 oz)	190	7	530	28	1
Buttermilk	2 (2.5 oz)	170	6	410	27	1
Cinnamon	2 (2.5 oz)	180	6	470	28	1
Oatmeal	2 (2.5 oz)	170	7	660	27	3
Whole Grain	2 (2.5 oz)	170	7	450	24	2
Belgian Chef						
Belgian	2 (2.5 oz)	140	3	340	24	1

FOOD	PORTION	CAL.	FAT	SOD.	CARB.	FIB.
Downyflake						
Blueberry	2	180	4	570	32	—
Buttermilk	2	190	5	750	32	—
Hot-N-Buttery	2	180	6	620	27	—
Multi-Grain	2	250	14	500	28	4
Oat Bran	2	260	13	650	30	3
Regular	2	120	3	420	20	—
Regular Jumbo	2	170	4	570	30	—
Rice Bran	2	210	11	230	25	4
Roman Meal	2	280	14	680	33	3
Eggo						
Apple Cinnamon	2 (2.7 oz)	220	8	450	33	0
Blueberry	2 (2.7 oz)	220	8	450	33	0
Buttermilk	2 (2.7 oz)	220	8	480	30	0
Common Sense Oat Bran	2 (2.7 oz)	200	7	350	27	3
Common Sense Oat Bran With Fruit & Nut	2 (2.9 oz)	220	8	340	32	4
Homestyle	2 (2.7 oz)	220	8	470	30	0
Minis Blueberry	12 (3 oz)	240	8	510	37	0
Minis Cinnamon Toast	12 (3.2 oz)	280	9	470	40	0
Minis Homestyle	12 (1.8 oz)	240	8	520	34	0
Nut & Honey	2 (2.7 oz)	240	10	480	32	0
Nutri-Grain	2 (2.7 oz)	190	6	430	30	4
Nutri-Grain Multi-Bran	2 (2.7 oz)	180	6	400	32	6
Nutri-Grain Raisin & Bran	2 (3 oz)	210	6	390	36	5
Special K	2 (2 oz)	140	0	250	29	0
Strawberry	2 (2.7 oz)	220	8	460	32	0
Great Starts						
Belgian Waffles And Sausage	2.85 oz	280	19	420	21	—
Belgian Waffles Strawberries And Sausage	3½ oz	210	8	240	31	—
Waffle With Bacon	2.2 oz	230	14	710	19	—
Van's						
Belgian 7 Grain	1	80	2	80	10	—
Belgian Original	1	73	2	46	12	—
Toaster Apple Cinnamon	1	75	2	68	9	3
Toaster Honey Almond	1	75	2	68	9	3
Toaster Multigrain	1	75	2	68	9	3
Toaster Wheat Free	1	110	3	195	16	3
Toaster Wheat Free Cinnamon Apple	1	110	3	195	16	3

FOOD	PORTION	CAL.	FAT	SOD.	CARB.	FIB.
Weight Watchers						
Belgian	1 (1.5 oz)	120	4	220	17	—
Multi-Grain Belgian	1 (1.5 oz)	120	4	200	16	—
buttermilk	1, 4 in sq (1.2 oz)	88	3	262	14	1
plain	1, 4 in sq (1.2 oz)	88	3	262	14	1
HOME RECIPE						
plain	1 (7 in diam)	218	11	383	25	—
MIX						
plain as prep	1, 7 in diam (2.6 oz)	218	10	458	26	1
WALNUTS						
Planters						
Black	1 pkg (2 oz)	340	31	0	8	3
Gold Measure Halves	1 pkg (2 oz)	380	38	0	8	2
Halves	⅓ cup (1.2 oz)	220	22	0	5	1
Pieces	¼ cup (1 oz)	190	20	0	4	1
black dried	1 oz	172	16	0	3	1
black dried chopped	1 cup	759	71	2	15	—
english dried	1 oz	182	18	3	5	1
english dried chopped	1 cup	770	74	12	22	6
WATER CHESTNUTS						
CANNED						
Empress						
Sliced	2 oz	14	0	10	3	—
Whole	2 oz	14	0	10	3	—
Ka-Me						
Whole In Water	½ cup (4.5 oz)	45	0	10	11	4
La Choy						
Sliced	¼ cup	18	tr	3	4	tr
Whole	4	14	tr	2	4	tr
chinese sliced	½ cup	35	tr	6	9	—
FRESH						
sliced	½ cup	66	tr	9	15	—
WATERCRESS						
(*see also* CRESS)						
FRESH						
raw chopped	½ cup	2	tr	7	tr	tr
WATERMELON						
FRESH						
cut up	1 cup	50	1	3	11	1
wedge	¹⁄₁₆	152	2	10	35	2
SEEDS						
dried	1 oz	158	13	28	4	—
dried	1 cup	602	51	28	17	—

FOOD	PORTION	CAL.	FAT	SOD.	CARB.	FIB.
WAX BEANS						
CANNED						
Del Monte						
Cut Golden	½ cup (4.3 oz)	20	0	360	4	2
Owatonna						
Cut	½ cup	20	0	—	—	—
S&W						
Golden Cut Premium	½ cup	20	0	385	5	—
Seneca						
Cuts Natural Pack	½ cup	25	0	0	6	2
Wax Beans	½ cup	25	0	360	6	2
WHALE						
raw	3.5 oz	134	3	100	0	—
WHEAT						
(*see also* BULGUR, BRAN, CEREAL, COUSCOUS, FLOUR, WHEAT GERM)						
Arrowhead						
Kamut Grain	¼ cup (1.7 oz)	140	1	0	32	5
Seitan Quick Mix	⅓ cup (1.4 oz)	150	1	20	14	2
Hodgson Mill						
Vital Wheat Gluten Plus Ascorbic Acid	1 tbsp (0.3 oz)	30	0	0	2	1
Near East						
Taboule Salad Mix as prep	⅔ cup	120	3	340	23	3
Wheat Pilaf as prep	1 cup	220	5	690	42	5
Sonoma						
Wheat Nuts Salted	2 tbsp (0.5 oz)	60	3	140	8	1
White Wave						
Seitan	½ pkg (4 oz)	140	0	240	4	1
Seitan Fajita Strips	⅓ cup (1.8 oz)	60	0	105	2	1
Seitan Marinated Slices	3 slices (1.8 oz)	60	0	105	2	1
sprouted	⅓ cup	71	tr	6	15	—
starch	3½ oz	348	tr	2	86	—
WHEAT GERM						
Arrowhead	3 tbsp (0.5 oz)	50	1	0	10	2
Hodgson Mill	2 tbsp (0.5 oz)	55	1	0	7	4
Kretschmer	¼ cup	103	3	2	12	3
Honey Crunch	¼ cup	105	3	2	15	3
Stone-Buhr						
Untoasted	2 tbsp (0.5 oz)	58	2	0	7	2
plain toasted	1 cup	431	12	4	56	—
plain toasted	¼ cup	108	3	1	14	4

FOOD	PORTION	CAL.	FAT	SOD.	CARB.	FIB.
plain untoasted	¼ cup	104	3	4	15	4
w/ brown sugar & honey toasted	1 cup	426	9	3	69	—
w/ brown sugar & honey toasted	1 oz	107	2	1	17	—

WHEY

acid dry	1 tbsp (3 g)	10	tr	28	2	—
acid fluid	1 cup (8 fl oz)	59	tr	118	13	—
sweet dry	1 tbsp (8 g)	26	tr	80	6	—
sweet fluid	1 cup (8 fl oz)	66	1	132	13	—
whey cheese	3.5 oz	440	27	511	33	0

WHIPPED TOPPINGS
(see also CREAM)

FOOD	PORTION	CAL.	FAT	SOD.	CARB.	FIB.
Cool Whip						
Extra Creamy	1 tbsp	13	1	3	1	—
Lite	1 tbsp	9	1	3	1	—
Non Dairy	1 tbsp	11	1	1	1	—
D-Zerta						
As prep	1 tbsp	7	1	6	0	—
Dream Whip						
As prep	1 tbsp	9	1	4	1	—
Estee						
Whipped Topping Sugar Free as prep	2 tbsp	10	1	5	1	—
Hood						
Instant	2 tbsp	20	2	0	1	0
Light Instant	2 tbsp	15	1	0	1	0
Kraft						
Real Cream	2 tbsp (0.4 oz)	20	2	0	1	0
Whipped Topping	2 tbsp (0.4 oz)	20	2	0	1	0
Pet						
Whip	1 tbsp	14	1	0	1	—
Reddiwip						
Lite	2 tbsp (8 g)	15	1	5	2	—
Non-Dairy	2 tbsp (8 g)	20	2	5	2	—
Real Whipped Heavy Cream	2 tbsp (8 g)	30	3	0	tr	—
Real Whipped Light Cream	2 tbsp (8 g)	20	2	0	tr	—
cream pressurized	1 tbsp	8	tr	4	tr	—
cream pressurized	1 cup	154	13	78	7	—
nondairy frzn	1 tbsp	13	1	1	1	—
nondairy powdered as prep w/ whole milk	1 cup	151	10	53	13	—

FOOD	PORTION	CAL.	FAT	SOD.	CARB.	FIB.
nondairy powdered as prep w/ whole milk	1 tbsp	8	tr	3	1	—
nondairy pressurized	1 cup	184	16	43	11	—
nondairy pressurized	1 tbsp	11	1	2	1	—

WHITE BEANS
CANNED
Goya

FOOD	PORTION	CAL.	FAT	SOD.	CARB.	FIB.
Spanish Style	7.5 oz	130	1	990	29	12
Progresso						
Cannellini	½ cup	80	tr	220	19	7
white beans	1 cup	306	1	13	58	—
DRIED						
regular cooked	1 cup	249	1	11	45	—
small cooked	1 cup	253	1	4	46	—

WHITEFISH

FOOD	PORTION	CAL.	FAT	SOD.	CARB.	FIB.
baked	3 oz	146	6	56	0	—
smoked	3 oz	92	1	866	0	—
smoked	1 oz	39	tr	285	0	—

WHITING

FOOD	PORTION	CAL.	FAT	SOD.	CARB.	FIB.
cooked	3 oz	98	1	113	0	—
raw	3 oz	77	1	61	0	—

WILD RICE

FOOD	PORTION	CAL.	FAT	SOD.	CARB.	FIB.
cooked	½ cup	83	tr	3	18	—

WINE
(*see also* CHAMPAGNE, WINE COOLERS)
Boone's

FOOD	PORTION	CAL.	FAT	SOD.	CARB.	FIB.
Country Kwencher	1 fl oz	24	0	1	3	—
Delicious Apple	1 fl oz	21	0	1	3	—
Sangria	1 fl oz	22	0	1	3	—
Snow Creek Berry	1 fl oz	18	0	tr	3	—
Strawberry Hill	1 fl oz	22	0	1	3	—
Sun Peak Peach	1 fl oz	18	0	1	3	—
Wild Island	1 fl oz	18	0	tr	3	—
Carlo Rossi						
Blush	1 fl oz	21	0	1	1	—
Burgundy	1 fl oz	22	0	1	tr	—
Chablis	1 fl oz	21	0	1	tr	—
Paisano	1 fl oz	23	0	3	tr	—
Red Sangria	1 fl oz	24	0	1	2	—
Rhine	1 fl oz	21	0	1	1	—
Vin Rose'	1 fl oz	21	0	1	1	—

FOOD	PORTION	CAL.	FAT	SOD.	CARB.	FIB.
Carlo Rossi (CONT.)						
White Grenache	1 fl oz	20	0	tr	1	—
Fairbanks						
Cream Sherry	1 fl oz	42	0	1	4	—
Port	1 fl oz	44	0	1	4	—
Sherry	1 fl oz	34	0	2	2	—
White Port	1 fl oz	44	0	1	4	—
Gallo						
Blush Chablis	1 fl oz	22	0	2	1	—
Burgundy	1 fl oz	22	0	1	tr	—
Cabernet Sauvignon	1 fl oz	22	0	tr	0	—
Chablis Blanc	1 fl oz	20	0	1	tr	—
Chardonnay	1 fl oz	23	0	1	tr	—
Classic Burgundy	1 fl oz	21	0	tr	0	—
French Colombard	1 fl oz	21	0	1	1	—
Hearty Burgundy	1 fl oz	22	0	1	tr	—
Johannisbery Riesling '88	1 fl oz	20	0	1	1	—
Pink Chablis	1 fl oz	20	0	1	1	—
Red Rose'	1 fl oz	23	0	2	1	—
Rhine	1 fl oz	22	0	1	1	—
Sauvignon Blanc '90	1 fl oz	20	0	1	tr	—
White Grenache '92	1 fl oz	20	0	1	1	—
White Grenache New Vintage	1 fl oz	20	0	tr	1	—
White Zinfandel '91	1 fl oz	18	0	1	tr	—
White Zinfandel New Vintage	1 fl oz	18	0	1	tr	—
Zinfandel '87	1 fl oz	23	0	tr	0	—
Ka-Me						
Chinese Cooking	2 tbsp (1 fl oz)	20	0	170	5	0
Sheffield Cellars						
Sherry	1 fl oz	44	0	1	4	—
Tawny Port	1 fl oz	45	0	2	4	—
Vermouth Extra Dry	1 fl oz	28	0	1	1	—
Vermouth Sweet	1 fl oz	43	0	2	4	—
Very Dry Sherry	1 fl oz	32	0	2	1	—
madeira	3.5 oz	169	0	—	10	0
port	3.5 oz	156	0	4	11	0
red	3.5 oz	74	0	6	2	—
rose	3.5 oz	73	0	5	2	—
sherry	2 oz	84	0	—	5	—
sweet dessert	2 oz	90	0	5	7	—
vermouth dry	3.5 oz	105	0	—	1	—

FOOD	PORTION	CAL.	FAT	SOD.	CARB.	FIB.
vermouth sweet	3.5 oz	167	0	—	12	—
white	3.5 oz	70	0	5	1	—

WINE COOLERS
Bartles & Jaymes
Berry	12 fl oz	210	0	0	32	—
Margarita	12 fl oz	260	0	40	46	—
Original	12 fl oz	190	0	10	28	—
Peach	12 fl oz	210	0	5	33	—
Pina Colada	12 fl oz	280	0	0	49	—
Planter's Punch	12 fl oz	230	0	0	36	—
Strawberry	12 fl oz	210	0	0	32	—
Strawberry Daquiri	12 fl oz	230	0	5	37	—
Tropical	12 fl oz	230	0	0	38	—

WINGED BEANS
dried cooked	1 cup	252	10	22	26	—

WOLFFISH
atlantic baked	3 oz	105	3	93	0	—

YAM
(*see also* SWEET POTATO)
CANNED
Allen
Cut	⅔ cup (5.8 oz)	160	1	35	40	3
Bruce						
Cut	½ cup	139	1	27	20	—
Mashed	½ cup	130	1	50	29	—
Vacuum Pack	½ cup	122	1	30	28	—
Whole	½ cup	139	1	27	31	—
Princella						
Cut	⅔ cup (5.8 oz)	160	1	40	40	—
Royal Prince						
Whole	4 pieces (5.9 oz)	200	1	40	48	4
S&W						
Candied	½ cup	180	0	355	44	—
Southern Whole In Extra Heavy Syrup	½ cup	139	1	27	31	—
Sugary Sam						
Cut	⅔ cup (5.8 oz)	160	1	35	40	3
Trappey						
Whole	4 pieces (5.9 oz)	200	1	40	48	4
FRESH						
mountain yam hawaii cooked	½ cup	59	tr	9	14	—
yam cubed cooked	½ cup	79	tr	6	19	—

FOOD	PORTION	CAL.	FAT	SOD.	CARB.	FIB.
YAM BEAN						
cooked	¾ cup	38	tr	4	9	—
YARDLONG BEANS						
dried cooked	1 cup	202	1	9	36	—
YEAST						
Fleischmann's						
Active Dry	1 pkg (¼ oz)	20	0	10	3	—
Fresh Active	1 pkg (0.6 oz)	15	0	5	2	—
Household Yeast	½ oz	15	0	5	2	—
RapidRise	1 pkg (¼ oz)	20	0	10	3	—
Red Star						
Small Flakes	3 tbsp (0.5 oz)	47	tr	5	5	4
Yeast Flakes	3 tbsp (0.5 oz)	47	tr	5	5	4
baker's compressed	1 cake (0.6 oz)	18	tr	5	3	2
baker's dry	1 pkg (¼ oz)	21	tr	—	3	—
baker's dry	1 tbsp	35	1	—	5	3
brewer's dry	1 tbsp	25	tr	10	3	—
YELLOW BEANS						
CANNED						
B&M						
Baked Beans	8 oz	326	7	770	50	—
DRIED						
cooked	1 cup	254	2	8	45	—
YELLOWEYE BEANS						
CANNED						
B&M						
Baked Beans	⅞ cup	290	7	—	—	—
DRIED						
Bean Cuisine	½ cup	115	1	5	—	5
YELLOWTAIL						
baked	3 oz	159	6	42	0	—
YOGURT						
(*see also* YOGURT FROZEN)						
Breyers						
1% Fat Black Cherry	8 oz	260	3	110	50	0
1% Fat Blueberry	8 oz	250	3	110	48	0
1% Fat Mixed Berry	8 oz	250	3	110	48	0
1% Fat Peach	8 oz	250	3	110	48	0
1% Fat Pineapple	8 oz	250	3	110	49	0
1% Fat Red Raspberry	8 oz	250	3	110	48	2
1% Fat Strawberry	8 oz	250	3	110	47	0

FOOD	PORTION	CAL.	FAT	SOD.	CARB.	FIB.
Breyers (CONT.)						
1% Fat Strawberry Banana	8 oz	250	3	115	50	tr
1.5% Fat Coffee	8 oz	220	3	135	38	0
1.5% Fat Plain	8 oz	130	3	150	15	0
1.5% Fat Vanilla	8 oz	220	3	135	38	0
Cabot						
All Flavors	8 oz	220	3	120	42	—
Plain	8 oz	140	4	160	16	—
Colombo						
Banana Strawberry	8 oz	210	4	110	39	0
Black Cherry	8 oz	200	4	115	36	0
Blueberry	8 oz	200	4	110	36	0
Fat Free Apples 'n Spice	8 oz	190	0	130	39	0
Fat Free Apricot	8 oz	190	0	130	39	0
Fat Free Banana Strawberry	8 oz	200	0	130	42	0
Fat Free Blueberry	8 oz	190	0	130	39	0
Fat Free Cappuccino	8 oz	180	0	140	35	0
Fat Free Cherry	8 oz	190	0	135	39	0
Fat Free Cranberry Strawberry	8 oz	200	0	120	43	0
Fat Free French Roast	8 oz	180	0	140	35	0
Fat Free Fruit Cocktail	8 oz	190	0	130	39	0
Fat Free Lemon	8 oz	170	0	150	33	0
Fat Free Peach	8 oz	190	0	130	33	0
Fat Free Plain	8 oz	110	0	170	16	0
Fat Free Raspberry	8 oz	190	0	130	39	0
Fat Free Strawberry	8 oz	190	0	130	39	0
Fat Free Strawberry Pineapple Orange	8 oz	190	0	125	38	0
Fat Free Vanilla	8 oz	170	0	150	32	0
French Vanilla	8 oz	180	4	130	29	0
Light 100 Blueberry	8 oz	100	0	140	16	0
Light 100 Cherry Vanilla	8 oz	100	0	120	16	0
Light 100 Coffee & Cream	8 oz	100	0	120	16	0
Light 100 Creamy Vanilla	8 oz	100	0	130	16	0
Light 100 Fruit Medley	8 oz	100	0	120	16	0
Light 100 Juicy Peach	8 oz	100	0	140	16	0
Light 100 Lemon Creme	8 oz	100	0	160	16	0
Light 100 Mandarin Orange	8 oz	100	0	120	16	0
Light 100 Mixed Berries	8 oz	100	0	110	16	0

FOOD	PORTION	CAL.	FAT	SOD.	CARB.	FIB.
Colombo (cont.)						
Light 100 Raspberry	8 oz	100	0	140	16	0
Light 100 Strawberry	8 oz	100	0	140	16	0
Peach Melba	8 oz	200	4	115	36	0
Plain	8 oz	120	5	150	12	0
Raspberry	8 oz	200	4	115	36	0
Strawberry	8 oz	200	4	110	36	0
Dannon						
Blended Nonfat Blueberry	6 oz	160	0	105	33	0
Blended Nonfat French Vanilla	6 oz	160	0	100	31	0
Blended Nonfat Lemon Chiffon	6 oz	150	0	110	31	0
Blended Nonfat Peach	6 oz	150	0	100	31	0
Blended Nonfat Raspberry	6 oz	160	0	100	32	0
Blended Nonfat Strawberry	6 oz	150	0	105	31	0
Blended Nonfat Strawberry Banana	6 oz	150	0	105	31	0
Danimals Lowfat Blueberry	4.4 oz	140	2	90	25	0
Danimals Lowfat Grape Lemonade	4.4 oz	130	2	80	23	0
Danimals Lowfat Lemon Ice	4.4 oz	130	2	90	22	0
Danimals Lowfat Orange Banana	4.4 oz	140	2	80	24	0
Danimals Lowfat Strawberry	4.4 oz	140	2	85	24	0
Danimals Lowfat Tropical Punch	4.4 oz	140	2	85	25	0
Danimals Lowfat Vanilla	4.4 oz	140	2	80	24	0
Danimals Lowfat Wild Raspberry	4.4 oz	130	2	80	22	0
Fruit On The Bottom Lowfat Apple Cinnamon	8 oz	240	3	140	46	1
Fruit On The Bottom Lowfat Blueberry	8 oz	240	3	140	46	1
Fruit On The Bottom Lowfat Boysenberry	8 oz	240	3	150	45	1
Fruit On The Bottom Lowfat Cherry	8 oz	240	3	135	46	1

FOOD	PORTION	CAL.	FAT	SOD.	CARB.	FIB.
Dannon (CONT.)						
Fruit On The Bottom Lowfat Mixed Berries	8 oz	240	3	150	45	1
Fruit On The Bottom Lowfat Orange	8 oz	240	3	135	45	0
Fruit On The Bottom Lowfat Peach	8 oz	240	3	140	45	1
Fruit On The Bottom Lowfat Pear	8 oz	240	3	135	45	0
Fruit On The Bottom Lowfat Raspberry	8 oz	240	3	150	45	1
Fruit On The Bottom Lowfat Strawberry	8 oz	240	3	135	46	1
Fruit On The Bottom Lowfat Strawberry Banana	8 oz	240	3	140	43	1
Light 'N Crunchy Nonfat Cappuccino w/ Chocolate	1 pkg	150	0	170	27	0
Light 'N Crunchy Nonfat Caramel Apple Crunch	1 pkg	150	0	180	28	0
Light 'N Crunchy Nonfat Lemon Chiffon w/ Blueberry	1 pkg	140	0	150	26	0
Light 'N Crunchy Nonfat Raspberry w/ Granola	1 pkg	150	0	135	17	0
Light 'N Crunchy Nonfat Vanilla w/ Chocolate	1 pkg	150	0	170	26	1
Light Nonfat Banana Cream Pie	4.4 oz	60	0	80	9	0
Light Nonfat Banana Cream Pie	8 oz	100	0	150	17	0
Light Nonfat Blueberry	8 oz	100	0	140	20	0
Light Nonfat Cherry Vanilla	1 cup (3.5 oz)	110	0	160	19	0
Light Nonfat Creme Caramel	8 oz	100	0	125	15	0
Light Nonfat Lemon	8 oz	100	0	140	17	0
Light Nonfat Lemon Chiffon	4.4 oz	60	0	75	9	0
Light Nonfat Peach	4.4 oz	50	0	70	8	0
Light Nonfat Peach	8 oz	100	0	140	18	0
Light Nonfat Raspberry	8 oz	100	0	150	18	0
Light Nonfat Strawberry	8 oz	100	0	140	18	0

FOOD	PORTION	CAL.	FAT	SOD.	CARB.	FIB.
Dannon (CONT.)						
Light Nonfat Strawberry Banana	8 oz	100	0	140	18	0
Light Nonfat Tropical Fruit	8 oz	100	0	140	19	0
Light Nonfat Vanilla	8 oz	100	0	140	17	0
Light Nonfat Strawberry	1 cup (3.5 oz)	110	0	160	19	0
Light Nonfat Strawberry	4.4 oz	50	0	70	8	0
Light Nonfat Vanilla	1 cup (3.5 oz)	110	0	160	18	0
Lowfat Coffee	8 oz	210	3	160	36	0
Lowfat Coffee	1 cup (8.7 oz)	230	4	170	39	0
Lowfat Cranberry Raspberry	8 oz	210	3	160	36	0
Lowfat Lemon	8 oz	210	3	160	36	0
Lowfat Lemon	1 cup (8.7 oz)	230	4	170	39	0
Lowfat Plain	8 oz	140	4	150	16	0
Lowfat Plain	1 cup (8.7 oz)	150	4	170	17	0
Lowfat Vanilla	1 cup (8.7 oz)	230	4	170	39	0
Lowfat Vanilla	8 oz	210	3	160	36	0
Minipack Blended Nonfat Blueberry	4.4 oz	120	0	105	23	0
Minipack Blended Nonfat Cherry	4.4 oz	110	0	75	23	0
Minipack Blended Nonfat Peach	4.4 oz	110	0	75	23	0
Minipack Blended Nonfat Raspberry	4.4 oz	120	0	75	23	0
Minipack Blended Nonfat Strawberry	4.4 oz	110	0	105	23	0
Minipack Blended Nonfat Strawberry Banana	4.4 oz	110	2	105	23	0
Nonfat Plain	1 cup (8.7 oz)	120	0	170	17	0
Nonfat Plain	8 oz	110	0	150	16	0
Nonfat Light Cherry Vanilla	8 oz	100	0	140	17	0
Nonfat Light Strawberry Fruit Cup	8 oz	100	0	140	18	0
Sprinkl'ins Banana	4.1 oz	140	3	85	24	0
Sprinkl'ins Cherry Vanilla	4.1 oz	140	3	95	24	0
Sprinkl'ins Crazy Crunch Cherry w/ Honey Grahams	4.4 oz	170	3	150	30	0

FOOD	PORTION	CAL.	FAT	SOD.	CARB.	FIB.
Dannon (CONT.)						
Sprinkl'ins Crazy Crunch Grape w/ Chocolate Grahams	4.4 oz	160	3	170	29	0
Sprinkl'ins Crazy Crunch Vanilla w/ Chocolate Grahams	4.4 oz	160	3	140	29	0
Sprinkl'ins Crazy Crunch Vanilla w/ Honey Grahams	4.4 oz	170	3	135	30	0
Sprinkl'ins Strawberry	4.1 oz	140	3	95	24	0
Sprinkl'ins Strawberry Banana	4.1 oz	140	3	95	24	0
Tropifruta Nonfat Banana	6 oz	150	0	105	31	0
Tropifruta Nonfat Guava	6 oz	150	0	105	29	0
Tropifruta Nonfat Mango	6 oz	150	0	105	31	0
Tropifruta Nonfat Papaya Pineapple	6 oz	150	0	105	30	0
Tropifruta Nonfat Pina Colada	6 oz	150	0	105	30	0
Tropifruta Nonfat Strawberry	6 oz	150	0	105	31	0
Tropifruta Nonfat Strawberry Banana	6 oz	150	0	105	31	0
Tropifruta Nonfat Strawberry Kiwi	6 oz	150	0	105	30	0
With Fruit Toppings Banana Creme Strawberry	6 oz	170	3	90	30	1
With Fruit Toppings Bavarian Creme Raspberry	6 oz	170	3	115	31	0
With Fruit Toppings Cheesecake Cherry	6 oz	170	3	90	31	0
With Fruit Toppings Cheesecake Strawberry	6 oz	170	3	90	30	1
With Fruit Toppings Vanilla Peach & Apricot	6 oz	170	3	90	30	0
With Fruit Toppings Vanilla Strawberry	6 oz	170	3	90	30	1
Friendship						
Coffee	8 oz	210	3	170	30	0

FOOD	PORTION	CAL.	FAT	SOD.	CARB.	FIB.
Friendship (CONT.)						
Fruit Crunch Blueberry	6 oz	190	4	125	32	0
Fruit Crunch Peach	6 oz	190	5	125	31	0
Fruit Crunch Strawberry	6 oz	190	5	125	31	0
Fruit Crunch Strawberry Banana	6 oz	190	4	125	32	0
Plain	8 oz	150	3	190	13	0
Hood						
Fat Free Blueberry	1 (8 oz)	190	0	120	40	1
Fat Free Cherry	1 (8 oz)	190	0	120	40	1
Fat Free Peach	1 (8 oz)	190	0	120	40	1
Fat Free Plain	1 (8 oz)	130	0	190	18	0
Fat Free Raspberry	1 (8 oz)	190	0	120	40	1
Fat Free Strawberry	1 (8 oz)	190	0	120	39	1
Fat Free Strawberry Banana	1 (8 oz)	190	0	120	40	1
Fat Free Vanilla	1 (8 oz)	190	0	170	34	1
Fat Free Swiss Blueberry	1 (8 oz)	210	0	110	45	0
Fat Free Swiss Lemon	1 (8 oz)	210	0	110	45	0
Fat Free Swiss Raspberry	1 (8 oz)	210	0	110	45	0
Fat Free Swiss Strawberry	1 (8 oz)	210	0	105	45	0
Fat Free Swiss Strawberry Banana	1 (8 oz)	210	0	110	45	0
Fat Free Swiss Vanilla	1 (8 oz)	210	0	105	45	0
Knudsen						
1.5% Fat Creamy Lemon	8 oz	220	3	140	38	0
70 Calories Black Cherry	6 oz	70	0	85	12	0
70 Calories Blueberry	6 oz	70	0	80	12	0
70 Calories Lemon	6 oz	70	0	100	11	tr
70 Calories Peach	6 oz	70	0	80	11	tr
70 Calories Pineapple	6 oz	70	0	80	11	0
70 Calories Red Raspberry	6 oz	70	0	75	11	0
70 Calories Strawberry	6 oz	70	0	85	11	0
70 Calories Strawberry Banana	6 oz	70	0	85	11	0
70 Calories Strawberry Fruit Basket	6 oz	70	0	90	11	0
70 Calories Vanilla	6 oz	70	0	80	11	0
Free Lemon	6 oz	160	0	105	33	0
Free Mixed Berry	6 oz	170	0	105	33	0
Free Peach	6 oz	170	0	105	33	0

FOOD	PORTION	CAL.	FAT	SOD.	CARB.	FIB.
Knudsen (CONT.)						
Free Red Raspberry	6 oz	170	0	105	31	0
Free Strawberry	6 oz	170	0	105	32	0
Free Vanilla	6 oz	170	0	100	32	0
La Yogurt						
French Style Banana	6 oz	180	3	100	32	0
French Style Blueberry	6 oz	180	3	100	32	1
French Style Cherry	6 oz	180	3	100	32	0
French Style Cherry Vanilla	6 oz	190	3	95	35	0
French Style Guava	6 oz	180	3	100	32	1
French Style Key Lime	6 oz	180	3	100	32	0
French Style Mango	6 oz	180	3	100	32	0
French Style Mixed Berry	6 oz	180	3	100	32	0
French Style Nonfat Blueberry	6 oz	70	0	90	12	0
French Style Nonfat Cherry	6 oz	75	0	90	13	0
French Style Nonfat Raspberry	6 oz	70	0	90	12	0
French Style Nonfat Strawberry	6 oz	70	0	90	12	0
French Style Nonfat Strawberry Banana	6 oz	70	0	90	12	0
French Style Peach	6 oz	180	3	100	32	0
French Style Pina Colada	6 oz	180	3	100	32	0
French Style Raspberry	6 oz	180	3	100	32	1
French Style Strawberry	6 oz	180	3	100	32	0
French Style Strawberry Banana	6 oz	180	3	100	32	0
French Style Strawberry Fruit Cup	6 oz	180	3	100	32	0
French Style Tropical Orange	6 oz	180	4	100	32	0
French Style Vanilla	6 oz	170	3	110	28	0
Latin Style Banana	6 oz	190	3	105	34	0
Latin Style Guava	6 oz	190	3	105	34	0
Latin Style Mango	6 oz	190	3	105	34	0
Latin Style Papaya	6 oz	190	3	105	34	0
Latin Style Passion Fruit	6 oz	190	3	105	34	0
Latin Style Strawberry Kiwi	6 oz	180	3	100	32	0
Light N'Lively						
Free Blueberry	6 oz	190	0	105	38	0

FOOD	PORTION	CAL.	FAT	SOD.	CARB.	FIB.
Light N'Lively (CONT.)						
Free Lemon	6 oz	170	0	105	35	0
Free Mixed Berry	6 oz	170	0	105	34	0
Free Peach	6 oz	170	0	105	35	0
Free Red Raspberry	6 oz	180	0	105	36	0
Free Strawberry	6 oz	180	0	105	36	0
Free Strawberry Fruit Cup	6 oz	170	0	105	35	0
Free Vanilla	6 oz	160	0	105	32	0
Free 50 Calories Blueberry	4.4 oz	50	0	60	8	0
Free 50 Calories Peach	4.4 oz	50	0	60	9	0
Free 50 Calories Red Raspberry	4.4 oz	50	0	60	8	0
Free 50 Calories Strawberry	4.4 oz	50	0	60	8	0
Free 50 Calories Strawberry Banana	4.4 oz	50	0	60	8	0
Free 50 Calories Strawberry Fruit Cup	4.4 oz	50	0	60	8	0
Free 70 Calories Black Cherry	6 oz	70	0	85	11	0
Free 70 Calories Blueberry	6 oz	70	0	80	11	0
Free 70 Calories Lemon	6 oz	70	0	120	12	0
Free 70 Calories Peach	6 oz	70	0	80	12	0
Free 70 Calories Red Raspberry	6 oz	70	0	80	11	0
Free 70 Calories Strawberry	6 oz	70	0	85	11	0
Free 70 Calories Strawberry Banana	6 oz	70	0	85	11	0
Free 70 Calories Strawberry Fruit Cup	6 oz	70	0	80	11	0
Kidpack Banana Berry	4.4 oz	130	1	65	24	0
Kidpack Berry Blue	4.4 oz	150	1	65	30	0
Kidpack Cherry	4.4 oz	140	1	65	27	0
Kidpack Grape	4.4 oz	130	1	65	24	0
Kidpack Outrageous Orange	4.4 oz	150	1	65	29	0
Kidpack Tropical Punch	4.4 oz	140	1	65	28	0
Kidpack Wild Berry	4.4 oz	140	1	65	27	0
Kidpack Wild Strawberry	4.4 oz	140	1	65	28	0
Multipack Blueberry	4.4 oz	140	1	65	27	0

FOOD	PORTION	CAL.	FAT	SOD.	CARB.	FIB.
Light N'Lively (CONT.)						
Multipack Peach	4.4 oz	140	1	65	27	0
Multipack Pineapple	4.4 oz	140	1	60	27	0
Multipack Red Raspberry	4.4 oz	130	1	65	24	0
Multipack Strawberry	4.4 oz	140	1	65	26	0
Multipack Strawberry Banana	4.4 oz	140	1	60	28	0
Multipack Strawberry Fruit Cup	4.4 oz	140	1	60	27	0
Lite Line						
Swiss Style Cherry Vanilla	1 cup	240	2	150	45	—
Swiss Style Peach	1 cup	230	2	150	42	—
Swiss Style Plain	1 cup	140	2	150	16	—
Swiss Style Strawberry	1 cup	240	2	150	46	—
Meadow Gold						
Plain	1 cup	160	5	160	16	—
Sundae Style Raspberry	1 cup	250	4	160	42	—
Mountain High						
Blueberry	1 cup	220	6	140	31	—
Plain	1 cup	200	9	140	16	—
Weight Watchers						
Nonfat Plain	1 cup	90	0	135	13	—
Ultimate 90 All Flavors	1 cup	90	0	120	13	—
Yoplait						
Custard Style Banana	6 oz	190	4	95	32	—
Custard Style Blueberry	6 oz	190	4	95	32	—
Custard Style Cherry	6 oz	180	4	95	30	—
Custard Style Lemon	6 oz	190	4	95	32	—
Custard Style Mixed Berry	6 oz	180	4	95	30	—
Custard Style Raspberry	6 oz	190	4	95	32	—
Custard Style Strawberry	4 oz	130	3	60	21	—
Custard Style Strawberry	6 oz	190	4	95	32	—
Custard Style Strawberry Banana	6 oz	190	4	95	32	—
Custard Style Strawberry Banana	4 oz	130	3	60	21	—
Custard Style Vanilla	4 oz	130	3	70	20	—
Custard Style Vanilla	6 oz	180	4	110	30	—
Fat Free Blueberry	6 oz	150	0	95	31	—
Fat Free Cherry	6 oz	150	0	95	31	—
Fat Free Mixed Berry	6 oz	150	0	95	31	—

FOOD	PORTION	CAL.	FAT	SOD.	CARB.	FIB.
Yoplait (CONT.)						
Fat Free Peach	6 oz	150	0	95	31	—
Fat Free Raspberry	6 oz	150	0	95	31	—
Fat Free Strawberry	6 oz	150	0	95	31	—
Fat Free Strawberry Banana	6 oz	150	0	95	31	—
Light Blueberry	4 oz	60	0	75	9	—
Light Blueberry	6 oz	80	0	80	13	—
Light Cherry	6 oz	80	0	80	13	—
Light Cherry	4 oz	60	0	75	9	—
Light Peach	4 oz	60	0	75	9	—
Light Peach	6 oz	80	0	80	13	—
Light Raspberry	6 oz	80	0	80	13	—
Light Raspberry	4 oz	60	0	75	9	—
Light Strawberry	6 oz	80	0	110	13	—
Light Strawberry	4 oz	60	0	75	9	—
Light Strawberry Banana	6 oz	80	0	80	13	—
Light Strawberry Banana	4 oz	60	0	75	9	—
Nonfat Plain	8 oz	120	0	160	18	—
Nonfat Vanilla	8 oz	180	0	140	35	—
Original Apple	6 oz	190	3	110	32	—
Original Blueberry	6 oz	190	3	110	32	—
Original Blueberry	4 oz	120	2	75	21	—
Original Boysenberry	6 oz	190	3	110	32	—
Original Cherry	6 oz	190	3	110	32	—
Original Lemon	6 oz	190	3	110	32	—
Original Mixed Berry	6 oz	190	3	110	32	—
Original Orange	6 oz	190	3	110	32	—
Original Peach	6 oz	190	3	110	32	—
Original Peach	4 oz	120	2	75	21	—
Original Pina Colada	6 oz	190	3	110	32	—
Original Pineapple	6 oz	190	3	110	32	—
Original Plain	6 oz	130	3	140	15	—
Original Raspberry	6 oz	190	3	110	32	—
Original Raspberry	4 oz	120	2	75	21	—
Original Strawberry	6 oz	190	3	110	32	—
Original Strawberry	4 oz	120	2	75	21	—
Original Strawberry Banana	6 oz	190	3	110	32	—
Original Strawberry Rhubarb	6 oz	190	3	110	32	—
Original Vanilla	6 oz	180	3	120	29	—
coffee lowfat	8 oz	194	3	149	31	—
fruit lowfat	4 oz	113	1	60	21	—

FOOD	PORTION	CAL.	FAT	SOD.	CARB.	FIB.
fruit lowfat	8 oz	225	3	121	42	—
plain	8 oz	139	7	105	11	—
plain lowfat	8 oz	144	4	159	16	—
plain no fat	8 oz	127	tr	174	17	—
vanilla lowfat	8 oz	194	3	149	31	—

YOGURT FROZEN
(*see also* TOFU YOGURT)

Bee-Lite

Chocolate	4 oz	100	tr	55	23	—
Vanilla	4 oz	110	tr	55	23	—

Ben & Jerry's

Cherry Garcia	½ cup (3.7 oz)	170	3	70	31	0
Chocolate Fudge Brownie	½ cup (3.7 oz)	190	4	130	35	2
Coffee Almond Fudge	½ cup (3.7 oz)	200	7	85	30	1
English Toffee Crunch	½ cup (3.7 oz)	190	6	110	32	0
No Fat Cappuccino	½ cup (3.3 oz)	140	0	85	32	0
Pop Cherry Garcia	1 (3.8 oz)	290	16	60	34	2

Borden

Strawberry	½ cup	100	2	50	19	—

Bresler's

All Flavors	5 oz	145	2	—	28	—
All Flavors Lite	5 oz	135	0	—	30	—

Breyers

Black Cherry	½ cup (2.7 oz)	140	3	40	25	0
Chocolate	½ cup (2.7 oz)	150	4	45	25	1
Chocolate Brownie	½ cup (2.7 oz)	170	5	45	29	1
Peach	½ cup (2.7 oz)	140	3	40	24	0
Red Raspberry	½ cup (2.7 oz)	140	4	40	24	0
Strawberry	½ cup (2.7 oz)	130	3	40	23	0
Strawberry Banana	½ cup (2.7 oz)	140	3	40	24	0
Strawberry Cheesecake	½ cup (2.7 oz)	160	5	60	26	0
Toffee Bar Crunch	½ cup (2.7 oz)	160	5	55	26	0
Vanilla	½ cup (2.7 oz)	140	4	45	24	0
Vanilla Chocolate Strawberry	½ cup (2.7 oz)	140	4	45	24	0
Vanilla Fudge Twirl	½ cup (2.7 oz)	150	4	45	25	1
Vanilla Raspberry Swirl	½ cup (2.7 oz)	140	4	45	24	0

Dannon

Coco-Nut Fudge	½ cup (3 oz)	160	3	70	28	0
Light Cappuccino	½ cup (2.8 oz)	80	0	70	19	0
Light Cherry Vanilla Swirl	½ cup (2.8 oz)	90	0	65	21	0

FOOD	PORTION	CAL.	FAT	SOD.	CARB.	FIB.
Dannon (CONT.)						
Light Chocolate	½ cup (2.7 oz)	80	0	60	21	1
Light Lemon Chiffon	½ cup (2.8 oz)	90	0	65	22	0
Light 'N Crunchy Banana Cream Pie	½ cup (2.8 oz)	110	1	65	24	0
Light 'N Crunchy Mocha Chocolate Chunk	½ cup (2.8 oz)	110	1	60	26	0
Light 'N Crunchy Peanut Chocolate Crunch	½ cup (2.8 oz)	110	0	65	29	0
Light 'N Crunchy Triple Chocolate	½ cup (2.8 oz)	110	0	60	28	0
Light 'N Crunchy Vanilla Blueberry Swirl	½ cup (2.8 oz)	110	1	65	26	0
Light Nonfat Cappuccino	8 oz	100	0	140	17	0
Light Peach Raspberry Melba	½ cup (2.8 oz)	90	0	65	21	0
Light Strawberry Cheesecake	½ cup (2.8 oz)	90	0	60	22	0
Light Vanilla	½ cup (2.8 oz)	80	0	65	21	0
Pure Indulgence Cherry Chocolate Cherry	½ cup (3 oz)	150	3	85	26	0
Pure Indulgence Chunky Chocolate Nut	½ cup (3 oz)	150	3	65	25	0
Pure Indulgence Cookies'n Cream	½ cup (3 oz)	150	3	105	24	0
Pure Indulgence Crunchy Expresso	½ cup (3 oz)	150	3	85	26	0
Pure Indulgence Heath Toffee Crunch	½ cup (3 oz)	150	3	105	25	0
Pure Indulgence Vanilla Raspberry Truffle	½ cup (3 oz)	150	3	70	25	1
Desserve						
All Flavors	4 oz	70	0	57	16	—
Dutch Chocolate	4 oz	80	0	62	18	—
Edy's						
Banana Strawberry	3 oz	80	1	40	15	—
Blueberry	3 oz	80	1	40	15	—
Cherry	3 oz	80	1	40	15	—
Chocolate	3 oz	80	1	40	15	—
Chocolate Chip	3 oz	100	1	55	20	—
Citrus Heights	3 oz	80	1	40	15	—
Cookies'N'Cream	3 oz	100	1	55	20	—
Marble Fudge	3 oz	100	1	55	20	—
Perfectly Peach	3 oz	80	1	40	15	—

FOOD	PORTION	CAL.	FAT	SOD.	CARB.	FIB.
Edy's (CONT.)						
Raspberry	3 oz	80	1	40	15	—
Raspberry Vanilla Swirl	3 oz	80	1	45	15	—
Strawberry	3 oz	80	1	40	15	—
Vanilla	3 oz	80	1	50	15	—
Elan						
Blueberry	4 oz	130	3	50	23	—
Caramel Almond Praline	4 oz	150	4	90	26	—
Chocolate	4 oz	130	3	50	24	—
Chocolate Almond	4 oz	160	6	50	22	—
Coffee	4 oz	130	3	60	22	—
Coffee Decaffeinated	4 oz	130	3	60	22	—
Peach	4 oz	130	3	50	23	—
Rum Raisin	4 oz	135	3	55	25	—
Strawberry	4 oz	125	3	50	22	—
Vanilla	4 oz	130	3	60	22	—
Fi-Bar						
Chocolate	1	190	7	160	26	4
Strawberry	1	190	7	150	26	4
Vanilla	1	190	7	150	26	4
Friendly's						
Apple Bettie	½ cup (2.6 oz)	140	3	75	25	0
Fabulous Fudge Swirl	½ cup (2.6 oz)	140	3	80	23	0
Fudge Berry Swirl	½ cup (2.6 oz)	150	4	75	25	0
Lowfat Perfectly Peach	½ cup (2.6 oz)	110	2	55	21	0
Lowfat Purely Chocolate	½ cup (2.6 oz)	120	3	65	20	0
Lowfat Raspberry Delight	½ cup (2.6 oz)	120	3	60	21	0
Lowfat Simply Vanilla	½ cup (2.6 oz)	120	3	70	19	0
Lowfat Strawberry Patch	½ cup (2.6 oz)	110	2	55	20	0
Mint Chocolate Chip	½ cup (2.6 oz)	130	4	65	21	0
Strawberry Cheesecake Blast	½ cup (2.6 oz)	140	4	75	22	0
Toffee Almond Crunch	½ cup (2.6 oz)	160	5	85	24	tr
Good Humor						
Creamsicle Raspberry	1 (2.8 oz)	100	1	20	23	0
Frista Cup	1 (6.2 oz)	220	5	125	38	1
Haagen-Dazs						
Banana Nut Blast	½ cup (3.5 oz)	220	8	65	29	1
Bars Cherry Chocolate Fudge	1 (2.6 oz)	240	13	45	26	1
Bars Peach	1 (2.5 oz)	90	1	20	19	0
Bars Pina Colada	1 (2.5 oz)	100	1	45	19	0
Bars Raspberry & Vanilla	1 (2.5 oz)	90	1	25	19	0

FOOD	PORTION	CAL.	FAT	SOD.	CARB.	FIB.
Haagen-Dazs (CONT.)						
Bars Strawberry Daiquiri	1 (2.5 oz)	90	1	20	18	0
Chocolate	½ cup (3.4 oz)	160	3	60	26	tr
Coffee	½ cup (3.4 oz)	160	3	55	26	0
Fat Free Bar Raspberry & Vanilla	1 (2.5 oz)	90	0	15	20	0
Fat Free Cherry Vanilla	½ cup (3.3 oz)	140	0	40	30	0
Fat Free Chocolate	½ cup (3.3 oz)	140	0	45	28	tr
Fat Free Coffee	½ cup (3.3 oz)	140	0	45	29	0
Fat Free Vanilla	½ cup (3.3 oz)	140	0	45	29	0
Fat Free Vanilla Fudge	½ cup (3.3 oz)	160	0	100	34	0
Orange Tango	½ cup (3.5 oz)	130	1	25	26	0
Pina Colada	½ cup (3.4 oz)	130	2	25	26	0
Raspberry Randevous	½ cup (3.5 oz)	130	2	25	26	1
Strawberry Cheesecake Craze	½ cup (3.6 oz)	220	8	140	31	0
Strawberry Duet	½ cup (3.4 oz)	130	2	25	26	tr
Vanilla	½ cup (3.4 oz)	160	3	55	26	0
Hood						
Bavarian Truffle & Twist	½ cup (2.6 oz)	150	4	60	26	0
Coffee Toffee Chunk Sundae	½ cup (2.6 oz)	150	4	75	27	0
Combo Bars	1 (2.2 oz)	90	2	40	17	0
Cookies & Cream	½ cup (2.6 oz)	140	4	75	25	0
Grandma's Raisin Oatmeal Cookie Dough	½ cup (2.6 oz)	140	3	75	25	0
Mixed Berry Swirl	½ cup (2.6 oz)	120	2	45	24	0
Natural Strawberry	½ cup (2.6 oz)	110	3	50	21	0
Natural Strawberry Banana	½ cup (2.6 oz)	110	3	50	21	0
Natural Vanilla	½ cup (2.6 oz)	120	3	55	22	0
Nonfat Caramel & Brownie Sundae	½ cup (2.6 oz)	120	0	60	28	0
Nonfat Chocolate Marshmallow	½ cup (2.6 oz)	110	0	60	26	0
Nonfat Double Raspberry	½ cup (2.6 oz)	120	0	55	26	0
Nonfat Mocha Fudge	½ cup (2.6 oz)	120	0	55	27	0
Nonfat Olde Fashioned Vanilla	½ cup (2.6 oz)	110	0	55	24	0
Nonfat Peach Cobbler A La Mode	½ cup (2.6 oz)	110	0	50	25	0
Nonfat Strawberry	½ cup (2.6 oz)	100	0	50	23	0

FOOD	PORTION	CAL.	FAT	SOD.	CARB.	FIB.
Hood (CONT.)						
Nonfat Vanilla Fudge	½ cup (2.6 oz)	120	0	55	27	0
Raspberry Swirl	½ cup (2.6 oz)	130	2	55	25	0
Sundae Cups Chocolate & Strawberry	1 (2.2 oz)	110	2	55	24	1
Vanilla Chocolate Strawberry	½ cup (2.6 oz)	120	3	50	22	0
Vanilla Swiss Almond Sundae	½ cup (2.6 oz)	150	4	60	25	0
Just 10						
All Flavors	1 oz	10	0	14	3	—
Kissed With Honey						
Chocolate	3.5 oz	100	3	50	18	—
Nonfat Chocolate	3.5 oz	85	tr	60	19	—
Nonfat Vanilla	3.5 oz	85	tr	50	18	—
Vanilla	3.5 oz	100	3	75	17	—
Meadow Gold						
Strawberry	½ cup	100	2	50	19	—
Sealtest						
Chocolate	½ cup (2.7 oz)	120	2	45	24	tr
Mocha Fudge	½ cup (2.6 oz)	130	2	45	25	tr
Vanilla	½ cup (2.6 oz)	120	2	45	24	0
Tofutti						
Beter Than Yogurt Passion Island Fruit	4 fl oz	100	1	100	21	0
Better Than Yogurt Chocolate Fudge	4 fl oz	120	2	98	25	0
Better Than Yogurt Coffee Mashmallow Swirl	4 fl oz	100	1	77	24	0
Better Than Yogurt Peach Mango	4 fl oz	100	1	102	23	0
Better Than Yogurt Strawberry Banana	4 fl oz	100	1	92	23	0
Better Than Yogurt Vanilla Fudge	4 fl oz	120	2	90	24	0
Turkey Hill						
Chocolate Cherry Cordial	½ cup (2.6 oz)	130	3	60	22	0
Chocolate Chip Cookie Dough	½ cup (2.6 oz)	140	5	120	23	0
Death By Chocolate	½ cup (2.6 oz)	150	4	90	25	0
Nonfat Chocolate Marshmallow	½ cup (2.4 oz)	130	0	40	30	0

FOOD	PORTION	CAL.	FAT	SOD.	CARB.	FIB.
Turkey Hill (CONT.)						
Nonfat Chocolate Cherry Cordial	½ cup (2.4 oz)	100	0	70	24	0
Nonfat Coffee Cappuccino	½ cup (2.4 oz)	110	0	60	23	0
Nonfat Mint Cookie 'N Cream	½ cup (2.4 oz)	110	0	80	24	0
Nonfat Neapolitan	½ cup (2.4 oz)	100	0	50	22	0
Nonfat Raspberry Chocolate Bliss	½ cup (2.4 oz)	110	0	100	25	0
Nonfat Southern Lemon Pie	½ cup (2.4 oz)	110	0	90	25	0
Nonfat Vanilla Fudge	½ cup (2.4 oz)	110	0	80	24	0
Peach Raspberry	½ cup (2.6 oz)	110	2	60	20	0
Strawberry	½ cup (2.6 oz)	110	2	60	20	0
Tin Roof Sundae	½ cup (2.6 oz)	140	5	100	21	0
Vanilla & Chocolate	½ cup (2.6 oz)	110	3	70	19	0
Vanilla Bean	½ cup (2.6 oz)	110	3	70	17	0
Weight Watchers						
Chocolate Shake	7.5 oz	220	1	140	44	—
chocolate soft serve	½ cup (4 fl oz)	115	4	71	18	—
vanilla soft serve	½ cup (4 fl oz)	114	4	63	17	—

ZABAGLIONE
(*see* CUSTARD)

ZUCCHINI
CANNED

FOOD	PORTION	CAL.	FAT	SOD.	CARB.	FIB.
Del Monte						
With Italian Tomato Sauce	½ cup (4.2 oz)	30	0	490	7	1
Progresso						
Italian Style	½ cup	50	2	540	8	2
S&W						
Italian Style	½ cup	45	1	467	7	—
italian style	½ cup	33	tr	427	8	—
FRESH						
baby raw	1 (½ oz)	3	tr	0	1	tr
raw sliced	½ cup	9	tr	2	2	1
sliced cooked	½ cup	14	tr	2	4	1
FROZEN						
Big Valley	¾ cup (3 oz)	10	0	0	2	1
Empire						
Breaded	1 (2.9 oz)	100	0	280	18	1
Southland						
Zucchini Sliced	3.2 oz	15	0	—	—	—
cooked	½ cup	19	tr	2	4	—